Emerging Protozoan Pathogens

Emerging Protozoan Pathogens

Editor: Stepanie Archer

AMERICAN
MEDICAL PUBLISHERS
www.americanmedicalpublishers.com

AMERICAN
MEDICAL PUBLISHERS
www.americanmedicalpublishers.com

Cataloging-in-Publication Data

Emerging protozoan pathogens / edited by Stepanie Archer.
p. cm.
Includes bibliographical references and index.
ISBN 979-8-88740-090-7
1. Protozoa, Pathogenic. 2. Protozoan diseases. 3. Emerging infectious diseases.
4. Host-parasite relationships. I. Archer, Stepanie.
QR251 .E44 2023
616.96--dc23

American Medical Publishers,
41 Flatbush Avenue,
1st Floor, New York,
NY 11217, USA

ISBN 979-8-88740-090-7 (Hardback)

Contents

Preface

This book was inspired by the evolution of our times; to answer the curiosity of inquisitive minds. Many developments have occurred across the globe in the recent past which has transformed the progress in the field.

Pathogenic protozoa consist of various eukaryotic microorganisms which cause a number of parasitic diseases. Some of these diseases have clinical significance as they affect humans and include diseases like trichomoniasis, malaria, giardiasis, toxoplasmosis, amebiasis, leishmaniasis and Chagas disease. A prominent example of pathogenic protozoa are free living amoebae (FLA). They comprise opportunistic parasitic protozoa causing infections in humans as well as animals. FLA cause infections like amoebic encephalitis and Acanthamoeba keratitis. Protozoan pathogens can be identified in clinical samples by identifying the causative agent or by identifying particular immune reactions in the host. The diagnosis of the parasitic diseases caused by the protozoan pathogens is majorly dependent on microscopy. However, other methods such as techniques based on polymerase chain reaction (PCR) have also gained significance. This book aims to shed light on some of the unexplored aspects of protozoan pathogens and the recent researches on them. It is appropriate for students seeking detailed information on these pathogens as well as for experts.

This book was developed from a mere concept to drafts to chapters and finally compiled together as a complete text to benefit the readers across all nations. To ensure the quality of the content we instilled two significant steps in our procedure. The first was to appoint an editorial team that would verify the data and statistics provided in the book and also select the most appropriate and valuable contributions from the plentiful contributions we received from authors worldwide. The next step was to appoint an expert of the topic as the Editor-in-Chief, who would head the project and finally make the necessary amendments and modifications to make the text reader-friendly. I was then commissioned to examine all the material to present the topics in the most comprehensible and productive format.

I would like to take this opportunity to thank all the contributing authors who were supportive enough to contribute their time and knowledge to this project. I also wish to convey my regards to my family who have been extremely supportive during the entire project.

Editor

1

Scrutinizing the Biomarkers for the Neglected Chagas Disease: How Remarkable!

*Rosa T. Pinho[1], Mariana C. Waghabi[2], Fabíola Cardillo[3], José Mengel[1,4] and Paulo R. Z. Antas[1]**

[1] Laboratório de Imunologia Clínica, Instituto Oswaldo Cruz, FIOCRUZ, Rio de Janeiro, Brazil, [2] Laboratório de Genômica Funcional e Bioinformática, Instituto Oswaldo Cruz, FIOCRUZ, Rio de Janeiro, Brazil, [3] Centro de Pesquisa Gonçalo Muniz, FIOCRUZ, Salvador, Brazil, [4] Faculdade de Medicina de Petropolis (FMP-FASE), Petrópolis, Brazil

***Correspondence:**
Paulo R. Z. Antas
pzuquim@ioc.fiocruz.br

Biomarkers or biosignature profiles have become accessible over time in population-based studies for Chagas disease. Thus, the identification of consistent and reliable indicators of the diagnosis and prognosis of patients with heart failure might facilitate the prioritization of therapeutic management to those with the highest chance of contracting this disease. The purpose of this paper is to review the recent state and the upcoming trends in biomarkers for human Chagas disease. As an emerging concept, we propose a classification of biomarkers based on plasmatic-, phenotype-, antigenic-, genetic-, and management-related candidates. The available data revisited here reveal the lessons learned thus far and the existing challenges that still lie ahead to enable biomarkers to be employed consistently in risk evaluation for this disease. There is a strong need for biomarker validation, particularly for biomarkers that are specific to the clinical forms of Chagas disease. The current failure to achieve the eradication of the transmission of this disease has produced determination to solve this validation issue. Finally, it would be strategic to develop a wide variety of biomarkers and to test them in both preclinical and clinical trials.

Keywords: Chagas disease, biomarkers for immune responsiveness, human experimentation, clinical forms, mini review

INTRODUCTION

Population-based studies have identified a range of biomarkers that indicate exposure to, effects of, and genetic susceptibility for different pathogen-related diseases. These biomarkers could potentially be applied for diagnostic and prognostic purposes in human Chagas disease. The available data reveal the lessons learned to date and the current challenges that still remain to enable biomarkers to be employed reliably in risk evaluation for this disease. Our main purpose here is to revisit the current evidence and future trends in biomarker research for human Chagas disease. And due to recent, elegant systematic reviews focusing on this important topic (see below), we instead present here a literature review.

Chagas disease, or American trypanosomiasis, is caused by the etiological agent *Trypanosoma cruzi* and affects at least eight million people in Central and South America (1). The morbidity is high. The acute phase of infection is followed by an asymptomatic phase, but ~30% of infected patients develop a symptomatic, chronic phase that is characterized by either severe cardiac or digestive forms of Chagas disease (2, 3). Hence, the identification of consistent and reliable indicators of Chagas disease pathology, namely biomarkers or biosignature profiles, might facilitate the prioritization of management to those with a chance of contracting Chagas disease. Biomarker candidates might be engaged for the determination of some forms of Chagas disease. It is difficult to predict features related to morbidity and mortality as well as disease evolution. This information would assist in the supervision, decision-making, and follow-up related to this complex disease. Hence, there is a need to discover simple and quantifiable biomarkers that are more reliable than conventional screening methods and can be applied to support the diagnosis and prognosis of patients with heart failure (4).

A total of two systematic reviews of prospective biomarker targets during the course of therapeutic chronic Chagas disease underlined the requirement for the development of unique biomarkers to assess prompt responses to therapeutic management of the disease (5, 6). There are several studies that are investing in new diagnostic approaches to cure Chagas disease, particularly regarding the identification of disease biomarkers. Data from forthcoming studies will assist the categorization of patients in terms of clinical aspects for initial follow-ups (6).

Some blood-derived biomarkers that have demonstrated the capacity to predict the progression of early Chagas disease cardiomyopathy have been engaged to assess the value of antiparasitic drugs and to identify initial cardiac and gastrointestinal injuries in asymptomatic patients. Nevertheless, future studies with extended follow-ups are required to establish biomarkers that are able to assess clinical or parasitological cures following therapy (6).

Biomarkers might be categorized based on biochemical configurations and major biological activities, such as inflammation and cellular injury biomarkers, metabolic biomarkers, prothrombotic biomarkers, and antigenic biomarkers (i.e., specific antigens of the parasite). Conversely, we propose a different classification. **Table 1** and the next sections of this review summarize the recent data related to biomarker research. Once the scientific data become more readily available, the future identification of critical and consistent biomarker candidates for human Chagas disease should be simplified.

PLASMATIC-RELATED CANDIDATES

Effectively treated and cured chagasic patients may be identified based on their patterns of circulating biomarkers (7). Recently, studies have indicated that serum markers, such as A- and B-type natriuretic peptides (ANP and BNP, respectively), N-terminal pro-BNP, troponin I, TGF-β, MMP-2, and TIMP-1 and -2, are higher during the severe stages of Chagas disease and represent cardiac damage and inflammation. However, several candidates are not disease specific. Hitherto, the levels of these aforementioned natriuretic peptides have been found to be higher in Chagas disease patients with cardiomyopathy than in those with different forms or other etiologies. Moreover, natriuretic peptide levels are increased in asymptomatic chagasic patients who exhibit no signs of ventricular dysfunction. Hence, natriuretic peptides showed a high predictive value for evaluated outcomes (4, 8). Both of the pioneering studies were performed in Brazilian cohorts. According to the data from these studies, BNP is comparable to echocardiogram in terms of the assessment of cardiological patients. To reinforce those prior findings, another study performed in an independent setting found that BNP, pro-BNP, creatine kinase (CK)-MB, and MMP-2 have high predictive values for short-term mortality even in the presence of a decreased ejection fraction and other clinical signs of congestive heart failure, which were all found to be associated with severe chagasic cardiomyopathy in a Bolivian cohort (9).

TABLE 1 | Summary of biomarker investigations related to Chagas disease.

Study	Source	Biomarker name	Result	Reference
Experimental, parasitemia-specific	Antigenic	Aptamer	Increased levels	(39, 40)
Chagasic cardiomyopathy	Genetic	CCL2 and MAL/TIRAP	Increased susceptibility	(41)
Chagasic cardiomyopathy	Genetic	CCR5	Protection	(41)
Chagasic cardiomyopathy	Phenotype	CD15s+ Treg cells	Protection	(35, 36)
Chagasic cardiomyopathy	Phenotype	CD27+CD28+CD8+ T cells	Protection	(37, 38)
Non-specific	Plasmatic	TIMP-1 and TIMP-2	Increased levels	(5, 6)
Non-specific	Plasmatic	Troponin I	Increased levels	(5, 6)
Non-specific	Plasmatic	TGF-β	Increased levels	(5, 6)
Asymptomatic	Plasmatic	IL-10	Increased levels	(11)
Non-specific	Plasmatic	APOA1	Decreased levels	(7)
Non-specific	Plasmatic	Fibronectin	Increased levels	(7)
Asymptomatic	Plasmatic	MMP-2	Increased levels	(14)
Chagasic cardiomyopathy	Plasmatic	MMP-9	Increased levels	(14)
Chagasic cardiomyopathy	Plasmatic	ANP, BNP, N-terminal pro-BNP, IFN-γ, TNF-α, IL-1β, and IL-6	Increased levels	(4, 8, 10, 11)
Chagasic cardiomyopathy	Plasmatic	miRNA-1, miRNA-133a and -133b, and miRNA-208a and -208b	Decreased levels	(13)
Experimental, chagasic cardiomyopathy	Plasmatic	PICP and PIIINP	Increased levels	(15)
Experimental, chagasic cardiomyopathy	Plasmatic	Syndecan-4, ICAM-1, and Galectin-3	Increased levels	(16)
Efficacy	Management	KMP11, HSP70, PAR2, and Tgp63	Increased Ab. levels	(5, 6)
Efficacy	Management	Antigen 13 and SAPA	Increased Ab. levels	(5, 6)
Efficacy	Management	Tc24	Increased Ab. levels	(43)

Because the BNP procedure is simple and quick, this biomarker can be used in endemic zones of Chagas disease with limited access to echocardiographic housing facilities. Finally, pro-BNP and *T. cruzi* DNA as detected by PCR are the only tests that have been found to have independent clinical value for disease staging in concert with electrocardiogram (ECG), echocardiogram, and clinical assessments (10). In a different study, the authors found that cytokine levels are related to cardiac injury in Chagas disease (11). Asymptomatic individuals exhibited high IL-10 levels that were associated with better prognosis. Conversely, IL-1β, IL-6, IFN-γ, and TNF-α reached the highest levels of expression in chagasic patients with cardiomyopathy. Overall, these findings sustain the perception that the balance between regulatory and inflammatory cytokines is associated with different forms of chronic Chagas disease (11, 12). Some micro (mi)RNAs, such as miRNA-1, miRNA-133, and miRNA-208, have been demonstrated to be involved with gene regulation properties and specific expression profiles, and imbalances can be found in chagasic cardiomyopathy (13). Recently, Santamaria and colleagues (7) pursued the identification of serum biomarkers that might be used as surrogates of therapeutic management in Chagas disease. APOA1 and specific fragments thereof and one fragment of fibronectin were uncovered. In chagasic samples, these biomarkers, excluding the full-length APOA1, are upregulated. These biomarkers revert to regular levels in 43% of cured patients. Notably, whenever serum MMP-9 levels are dominant, cardiac remodeling is strengthened and the advance of the cardiac form of Chagas disease is favored. Conversely, when serum MMP-2 levels prevail, patients persist as clinically asymptomatic. These processes might be IL-1β- and TNF-α dependent (14). In a particular model of infection, the cardiac levels of collagen I, III, and IV rise steadily and reach a peak during the chronic phase of Chagas disease. Thereafter, high serum levels of procollagen type I carboxy-terminal propeptide (PICP) and procollagen type III amino-terminal propeptide (PIIINP) are also observed. Given that increased PICP and PIIINP levels may indicate cardiac fibrosis, it is tempting to speculate that both biomarkers are suitable for detecting fibrosis during cardiac remodeling associated with *T. cruzi* infection (15). ICAM-1, galectin-3, and syndecan-4 have been found to be overexpressed in the hearts of mice chronically infected with *T. cruzi* (16). High levels of expression of galectin-3 in inflammatory cells have also been uncovered, and these levels are correlated with a decline in inflammation. A reduction in syndecan-4 and ICAM-1 might indirectly reduce cell migration into the myocardium and, thus, decrease inflammation (17). By contrast, in attempts to the uncover critical aspects of TGF-β as a candidate with prognostic value, several studies have demonstrated the influence of this anti-inflammatory cytokine on the development of chagasic cardiomyopathy by facilitating parasite cell invasion and its cycle (18, 19), improving parasite survival (20, 21), inducing exacerbated heart fibrosis and remodeling (22, 23), downregulating cardiac gap junctions (24), and mediating hypertrophy of the surviving cardiomyocytes (25). Increased circulating levels of TGF-β are observed in chronic Chagas disease patients (22, 26), and its active form is observed in the myocardia of chronic patients (27, 28). Moreover, due to the substantial involvement of TGF-β in the development of cardiac damage observed in Chagas disease, active compounds targeting TGF-β are currently under study as alternative treatments for the symptomatic cardiac form of Chagas disease (24, 29). Recently, the major cysteine protease from *T. cruzi*, cruzipain, has been observed to be capable of directly activating latent TGF-β, which favors parasite invasion into host cells (30). New therapeutic approaches for Chagas disease using anti-cruzipain compounds would be of beneficial not only due to their trypanocidal effect but also because they indirectly inhibit different TGF-β activities that are crucial for the development of Chagas disease. A retrospective study reported evidence supporting the clinical prognostic value of TGF-β as a biomarker for Chagas disease by demonstrating an association between its serological levels and clinical outcomes after 10 years of follow-up (31). Accordingly, TGF-β has demonstrated prognostic value as an independent predictor of all-cause mortality in patients without heart failure and with an ejection fraction above 45%. The optimal TGF-β cutoff for identifying patients who presented with all-cause mortality was 12.9 ng/ml. A further prospective study is clearly necessary to validate these data. Thus, the serological levels of TGF-β could be considered one potential biomarker for the outcome of Chagas disease and, moreover, could be used to follow the effects of treatments and interventions.

PHENOTYPE-RELATED CANDIDATES

First, we would like to propose the regulatory T cell (Treg) axis as a biomarker for Chagas disease progression. As discussed elsewhere, a malfunction of regulatory immune mechanisms may also be involved in the pathogenesis of Chagas disease (32). This malfunction may be due to the action of Treg cells that have the potential to curb effector responses, allow a partially effective anti-parasite immune response, and therefore enable the establishment and maintenance of chronic Chagas infection (32). By contrast, recent findings in humans have demonstrated an increased rate of Treg cells in chagasic patients in the indeterminate chronic phase (free of disease) compared with those with heart damage, which suggests an important role for Treg cells in the control of the inflammatory response during Chagas disease (33). Additionally, using a non-depleting monoclonal antibody to CD25, it was recently demonstrated that Treg cells bearing the CD4+CD25+Foxp3+ phenotype may also help to control the inflammatory immune response in mice that are chronically infected with *T. cruzi* (34). Therefore, there is a clear indication that the functional activity of Treg cells might be of crucial importance during the chronic phase of the infection due to their potential to decrease tissue damage and pathology. Recently, the expression of CD15s (Sialyl Lewis x) was described to identify the majority of suppressive Treg cells in humans (35). Thus, this biomarker discriminates suppressive from effector CD4+CD25+Foxp3+ T cells in humans (35). Interestingly, a previous study reported that the expression of CD15s is decreased in peripheral blood lymphocytes from patients with severe Chagas disease (36). Although additional studies are urgently required to uncover the critical aspects of both phenotypes, the expression of CD15s in Treg cells may be a reliable biomarker for the prediction of the progression to pathology of chagasic patients. Additionally, another distinct phenotype, i.e., fully differentiated memory CD8 T cells (CD27−CD28−) bearing increased CCR7 expression, has been related to Chagas disease outcome (37). This study demonstrated an increase in total effector/memory CD8+ T cells in *T. cruzi*-infected individuals with mild heart disease compared with otherwise healthy controls. The study was based on the combined expression of CD27 and CD28 as previously proposed by Appay and colleagues (38), being related to a linear differentiation model for memory CD8+ T cells (38). This study suggested different fates of the T cell lineage, including early, intermediate, and late stages of cell-memory as follows: CD27+CD28+, CD27−CD28+ (or CD27+CD28−), and CD27−CD28− cells, respectively. As has previously been recognized, the proportion of fully differentiated memory (CD27−CD28−) in the total amount of CD8+ T cells is increased in mild Chagas disease. Conversely, the frequency of CD27+CD28+CD8+ T cells in the total memory CD8+ T cell population decreases as the disease becomes more severe. Albareda and colleagues (37) hypothesized that this pattern could be a consequence of the gradual clonal exhaustion of the CD8+ T cell population during infection. Analysis of the chemokine receptor CCR7 for lymph node homing (CCR7 expression) also revealed a significant increase in total effector/memory CD8 T cells in subjects with mild heart disease compared with healthy controls (37).

ANTIGENIC-RELATED CANDIDATES

A correlated ELISA approach to the detection of aptamers in mouse plasma that is highly specific for circulating parasite excreted-secreted antigens (TESA) has been developed for biomarkers of *T. cruzi* infection (39, 40). An aptamer exhibited specific binding to TESA and trypomastigote extract, but it did not bind to self-proteins or *Leishmania donovani* proteins. Infected mice have exhibited increased levels of aptamer binding compared with control littermates, which suggests this aptamer as a potential candidate for a future biomarker of *T. cruzi* infection. Furthermore, this aptamer might sense circulating biomarkers in both acute and chronic phases of Chagas disease (39). Recently, the same group confirmed that *T. cruzi*-infected mice have considerably higher biomarker levels than their non-infected counterparts. This study found that the biomarker levels are also diminished upon therapy (40). However, the biomarker levels in the infected and treated group did not decrease entirely and persisted above the assay cutoff point, which suggests that parasitemia was reduced, but a cure was not achieved. The test was capable of distinguishing circulating biomarkers in animals infected with several subpopulations of *T. cruzi*.

GENETIC-RELATED CANDIDATES

Genetic markers can provide evidence of the pathogenesis of Chagas disease and also have the potential to be utilized to identify new therapeutic targets. Frade and colleagues (41) studied genetic predispositions that influenced left ventricular ejection fractions in a Brazilian cohort. The authors found that CCL2 and MAL/TIRAP, but not CCR5, were linked to an increased susceptibility to chagasic cardiomyopathy.

MANAGEMENT-RELATED CANDIDATES

Regardless of most recent advances in drug development, there is virtually no consensus regarding the use of biomarkers to assess the efficacies of new drugs. Between the two main classes of recombinant proteins that are active during distinct ages and stages of Chagas disease, a 16-protein group and a combination of four recombinant proteins, namely KMP11, HSP70, PAR2, and Tgp63, have been identified (5). That combination could potentially serve as biomarkers candidates. Similarly, antibodies against antigen 13, among 5 others comprising the shed acute phase antigen (SAPA), have been demonstrated to be potential markers of cure efficacy [reviewed in Ref. (5)]. Additionally, a complement-mediated lysis test and an ELISA method based on Tc24 have also been created and the latter found to be a reliable candidate for a helpful parasite biomarker (42, 43).

FUTURE TRENDS

Researchers agree that the use of biomarkers in human Chagas disease will foster the progressing steps during the clinical assessment and also assist in the development of consistent diagnostic tools to lessen the time gap between the progression and detection of disease-relevant measures. Additionally, such biomarkers will allow for the prediction of both primary (genetic) and secondary (acquired factors) immunodeficiencies related to individual susceptibility. The deficiency of biomarkers in the prediction of parasitological outcome status and cure represents a main hurdle for the development of new drugs for Chagas disease. Thus, it is crucial to develop a reliable method to assess the cure of this disease. The aforementioned classes of biomarkers could yield uninterrupted longitudinal results related to Chagas disease management. Processes that are commonly used to identify biomarkers cannot be employed as endpoint evaluations in human clinical trials for ethical reasons. Some existing studies aim to develop alternative, emerging applications for biotechnologies based on the results of chagasic biomarker research. Furthermore, data from biomarker discovery research, such as the presence of TESA, could be used in vaccine development. In parasite-challenged vaccinated animals, TESA positivity could be an indication that the immune response was not appropriate to control the infection (39, 40). As a result of these struggles, the success of biomarker research in Chagas disease has not yet allowed for a better understanding of the disease risk from the clinical perspective. A range of issues exacerbates this frustration. One such issue is the incomplete validations of many biomarker candidates. Before conducting human trials, it is essential to identify and validate biomarkers that indicate cured patients. It is also necessary to evaluate the risks associated with the use of new agents in larger cohorts; thus, high-throughput biomarker procedures are needed. Ideally, approaching an accurate, rapid, and reliable point-of-care diagnostic tool in resource-limited, high-burden settings for Chagas disease through evaluation of biomarkers across that clinical spectrum in order to detect relevant pathogen-specific fingerprints will be of communal benefits, which undoubtedly outweigh the costs. The WHO predicted the eradication of

Chagas disease transmission by the year 2010, but this goal has not yet been achieved. Indeed, the disease is spreading beyond locations in which it was originally endemic (1). It is crucial to understand the partial corroboration of simple biomarker technologies to avoid generating data that exceeds our ability to analyze the applications of novel technologies that are emerging from population studies. Finally, it would be strategic to develop a wide variety of biomarkers and to test them during preclinical and clinical trials.

AUTHOR CONTRIBUTIONS

RP and PA conceived and participated in the design and coordination of the manuscript. MW, FC, and JM provided helpful discussions and edited the manuscript. All authors wrote, read, and approved the final manuscript.

ACKNOWLEDGMENTS

The authors are grateful to Mr. Patrick Salinas and to Mrs. Veronica Antas for text editing. We also thank the laboratory staff for their help during the writing of the manuscript.

REFERENCES

1. WHO. *Chagas Disease (American trypanosomiasis) Fact Sheet 340*. World Health Organization (2012). Available from: http://www.who.int/mediacentre/factsheets/fs340/en/index.html
2. Punukollu G, Gowda RM, Khan IA, Navarro VS, Vasavada BC. Clinical aspects of the Chagas' heart disease. *Int J Cardiol* (2007) 115:279–83. doi:10.1016/j.ijcard.2006.03.004
3. Pinazo MJ, Canas E, Elizalde JI, Garcia M, Gascon J, Gimeno F, et al. Diagnosis, management and treatment of chronic Chagas' gastrointestinal disease in areas where *Trypanosoma cruzi* infection is not endemic. *Gastroenterol Hepatol* (2010) 33:191–200. doi:10.1016/j.gastrohep.2009.07.009
4. Wang Y, Moreira Mda C, Heringer-Walther S, Ebermann L, Schultheiss HP, Wessel N, et al. Plasma ACE 2 activity is an independent prognostic marker in Chagas' disease and equally potent as BNP. *J Card Fail* (2010) 16(2):157–63. doi:10.1016/j.cardfail.2009.09.005
5. Requena-Mendez A, Lopez MC, Angheben A, Izquierdo L, Ribeiro I, Pinazo MJ, et al. Evaluating Chagas' disease progression and cure through blood-derived biomarkers: a systematic review. *Expert Rev Anti Infect Ther* (2013) 11(9):957–76. doi:10.1586/14787210.2013.824718
6. Pinazo MJ, Thomas MC, Bua J, Perrone A, Schijman AG, Viotti RJ, et al. Biological markers for evaluating therapeutic efficacy in Chagas' disease, a systematic review. *Expert Rev Anti Infect Ther* (2014) 12(4):479–96. doi:10.1586/14787210.2014.899150
7. Santamaria C, Chatelain E, Jackson Y, Miao Q, Ward BJ, Chappuis F, et al. Serum biomarkers predictive of cure in Chagas' disease patients after nifurtimox treatment. *BMC Infect Dis* (2014) 14:302. doi:10.1186/1471-2334-14-302
8. Ribeiro AL, Dos Reis AM, Barros MV, Rocha MOC. Brain natriuretic peptide and left ventricular dysfunction in Chagas' disease. *Lancet* (2002) 360(9331):461–2. doi:10.1016/S0140-6736(02)09638-1
9. Sherbuk JE, Okamoto EE, Marks MA, Fortuny E, Clark EH, Galdos-Cardenas G, et al. Biomarkers and mortality in severe Chagas cardiomyopathy. *Glob Heart* (2015) 10(3):173–80. doi:10.1016/j.gheart.2015.07.003
10. Keating SM, Deng X, Fernandes F, Cunha-Neto E, Ribeiro AL, Adesina B, et al. Inflammatory and cardiac biomarkers are differentially expressed in clinical stages of Chagas disease. *Int J Cardiol* (2015) 15(199):451–9. doi:10.1016/j.ijcard.2015.07.040
11. Sousa GR, Gomes JA, Fares RC, Damasio MP, Chaves AT, Ferreira KS, et al. Plasma cytokine expression is associated with cardiac morbidity in Chagas' disease. *PLoS One* (2014) 9(3):e87082. doi:10.1371/journal.pone.0087082
12. Guedes PM, Gutierrez FR, Silva GK, Dellalibera-Joviliano R, Rodrigues GJ, Bendhack LM, et al. Deficient regulatory T cell activity and low frequency of IL-17-producing T cells correlate with the extent of cardiomyopathy in human Chagas' disease. *PLoS Negl Trop Dis* (2012) 6(4):e1630. doi:10.1371/journal.pntd.0001630
13. Ferreira LR, Frade AF, Santos RH, Teixeira PC, Baron MA, Navarro IC, et al. MicroRNAs miR-1, miR-133a, miR-133b, miR-208a and miR-208b are dysregulated in chronic Chagas disease cardiomyopathy. *Int J Cardiol* (2014) 175(3):409–17. doi:10.1016/j.ijcard.2014.05.019
14. Fares RC, Gomes Jde A, Garzoni LR, Waghabi MC, Saraiva RM, Medeiros NI, et al. Matrix metalloproteinases 2 and 9 are differentially expressed in patients with indeterminate and cardiac clinical forms of Chagas' disease. *Infect Immun* (2013) 81(10):3600–8. doi:10.1128/IAI.00153-13
15. Castro-Sesquen YE, Gilman RH, Paico H, Yauri V, Angulo N, Ccopa F, et al. Cell death and serum markers of collagen metabolism during cardiac remodeling in *Cavia porcellus* experimentally infected with *Trypanosoma cruzi*. *PLoS Negl Trop Dis* (2013) 7(2):e1996. doi:10.1371/journal.pntd.0001996
16. Soares MB, de Lima RS, Rocha LL, Vasconcelos JF, Rogatto SR, dos Santos RR, et al. Gene expression changes associated with myocarditis and fibrosis in hearts of mice with chronic chagasic cardiomyopathy. *J Infect Dis* (2010) 202(3):416–26. doi:10.1086/653481
17. Vasconcelos JF, Souza BS, Lins TF, Garcia LM, Kaneto CM, Sampaio GP, et al. Administration of granulocyte colony-stimulating factor induces immunomodulation, recruitment of T regulatory cells, reduction of myocarditis and decrease of parasite load in a mouse model of chronic Chagas disease cardiomyopathy. *FASEB J* (2013) 27(12):4691–702. doi:10.1096/fj.13-229351
18. Waghabi MC, Keramidas M, Bailly S, Degrave W, Mendonça-Lima L, Soeiro MN, et al. Uptake of host cell transforming growth factor-beta by *Trypanosoma cruzi* amastigotes in cardiomyocytes: potential role in parasite cycle completion. *Am J Pathol* (2005) 167(4):993–1003. doi:10.1016/S0002-9440(10)61189-3
19. Waghabi MC, Keramidas M, Feige JJ, Araujo-Jorge TC, Bailly S. Activation of transforming growth factor beta by *Trypanosoma cruzi*. *Cell Microbiol* (2005) 7(4):511–7. doi:10.1111/j.1462-5822.2004.00481.x
20. Silva JS, Twardzik DR, Reed SG. Regulation of *Trypanosoma cruzi* infections in vitro and in vivo by transforming growth factor beta (TGF-beta). *J Exp Med* (1991) 174(3):539–45. doi:10.1084/jem.174.3.539
21. dos Reis GA. Evasion of immune responses by *Trypanosoma cruzi*, the etiological agent of Chagas disease. *Braz J Med Biol Res* (2011) 44:84–90. doi:10.1590/S0100-879X2011007500005
22. Araújo-Jorge TC, Waghabi MC, Hasslocher-Moreno AM, Xavier SS, Higuchi ML, Keramidas M, et al. Implication of transforming growth factor-beta1 in Chagas disease myocardiopathy. *J Infect Dis* (2002) 186(12):1823–8. doi:10.1086/345882
23. Rossi MA. The pattern of myocardial fibrosis in chronic Chagas' heart disease. *Int J Cardiol* (1991) 30(3):335–40. doi:10.1016/0167-5273(91)90012-E
24. Waghabi MC, Coutinho-Silva R, Feige JJ, Higuchi Mde L, Becker D, Burnstock G, et al. Gap junction reduction in cardiomyocytes following transforming growth factor-beta treatment and *Trypanosoma cruzi* infection. *Mem Inst Oswaldo Cruz* (2009) 104(8):1083–90.
25. Rosenkranz S. TGF-beta1 and angiotensin networking in cardiac remodeling. *Cardiovasc Res* (2004) 63(3):423–32. doi:10.1016/j.cardiores.2004.04.030
26. Perez AR, Silva-Barbosa SD, Berbert LR, Revelli S, Beloscar J, Savino W, et al. Immunoneuroendocrine alterations in patients with progressive forms of chronic Chagas disease. *J Neuroimmunol* (2011) 235(1–2):84–90. doi:10.1016/j.jneuroim.2011.03.010

27. Araujo-Jorge TC, Waghabi MC, Soeiro MN, Keramidas M, Bailly S, Feige JJ. Pivotal role for TGF-beta in infectious heart disease: the case of *Trypanosoma cruzi* infection and consequent chagasic myocardiopathy. *Cytokine Growth Factor Rev* (2008) 19(5–6):405–13. doi:10.1016/j.cytogfr.2008.08.002
28. Araujo-Jorge TC, Waghabi MC, Bailly S, Feige JJ. The TGF-β pathway as an emerging target for Chagas disease therapy. *Clin Pharmacol Ther* (2012) 92(5):613–21. doi:10.1038/clpt.2012.102
29. de Oliveira FL, Araujo-Jorge TC, de Souza EM, de Oliveira GM, Degrave WM, Feige JJ, et al. Oral administration of GW788388, an inhibitor of transforming growth factor beta signaling, prevents heart fibrosis in Chagas disease. *PLoS Negl Trop Dis* (2012) 6(6):e1696. doi:10.1371/journal.pntd.0001696
30. Ferrao PM, d'Avila-Levy CM, Araujo-Jorge TC, Degrave WM, Gonçalves AS, Garzoni LR, et al. Cruzipain activates latent TGF-β from host cells during *T. cruzi* invasion. *PLoS One* (2015) 10(5):e0124832. doi:10.1371/journal.pone.0124832
31. Saraiva RM, Waghabi MC, Vilela MF, Madeira FS, Sperandio da Silva GM, Xavier SS, et al. Predictive value of transforming growth factor-β1 in Chagas disease: towards a biomarker surrogate of clinical outcome. *Trans R Soc Trop Med Hyg* (2013) 107(8):518–25. doi:10.1093/trstmh/trt050
32. Cardillo F, de Pinho RT, Antas PR, Mengel J. Immunity and immune modulation in *Trypanosoma cruzi* infection. *Pathog Dis* (2015) 73(9):ftv082. doi:10.1093/femspd/ftv082
33. de Araujo FF, Vitelli-Avelar DM, Teixeira-Carvalho A, Antas PR, Assis Silva Gomes J, Sathler-Avelar R, et al. Regulatory T cells phenotype in different clinical forms of Chagas disease. *PLoS Negl Trop Dis* (2011) 5(5):e992. doi:10.1371/journal.pntd.0000992
34. Nihei J, Cardillo F, Dos Santos WL, Pontes-de-Carvalho L, Mengel J. Administration of a nondepleting anti-CD25 monoclonal antibody reduces disease severity in mice infected with *Trypanosoma cruzi*. *Eur J Microbiol Immunol (Bp)* (2014) 4(2):128–37. doi:10.1556/EuJMI.4.2014.2.6
35. Miyara M, Chader D, Sage E, Sugiyama D, Nishikawa H, Bouvry D, et al. Sialyl Lewis x (CD15s) identifies highly differentiated and most suppressive FOXP3high regulatory T cells in humans. *Proc Natl Acad Sci U S A.* (2015) 112(23):7225–30. doi:10.1073/pnas.1508224112
36. Laucella SA, Riarte A, Prado N, Zapata J, Segura EL. alpha 4 integrins and sialyl Lewis x modulation in chronic Chagas disease: further evidence of persistent immune activation. *Scand J Immunol* (2001) 53(5):514–9. doi:10.1046/j.1365-3083.2001.00916.x
37. Albareda MC, Laucella SA, Alvarez MG, Armenti AH, Bertochi G, Tarleton RL, et al. *Trypanosoma cruzi* modulates the profile of memory CD8 T cells in chronic Chagas disease patients. *Int Immunol* (2006) 18(3):465–71. doi:10.1093/intimm/dxh387
38. Appay V, Dunbar PR, Callan M, Klenerman P, Gillespie GM, Papagno L, et al. Memory CD8+ T cells vary in differentiation phenotype in different persistent virus infections. *Nat Med* (2006) 8:379. doi:10.1038/nm0402-379
39. Nagarkatti R, de Araujo FF, Gupta C, Debrabant A. Aptamer based, non-PCR, non-serological detection of Chagas' disease biomarkers in *Trypanosoma cruzi* infected mice. *PLoS Negl Trop Dis* (2014) 8(1):e2650. doi:10.1371/journal.pntd.0002650
40. de Araujo FF, Nagarkatti R, Gupta C, Marino AP, Debrabant A. Aptamer-based detection of disease biomarkers in mouse models for Chagas drug discovery. *PLoS Negl Trop Dis* (2015) 9(1):e3451. doi:10.1371/journal.pntd.0003451
41. Frade AF, Pissetti CW, Ianni BM, Saba B, Lin-Wang HT, Nogueira LG, et al. Genetic susceptibility to Chagas disease cardiomyopathy: involvement of several genes of the innate immunity and chemokine-dependent migration pathways. *BMC Infect Dis* (2013) 13:587. doi:10.1186/1471-2334-13-587
42. Galvao LM, Nunes RM, Cançado JR, Brener Z, Krettli AU. Lytic antibody titre as a means of assessing cure after treatment of Chagas' disease: a 10 years follow-up study. *Trans R Soc Trop Med Hyg* (1993) 87(2):220–3. doi:10.1016/0035-9203(93)90501-G
43. Krautz GM, Galvão LM, Cançado JR, Guevara-Espinoza A, Ouaissi A, Krettli AU. Use of a 24-kilodalton *Trypanosoma cruzi* recombinant protein to monitor cure of human Chagas' disease. *J Clin Microbiol* (1995) 33(8):2086–90.

2

Malaria Parasites: The Great Escape

Laurent Rénia* and Yun Shan Goh

*Singapore Immunology Network, Agency for Science, Technology and Research (A*STAR), Singapore*

***Correspondence:**
Laurent Rénia
renia_laurent@immunol.a-star.edu.sg

Parasites of the genus *Plasmodium* have a complex life cycle. They alternate between their final mosquito host and their intermediate hosts. The parasite can be either extra- or intracellular, depending on the stage of development. By modifying their shape, motility, and metabolic requirements, the parasite adapts to the different environments in their different hosts. The parasite has evolved to escape the multiple immune mechanisms in the host that try to block parasite development at the different stages of their development. In this article, we describe the mechanisms reported thus far that allow the *Plasmodium* parasite to evade innate and adaptive immune responses.

Keywords: malaria, vaccine, escape mechanism, antibodies, T cells, immunosuppression, antigenic polymorphism, antigenic variation

INTRODUCTION

Malaria, a disease caused by *Plasmodium* parasites and transmitted by *Anopheles* mosquitoes, remains one of the most deadly diseases. There are six species able to infect humans, namely, *Plasmodium falciparum*, *Plasmodium vivax*, *Plasmodium ovale*, *Plasmodium malariae*, and the zoonotic monkey malaria species *Plasmodium knowlesi* (1) and *Plasmodium cynomolgi* (2). Around 300 million cases of clinical malaria are recorded every year. Approximately, half a million deaths occur in Africa and are mainly due to *P. falciparum* infections (3).

Plasmodium parasites have a complex life cycle. It starts when sporozoites are inoculated into the dermis of the mammalian host by infected mosquitoes. Sporozoites are highly motile and a majority of them migrate from the skin to the capillaries for dissemination by the bloodstream (4, 5). They are retained in the liver where they transmigrate through Kupffer cells and hepatocytes before seeding in final hepatocytes (6, 7). Depending on the species of their mammalian hosts, sporozoites mature in 2–14 days. At maturity, budding vesicles called merosomes are released and are ruptured in the lung circulation where the merozoites are released, ready to infect red blood cells (RBC) (8). During the erythrocytic cycle, a fraction of parasites differentiates into male and female gametocytes which can be taken up during the feeding of an *Anopheles* mosquito. In the mosquito midgut, ookinetes, generated by the gametocyte fusion, cross the mosquito midgut wall and develop into oocysts. Sporozoites released from mature oocyst then migrate to the salivary gland, ready for the next round of infection during the mosquito's next blood meal.

Malaria is a disease characterized by fever, headache, chills, sweating, and vomiting (9). Unlike viral or bacterial infections, the main indication of clinical malaria is the recurrent fever which varies between species. This is due to the release of parasite toxins into the bloodstream during the erythrocytic cycles of merozoite egress and reinvasion of erythrocytes. As the infection progresses, the number of RBC decreases and this may lead to severe anemia (10). In addition, RBC containing parasites such as *P. falciparum* can also sequester in deep tissues by cytoadhering to endothelial cells (11). This may cause organ failure, and is partly responsible for cerebral malaria. All these pathologies can eventually lead to death (9, 12, 13).

In the last two decades, the mortality to malaria has decreased substantially (3). This results from the combined efficacy of prevention measures, such as the use of insecticide-impregnated bednets, the development and use of rapid and easy to use diagnostic tools, and the potent artemisinin-based combinations therapies against the malaria parasites (14). However, this gain of lives might be temporary. In the recent years, all these interventions have shown some limitations. With the advent of decreased efficacy of artemisinin (15, 16), it is now clear that new drugs and other interventions should be developed (9, 17, 18). New drug families, such as spiroindolones (19, 20) and imidalopiperazines (21, 22) compounds, have shown promising results in phase II clinical trials in the recent years and have a great future ahead. However, a vaccine would be the most important tool in the armamentarium against malaria.

While vaccines have been readily developed for many bacterial and viral infections, there are currently no vaccines to protect against human parasites. The need to develop a vaccine to protect against malaria has been highlighted as early as the identification of the parasite in 1897 (23). There have been two schools of thought for the development an antimalarial vaccine. The first is based on the fact that naturally acquired immunity is often observed under field conditions. However, this immunity requires long period of time to develop. It first targets the disease and then the parasite (24). This immunity has been called premonition or relative immunity. It has been defined by Edmond Sergent in 1935 as "*a special type of immunity connected with the persistence of living germs in the organs of the immunized host*" (25). In other words, immunity is maintained as long as the host immunity is stimulated by the continuous or repeated parasite exposure. Understanding the mechanisms responsible for this premonition will help to develop a vaccine.

The other approach is based on the Jenner principle of vaccination, which was further exemplified by Louis Pasteur. Instead of letting Nature takes its course, this approach uses an inoffensive target as a formulation to induce an immune response in healthy individuals to protect against a subsequent infection. It might not be surprising, that the first attempt was reported by the same Sergent mentioned above, who was working in the Pasteur Institute in Algiers in Algeria. Sergent was able to partially protect birds from *Plasmodium lophurae*, an avian malaria parasite, using inactivated sporozoites (26). Decades later, in 1946, the first attempt in human was done by Heidelberger et al. using formalin-inactivated *P. vivax*-infected blood to immunize volunteers, however no protection was induced (27, 28). Jules Freund took it one step further by inventing the Freund adjuvant and combining the adjuvant with formalin-inactivated-blood infected with *P. lophurae* or *P. knowlesi*, a monkey malaria parasite. Freund was more successful in protecting ducks or rhesus monkeys, respectively (29, 30). However, because of its toxic side effects, the adjuvant could not be used in humans. Since then, various approaches and technologies have been used for vaccine development against the malaria parasites. Purified parasite preparation has been used as immunogens. Peptides, recombinant proteins, DNA plasmids, bacterial and viral vectors, and genetically modified malaria parasites, in combination with new adjuvants, have also been used as vaccine delivery systems (31). However, despite having more than thousands of pre-clinical trials in rodent and monkey models and more than 200 trials in humans, very few vaccine candidates have shown vaccine efficacy in human. The subunit vaccine, RTS,S, a chimeric molecule based on a large part of the circumsporozoite (CS) protein, the major surface protein of the sporozoite, fused to the S antigen of the hepatitis B virus, together with a strong adjuvant in the formulation, is the only candidate that has moved to Phase III clinical trials. However its efficacy was at best ~50% against infection or clinical disease (32, 33). So far, only whole-parasite based approaches have repeatedly shown high efficacy (34–36).

MECHANISMS OF IMMUNITY AGAINST THE MALARIA PARASITE

The parasite has a complex life cycle. Depending on the stage of development in its mammalian host, the parasite can be extracellular or intracellular. The parasite exists in different forms and shapes, possibly expressing different sets of its ~ 5000 gene pool (37) at a particular time. The parasite also has different localizations during development, infecting different cell types. Hence, various innate and adaptive immune mechanisms are involved in parasite control and elimination (38, 39). Thus, for any vaccine development, it is important to know the protective immune mechanisms to induce.

Immunity to the Pre-Erythrocytic Stage

During the pre-erythrocytic stage, antibodies can (i) inhibit sporozoite motility in the dermis or in the liver (40), (ii) bind to sporozoite and facilitate phagocytosis by monocytes or macrophages in the spleen or the liver (41), (iii) block sporozoite invasion into hepatocytes by preventing the sporozoite ligand to interact with the hepatocyte receptor(s) (42), and (iv) inhibit sporozoite development inside the hepatocytes (42). Antibodies can also recognize parasite neo-antigens such as heat-shock protein expressed at the surface of infected hepatocytes and induce liver parasite killing through an antibody-dependent cell-mediated mechanism likely involving Kuppfer cells or NK cells (43). The production of high levels of antibodies is dependent of CD4 T cell help, preferably by recognizing (an) epitope(s) present in the sporozoite to facilitate boosting of the antibody during natural infection with the parasite. When the parasite is inside the hepatocytes, it can become the target of CD4 or CD8 T cells (44–46). Hepatocytes express MHC Class I and Class II molecules that can be loaded with parasite antigen-derived epitopes following the TAP or the endosomal pathways (44–47). T cells kill the parasite either directly or through the action of cytokines, such as IFN-γ. IFN-γ induces the inducible nitric oxide enzyme to produce nitric oxide which directly kills the liver parasites (48–51). Innate immune mechanisms involving type I interferon pathway induced by the parasite infection and active against late schizonts or against reinfection have been recently uncovered (52–54).

Immunity against the Erythrocytic Stage

Adaptive immunity against the blood stage is more complex than in the liver stage. Merozoite-specific antibodies can (i) prevent merozoites from invading RBC alone (55–57) or, in conjunction with complement factors, (ii) prevent merozoite egress from RBC, (iii) agglutinate released merozoites, (iv) promote phagocytosis of merozoites, and (v) facilitate clearance of infected RBC (iRBC) by phagocytic cells through a mechanism called antibody cell-dependent inhibition (ADCI) (58). In ADCI, anti-merozoite cryophilic (IgG1 or IgG3) antibodies bind to merozoites and the immune complexes stimulate phagocytes to release cytokines such as TNF-α, which in turn stimulate the phagocytes to produce mediators that lead to the killing of intra-erythrocytic parasites (59, 60). *Plasmodium* parasites express antigens at the surface of iRBC (61). These antigens are mainly encoded by multigene families such as the *var* (62), *stevor* (63), and *rifins* gene families (64, 65) for *P. falciparum* or the *pir* gene family for *P. vivax*, *P. knowlesi*, and the rodent malaria species (66). The antigens they encoded have been implicated in the cytoadherence phenotype to endothelial cells in deep tissues in order to avoid splenic clearance (67, 68). They are also involved in other adhesive phenomena, such as rosetting (the binding of an iRBC to non-infected RBC) (69–72) and agglutination (the binding to iRBC to iRBC through bridging by platelets) (73, 74). The cytoadherence abilities of the malaria parasites have been proposed to be responsible for some of the pathologies during malaria infection. Antibodies targeting the surface antigens are thought to act through preventing cytoadherence, promoting iRBC phagocytosis, or iRBC agglutination (74, 75).

Antibodies targeting the parasite toxins could also protect from disease. During infection, multiple parasite toxins are released at the time of iRBC rupture. These toxins include the malaria pigment, a by-product of heme degradation by the parasite (76–78), glycophosphatidylinositol (GPI) moieties that are present in many merozoite proteins, a TatD-like DNase (79), a tyrosine-tRNA synthase (80), or lipids extracted from *P. vivax* schizonts (81). Protection from disease by anti-toxins antibodies has been demonstrated experimentally using synthetic glycans mimicking GPI (82).

T cells are also critical effectors in the immunity against blood-stage malaria infections, despite the lack of MHC antigens on the surface of iRBC. First and foremost, blood-stage parasite-specific antibodies secreted by B cells depend on $CD4^+$ T helper cells enhancement for optimal production (39). Cytokines released by CD4 T cells are important for multiplication and maturation of B cells. The cytokines produced by malaria-specific T cells influence the isotype of the antibodies produced (83, 84) and thus possibly affecting the type of antibody-mediated responses induced. It has been shown that ADCI against *P. falciparum* is mediated by human IgG3 (induced by a Th1 response) and antagonized by IgG2 and IgG4 (induced by a Th2 response) (59, 85). Inducing the right isotype is thus important for an antibody-based vaccine. Recent studies have shown that inducing an immune response skewed toward the IgG3 could be achieved through the use of the right adjuvant (86). CD8 T cells were once thought to have only a minimal role in blood-stage immunity (87, 88). However, there is now evidence that these cells can inhibit blood-stage infection (89, 90). In particular, IFNγ-secreting CD8 T cells are important for preventing chronic blood-stage infection in mice (91).

Immunity against the Sexual Stages

The sexual forms of *Plasmodium* parasites, gametocytes, are also targets of the immunity against the disease. They are targeted by antibodies which can induce complement-mediated killing of the gametocytes in the host blood (92, 93). In the mosquito, antibodies can (i) prevent gamete fusion (94), (ii) induce complement-killing of gametes or ookinetes (95), and (ii) prevent ookinete motility, penetration of the midgut wall and formation of oocyst (96–99). Sexual-stage parasite-specific antibodies depend on CD4 T helper cells for optimal production. However, although antibodies specific for gametes or ookinetes can be produced by vaccination, the humoral immune response cannot be boosted by repeated infections since these forms are not present during infection in the mammalian hosts. Monocytes/macrophages stimulated during infection by the parasites produce cytokines such as TNF-α which in turn stimulates the monocytes/macrophages to produce nitric oxide, a potent inhibitor of gametocytes (100).

MECHANISMS OF IMMUNE EVASION

To avoid being eliminated by the host immunity, the parasite has developed many escape strategies (**Table 1**).

EVASION OF THE COMPLEMENT SYSTEM

The complement system is one of the first innate immune defense mechanisms against pathogens. Many proteins are involved in the activation or the regulation of its lytic activity (101). During the blood-stage, the parasite has developed multiple ways of evading the action of complement. *P. falciparum* merozoites and iRBC bind to the factor H (fH), a complement regulator factor, and its alternatively spliced form fH-like protein 1 through its surface molecule Pf92. In the mosquito, gametes bind the fH through PfGAP50 (102). In both situations, this allows protection against the activation of complement-mediated lysis. In addition, ookinetes express Pfs47, which disrupts the c-Jun N-terminal kinase pathway and prevents mosquito midgut epithelial nitration, making the parasite undetectable by complement system (103).

ANTIBODY-DEPENDENT ENHANCEMENT OF INFECTION

Antibody-dependent enhancement of infection was first described for viruses (104). Similarly, antibody-dependent enhancement of infection has been described for all stages of parasite development in the mammalian host. It was first reported in the early 1990s that antibodies against the repeat region of the CS protein enhance sporozoite entry and development in hepatocytes for both rodent (42, 43) and human parasites (105). Antibodies against the *P. falciparum* asparagine-rich protein enhance merozoite invasion of RBC *in vitro* (106). Merozoite-specific antibodies in conjunction with complement can also facilitate RBC invasion (107). Antibody-dependent enhancement of infection was also observed *in vivo* after immunization with a *Plasmodium berghei* parasite blood-stage preparation

TABLE 1 | Host immunity and parasite immune escape strategies.

Host immunity	Parasite stage	Parasite evasion strategy	Outcome
Complement	AS, S	Bind complement regulatory factor, factor H Disrupt c-Jun kinase pathway	Prevent complement activation system Avoid recognition by complement
Monocytes/macrophages	AS	Subvert or kill phagocytes by (1) inhibiting phagocytosis and (2) inducing apoptosis	Prevent parasite elimination by (1) inhibiting phagocyte function and (2) reducing phagocyte numbers
Dendritic cells (DC)	AS	Subvert or kill DC by (1) inhibiting DC maturation and (2) engaging apoptosis receptor, Fas	Decrease DC functions by (1) preventing T cell priming and expansion and (2) inducing immunosuppression through decreased pro-inflammatory (IL12) cytokine production and increased immunosuppressive (IL10) cytokine production
Antibodies/B cells	Spz, AS, S	Antibody enhancement invasion and/or growth	Expansion of parasite in host
	Spz, AS, S	Antigen polymorphism	Avoid recognition by antibody
	AS	Antigenic variation	Avoid recognition by antibody
	AS	Antigenic diversion	Prevent the action of neutralizing antibodies
	AS	Epitope masking	Prevent the action of neutralizing antibodies
	AS	Smoke-screen strategy	Avoid antibody recognition by diverting neutralizing antibody from their target
	AS	B cell dysregulation	Poor or limited B cell memory
	Spz, AS, S	Homology with host proteins	Poor or no antibody response by inducing immunological tolerance
	AS	B cell apoptosis	Poor antibody response
	AS	Redundancy in cell invasion pathways	Allow continued invasion and expansion of parasite even when one invasion pathway is inhibited by antibody
T cells	LS	T cell epitope polymorphism	Avoid T cell recognition prevent T cell priming and activity, and interfere with memory T cell development
	AS	Apoptosis	Poor T cell response
	AS	Induction of expression of check-point inhibitors	Anergy and/or T cell exhaustion
	AS	Regulatory T cells	Negative regulation of immune responses
Hepatocytes	LS	Cellular shelter	Avoid immune surveillance due to intracellular niche

Spz, sporozoite; LS, liver stage; AS, asexual blood stage; S, sexual stage.

which led to increased death after challenge (108). In the sexual stage, anti-gamete antibodies were shown to enhance transmission to the mosquito (109).

Antibodies against proteins expressed in one stage of the parasite's development might mediate an enhancement effect in another stage of the parasite's development. This was observed for antibodies against two antigens, the CS protein and heat-shock protein 1 (HSP-1) (110). The CS protein is expressed during sporogony in the mosquito and in the subsequent sporozoite stage. Do Rosario et al. showed that sporozoites generated during sporogony in the presence of anti-CS protein antibodies cannot be inhibited by human polyclonal anti-CS (sporozoite CS) protein (111). HSP70-1 is expressed by the liver stage and the blood stages (43, 110). HSP70-1 antibodies have no effect against the blood-stage parasites but they can partially mediate inhibition of liver-stage development through ADCI (43). However, vaccination with a recombinant protein against the C-terminal fragment of HSP70-1 increased the number of gametocytes generated and the subsequent transmission to mosquito (112). Thus, it was proposed that antibodies against the liver-stage parasites can drive merozoites to differentiate into gametocytes and facilitate transmission (112). Immune cross-talk between the different stages of the infection has not been extensively studied beyond the two reports mentioned above. This cross-talk has wider implications. Indeed vaccination against one stage may influence the subsequent stages positively or negatively. For any vaccine against the pre-erythrocytic or blood stages, there will be a need for follow-up studies on the effect on transmission and development of the parasite in the mosquitoes.

ANTIGENIC POLYMORPHISM

Similar to all other organisms, the parasite is prone to mutation since the replicative machinery is not error free. In its mammalian host, the parasite is haploid and the mutation rate is $\sim 1–0.7 \times 10^{-9}$ mutations per base per generation (113). Since the *Plasmodium* parasites have a 24- to 72-h blood cycle, there is a high probability that mutation can occur and generate different parasite clones. In the mosquito host, the parasite undergoes sexual reproduction where two haploid gametocytes will generate four haploid sporozoite progenies. Recombination does occur in the mosquito stage, and, thus, it will increase the occurrence of gene polymorphism. For some antigens, hundreds of haplotypes have been observed (114). Polymorphism in the coding sequence can be due to point mutations, insertions, or deletions. Interestingly, many *Plasmodium* antigens possess regions of repeats which can vary in size and number of repetitive units (115). Such diversity is, in most cases, the result of immune pressure since mutations often occur in regions which can be recognized by antibodies or T cells. Mutations in B epitopes abolish the recognition of parasites by antibodies and may lead to the selection of parasites with a different haplotype. This is important for vaccine development since antibody-based vaccine formulation targeting polymorphic epitopes may either have limited efficacy or select for vaccine-resistant parasite. One such example is the vaccine based on the AMA-1 protein, a highly polymorphic antigen (116–118). However, it is possible to envisage that immunogen(s) inducing broadly inhibitory antibodies recognizing multiple variants may circumvent polymorphism. Studies to identify structural conserved constraints in different variants may pave the way for new vaccines against polymorphic antigens (56).

Polymorphism in T cell epitopes may have profound consequences in T cell responses and have shown to limit the efficacy of the RTS,S vaccine (119). T cell epitopes are, in general, 8–11 amino acid (aa) and 11–25 aa in length for CD8 T cell and CD4 T cells, respectively (120). After the digestion of parasite protein in the cytoplasm, CD8 antigenic peptides are generated and transported to endoplasmic reticulum by the transporter antigenic peptide protein in the endoplasmic reticulum where they are loaded onto MHC class I molecules and beta 2-microglobulin. CD4 epitopes are generated in endosomes after phagocytosis and protease digestion where they meet MHC class II. Peptide–MHC complexes are then expressed in the surface. Exogenous antigens can also be presented by cross-presentation by MHC class I (121). These complexes can be recognized by the T cell receptor (122). Mutations in the amino acids that anchor the epitope to the MHC grove can prevent binding of the peptides to the MHC or recognition by the TCR and thus abrogate T cell activity (123, 124). This was demonstrated for the CS protein (125). Altered peptide ligand (APL) can still bind to the MHC molecules; however, they prevent T cell proliferation, no matter if it was used singly or concurrently with a wild-type peptide. They can also prevent cytokine production (126) or change their production pattern, i.e., from IFN-γ to the immunosuppressive cytokine interleukin-10 (127). These APL can also interfere with induction of memory T cells from naïve T cells (128). This potent mechanism of immune escape is a major hurdle for vaccine development. For any T cell-based vaccine to succeed, a thorough analysis of T cell polymorphism and their effect should be performed.

ANTIGENIC VARIATION

Antigenic variation was first described by Neil Brown during *P. knowlesi* chronic relapsing infection in Rhesus monkeys induced by sub-curative drug treatment (129). In an agglutination assay, antibodies produced against different relapse parasite broods agglutinated only schizonts of the immunizing brood but not the other broods. It was further shown that antibodies (130) and spleen could induce antigenic variation in Rhesus monkey infected with a cloned line of *P. knowlesi* (67) or monkey infected with cloned lines of *P. falciparum* (131). The latter experiments suggested that, contrary to antigenic polymorphism where parasites have different alleles and can be categorized as genomic clones, antigenic variation is a phenotypic variation occurring with the same genomic clone of the parasite. The molecular basis of this phenomenon was elucidated with the sequencing of large segments of the *P. falciparum* and *P. knowlesi* genomes and the subsequent complete sequencing of the genome of many *Plasmodium* species. Antigens prone to antigenic variation are often expressed on the surface of iRBC. Examples includes the multigene family, such the *var* genes (62), the *stevor* gene family, the *rifin* gene family (63), the *surfin* gene family (132), the *sicavar* gene family (133), and the *Plasmodium* interspersed repeats (*pir*) genes. The *var* gene family is the most studied and has been shown to be the target of protective anti-blood-stage antibodies (134, 135). It is also involved in many of malaria pathologies due to parasite sequestration resulting from iRBC cytoadherence (136). PfEMP1 proteins, encoded by the *var* gene family, are highly polymorphic and have different variable domains, called Duffy binding-like domain, which determine their binding specificities to various ligands on endothelial cells such as thrombospondin (137), CD36 (138), ICAM-1/CD54 (139), chondroitin sulfate A (140–142), VCAM-1, E-selectin (143), αvβ3 integrin (144), hyaluronic acid (145), PECAM-1/CD31 (146), gC1qR/HABP1/p32 (147), or endothelial protein C receptor (148). PfEMP-1 proteins bind also to RBC through complement receptor 1 to form rosettes (149). *P. falciparum* parasites possess ~60 var genes distributed over the 14 chromosomes of the parasite (37). *Var* genes expression is extremely regulated and only one PfEMP1 type is produced and displayed on the surface of iRBC (150). At each cycle, the parasite switches the expression of the *var* gene at a rate of 2% *in vitro*, generating new clones with new antigenic and adhesive phenotype (151, 152). Vir proteins, members of a superfamily of the *pir* multigene superfamily, also mediate cytoadherence of *P. vivax* iRBC to endothelial cells (153), resulting to sequestration of mature iRBC (154). There are ~350 *vir* genes, and they are also highly polymorphic (155, 156). Stevor and Rifin proteins are involved in cytoadherence processes and are also highly polymorphic (70, 71). In the recent years, it has become clear that some members of these multigene family has a particular role and may be involved in certain pathology. As example, *var2*CSA mediated the specific cytoadherence of iRBC to placenta (142) and is associated with placental pathology, such as still birth and fetus growth retardation Vaccination using immunogens based on *var2*CSA will thus induce inhibitory antibodies, preventing cytoadherence (157, 158) and placental sequestration. Thus defining the role of members of these multigene families may lead to tailored immune intervention.

ANTIGENIC DIVERSION

Antigenic diversion occurs when non-inhibitory anti-parasite antibodies prevent the action of inhibitory antibodies. Antigenic diversion has been observed with the merozoite surface protein (MSP)-1. MSP-1 is a surface protein which binds to glycophorin A, a molecule present on the surface of RBC, and thus is essential for merozoite invasion (159, 160). MSP-1 is cleaved at the time of invasion. Neutralizing antibodies, which block the proteolytic cleavage in the C-terminal part (MSP-1_{19}) of the protein (antibodies), can prevent invasion (152, 161). However, antibodies against the adjacent or overlapping region can block the effect of MSP1_{19}-inhibitory antibodies (blocking antibodies) and thus allowing invasion to occur (162). One possibility to overcome this phenomenon is to design immunogen(s) that either induce(s) neutralizing but not blocking antibodies in naïve individuals or tip the balance to greater production of neutralizing antibodies over blocking antibodies in naturally exposed individuals. So far, there has been limited success with MSP-1 (159, 163).

EPITOPE MASKING

Epitope masking is the capacity of non-parasite-specific antibodies to prevent parasite-specific inhibitory antibodies to react with their epitopes. During the establishment of an antibody response, IgM precedes IgG production and thus are the first line of humoral response either alone or in combination with complement (164). Malaria-specific IgM have been shown to have efficient inhibitory activity against sporozoite and iRBC (165). However, IgM with different specificities can also bind to PfEMP-1 molecules expressed at the surface of iRBC through their Fc portion (Fc) (166). Non-parasite-specific IgM (NpsIgM) promote rosetting and thus may facilitate sequestration, in order to avoid splenic elimination. NpsIgM binding to the PfEMP-1 VARCSA2, which is involved in the binding of iRBC to chondroitin sulfate in the placenta, appears to protect iRBC from phagocytosis mediated by IgG (167). NpsIgM also binds to the MSP DBLMSP and DBLMSP2 and prevents IgG binding to these molecules by masking epitopes (168). The role of these two molecules in merozoite biology is still unclear but non-specific IgM epitope masking may be important for protecting the parasite against a specific IgG inhibitory response.

SMOKE-SCREEN STRATEGY BY CROSS-REACTIVITY

Smoke-screen strategy is often used by the parasite to divert the antibodies specific for one antigen (antigen A, e.g., an epitope of inhibitory antibodies) to react against another antigen (antigen B, e.g., an epitope of non-inhibitory antibodies) which possess regions homologous to antigen A. Antibody reactivity to segments shared by the two proteins will decrease the amount of antibodies reacting to antigen A and thus reducing efficacy of inhibitory antibodies that can inhibit parasite invasion or development. Many *Plasmodium* antigens contain repeats, and it was shown that cross-reactivity can occur between different blocks of repeats (169). Cross-reactivity has been observed: (i) between different epitopes from the same block of repeats [i.e., within the same block of repeats in the CS protein, or Ring-erythrocyte surface (RESA), or S-antigen or falciparum interspersed repeat antigen (FIRA)]; (ii) between epitopes present in different blocks of the same antigen (i.e., RESA or FIRA), between repeats of different antigens [between the CS protein and the cross-reactive antigen (CRA), between the histidine-rich proteins]. So far, the importance of this mechanism in the immune response evasion has remained uncertain.

DYSREGULATION OF B CELLS

Atypical memory B cells are a population of hypo-responsive memory cells which have been first described in chronic HIV infections (170). They increase in numbers during chronic exposure to malaria and are poor responders to antigen restimulation (171). However, they are able to produce neutralizing antibodies (172). These cells might be important during repeated stimulation due to constant exposure and help to control parasite density. However, in regions with lower exposure or in the absence of reinfection, immunity might wane rapidly.

As mentioned in the previous section, many *Plasmodium* antigens contain repeats. Similar to many viral antigens (173) and haptenated polymers (174), repeats-containing *Plasmodium* antigens can stimulate B cell independently of T cell help. However, this often leads to the production of mainly IgM and limited B cell memory (175). In addition, exposure to antigens containing repeated motifs can result in the suppression of an ongoing T cell response (176, 177).

HOMOLOGIES WITH HOST PROTEINS

Many *Plasmodium* antigens involved in the invasion of host cells have regions which strong homologies with host proteins involved in protein–protein interactions. Thrombospondin type-1 repeat (TSR) domains and von Willebrand factor (vWF)-like A domains are present in the CS protein, thrombospondin-related anonymous protein (TRAP) (178, 179), CS protein TRAP-related protein (CTRP) sporozoite surface protein (180), secreted protein with an altered thrombospondin (SPATR) (181), and thrombospondin-related apical merozoite protein (TRAMP) (182). These molecules are involved in different stages of parasite development, in sporozoite and merozoite motility, and in invasion of mosquito midguts, salivary glands, hepatocytes, and RBC. Many merozoite proteins such as MSP-1, MSP-4, MSP-5, MSP-8, and MSP-10 (183), PfRipr (184) and sexual-stage protein, such as P25 or P28 (185, 186), have been found to contain an epidermal growth factor domain that is involved in its binding to their receptor. Due to the homology to the host protein, the induction of antibodies to epitopes contained in these homologous regions is difficult since the host is tolerized against its own proteins. Immunization with immunogens containing these motifs with strong adjuvants could possibly escape immunological tolerance but may have the risk of inducing auto-immunity.

IMMUNOSUPPRESSION

Myeloid cells are essential mediators of an efficient immune response against the malaria parasites. Monocytes, macrophages, and neutrophils phagocytose iRBC, which eventually leads to the elimination of the parasites (187). Phagocytosis by monocytes/macrophages can be mediated through the interactions of PfEMP-1 and CD36 without inducing or increasing a protective pro-inflammatory response (188). However, during infection, phagocyte functions can be diminished after the ingestion of the malaria pigment or hemozoin (the digested product of hemoglobin by the parasites) (189, 190). Pigment-loaded macrophages cannot phagocytose more iRBC, and their capacity to generate radical oxygen intermediates is also reduced (191).

Dendritic cells (DCs) are essential to induce adaptive immune responses (192). Engagement of CD36 and CD51 (the αv integrin chain) on DCs by PfEMP-1-expressing parasites impair DC maturation and its capacity to prime T cell responses, leading to reduced production of pro-inflammatory cytokines such as IL-12 and increased production of immunosuppressive cytokines such as IL-10 (193).

Acute blood-stage infection induces a strong activation of mononuclear cells. This can result in apoptosis in monocytes, B cells, T cells, and DCs (194–199). Acute infection can also lead to thymus apoptosis and depletion, thereby diminishing the output of new naïve T cells (200). On the other hand, chronically activated T cells (both αβ and γδ) during lingering blood infection or multiple reinfections can also enter a phase of anergy (201–203) and/or exhaustion (204). *Plasmodium* infection activates check-point inhibitors molecules such as program cell death protein 1 (PD-1), program death ligand 1 (PD-L1), PD-L2, lymphocyte-activation gene 3 (LAG-3), and cytotoxic T lymphocyte antigen-4 (CTLA-4) in CD4 and CD8 T cells. In rodent models, blockade of these molecules facilitates the elimination of blood parasites (91, 205, 206) and the establishment of T cell memory (207). Regulatory T cells often expand during infection (208). Their principal role is to control the excessive pro-inflammatory response which depending on the parasite species may be beneficial or detrimental (209–211). Taken together, these mechanisms leading to immunosuppression are likely to favor survival of the parasite in the host and prevent the establishment of an efficient memory response. In addition, while it might also be beneficial for the host to prevent immunopathogenesis (212), ensuring host survival is advantageous to parasite survival.

REDUNDANT PATHWAYS OF RED BLOOD CELL INVASION

Invasion of RBC by merozoites is a complex process. It involves a precise and coordinated expression of different sets of proteins which are either expressed on the surface of the merozoite or in the organelles such as rhoptries, micronemes, and dense granules located at the apical end of the merozoite (183). The invasion process has been amply studied for *P. falciparum*. It was shown that the parasites can use multiple pathways involving at least nine ligand/receptor combinations to invade a RBC. There are two parasite protein families involved in the host-cell selection and invasion process; the reticulocyte-binding protein homologs (Rh) and the erythrocyte binding-like proteins (EBL) (213). These proteins are polymorphic, and their expression varies depending on parasite clones. Polymorphisms in a *P. falciparum* EBL have been shown to result in a change in their receptor specificity (214) or in a switch to Rh-dependent invasion, a different invasion pathway for RBC invasion (215). Variation in the use of erythrocyte invasion pathways results in evasion of human inhibitory antibodies (216). Thus, this suggests that vaccines targeting only one pathway will select parasite using other pathways. However, so far, the pathway involving Rh5 and its ligand Basigin/CD147 has been shown to be required for all parasites clones and isolates tested so far and has shown limited polymorphism (217). It thus represents a promising vaccine candidate (218, 219).

Contrary to *P. falciparum*, *P. vivax* was thought to use only one pathway to invade RBC (220). *P. vivax* merozoites only invade reticulocytes, the immature RBC. Since people in West Africa or with West African origins naturally lack the Duffy antigen, they are resistant to *P. vivax* blood infection (221, 222). This serves as a strong argument for the existence of only one invasion pathway for *P. vivax*. However, in the recent years, many studies have reported *P. vivax* infections in Duffy-negative patients (220, 222–228), suggesting that *P. vivax* merozoites may use another pathway to invade reticulocytes (229). This may limit the efficacy of vaccine based on the Duffy-binding protein, the ligand of the Duffy antigen (230), by selecting for parasites that are able to invade *via* this alternative pathway.

SHELTERS

Infection with sporozoites from some human/primate parasites, such as *P. vivax*, *P. ovale*, *P. cynomolgi*, *Plasmodium simiovale*, and *Plasmodium fieldi*, may lead to relapse (231). After a patent blood infection is completely cleared by the immune system or by drug treatment, blood parasites may reappear and induce new clinical attacks (232). This new infection originates from long-lasting liver forms, called hypnozoites (233). These non-dividing and metabolically active forms (234) can persist in the liver of their infected hosts for long period of time. Histological analysis on liver from infected rhesus monkeys did not show any signs of cellular immune responses against hypnozoites or late-developing schizonts originating from these forms (235, 236). This suggests that hypnozoites do not trigger any immune response, and do not lead to the expression of MHC molecules containing parasites-derived peptides. Due to the difficulty in studying these forms *in vitro* and *in vivo* (237), the mechanisms by which the parasite subverts immune recognition is unknown. Vaccine development against the pre-erythrocytic of *P. vivax* has been limited, and formulations targeting the liver forms may not work against the hypnozoites.

As mentioned above, during primary sporozoite-induced infection in natural hosts, no cellular immune responses are observed (8, 238–240). The liver is rich in macrophages and Kupffer cells, which can phagocytose emerging hepatic merozoites. To avoid being recognized by phagocytes, merozoites are released inside vesicles called merosomes in to the sinusoid lumen. Merosomes do not express macrophage-recognition signal such as phosphatidyl-serine and thus escape being phagocytosed (8). Merosomes are carried to the lung vasculature where blood circulation is low (241) before releasing their merozoite cargo (242).

Vesicles containing merozoites have been observed inside other cell types other than RBC, such as platelets (243), in macrophages (244), and in DCs (245, 246). It has been shown that merozoites can also divide in the DCs expressing CD317/tetherin, and eventually initiate new infections (245). It is not yet known how the phagocytosed parasites evade digestion or if a population of merozoites can infect and multiply in these cells. Free merozoite-containing vesicles, called merophores, have also been observed in the lymph circulation during rodent malaria infection (247, 248). This could explain recrudescence or latency of infection. However, as for the merosomes, these vesicles may be devoid of recognition signals for phagocyte uptake and may not express parasite antigens on their surface.

CONCLUSION

Malaria parasites have been interacting with its mammalian hosts for more than 150 million years (249) and have efficiently evolved to survive under the pressure of the host immune system. The parasite has developed numerous immune evasion mechanisms. Since new host immune mechanisms against the parasite are constantly being discovered, it will be of no surprise that new immune escape mechanisms by the parasite will be uncovered. For example, there is still little known on how innate immunity are induced during infection and on how protective epitopes are generated. The ultimate goal of understanding the immune responses to the malaria parasites is the development of vaccines. The selection of antigens and delivery system is governed by the target. Historically, before the whole genome was sequenced, the first malarial antigens, that were cloned and sequenced, have been assumed to be good vaccine candidates (250). However, all these antigens are immunodominant and are involved in immune escape. For vaccines to develop in a timely manner, the selection criteria should involve a more stringent GO-NO Go selection based on the analysis of the potential of the vaccine candidate to avoid immune escape. This also calls for an immunological approach to define correlates of protection to guide vaccine development. The development of the experimental human malarial challenge model, where complete sterile protection can be obtained (34, 35), is strong evidence that a vaccine against malaria can be obtained. Together with parasite genetics, the development of the rodent models and the experimental human challenge model would greatly assist in making the critical GO-NO Go decisions and facilitate the development of an efficacious vaccine against malaria in the foreseeable future.

AUTHOR CONTRIBUTIONS

Both the authors listed have made substantial, direct, and intellectual contribution to the work and approved it for publication.

REFERENCES

1. Millar SB, Cox-Singh J. Human infections with *Plasmodium knowlesi* – zoonotic malaria. *Clin Microbiol Infect* (2015) 21:640–8. doi:10.1016/j.cmi.2015.03.017
2. Ta TH, Hisam S, Lanza M, Jiram AI, Ismail N, Rubio JM. First case of a naturally acquired human infection with *Plasmodium cynomolgi*. *Malar J* (2014) 13:68. doi:10.1186/1475-2875-13-68
3. World Health Organisation. *World Malaria Report*. Geneva: World Health Organisation (2015).
4. Amino R, Thiberge S, Martin B, Celli S, Shorte S, Frischknecht F, et al. Quantitative imaging of *Plasmodium* transmission from mosquito to mammal. *Nat Med* (2006) 12:220–4. doi:10.1038/nm1350
5. Amino R, Giovannini D, Thiberge S, Gueirard P, Boisson B, Dubremetz JF, et al. Host cell traversal is important for progression of the malaria parasite through the dermis to the liver. *Cell Host Microbe* (2008) 3:88–96. doi:10.1016/j.chom.2007.12.007
6. Mota MM, Pradel G, Vanderberg JP, Hafalla JCR, Frevert U, Nussenzweig RS, et al. Migration of *Plasmodium* sporozoites through cells before infection. *Science* (2001) 291:141–4. doi:10.1126/science.291.5501.141
7. Tavares J, Formaglio P, Thiberge S, Mordelet E, van Rooijen N, Medvinsky A, et al. Role of host cell traversal by the malaria sporozoite during liver infection. *J Exp Med* (2013) 210:905–15. doi:10.1084/jem.20121130
8. Sturm A, Amino R, Van De Sand C, Regen T, Retzlaff S, Rennenberg A, et al. Manipulation of host hepatocytes by the malaria parasite for delivery into liver sinusoids. *Science* (2006) 313:1287–90. doi:10.1126/science.1115257
9. White NJ, Pukrittayakamee S, Hien TT, Faiz MA, Mokuolu OA, Dondorp AM. Malaria. *Lancet* (2013) 383:7223. doi:10.1016/S0140-6736(13)60024-0
10. Pathak VA, Ghosh K. Erythropoiesis in malaria infections and factors modifying the erythropoietic response. *Anemia* (2016) 2016:9310905. doi:10.1155/2016/9310905
11. Storm J, Craig AG. Pathogenesis of cerebral malaria-inflammation and cytoadherence. *Front Cell Infect Microbiol* (2014) 4:100. doi:10.3389/fcimb
12. Haldar K, Murphy SC, Milner DA, Taylor TE. Malaria: mechanisms of erythrocytic infection and pathological correlates of severe disease. *Annu Rev Pathol* (2007) 2:217–49. doi:10.1146/annurev.pathol.2.010506.091913
13. Milner DA Jr, Whitten RO, Kamiza S, Carr R, Liomba G, Dzamalala C, et al. The systemic pathology of cerebral malaria in African children. *Front Cell Infect Microbiol* (2014) 4:104. doi:10.3389/fcimb.2014.00104
14. Kanyuka M, Ndawala J, Mleme T, Chisesa L, Makwemba M, Amouzou A, et al. Malawi and millennium development goal 4: a countdown to 2015 country case study. *Lancet Glob Health* (2016) 4:e201–2124. doi:10.1016/S2214-109X(15)00294-6
15. Dondorp AM, Yeung S, White L, Nguon C, Day NP, Socheat D, et al. Artemisinin resistance: current status and scenarios for containment. *Nat Rev Microbiol* (2010) 8:272–80. doi:10.1038/nrmicro2331
16. White LJ, Flegg JA, Phyo AP, Wiladpai-Ngern JH, Bethell D, Plowe CV, et al. Defining the *in vivo* phenotype of artemisinin-resistant falciparum malaria: a modelling approach. *PLoS Med* (2015) 12:e1001823. doi:10.1371/journal.pmed.1001823
17. Canavati SE, Lawford HL, Fatunmbi BS, Lek D, Top-Samphor N, Leang R, et al. Establishing research priorities for malaria elimination in the context of the emergency response to artemisinin resistance framework-the Cambodian approach. *Malar J* (2016) 15:120. doi:10.1186/s12936-016-1117-9
18. von Seidlein LV, Dondorp AM. Fighting fire with fire: mass antimalarial drug administrations in an era of antimalarial resistance. *Expert Rev Anti Infect Ther* (2015) 13:715–30. doi:10.1586/14787210.2015.1031744
19. White NJ, Pukrittayakamee S, Phyo AP, Rueangweerayut R, Nosten F, Jittamala P, et al. Spiroindolone KAE609 for falciparum and vivax malaria. *N Engl J Med* (2014) 371:403–10. doi:10.1056/NEJMoa1315860
20. Rottmann M, McNamara C, Yeung BK, Lee MC, Zou B, Russell BM, et al. Spiroindolones, a potent compound class for the treatment of malaria. *Science* (2010) 329:1175–80. doi:10.1126/science.1193225
21. White NJ, Duong TT, Uthaisin C, Nosten F, Phyo AP, Hanboonkunupakarn B, et al. Antimalarial activity of KAF156 in falciparum and vivax malaria. *N Engl J Med* (2016) 375:1152–60. doi:10.1056/NEJMoa1602250
22. McNamara CW, Lee MC, Lim CS, Lim SH, Roland J, Nagle A, et al. Targeting *Plasmodium* PI(4)K to eliminate malaria. *Nature* (2013) 504:248–53. doi:10.1038/nature1278
23. Celli A, Santori FS. Intorno alla siero-profilassi della malaria. 1a comunicazione. *Annali d'Igiene Sperimentale* (1897) 7:183–90.
24. McGregor IA. Malarial immunity: current trends and prospects. *Ann Trop Med Parasitol* (1987) 81:647–56.
25. Sergent E, Parrot L. L'immunite, la premunition et la resistance. *Ann Inst Pasteur Algers* (1935) 13:279–315.
26. Sergent E. Sur l'immunite dans le paludisme des oiseaux. Conservation *in vitro* des sporozoites de *Plasmodium relictum*. Immunite relative obtenue par inoculation de ces sporozoites. *C R Acad Sci* (1910) 151:407–9.
27. Heidelberger M, Mayer MM, Alving AS, Craige BJ, Jones R Jr, Pullman TN, et al. Studies in human malaria. IV. An attempt at vaccination of volunteers against mosquito-borne infection with *Plasmodium vivax*. *J Immunol* (1946) 53:113–8.

28. Heidelberger M, Mayer MM, Demarest CR. Studies in human malaria. I. The preparation of vaccines and suspensions containing plasmodia. *J Immunol* (1946) 52:325–30.
29. Freund J, Sommer HE, Walter AW. Immunization against malaria: vaccination of ducks with killed parasites incorporated with adjuvants. *Science* (1945) 102:200–2. doi:10.1126/science.102.2643.200
30. Freund J, Thomson KJ, Sommer HE, Walter AW, Schenkein EL. Immunization of rhesus monkeys against malarial infection (*P. knowlesi*) with killed parasites and adjuvants. *Science* (1945) 102:202–4. doi:10.1126/science.102.2643.202
31. Halbroth BR, Draper SJ. Recent developments in malaria vaccinology. *Adv Parasitol* (2015) 88:1–49. doi:10.1016/bs.apar.2015.03.001
32. Kaslow DC, Biernaux S. RTS,S: toward a first landmark on the malaria vaccine technology roadmap. *Vaccine* (2015) 33:7425–32. doi:10.1016/j
33. Olotu A, Fegan G, Wambua J, Nyangweso G, Awuondo KO, Leach A, et al. Four-year efficacy of RTS,S/AS01E and its interaction with malaria exposure. *N Engl J Med* (2013) 368:1111–20. doi:10.1056/NEJMoa1207564
34. Roestenberg M, McCall M, Hopman J, Wiersma J, Luty AJF, van Gemert GJ, et al. Protection against a malaria challenge by sporozoite inoculation. *N Engl J Med* (2009) 361:468–77. doi:10.1056/NEJMoa0805832
35. Seder RA, Chang LJ, Enama ME, Zephir KL, Sarwar UN, Gordon IJ, et al. Protection against malaria by intravenous immunization with a non-replicating sporozoite vaccine. *Science* (2013) 341:1359–65. doi:10.1126/science.1241800
36. Ishizuka AS, Lyke KE, DeZure A, Berry AA, Richie TL, Mendoza FH, et al. Protection against malaria at 1 year and immune correlates following PfSPZ vaccination. *Nat Med* (2016) 22:614–23. doi:10.1038/nm.4110
37. Gardner MJ, Hall N, Fung E, White O, Berriman M, Hyman RW, et al. Genome sequence of the human malaria parasite *Plasmodium falciparum*. *Nature* (2002) 419:498–511. doi:10.1038/nature01097
38. Stevenson MM, Riley EM. Innate immunity to malaria. *Nat Rev Immunol* (2004) 4:169–80. doi:10.1038/nri1311
39. Langhorne J, Ndungu FM, Sponaas AM, Marsh K. Immunity to malaria: more questions than answers. *Nat Immunol* (2008) 9:725–32. doi:10.1038/ni.f.205
40. Vanderberg JP, Frevert U. Intravital microscopy demonstrating antibody-mediated immobilisation of *Plasmodium berghei* sporozoites injected into skin by mosquitoes. *Int J Parasitol* (2004) 34:991–6. doi:10.1016/j.ijpara.2004.05.005
41. Schwenk R, Lumsden JM, Rein LE, Juompan L, Kester KE, Heppner DG Jr, et al. Immunization with the RTS,S/AS malaria vaccine induces IFN-gamma+ CD4 T cells that recognize only discrete regions of the circumsporozoite protein and these specificities are maintained following booster immunizations and challenge. *Vaccine* (2011) 29:8846–54. doi:10.1016/j.vaccine.2011.09.098
42. Nudelman S, Renia L, Charoenvit Y, Yuan L, Miltgen F, Beaudoin RL, et al. Dual action of anti-sporozoite antibodies in vitro. *J Immunol* (1989) 143:996–1000.
43. Renia L, Mattei DM, Goma J, Pied S, Dubois P, Miltgen F, et al. A malaria heat-shock-like determinant expressed on the infected hepatocyte surface is the target of antibody-dependent cell-mediated cytotoxic mechanisms by nonparenchymal liver cells. *Eur J Immunol* (1990) 20:1445–9. doi:10.1002/eji.1830200706
44. Renia L, Marussig MS, Grillot D, Pied S, Corradin G, Miltgen F, et al. *In vitro* activity of CD4+ and CD8+ T lymphocytes from mice immunized with a synthetic malaria peptide. *Proc Natl Acad Sci U S A* (1991) 88:7963–7. doi:10.1073/pnas.88.18.7963
45. Renia L, Grillot DA, Marussig M, Corradin G, Miltgen F, Lambert PH, et al. Effector functions of circumsporozoite peptide-primed $CD4^+$ T cell clones against *Plasmodium yoelii* liver stages. *J Immunol* (1993) 150:1471–8.
46. Bongfen SE, Torgler R, Romero JF, Renia L, Corradin G. *Plasmodium berghei*-infected primary hepatocytes process and present the circumsporozoite protein to specific CD8+ T cells *in vitro*. *J Immunol* (2007) 178:7054–63. doi:10.4049/jimmunol.178.11.7054
47. Pichugin A, Steers N, De la Vega P, Zarling S, Chalom I, Krzych U. TAP-mediated processing of exoerythrocytic antigens is essential for protection induced with radiation-attenuated *Plasmodium* sporozoites. *Eur J Immunol* (2016) 46:885–96. doi:10.1002/eji.201545748
48. Mellouk S, Hoffman SL, Liu ZZ, de la Vega P, Billiar TR, Nussler AK. Nitric oxide-mediated antiplasmodial activity in human and murine hepatocytes induced by gamma interferon and the parasite itself: enhancement by exogenous tetrahydrobiopterin. *Infect Immun* (1994) 62:4043–6.
49. Nussler AK, Renia L, Pasquetto V, Miltgen F, Matile H, Mazier D. *In vivo* induction of the nitric oxide pathway in hepatocytes after injection with irradiated malaria sporozoites, malaria blood parasites or adjuvants. *Eur J Immunol* (1993) 23:882–7. doi:10.1002/eji.1830230417
50. Seguin MC, Klotz FW, Schneider I, Weir JP, Goodbary M, Slayter M, et al. Induction of nitric oxide synthase protects against malaria in mice exposed to irradiated *Plasmodium berghei* infected mosquitoes: involvement of interferon-gamma and CD8+ T cells. *J Exp Med* (1994) 180:353–8. doi:10.1084/jem.180.1.353
51. Cockburn IA, Amino R, Kelemen RK, Kuo SC, Tse SW, Radtke A, et al. *In vivo* imaging of CD8+ T cell-mediated elimination of malaria liver stages. *Proc Natl Acad Sci U S A* (2013) 110:9090–5. doi:10.1073/pnas.1303858110
52. Liehl P, Meireles P, Albuquerque IS, Pinkevych M, Baptista F, Mota MM, et al. Innate immunity induced by *Plasmodium* liver infection inhibits malaria reinfections. *Infect Immun* (2015) 83:1172–80. doi:10.1128/IAI.02796-14
53. Liehl P, Zuzarte-Luis V, Chan J, Zillinger T, Baptista F, Carapau D, et al. Host-cell sensors for *Plasmodium* activate innate immunity against liver-stage infection. *Nat Med* (2013) 20:47–53. doi:10.1038/nm.3424
54. Miller JL, Sack BK, Baldwin M, Vaughan AM, Kappe SH. Interferon-mediated innate immune responses against malaria parasite liver stages. *Cell Rep* (2014) 7:436–47. doi:10.1016/j.celrep.2014.03.018
55. Reiling L, Richards JS, Fowkes FJ, Barry AE, Triglia T, Chokejindachai W, et al. Evidence that the erythrocyte invasion ligand PfRh2 is a target of protective immunity against *Plasmodium falciparum* malaria. *J Immunol* (2010) 185:6157–67. doi:10.4049/jimmunol.1001555
56. Dutta S, Lee SY, Batchelor AH, Lanar DE. Structural basis of antigenic escape of a malaria vaccine candidate. *Proc Natl Acad Sci U S A* (2007) 104:12488–93. doi:10.1073/pnas.0701464104
57. Jiang L, Gaur D, Mu J, Zhou H, Long CA, Miller LH. Evidence for erythrocyte-binding antigen 175 as a component of a ligand-blocking blood-stage malaria vaccine. *Proc Natl Acad Sci USA* (2011) 108:7553–8. doi:10.1073/pnas.1104050108
58. Marsh K, Kinyanjui SM. Immune effector mechanisms in malaria. *Parasite Immunol* (2006) 28:51–60. doi:10.1111/j.1365-3024.2006.00808.x
59. Bouharoun-Tayoun H, Attanath P, Sabchareon A, Chongsuphajaisiddhi T, Druilhe P. Antibodies that protect humans against *Plasmodium falciparum* blood stages do not on their own inhibit parasite growth and invasion *in vitro*, but act in cooperation with monocytes. *J Exp Med* (1990) 172:1633–41. doi:10.1084/jem.172.6.1633
60. Bouharoun-Tayoun H, Oeuvray C, Lunel F, Druilhe P. Mechanisms underlying the monocyte-mediated antibody-dependent killing of *Plasmodium falciparum* asexual blood stages. *J Exp Med* (1995) 182:409–18. doi:10.1084/jem.182.2.409
61. Frech C, Chen N. Variant surface antigens of malaria parasites: functional and evolutionary insights from comparative gene family classification and analysis. *BMC Genomics* (2013) 14:427. doi:10.1186/1471-2164-14-427
62. Su XZ, Heatwole VM, Wertheimer SP, Guinet F, Herrfeldt JA, Peterson DS, et al. The large diverse gene family var encodes proteins involved in cytoadherence and antigenic variation of *Plasmodium falciparum*-infected erythrocytes. *Cell* (1995) 82:89–100. doi:10.1016/0092-8674(95)90055-1
63. Cheng Q, Cloonan N, Fischer K, Thompson J, Waine GJ, Lanzer MP, et al. Stevor and rif are *Plasmodium falciparum* multicopy gene families which potentially encode variant antigens. *Mol Biochem Parasitol* (1998) 97:161–76. doi:10.1016/S0166-6851(98)00144-3
64. Wang CW, Hviid L. Rifins, rosetting, and red blood cells. *Trends Parasitol* (2015) 31:285–6. doi:10.1016/j.pt.2015.04.009
65. Kyes SA, Rowe JA, Kriek N, Newbold CI. Rifins: a second family of clonally variant proteins expressed on the surface of red cells infected with *Plasmodium falciparum*. *Proc Natl Acad Sci U S A* (1999) 96:9333–8. doi:10.1073/pnas.96.16.9333
66. Janssen CS, Phillips RS, Turner CM, Barrett MP. *Plasmodium* interspersed repeats: the major multigene superfamily of malaria parasites. *Nucleic Acids Res* (2004) 32:5712–20. doi:10.1093/nar/gkh907

67. Barnwell JW, Howard RJ, Coon HG, Miller LH. Splenic requirement for antigenic variation and expression of the variant antigen on the erythrocyte membrane in cloned *Plasmodium knowlesi* malaria. *Infect Immun* (1983) 40:985–94.
68. David PH, Hommel M, Miller LH, Udeinya IJ, Oligino LD. Parasite sequestration in *Plasmodium falciparum* malaria: spleen and antibody modulation of cytoadherence of infected erythrocytes. *Proc Natl Acad Sci U S A* (1983) 80:5075–9. doi:10.1073/pnas.80.16.5075
69. Udomsangpetch R, Wahlin B, Carlson J, Berzins K, Torii M, Aikawa M, et al. *Plasmodium falciparum*-infected erythrocytes form spontaneous erythrocytes rosettes. *J Exp Med* (1987) 169:1835–40. doi:10.1084/jem.169.5.1835
70. Niang M, Yan YX, Preiser PR. The *Plasmodium falciparum* STEVOR multigene family mediates antigenic variation of the infected erythrocyte. *PLoS Pathog* (2009) 5:e1000307. doi:10.1371/annotation/c58250db-8cce-40c5-b7ac-42204050069a
71. Goel S, Palmkvist M, Moll K, Joannin N, Lara P, Akhouri R, et al. RIFINs are adhesins implicated in severe *Plasmodium falciparum* malaria. *Nat Med* (2015) 21:314–7. doi:10.1038/nm.3812
72. Lee WC, Malleret B, Lau YL, Mauduit M, Fong MY, Cho JS, et al. Glycophorin C (CD236R) mediates vivax malaria parasite rosetting to normocytes. *Blood* (2014) 123:e100–9. doi:10.1182/blood-2013-12-541
73. Pain A, Ferguson DJP, Kai O, Urban BC, Lowe B, Marsh K, et al. Platelet-mediated clumping of *Plasmodium falciparum*-infected erythrocytes is a common adhesive phenotype and is associated with severe malaria. *Proc Natl Acad Sci U S A* (2001) 98:1805–10. doi:10.1073/pnas.98.4.1805
74. Tan J, Pieper K, Piccoli L, Abdi A, Foglierini M, Geiger R, et al. A LAIR1 insertion generates broadly reactive antibodies against malaria variant antigens. *Nature* (2016) 529:105–9. doi:10.1038/nature16450
75. Chan JA, Fowkes FJ, Beeson JG. Surface antigens of *Plasmodium falciparum*-infected erythrocytes as immune targets and malaria vaccine candidates. *Cell Mol Life Sci* (2014) 71:3633–57. doi:10.1007/s00018-014-1614-3
76. Olivier M, Van Den Ham KM, Shio MT, Kassa FA, Fougeray S. Malarial pigment hemozoin and the innate inflammatory response. *Front Immunol* (2014) 5:25. doi:10.3389/fimmu.2014.00025
77. Corbett Y, Parapini S, D'Alessandro S, Scaccabarozzi D, Rocha BC, Egan TJ, et al. Involvement of Nod2 in the innate immune response elicited by malarial pigment hemozoin. *Microbes Infect* (2015) 17:184–94. doi:10.1016/j.micinf.2014.11.001
78. Boura M, Frita R, Gois A, Carvalho T, Hanscheid T. The hemozoin conundrum: is malaria pigment immune-activating, inhibiting, or simply a bystander? *Trends Parasitol* (2013) 29:469–76. doi:10.1016/j.pt.2013.07.005
79. Chang Z, Jiang N, Zhang Y, Lu H, Yin J, Wahlgren M, et al. The TatD-like DNase of *Plasmodium* is a virulence factor and a potential malaria vaccine candidate. *Nat Commun* (2016) 7:11537. doi:10.1038/ncomms11537
80. Bhatt TK, Khan S, Dwivedi VP, Banday MM, Sharma A, Chandele A, et al. Malaria parasite tyrosyl-tRNA synthetase secretion triggers pro-inflammatory responses. *Nat Commun* (2011) 2:530. doi:10.1038/ncomms1522
81. Wijesekera SK, Carter RL, Rathnayaka L, Mendis KN. A malaria parasite toxin associated with *Plasmodium vivax* paroxysms. *Clin Exp Immunol* (1996) 104:221–7. doi:10.1046/j.1365-2249.1996.07699.x
82. Schofield L, Hewitt MC, Evans K, Siomos MA, Seeberger PH. Synthetic GPI as a candidate anti-toxic vaccine in a model of malaria. *Nature* (2002) 418:785–9. doi:10.1038/nature00937
83. von der Weid T, Kopf MA, Kohler G, Langhorne J. The immune response to *Plasmodium chabaudi* malaria in interleukin-4-deficient mice. *Eur J Immunol* (1994) 24:2285–93. doi:10.1002/eji.1830241004
84. Seixas EM, Fonseca L, Langhorne J. The influence of gammadelta T cells on the CD4+ T cell and antibody response during a primary *Plasmodium chabaudi chabaudi* infection in mice. *Parasite Immunol* (2002) 24:131–40. doi:10.1046/j.1365-3024.2002.00446.x
85. Bouharoun-Tayoun H, Druilhe P. *Plasmodium falciparum* malaria: evidence for an isotype imbalance which may be responsible for delayed acquisition of protective immunity. *Infect Immun* (1992) 60:1473–81.
86. Chitnis CE, Mukherjee P, Mehta S, Yazdani SS, Dhawan S, Shakri AR, et al. Phase I clinical trial of a recombinant blood stage vaccine candidate for *Plasmodium falciparum* malaria based on MSP1 and EBA175. *PLoS One* (2015) 10:e0117820. doi:10.1371/journal.pone.0137816
87. Suss G, Eichmann K, Kury E, Linke A, Langhorne J. Roles of CD4 and CD8 bearing T lymphocytes in the immune response to the erythrocytic stages of *Plasmodium chabaudi*. *Infect Immun* (1988) 56:3081–8.
88. Podoba JE, Stevenson MM. CD4+ and CD8+ T lymphocytes both contribute to acquired immunity to blood-stage *Plasmodium chabaudi* AS. *Infect Immun* (1991) 59:51–8.
89. Imai T, Ishida H, Suzue K, Taniguchi T, Okada H, Shimokawa C, et al. Cytotoxic activities of CD8+ T cells collaborate with macrophages to protect against blood-stage murine malaria. *Elife* (2015) 4:e04232. doi:10.7554/eLife.04232
90. Imai T, Shen J, Chou B, Duan X, Tu L, Tetsutani K, et al. Involvement of CD8+ T cells in protective immunity against murine blood-stage infection with *Plasmodium yoelii* 17XL strain. *Eur J Immunol* (2010) 40:1053–61. doi:10.1002/eji.200939525
91. Horne-Debets JM, Faleiro R, Karunarathne DS, Liu XQ, Lineburg KE, Poh CM, et al. PD-1 dependent exhaustion of CD8 T cells drives chronic malaria. *Cell Rep* (2013) 5:1204–13. doi:10.1038/srep26210
92. Read D, Lensen AHW, Begarnie S, Haley S, Raza A, Carter RL. Transmission-blocking antibodies against multiple, non-variant target epitopes of the *Plasmodium falciparum* gamete surface antigen Pfs230 are all complement-fixing. *Parasite Immunol* (1994) 16:511–9. doi:10.1111/j.1365-3024.1994.tb00305.x
93. Margos G, Navarette S, Butcher GA, Davies A, Willers C, Sinden RE, et al. Interaction between host complement and mosquito-midgut-stage *Plasmodium berghei*. *Infect Immun* (2001) 69:5064–71. doi:10.1128/IAI.69.8.5064-5071.2001
94. Blagborough AM, Sinden RE. *Plasmodium berghei* HAP2 induces strong malaria transmission-blocking immunity *in vivo* and *in vitro*. *Vaccine* (2009) 27:5187–94. doi:10.1016/j.vaccine.2009.06.069
95. Volohonsky G, Steinert S, Levashina EA. Focusing on complement in the antiparasitic defense of mosquitoes. *Trends Parasitol* (2010) 26:1–3. doi:10.1016/j.pt.2009.10.003
96. Sieber KP, Huber M, Kaslow DC, Banks SM, Torii M, Aikawa M, et al. The peritrophic membrane as a barrier: its penetration by *Plasmodium gallinaceum* and the effect of a monoclonal antibody to ookinetes. *Exp Parasitol* (1991) 72:145–56. doi:10.1016/0014-4894(91)90132-G
97. Duffy PE, Pimenta P, Kaslow DC. Pgs28 belongs to a family of epidermal growth factor-like antigens that are targets of malaria transmission-blocking antibodies. *J Exp Med* (1993) 177:505–10. doi:10.1084/jem.177.2.505
98. Ranawaka GR, Fleck SL, Blanco AR, Sinden RE. Characterization of the modes of action of anti-Pbs21 malaria transmission-blocking immunity: ookinete to oocyst differentiation in vivo. *Parasitology* (1994) 109:403–11. doi:10.1017/S0031182000080653
99. Baton LA, Ranford-Cartwright LC. Do malaria ookinete surface proteins P25 and P28 mediate parasite entry into mosquito midgut epithelial cells? *Malar J* (2005) 4:15. doi:10.1186/1475-2875-4-15
100. Naotunne TS, Karunaweera ND, Mendis KN, Carter RL. Cytokine-mediated inactivation of malarial gametocytes is dependent on the presence of white blood cells and involves reactive nitrogen intermediates. *Immunology* (1993) 78:555–62.
101. Dunkelberger JR, Song WC. Complement and its role in innate and adaptive immune responses. *Cell Res* (2010) 20:34–50. doi:10.1038/cr.2009.139
102. Simon N, Lasonder E, Scheuermayer M, Kuehn A, Tews S, Fischer R, et al. Malaria parasites co-opt human factor H to prevent complement-mediated lysis in the mosquito midgut. *Cell Host Microbe* (2013) 13:29–41. doi:10.1016/j.chom.2012.11.013
103. Ramphul UN, Garver LS, Molina-Cruz A, Canepa GE, Barillas-Mury C. *Plasmodium falciparum* evades mosquito immunity by disrupting JNK-mediated apoptosis of invaded midgut cells. *Proc Natl Acad Sci U S A* (2015) 112:1273–80. doi:10.1073/pnas.1423586112
104. Morens DM. Antibody-dependent enhancement of infection and the pathogenesis of viral disease. *Clin Infect Dis* (1994) 19:500–12. doi:10.1093/clinids/19.3.500
105. Hollingdale MR, Appiah A, Leland P, Do Rosario VE, Mazier D, Pied S, et al. Activity of human volunteer sera to candidate *Plasmodium falciparum* circumsporozoite vaccines in the inhibition of sporozoite invasion (ISI) of human hepatoma cells and hepatocytes assays. *Trans R Soc Trop Med Hyg* (1990) 84:325–9. doi:10.1016/0035-9203(90)90303-V

106. Franzen L, Wahlin B, Wahlgren M, Aslund L, Perlmann P, Wigzell H, et al. Enhancement or inhibition of *Plasmodium falciparum* erythrocyte reinvasion *in vitro* by antibodies to an asparagine rich protein. *Mol Biochem Parasitol* (1989) 32:201–11. doi:10.1016/0166-6851(89)90071-6
107. Biryukov S, Angov E, Landmesser ME, Spring MD, Ockenhouse CF, Stoute JA. Complement and antibody-mediated enhancement of red blood cell invasion and growth of malaria parasites. *EBioMedicine* (2016) 9:207–16. doi:10.1016/j.ebiom.2016.05.015
108. Jerusalem CR, Weiss ML, Poels LG. Immunologic enhancement in malaria infection (*Plasmodium berghei*). *J Immunol* (1971) 107:260–8.
109. Mendis KN, Peiris JSM, Premawansa S, Udagama PV, Munesinghe YD, Ranawaka MB, et al. Immune modulation of parasite transmission in *Plasmodium vivax* malaria. Anti-gamete antibodies can both block and enhance transmission. In: Agabian N, Goodman H, Nogueira N, editors. *Molecular Strategies of Parasite invasion. UCLA symposium on Molecular and Cellular Biology*. New York: Alan R. Liss, Inc. (1987) 42:417–26.
110. Mattei DM, Sherf A, Bensaude O, Pereira da Silva LH. A heat shock-like protein from the human malaria parasite *Plasmodium falciparum* induces autoantibodies. *Eur J Immunol* (1989) 19:1823–8. doi:10.1002/eji.1830191010
111. Do Rosario VE, Appiah A, Vaughan JA, Hollingdale MR. *Plasmodium falciparum*: administration of anti-sporozoite antibodies during sporogony results in production of sporozoites which are not neutralized by human anti-circumsporozoite protein sera. *Trans R Soc Trop Med Hyg* (1989) 83:305–7. doi:10.1016/0035-9203(89)90481-1
112. Motard A, Marussig M, Renia L, Baccam D, Landau I, Mattei DM, et al. Immunization with the malaria heat shock like protein hsp70-1 enhances transmission to the mosquito. *Int Immunol* (1995) 7:147–50. doi:10.1093/intimm/7.1.147
113. Bopp SE, Manary MJ, Bright AT, Johnston GL, Dharia NV, Luna FL, et al. Mitotic evolution of *Plasmodium falciparum* shows a stable core genome but recombination in antigen families. *PLoS Genet* (2013) 9:e1003293. doi:10.1371/journal.pgen.1003293
114. Anders RF, Smythe JA. Polymorphic antigens in *Plasmodium falciparum*. *Blood* (1989) 74:1865–75.
115. Anders RF, Brown GV, Coppel RL, Kemp DJ. Repeat structures in malaria antigens. *PNG Med J* (1986) 29:87–93.
116. Thera MA, Doumbo OK, Coulibaly D, Laurens MB, Ouattara A, Kone AK, et al. A field trial to assess a blood-stage malaria vaccine. *N Engl J Med* (2011) 365:1004–13. doi:10.1056/NEJMoa1008115
117. Takala SL, Coulibaly D, Thera MA, Batchelor AH, Cummings MP, Escalante AA, et al. Extreme polymorphism in a vaccine antigen and risk of clinical malaria: implications for vaccine development. *Sci Transl Med* (2009) 1:2ra5. doi:10.1126/scitranslmed.3000257
118. Drew DR, Wilson DW, Elliott SR, Cross N, Terheggen U, Hodder AN, et al. A novel approach to identifying patterns of human invasion-inhibitory antibodies guides the design of malaria vaccines incorporating polymorphic antigens. *BMC Med* (2016) 14:144. doi:10.1186/s12916-016-0691-6
119. Neafsey DE, Juraska M, Bedford T, Benkeser D, Valim C, Griggs A, et al. Genetic diversity and protective efficacy of the RTS,S/AS01 malaria vaccine. *N Engl J Med* (2015) 373:2025–37. doi:10.1056/NEJMoa1505819
120. Yaneva R, Schneeweiss C, Zacharias M, Springer S. Peptide binding to MHC class I and II proteins: new avenues from new methods. *Mol Immunol* (2010) 47:649–57. doi:10.1016/j.molimm.2009.10.008
121. Blum JS, Wearsch PA, Cresswell P. Pathways of antigen processing. *Annu Rev Immunol* (2013) 31:443–73. doi:10.1016/j.vaccine.2009.06.069
122. Hennecke J, Wiley DC. T cell receptor-MHC interactions up close. *Cell* (2001) 104:1–4. doi:10.1016/S0092-8674(01)00185-4
123. De la Cruz VF, Maloy WL, Miller LH, Lal AA, Good MF, McCutchan TF. Lack of cross-reactivity between variant T cell determinants from malaria circumsporozoite protein. *J Immunol* (1988) 141:2456–60.
124. Zevering Y, Khamboonruang C, Good MF. Natural amino acid polymorphisms of the circumsprozoite protein of *Plasmodium falciparum* abrogate specific human CD4+ T cell responsiveness. *Eur J Immunol* (1994) 24:1418–25. doi:10.1002/eji.1830240627
125. Plebanski M, Lee EA, Hill AVS. Immune evasion in malaria: altered peptide ligands of the circumsporozoite protein. *Parasitology* (1997) 115:S55–66. doi:10.1017/S0031182097002035
126. Gilbert SC, Plebanski M, Gupta S, Morris J, Cox M, Aidoo MA, et al. Association of malaria parasite population structure, HLA, and immunological antagonism. *Science* (1998) 279:1173–7. doi:10.1126/science.279.5354.1173
127. Plebanski M, Flanagan KL, Lee EA, Reece WH, Hart K, Gelder C, et al. Interleukin 10-mediated immunosuppression by a variant CD4 T cell epitope of *Plasmodium falciparum*. *Immunity* (1999) 10:651–60. doi:10.1016/S1074-7613(00)80064-3
128. Plebanski M, Lee AM, Hanan CM, Flanagan KL, Gilbert SC, Gravenor MB, et al. Altered peptide ligands narrow the repertoire of cellular immune responses by interfering with T-cell priming. *Nat Med* (1999) 5:565–71. doi:10.1038/8444
129. Brown KN, Brown IN. Immunity to malaria: antigenic variation in chronic infections of *Plasmodium knowlesi*. *Nature* (1965) 208:1286–8. doi:10.1038/2081286a0
130. Brown KN. Antibody induced variation in malaria parasites. *Nature* (1973) 242:49–50. doi:10.1038/242049a0
131. Hommel M, David PH, Oligino LD. Surface alterations of erythrocytes in *Plasmodium falciparum* malaria antigenic variation, antigenic diversity, and the role of the spleen. *J Exp Med* (1983) 157:1137–48. doi:10.1084/jem.157.4.1137
132. Winter G, Kawai S, Haeggstrom M, Kaneko O, von Eule A, Kawazu S, et al. SURFIN is a polymorphic antigen expressed on *Plasmodium falciparum* merozoites and infected erythrocytes. *J Exp Med* (2005) 201:1853–63. doi:10.1084/jem.20041392
133. al-Khedery B, Barnwell JW, Galinski MR. Antigenic variation in malaria: a 3' genomic alteration associated with the expression of a *Plasmodium knowlesi* variant antigen. *Mol Cell* (1999) 3:131–41. doi:10.1016/S1097-2765(00)80304-4
134. Chan JA, Howell KB, Reiling L, Ataide R, Mackintosh CL, Fowkes FJ, et al. Targets of antibodies against *Plasmodium falciparum*-infected erythrocytes in malaria immunity. *J Clin Invest* (2012) 122:3227–38. doi:10.1172/JCI62182
135. Beeson JG, Chan JA, Fowkes FJ. PfEMP1 as a target of human immunity and a vaccine candidate against malaria. *Expert Rev Vaccines* (2013) 12:105–8. doi:10.1038/71582
136. Smith JD, Chitnis CE, Craig AG, Roberts DJ, Hudson-Taylor DE, Peterson DS, et al. Switches in expression of *Plasmodium falciparum var* genes correlate with changes in antigenic and cytoadherent phenotypes of infected erythrocytes. *Cell* (1995) 82:101–10. doi:10.1016/0092-8674(95)90056-X
137. Roberts DD, Sherwood JA, Spitalnik SL, Panton LJ, Howard RJ, Dixit VM, et al. Thrombospondin binds falciparum malaria parasitized erythrocytes and may mediate cytoadherence. *Nature* (1985) 318:64–6. doi:10.1038/318064a0
138. Oquendo P, Hundt E, Lawler JW, Seed B. CD36 directly mediates cytoadherence of *Plasmodium falciparum* parasitized erythrocytes. *Cell* (1989) 58:95–101. doi:10.1016/0092-8674(89)90406-6
139. Berendt AR, Simmons DL, Tansey J, Newbold C, Marsh K. Intercellular adhesion molecule-1 is an endothelial cell adhesion receptor for *Plasmodium falciparum*. *Nature* (1989) 341:57–9. doi:10.1038/341057a0
140. Fried M, Duffy PE. Adherence of *Plasmodium falciparum* to chondroitin sulfate A in the human placenta. *Science* (1996) 272:1502–4. doi:10.1126/science.272.5267.1502
141. Reeder JC, Cowman AF, Davern KM, Beeson JG, Thompson JK, Rogerson SJ, et al. The adhesion of *Plasmodium falciparum*-infected erythrocytes to chondroitin sulfate A is mediated by *P. falciparum* erythrocyte membrane protein 1. *Proc Natl Acad Sci U S A* (1999) 96:5198–202. doi:10.1073/pnas.96.9.5198
142. Buffet PA, Gamain B, Scheidig C, Baruch DI, Smith JD, Hernandez-Rivas R, et al. *Plasmodium falciparum* domain mediating adhesion to chondroitin sulfate A: a receptor for human placental infection. *Proc Natl Acad Sci U S A* (1999) 96:12743–8. doi:10.1073/pnas.96.22.12743
143. Ockenhouse CF, Tegoshi T, Maeno Y, Benjamin C, Ho M, Kan KE, et al. Human vascular endothelial cell adhesion receptors for *Plasmodium falciparum*-infected erythrocytes: roles for endothelial leukocyte adhesion molecule 1 and vascular cell adhesion molecule 1. *J Exp Med* (1992) 176:1183–9. doi:10.1084/jem.176.4.118
144. Siano JP, Grady KK, Millet P, Wick TM. *Plasmodium falciparum*: cytoadherence to alpha v beta3 on human microvascular endothelial cells. *Am J Trop Med Hyg* (1998) 59:77–9.

145. Beeson JG, Rogerson SJ, Cooke BM, Reeder JC, Chai W, Lawson AM, et al. Adhesion of *Plasmodium falciparum*-infected erythrocytes to hyaluronic acid in placental malaria. *Nat Med* (2000) 6:86–90. doi:10.1038/71582
146. Treutiger CJ, Heddini A, Fernandez V, Muller WA, Wahlgren M. PECAM-1/CD31, an endothelial receptor for binding *Plasmodium falciparum*-infected erythrocytes. *Nat Med* (1997) 3:1405–8. doi:10.1038/nm1297-1405
147. Biswas AK, Hafiz A, Banerjee B, Kim KS, Datta K, Chitnis CE. *Plasmodium falciparum* uses gC1qR/HABP1/p32 as a receptor to bind to vascular endothelium and for platelet-mediated clumping. *PLoS Pathog* (2007) 3:1271–80. doi:10.1371/journal.ppat.0030130
148. Turner L, Lavstsen T, Berger SS, Wang CW, Petersen JE, Avril M, et al. Severe malaria is associated with parasite binding to endothelial protein C receptor. *Nature* (2013) 499:223–7. doi:10.1038/nature12361
149. Rowe JA, Moulds JM, Newbold CI, Miller LH. *Plasmodium falciparum* rosetting mediated by a parasite-variant erythrocyte membrane protein and complement-receptor 1. *Nature* (1997) 388:292–5. doi:10.1038/40888
150. Chen Q, Fernandez V, Sundstrom A, Schlichtherle M, Datta S, Hagblom P, et al. Developmental selection of *var* gene expression in *Plasmodium falciparum. Nature* (1998) 394:392–5. doi:10.1038/28660
151. Roberts DJ, Craig AG, Berendt AR, Pinches RA, Nash GB, Marsh K, et al. Rapid switching to multiple antigenic and adhesive phenotypes in malaria. *Nature* (1992) 357:689–92. doi:10.1038/357689a0
152. Blackman MJ, Scott-Finnigan TJ, Shai S, Holder AA. Antibodies inhibit the protease-mediated processing of a malaria merozoite surface protein. *J Exp Med* (1994) 180:389–93. doi:10.1084/jem.180.1.389
153. Carvalho BO, Lopes SC, Nogueira PA, Orlandi PP, Bargieri DY, Blanco YC, et al. On the cytoadhesion of *Plasmodium vivax*-infected erythrocytes. *J Infect Dis* (2010) 202:638–47. doi:10.1086/654815
154. Lopes SC, Albrecht L, Carvalho BO, Siqueira AM, Thomson-Luque R, Nogueira PA, et al. Paucity of *Plasmodium vivax* mature schizonts in peripheral blood is associated with their increased cytoadhesive potential. *J Infect Dis* (2014) 209:1403–7. doi:10.1093/infdis/jiu018
155. Carlton JMR, Adams JH, Silva JC, Bidwell SL, Lorenzi H, Caler E, et al. Comparative genomics of the neglected human malaria parasite *Plasmodium vivax. Nature* (2008) 455:757–63. doi:10.1038/nature07327
156. Neafsey DE, Galinsky K, Jiang RH, Young L, Sykes SM, Saif S, et al. The malaria parasite *Plasmodium vivax* exhibits greater genetic diversity than *Plasmodium falciparum. Nat Genet* (2012) 44:1046–50. doi:10.1038/ng.2373
157. Srivastava A, Gangnard S, Round A, Dechavanne S, Juillerat A, Raynal B, et al. Full-length extracellular region of the var2CSA variant of PfEMP1 is required for specific, high-affinity binding to CSA. *Proc Natl Acad Sci U S A* (2010) 107:4884–9. doi:10.1073/pnas.1000951107
158. Gangnard S, Lewit-Bentley A, Dechavanne S, Srivastava A, Amirat F, Bentley GA, et al. Structure of the DBL3X-DBL4epsilon region of the VAR2CSA placental malaria vaccine candidate: insight into DBL domain interactions. *Sci Rep* (2015) 5:14868. doi:10.1038/srep14868
159. Holder AA. The carboxy-terminus of merozoite surface protein 1: structure, specific antibodies and immunity to malaria. *Parasitology* (2009) 136: 1445–56. doi:10.1017/S0031182009990515
160. Ayi K, Turrini F, Piga A, Arese P. Enhanced phagocytosis of ring-parasitized mutant erythrocytes: a common mechanism that may explain protection against falciparum malaria in sickle trait and beta-thalassemia trait. *Blood* (2004) 104:3364–71. doi:10.1182/blood-2003-11-3820
161. Blackman MJ, Heidrich HG, Donachie S, McBride JS, Holder AA. A single fragment of a malaria merozoite surface protein remains on the parasite during red cell invasion and is the target of invasion-inhibiting antibodies. *J Exp Med* (1990) 172:379–82. doi:10.1084/jem.172.1.379
162. Guevara-Patino JA, Holder AA, McBride JS, Blackman MJ. Antibodies that inhibit malaria merozoite surface protein-1 processing and erythrocyte invasion are blocked by naturally acquired human antibodies. *J Exp Med* (1997) 186:1689–99. doi:10.1084/jem.186.10.1689
163. Okafor CM, Anumudu CI, Omosun YO, Uthaipibull C, Ayede I, Awobode HO, et al. Cellular response to modified *Plasmodium falciparum* MSP119 antigens in individuals previously exposed to natural malaria infection. *Malar J* (2009) 8:263. doi:10.1186/1475-2875-8-263
164. Ehrenstein MR, Notley CA. The importance of natural IgM: scavenger, protector and regulator. *Nat Rev Immunol* (2010) 10:778–86. doi:10.1038/nri2849
165. Pleass RJ, Moore SC, Stevenson L, Hviid L. Immunoglobulin M: restrainer of inflammation and mediator of immune evasion by *Plasmodium falciparum* malaria. *Trends Parasitol* (2016) 32:108–19. doi:10.1016/j.pt.2015.09.007
166. Ghumra A, Semblat JP, McIntosh RS, Raza A, Rasmussen IB, Braathen R, et al. Identification of residues in the Cmu4 domain of polymeric IgM essential for interaction with *Plasmodium falciparum* erythrocyte membrane protein 1 (PfEMP1). *J Immunol* (2008) 181:1988–2000. doi:10.4049/jimmunol.181.3.1988
167. Barfod LK, Dalgaard MB, Pleman ST, Ofori MF, Pleass RJ, Hviid L. Evasion of immunity to *Plasmodium falciparum* malaria by IgM masking of protective IgG epitopes in infected erythrocyte surface-exposed PfEMP1. *Proc Natl Acad Sci U S A* (2011) 108:12485–90. doi:10.1073/pnas.1103708108
168. Crosnier C, Iqbal Z, Knuepfer E, Maciuca S, Perrin AJ, Kamuyu G, et al. Binding of *Plasmodium falciparum* merozoite surface proteins DBLMSP and DBLMSP2 to human immunoglobulin M is conserved amongst broadly diverged sequence variants. *J Biol Chem* (2016) 291:14285–99. doi:10.1074/jbc.M116.722074
169. Anders RF. Multiple cross-reactivities amongst antigens of *Plasmodium falciparum* impair the development of protective immunity against malaria. *Parasite Immunol* (1986) 8:529–35. doi:10.1111/j.1365-3024.1986.tb00867.x
170. Moir S, Ho J, Malaspina A, Wang W, DiPoto AC, O'Shea MA, et al. Evidence for HIV-associated B cell exhaustion in a dysfunctional memory B cell compartment in HIV-infected viremic individuals. *J Exp Med* (2008) 205:1797–805. doi:10.1084/jem.20072683
171. Portugal S, Tipton CM, Sohn H, Kone Y, Wang J, Li S, et al. Malaria-associated atypical memory B cells exhibit markedly reduced B cell receptor signaling and effector function. *Elife* (2015) 4:e07218. doi:10.7554/eLife.07218
172. Muellenbeck MF, Ueberheide B, Amulic B, Epp A, Fenyo D, Busse CE, et al. Atypical and classical memory B cells produce *Plasmodium falciparum* neutralizing antibodies. *J Exp Med* (2013) 210:389–99. doi:10.1084/jem.20121970
173. Fehr T, Bachmann MF, Bucher E, Kalinke U, Padova FED, Lang AB, et al. Role of repetitive antigen patterns for induction of antibodies against antibodies. *J Exp Med* (1997) 185:1785–92. doi:10.1084/jem.185.10.1785
174. Dintzis RZ, Okajima M, Middleton MH, Greene G, Dintzis HM. The immunogenicity of soluble haptenated polymers is determined by molecular mass and hapten valence. *J Immunol* (1989) 143:1239–44.
175. Zubler RH. Naive and memory B cells in T-cell-dependent and T-independent responses. *Springer Semin Immunopathol* (2001) 23:405–19. doi:10.1007/s281-001-8167-7
176. Symer DE, Reim J, Dintzis RZ, Voss EW Jr, Dintzis HM. Durable elimination of high affinity, T cell-dependent antibodies by low molecular weight antigen arrays in vivo. *J Immunol* (1995) 155:5608–16.
177. Puentes F, Dickhaut K, Hofstatter M, Pfeil J, Lauer U, Hamann A, et al. Immune modulation and prevention of autoimmune disease by repeated sequences from parasites linked to self antigens. *J Neuroimmune Pharmacol* (2016). doi:10.1007/s11481-016-9701-x
178. Robson KJH, Hall JR, Davies LC, Crisanti A, Hill AVS, Wellems TE. Polymorphism of the TRAP gene of *Plasmodium falciparum. Proc Biol Sci* (1990) 242:205–16. doi:10.1098/rspb.1990.0126
179. Muller HM, Scarselli E, Crisanti A. Thrombospondin related anonymous protein (TRAP) of *Plasmodium falciparum* in parasite-host cell interactions. *Parassitologia* (1993) 35:69–72.
180. Trottein F, Triglia T, Cowman AF. Molecular cloning of a gene from *Plasmodium falciparum* that codes for a protein sharing motifs found in adhesive molecules from mammals and plasmodia. *Mol Biochem Parasitol* (1995) 74:129–41. doi:10.1016/0166-6851(95)02489-1
181. Chattopadhyay R, Rathore D, Fujioka H, Kumar S, De la Vega P, Haynes D, et al. PfSPATR – a *Plasmodium falciparum* protein containing an altered thrombospondin type I repeat domain is expressed at several stages of the parasite life cycle and is the target of inhibitory antibodies. *J Biol Chem* (2003) 278:25977–81. doi:10.1074/jbc.M300865200
182. Siddiqui FA, Dhawan S, Singh S, Singh B, Gupta P, Pandey A, et al. A thrombospondin structural repeat containing rhoptry protein from *Plasmodium falciparum* mediates erythrocyte invasion. *Cell Microbiol* (2013) 15:1341–56. doi:10.1111/cmi.12118

183. Cowman AF, Berry D, Baum J. The cell biology of disease: the cellular and molecular basis for malaria parasite invasion of the human red blood cell. *J Cell Biol* (2012) 198:961–71. doi:10.1083/jcb.201206112
184. Chen L, Lopaticki S, Riglar DT, Dekiwadia C, Uboldi AD, Tham WH, et al. An EGF-like protein forms a complex with PfRh5 and is required for invasion of human erythrocytes by *Plasmodium falciparum*. *PLoS Pathog* (2011) 7:e1002199. doi:10.1371/journal.ppat.1002199
185. Kaslow DC, Quakyi IA, Syin C, Raum MG, Keister DB, Coligan JE, et al. A vaccine candidate from the sexual stage of human malaria that contains EGF-like domains. *Nature* (1988) 333:74–6. doi:10.1038/333074a0
186. Duffy PE, Kaslow DC. A novel malaria protein, Pfs28, and Pfs25 are genetically linked and synergistic as falciparum malaria transmission-blocking vaccines. *Infect Immun* (1997) 65:1109–13.
187. Urban BC, Roberts DJ. Malaria, monocytes, macrophages and myeloid dendritic cells: sticking of infected erythrocytes switches off host cells. *Curr Opin Immunol* (2002) 14:458–65. doi:10.1016/S0952-7915(02)00368-0
188. McGilvray ID, Serghides L, Kapus A, Rotstein OD, Kain KC. Nonopsonic monocyte/macrophage phagocytosis of *Plasmodium falciparum*-parasitized erythrocytes: a role for CD36 in malarial clearance. *Blood* (2000) 96:3231–40.
189. Schwarzer E, Turrini F, Ulliers D, Giribaldi G, Ginsburg HD, Arese P. Impairment of macrophage functions after ingestion of *Plasmodium falciparum*-infected erythrocytes or isolated malarial pigment. *J Exp Med* (1992) 176:1033–41. doi:10.1084/jem.176.4.1033
190. Cunnington AJ, Njie M, Correa S, Takem EN, Riley EM, Walther M. Prolonged neutrophil dysfunction after *Plasmodium falciparum* malaria is related to hemolysis and heme oxygenase-1 induction. *J Immunol* (2012) 189:5336–46. doi:10.4049/jimmunol.1201028
191. Schwarzer E, Arese P. Phagocytosis of malarial pigment hemozoin inhibits NADPH-oxidase activity in human monocyte-derived macrophages. *Biochim Biophys Acta* (1996) 1316:169–75. doi:10.1016/0925-4439(96)00021-X
192. Steinman RM. Decisions about dendritic cells: past, present, and future. *Annu Rev Immunol* (2012) 30:1–22. doi:10.1146/annurev-immunol-100311-102839
193. Urban BC, Ferguson DJP, Pain A, Willcox N, Plebanski M, Austyn JM, et al. *Plasmodium falciparum*-infected erythrocytes modulate the maturation of dendritic cells. *Nature* (1999) 400:73–7. doi:10.1038/21900
194. Toure Balde A, Sarthou JL, Aribot G, Michel P, Trape JF, Rogier C, et al. *Plasmodium falciparum* induces apoptosis in human mononuclear cells. *Infect Immun* (1996) 64:744–50.
195. Helmby H, Jonsson G, Troye-Blomberg M. Cellular changes and apoptosis in the spleens and peripheral blood of mice infected with blood-stage *Plasmodium chabaudi chabaudi* AS. *Infect Immun* (2000) 68:1485–90. doi:10.1128/IAI.68.3.1485-1490.2000
196. Wykes MN, Zhou YH, Liu XQ, Good MF. *Plasmodium yoelii* can ablate vaccine-induced long-term protection in mice. *J Immunol* (2005) 175: 2510–6. doi:10.4049/jimmunol.175.4.2510
197. Woodberry T, Minigo G, Piera KA, Amante FH, Pinzon-Charry A, Good MF, et al. Low-level *Plasmodium falciparum* blood-stage infection causes dendritic cell apoptosis and dysfunction in healthy volunteers. *J Infect Dis* (2012) 206:333–40. doi:10.1093/infdis/jis366
198. Matsumoto J, Kawai S, Terao K, Kirinoki M, Yasutomi Y, Aikawa M, et al. Malaria infection induces rapid elevation of the soluble Fas ligand level in serum and subsequent T lymphocytopenia: possible factors responsible for the differences in susceptibility of two species of *Macaca* monkeys to *Plasmodium coatneyi* infection. *Infect Immun* (2000) 68:1183–8. doi:10.1128/IAI.68.3.1183-1188.2000
199. Pinzon-Charry A, Woodberry T, Kienzle V, McPhun V, Minigo G, Lampah DA, et al. Apoptosis and dysfunction of blood dendritic cells in patients with falciparum and vivax malaria. *J Exp Med* (2013) 210:1635–46. doi:10.1084/jem.20121972
200. Carvalho LJ, Ferreira-da-Cruz MF, Daniel-Ribeiro CT, Pelajo-Machado M, Lenzi HL. *Plasmodium berghei* ANKA infection induces thymocyte apoptosis and thymocyte depletion in CBA mice. *Mem Inst Oswaldo Cruz* (2006) 101:523–8. doi:10.1590/S0074-02762006000500007
201. Theander TG, Bygbjerg IC, Jacobsen L, Jepsen S, Larsen PB, Kharazmi A. Low parasite specific T cell response in clinically immune individuals with low grade *Plasmodium falciparum* parasitaemia. *Trans R Soc Trop Med Hyg* (1986) 80:1000–1. doi:10.1016/0035-9203(86)90295-6
202. Martini F, Paglia MG, Montesano C, Enders PJ, Gentile M, Pauza CD, et al. Vgamma9Vdelta2 T-cell anergy and complementarity-determining region 3-specific depletion during paroxysm of nonendemic malaria infection. *Infect Immun* (2003) 71:2945–9. doi:10.1128/IAI.71.5.2945-2949.2003
203. Alves FA, Pelajo-Machado M, Totino PR, Souza MT, Goncalves EC, Schneider MP, et al. Splenic architecture disruption and parasite-induced splenocyte activation and anergy in *Plasmodium falciparum*-infected *Saimiri sciureus* monkeys. *Malar J* (2015) 14:128. doi:10.1186/s12936-015-0641-3
204. Illingworth J, Butler NS, Roetynck S, Mwacharo J, Pierce SK, Bejon P, et al. Chronic exposure to *Plasmodium falciparum* is associated with phenotypic evidence of B and T cell exhaustion. *J Immunol* (2012) 190:1038–47. doi:10.4049/jimmunol.1202438
205. Butler NS, Moebius J, Pewe LL, Traore B, Doumbo OK, Tygrett LT, et al. Therapeutic blockade of PD-L1 and LAG-3 rapidly clears established blood-stage *Plasmodium* infection. *Nat Immunol* (2012) 13:188–95. doi:10.1038/ni.2180
206. Karunarathne DS, Horne-Debets JM, Huang JX, Faleiro R, Leow CY, Amante FH, et al. Programmed death-1 ligand 2-mediated regulation of the PD-L1 to PD-1 axis is essential for establishing CD4+ T cell immunity. *Immunity* (2016) 45:333–45. doi:10.1016/j.immuni.2016.07.017
207. Horne-Debets JM, Karunarathne DS, Faleiro RJ, Poh CM, Renia L, Wykes MN. Mice lacking programmed cell death-1 show a role for CD8+ T cells in long-term immunity against blood-stage malaria. *Sci Rep* (2016) 6:26210. doi:10.1038/srep26210
208. Kho S, Marfurt J, Handayuni I, Pava Z, Noviyanti R, Kusuma A, et al. Characterization of blood dendritic and regulatory T cells in asymptomatic adults with sub-microscopic *Plasmodium falciparum* or *Plasmodium vivax* infection. *Malar J* (2016) 15:328. doi:10.1186/s12936-016-1382-7
209. Cambos M, Belanger B, Jacques A, Roulet A, Scorza T. Natural regulatory CD4+CD25+FOXP+ T cells control the production of pro-inflammatory cytokines during *Plasmodium chabaudi adami* infection and do not contribute to immune evasion. *Int J Parasitol* (2008) 38:229–38. doi:10.1016/j.ijpara.2007.07.006
210. Hisaeda H, Tetsutani K, Imai T, Moriya C, Tu L, Hamano S, et al. Malaria parasites require TLR9 signaling for immune evasion by activating regulatory T cells. *J Immunol* (2008) 180:2496–503. doi:10.4049/jimmunol.180.4.2496
211. Kho S, Marfurt J, Noviyanti R, Kusuma A, Piera KA, Burdam FH, et al. Preserved dendritic cell HLA-DR expression and reduced regulatory T cell activation in asymptomatic *Plasmodium falciparum* and *P. vivax* Infection. *Infect Immun* (2015) 83:3224–32. doi:10.1128/IAI.00226-15
212. Hafalla JCR, Claser C, Couper KN, Grau GE, Renia L, De Souza JB, et al. The CTLA-4 and PD-1/PD-L1 inhibitory pathways independently regulate host resistance to *Plasmodium*-induced acute immune pathology. *PLoS Pathog* (2012) 8:e1002504. doi:10.1371/journal.ppat.1002504
213. Iyer JK, Gruner AC, Renia L, Snounou G, Preiser PR. Invasion of host cells by malaria parasites: a tale of two protein families. *Mol Microbiol* (2007) 65:231–49. doi:10.1111/j.1365-2958.2007.05791.x
214. Mayer DCG, Mu JB, Feng X, Su XZ, Miller LH. Polymorphism in a *Plasmodium falciparum* erythrocyte-binding ligand changes its receptor specificity. *J Exp Med* (2002) 196:1523–8. doi:10.1084/jem.20020750
215. Stubbs J, Simpson KM, Triglia T, Plouffe D, Tonkin CJ, Duraisingh MT, et al. Molecular mechanism for switching of *Plasmodium falciparum* invasion pathways into human erythrocytes. *Science* (2005) 309:1384–7. doi:10.1126/science.1115257
216. Persson KE, McCallum FJ, Reiling L, Lister NA, Stubbs J, Cowman AF, et al. Variation in use of erythrocyte invasion pathways by *Plasmodium falciparum* mediates evasion of human inhibitory antibodies. *J Clin Invest* (2008) 118:342–51. doi:10.1172/JCI32138
217. Crosnier C, Bustamante LY, Bartholdson SJ, Bei AK, Theron M, Uchikawa M, et al. Basigin is a receptor essential for erythrocyte invasion by *Plasmodium falciparum*. *Nature* (2011) 480:534–7. doi:10.1038/nature10606
218. Douglas AD, Baldeviano GC, Lucas CM, Lugo-Roman LA, Crosnier C, Bartholdson SJ, et al. A PfRH5-based vaccine is efficacious against heterologous strain blood-stage infection in *Aotus* monkeys. *Cell Host Microbe* (2015) 17:130–9. doi:10.1016/j.chom.2014.11.017
219. Douglas AD, Williams AR, Illingworth JJ, Kamuyu G, Biswas S, Goodman AL, et al. The blood-stage malaria antigen PfRH5 is susceptible to vaccine-

inducible cross-strain neutralizing antibody. *Nat Commun* (2011) 2:601. doi:10.1038/ncomms1615
220. Zimmerman PA, Ferreira MU, Howes RE, Mercereau-Puijalon O. Red blood cell polymorphism and susceptibility to *Plasmodium vivax*. *Adv Parasitol* (2013) 81:27–76. doi:10.1016/B978-0-12-407826-0.0000
221. Miller LH, Mason SJ, Clyde DF, McGinniss MH. The resistance factor to *Plasmodium vivax* in blacks. The Duffy-blood-group genotype, FyFy. *N Engl J Med* (1976) 295:302–4. doi:10.1056/NEJM197608052950602
222. Livingstone FB. The Duffy blood groups, vivax malaria, and malaria selection in human populations: a review. *Hum Biol* (1984) 56:413–25.
223. Menard D, Barnadas C, Bouchier C, Henry-Halldin CN, Gray LR, Ratsimbasoa A, et al. *Plasmodium vivax* clinical malaria is commonly observed in Duffy-negative Malagasy people. *Proc Natl Acad Sci U S A* (2010) 107:5967–71. doi:10.1073/pnas.0912496107
224. Mendes C, Dias F, Figueiredo J, Mora VG, Cano J, de Sousa B, et al. Duffy negative antigen is no longer a barrier to *Plasmodium vivax*-molecular evidences from the African West Coast (Angola and Equatorial Guinea). *PLoS Negl Trop Dis* (2011) 5:e1192. doi:10.1371/journal.pntd.0001192
225. Abdelraheem MH, Albsheer MM, Mohamed HS, Amin M, Abdel Hamid MM. Transmission of *Plasmodium vivax* in Duffy-negative individuals in central Sudan. *Trans R Soc Trop Med Hyg* (2016) 110:258–60. doi:10.1093/trstmh/trw014
226. Lo E, Yewhalaw D, Zhong D, Zemene E, Degefa T, Tushune K, et al. Molecular epidemiology of *Plasmodium vivax* and *Plasmodium falciparum* malaria among Duffy-positive and Duffy-negative populations in Ethiopia. *Malar J* (2015) 14:84. doi:10.1186/s12936-015-0596-4
227. Ngassa Mbenda HG, Das A. Molecular evidence of *Plasmodium vivax* mono and mixed malaria parasite infections in Duffy-negative native Cameroonians. *PLoS One* (2014) 9:e103262. doi:10.1371/journal.pone.0103262
228. Rosenberg RL. *Plasmodium vivax* in Africa: hidden in plain sight? *Trends Parasitol* (2007) 23:193–6. doi:10.1016/j.pt.2007.02.009
229. Ntumngia FB, Thomson-Luque R, de Menezes Torres L, Gunalan K, Carvalho LH, Adams JH. A novel erythrocyte binding protein of *Plasmodium vivax* suggests an alternate invasion pathway into Duffy-Positive reticulocytes. *MBio* (2016) 7:e1261. doi:10.1128/mBio.01261-16
230. Fang XD, Kaslow DC, Adams JH, Miller LH. Cloning of the *Plasmodium vivax* Duffy receptor. *Mol Biochem Parasitol* (1991) 44:125–32. doi:10.1016/0166-6851(91)90228-X
231. Cogswell FB. The hypnozoite and relapse in primate malaria. *Clin Microbiol Rev* (1992) 5:26–35. doi:10.1128/CMR.5.1.26
232. Fairley NH. Chemotherapeutic suppression and prophylaxis in malaria. An experimental investigation undertaken by medical research teams in Australia. *Trans R Soc Trop Med Hyg* (1945) 38:311–65. doi:10.1016/0035-9203(45)90038-1
233. Krotoski WA, Garnham PCC, Bray RS, Krotoski DM, Killick-Kendrick R, Draper CC, et al. Observations on early and late post-sporozoite tissue stages in primate malaria. I. The discovery of a new latent form of *Plasmodium cynomolgi* (the hypnozoite), and failure to detect forms within the first 24 hours after infection. *Am J Trop Med Hyg* (1982) 31:24–35.
234. Mikolajczak SA, Vaughan AM, Kangwanrangsan N, Roobsoong W, Fishbaugher M, Yimamnuaychok N, et al. *Plasmodium vivax* liver stage development and hypnozoite persistence in human liver-chimeric mice. *Cell Host Microbe* (2015) 16:526–35. doi:10.1016/j.chom.2015.02.011
235. Krotoski WA, Bray RS, Garnham PCC, Gwadz RW, Killick-Kendrick R, Draper CC, et al. Observations on early and late post-sporozoite tissue stages in primate malaria. II. The hypnozoite of *Plasmodium cynomolgi bastianellii* from 3 to 105 days after infection, and detection of 36- to 40-hour pre-erythrocytic forms. *Am J Trop Med Hyg* (1982) 31:211–25.
236. Krotoski WA, Krotoski DM, Garnham PCC, Bray RS, Killick-Kendrick R, Draper CC, et al. Relapses in primate malaria: discovery of two populations of exoerythrocytic stages. Preliminary note. *Br Med J* (1980) 280:153–4. doi:10.1136/bmj.280.6208.153-a
237. Mazier D, Renia L, Snounou G. A pre-emptive strike against malaria's stealthy hepatic forms. *Nat Rev Drug Discov* (2009) 8:854–64. doi:10.1038/nrd29
238. Garnham PCC, Bray RS. The influence of immunity upon the stages (including late exo-erythrocytic schizonts) of mammalian malaria parasites. *Rev Bras Malariol Doencas Trop* (1956) 8:151–60.
239. Shortt HE, Garnham PCC. The pre-erythrocytic stage of human malaria, *Plasmodium vivax*. *Br Med J* (1948) 1:547. doi:10.1136/bmj.1.4550.547
240. Shortt HE, Fairley NH. The pre-erythrocytic stage of *Plasmodium falciparum*; a preliminary note. *Br Med J* (1949) 2:1006–8. doi:10.1136/bmj.2.4635.1006
241. Coquelin F, Boulard Y, Mora-Silvera E, Richard F, Chabaud AG, Landau I. Final stage of maturation of the erythrocytic schizonts of rodent *Plasmodium* in the lungs. *C R Acad Sci* (1999) 322:55–62. doi:10.1016/S0764-4469(99)80017-1
242. Baer K, Klotz C, Kappe SH, Schnieder T, Frevert U. Release of hepatic *Plasmodium yoelii* merozoites into the pulmonary microvasculature. *PLoS Pathog* (2007) 3:e171. doi:10.1371/journal.ppat.0030171
243. Fajardo LF. The role of platelets in infections. I. Observations in human and murine malaria. *Arch Pathol Lab Med* (1979) 103:131–4.
244. Mora-Silvera E, Coquelin F, Vuong P, Deharo E, Gautret P, Renia L, et al. Role of macrophages as possible transporters of *Plasmodium yoelii nigeriensis* merozoites through the lymphatic system. Preliminary note. *Parasite* (1997) 4:83–5. doi:10.1051/parasite/1997041083
245. Wykes MN, Kay JG, Manderson A, Liu XQ, Brown DL, Richard DJ, et al. Rodent blood-stage *Plasmodium* survive in dendritic cells that infect naive mice. *Proc Natl Acad Sci U S A* (2011) 108:11205–10. doi:10.1073/pnas.1108579108
246. Boulard Y, Coquelin F, Mora-Silvera E, Renia L, Gautret P, Deharo E, et al. Dendritic leucocytes as possible carriers of murine *Plasmodium* merozoites. *Parasite* (1996) 3:383–6. doi:10.1051/parasite/1996034383
247. Landau I, Chabaud AG, Vuong PN, Deharo E, Gautret P. Circulation in the lymphatic system and latency of *Plasmodium* merozoites. Preliminary note. *Parasite* (1995) 2:185–6. doi:10.1051/parasite/1995022185
248. Landau I, Chabaud AG, Mora-Silvera E, Coquelin F, Boulard Y, Renia L, et al. Survival of rodent malaria merozoites in the lymphatic network: potential role in chronicity of the infection. *Parasite* (1999) 6:311–22. doi:10.1051/parasite/1999064311
249. Carter RL, Mendis KN. Evolutionary and historical aspects of the burden of malaria. *Clin Microbiol Rev* (2002) 15:564–94. doi:10.1128/CMR.15.4.564-594.2002
250. Cox FEG. Malaria. Cloning genes for antigens of *Plasmodium falciparum*. *Nature* (1983) 304:13–4. doi:10.1038/304013a0

3

Interleukin-27 Early Impacts *Leishmania infantum* Infection in Mice and Correlates with Active Visceral Disease in Humans

Begoña Pérez-Cabezas[1,2], Pedro Cecílio[1,2], Ana Luisa Robalo[1,2], Ricardo Silvestre[3,4], Eugenia Carrillo[5], Javier Moreno[5], Juan V. San Martín[6], Rita Vasconcellos[7] and Anabela Cordeiro-da-Silva[1,2,8]*

[1] i3S – Instituto de Investigação e Inovação em Saúde, Universidade do Porto, Porto, Portugal, [2] IBMC – Instituto de Biologia Molecular e Celular, Universidade do Porto, Porto, Portugal, [3] ICVS – Instituto de Investigação em Ciências da Vida e Saúde, Escola de Ciências da Saúde, Universidade do Minho, Braga, Portugal, [4] ICVS/3B's – Laboratório Associado, Braga, Portugal, [5] WHO Collaborating Centre for Leishmaniasis, Centro Nacional de Microbiología, Instituto de Salud Carlos III, Madrid, Spain, [6] Hospital Universitario de Fuenlabrada, Madrid, Spain, [7] Departamento de Imunobiologia, Instituto de Biologia, Universidade Federal Fluminense, Niterói, Brazil, [8] Faculdade de Farmácia, Departamento de Ciências Biológicas, Universidade do Porto, Porto, Portugal

***Correspondence:**
Anabela Cordeiro-da-Silva
cordeiro@ibmc.up.pt

The complexity of *Leishmania*–host interactions, one of the main leishmaniasis issues, is yet to be fully understood. We detected elevated IL-27 plasma levels in European patients with active visceral disease caused by *Leishmania infantum*, which returned to basal levels after successful treatment, suggesting this cytokine as a probable infection mediator. We further addressed this hypothesis recurring to two classical susceptible visceral leishmaniasis mouse models. BALB/c, but not C57BL/6 mice, showed increased IL-27 systemic levels after infection, which was associated with an upregulation of IL-27p28 expression by dendritic cells and higher parasite burdens. Neutralization of IL-27 in acutely infected BALB/c led to decreased parasite burdens and a transient increase in IFN-γ^+ splenic T cells, while administration of IL-27 to C57BL/6 promoted a local anti-inflammatory cytokine response at the site of infection and increased parasite loads. Overall, we show that, as in humans, BALB/c IL-27 systemic levels are infection dependently upregulated and may favor parasite installation by controlling inflammation.

Keywords: IL-27, *Leishmania infantum*, human, mouse models, immune regulation

INTRODUCTION

The 2013 Global Burden of Disease reveals leishmaniasis as one of the deadliest neglected tropical infectious diseases, affecting millions of people worldwide (1). It is caused by the sandfly transmitted protozoan parasite *Leishmania*. The infection can be asymptomatic or manifest in cutaneous, mucosal, and visceral forms, the last one being fatal if left untreated (2). These forms depend mostly on the infecting parasite species but also on the efficiency of the host immune response, especially during the first moments after parasite inoculation (3). Phagocytic cells are rapidly recruited upon *Leishmania* deposition in the skin by the sandfly, but the parasite is able to manipulate them using different strategies. One of the effects of this immunomodulation is the alteration of cytokines secretion in the infection microenvironment. Interferences with receptors and signaling pathways prevent the production and the function of pro-inflammatory cytokines such as IL-12 and IFN-γ and favors anti-inflammatory IL-10 and TGF-β contributing to parasite survival [reviewed in Ref. (4)].

Interleukin-27 is composed of the subunits p28 and EBV-induced protein 3 (EBI3) that interacts with a receptor comprising the glycoprotein 130 (gp130) and IL-27Rα or WSX-1. Interleukin-27 is mainly produced by macrophages and dendritic cells (DCs) after the stimulation of surface receptors such as TLRs or CD40 and following IFNs signaling (5, 6). Although this cytokine was initially described as pro-inflammatory, numerous anti-inflammatory and immunomodulatory properties are recognized today [reviewed in Ref. (5, 6)].

In the past few years, several reports have contributed to the understanding of the IL-27 role during *Leishmania* infection. Active visceral leishmaniasis (VL) patients from India (7) and Brazil (8) present increased IL-27 in plasma. In mice, IL-27 appears to be essential to prevent severe immunopathology after infection with both cutaneous (9) and visceral (10) strains, mainly through the effects of IL-10. However, whether IL-27 directly affects parasite burdens (9, 11) or if IL-10 appears as a consequence of inflammatory (7, 12) or suppressor (13) events is still unclear.

In the present study, we report elevated IL-27 plasma levels in *Leishmania infantum*-infected European patients with active VL, which normalized after successful treatment. Curiously, IL-27 increased early after *L. infantum* infection in the serum of BALB/c, but not in C57BL/6 mice. We took advantage of this dichotomy to understand the mechanisms underlying the effects of IL-27 in visceral *Leishmania* infection. Early blocking of IL-27 in BALB/c mice decreased parasite loads, while IL-27 administration in C57BL/6 augmented parasite burdens. Immunological studies suggested that IL-27 is produced as a consequence of parasite subversion of the host immune response, resulting in a control of inflammation beneficial for parasite installation.

MATERIALS AND METHODS

Ethics Statement

Human sample collection was in accordance with Good Clinical Practice guidelines. The study was approved by the Ethics Committee of the University Hospital of Fuenlabrada (Madrid, Spain). All subjects provided their written informed consent.

Animal experiments were performed in accordance with the IBMC.INEB Animal Ethics Committees and the Portuguese National Authorities for Animal Health guidelines (directive 2010/63/EU). Begoña Pérez-Cabezas and Anabela Cordeiro-da-Silva are accredited for animal research (Portuguese Veterinary Direction, Ministerial Directive 113/2013).

Human Studies

Diagnosed VL patients were treated with liposomal Amphotericin B (21 mg/kg). Cure was 100% in 3 months after diagnosis. Subjects without previous VL symptomology were included as negative controls. Plasma was recovered from heparinized blood and stored at −20°C for posterior IL-27 determination using MILLIPLEX MAP (Millipore, Germany) and analyzed on a Bio-Plex-200 Luminex (Bio-Rad, CA, USA) (minimum detectable concentration 0.063 ng/mL).

Parasites and Mice

A clone of virulent *L. infantum* (MHOM/MA/67/ITMAP-263) was maintained by weekly subpassages at 26°C in RPMI 1640 medium supplemented with 10% heat-inactivated fetal bovine serum (FBS), 2 mM L-glutamine, 100 U/mL penicillin, 100 microgram/mL streptomycin, and 20 mM HEPES buffer (all from BioWhittaker, Lonza, Switzerland). Promastigotes from 4 to 10 passages were used in these experiments.

Six- to eight-week-old male BALB/c and C57BL/6 mice (Charles River Laboratories, France) were maintained under specific pathogen-free conditions at the IBMC facilities. Animals were infected i.p. with 1×10^8 stationary promastigotes from 5 culture days.

Mice Sera Collection

Blood from mice was collected through intracardiac puncture under isoflurane anesthesia. Serum was collected and stored at −80°C for posterior analysis.

Splenic Dendritic Cells and Macrophages Cell Sorting and Hepatic Kupffer Cell Enrichment Procedure

Spleen and Liver were aseptically collected from 24 h infected mice. Splenocytes were obtained and labeled to distinguish DCs ($CD11b^+/CD11c^{high}$) and macrophages ($CD11b^+/Ly6G^-/Ly6C^+/F4\text{-}80^+$), and sorted using a FACSAria and the FACSDiva software (BD Biosciences, NJ, USA) for posterior RNA analysis. Sorted cells purity was >95%.

Enriched Kupffer cells were obtained after hepatic collagenase digestion, followed by a Percoll density gradient centrifugation (Sigma-Aldrich, MO, USA) and a brief adhesion step, as described elsewhere (14). The percentage of Kupffer cells was determined by flow cytometry ($F4/80^+/CD11b^{variable}$). Cells were resuspended in lysis buffer and frozen for posterior RNA analysis.

RNA Extraction and Quantitative RT-PCR

Total RNA was extracted (RNeasy Mini Kit, Qiagen, CA, USA), quantified (NanoDrop1000, Thermo Scientific, MA, USA), and reversely transcribed (NZY-First-Strand cDNA synthesis Kit, NZYTech, Portugal). Quantitative RT-PCRs were run on an iQ5 iCycler thermal cycler (Bio-Rad) (15). Results were analyzed (built-in iQ5 v2, Bio-Rad) and normalized using the reference gene GAPDH. The sequences of the primers used were *IL-27p28* Forward TCGATTGCCAGGAGTGAACC, Reverse CGAAG TGGTAGCGAGGAAG; *EBI3* Forward AGCAGCAGCCTCC TAGCCT, Reverse ACGCCTTCCGGAGGGTC; and *GAPDH* Forward CTGGTCCTGAGTGTAGCCCAA, Reverse CATGGC CTTCCGTGTTCCTA.

In Vitro Differentiation and Infection of Bone Marrow-Derived DCs and Macrophages

For bone marrow-derived DCs (BMDCs) differentiation, 6×10^6 bone marrow cells were seeded in 25 mL of complete RPMI supplemented with 50 μM 2-mercaptoethanol (Sigma-Aldrich) and 10% of GM-CSF-containing supernatant from J558 cell conditioned medium (DC medium) (16). Cells were cultured at 37°C and 5% CO_2 for 3 days, after which the same amount of DC medium was added to each flask. At day 6, half of the culture supernatant was replaced with fresh DC medium. At day 8, cells were thoroughly resuspended, recovered, counted, and, finally, plated in 96 round-bottom culture plates at 1×10^5 cells/well in 200 μL of DC medium. Bone marrow-derived macrophages (BMMØ) were obtained from non-adherent bone marrow cells collected after an initial overnight incubation (37°C and 5% CO_2) in complete Dulbecco's modified Eagle's medium (DMEM) (Lonza). Non-adherent cells were counted and distributed in 96 flat-bottom well culture plates at 1×10^5 cells/well in 100 μL of complete DMEM supplemented with 5% of L-929 cell conditioned medium (LCCM). After 3 days of culture, 100 μL of DMEM + 5% LCCM were added per well. Half of the media volume was renewed at day 6 of culture. BMMØ acquired a definitive differentiation status at day 8.

Stationary promastigotes from 5 culture days (cultured as described in Section "Parasites and Mice") were added to BMDC or BMMØ at a 10:1 ratio. Non-internalized parasites were washed after 4 h incubation (37°C and 5% CO_2). Non-infected cells were stimulated with 1 μg/mL LPS (Sigma-Aldrich) as positive control, or received complete medium as negative control. Supernatants were recovered 24 h post-infection for cytokine quantification.

In Vivo IL-27 Modulation

Twenty-four hours after infection, BALB/c mice were i.p. treated with 20 μg of goat anti-mouse IL-27p28 neutralizing antibody (a-IL-27) and C57BL/6 with 1 μg of mouse recombinant IL-27 (rIL-27) (both from R&D Systems), as previously reported (17, 18). As controls, BALB/c and C57BL/6 received 20 μg of goat IgG (isotype control) and PBS (mock), respectively.

Determination of Parasite Burdens

Spleen and liver were aseptically collected, weighted, and disrupted. Splenic and hepatic parasite burdens were assessed by the limit dilution method. The parasite titer was considered as the last dilution with >1 motile parasite. The number of parasites per gram of organ was calculated, as discussed previously (19). Peritoneal cells were recovered and 2×10^5 cells from each exudate were subjected to cytospin in 200 μL of PBS during 5 min at 1000 rpm using a Shandon Cytospin II (GMI, MN, USA). Cell preparations were fixed with 2% paraformaldehyde (PFA) for 20 min. Afterward, an adapted staining protocol was performed (20) by 2 min immersion in Kaplow modified solution, followed by 45 s immersions in Hemacolor reagent 1 and reagent 2 (Merk Millipore, Germany). Finally, slides were washed with distilled water, air dried, and observed by optical microscopy (100× magnification). For determination of the percentage of infected cells, 200 consecutive cells were differentially counted (infected versus non-infected) in 3 different areas of the same preparation and the mean of the 3 areas was calculated. The number of parasites per infected cells was assessed by counting 100 different infected cells from which the mean was calculated.

Flow Cytometry

The anti-mouse monoclonal antibodies used to perform this study were all purchased to BioLegend (CA, USA) except if otherwise stated: FITC-labeled anti-IgM (R6-60.2, BD Biosciences, NJ, USA), anti-MHC-II(I-Ad) (AMS-32.1, BD), anti-MHC-II(I-A/I-E) (M5114.15.2), anti-IFN-γ (XMG1.2), and anti-IL-17A (TC11-18H10.1); PE-labeled anti-CD8 (53-6.7, BD), anti-CD11b (M1/70), anti-Siglec-F (E50-2440, BD), anti-F4/80 (BM8), anti-IL-4 (11B11), and anti-IL-6 (MP5-20F3); PerCP-labeled anti-CD11b (M1/70); PerCP-Cy5.5-labeled anti-Ly6C (HK1.4), anti-F4-80 (BM8), and anti-TNFα (MP6-XT22); PE-Cy7-labeled anti-CD3 (HA2) and anti-CD11b (M1/70); APC-Cy7-labeled anti-CD11c (N418); APC-labeled anti-CD19 (6D5), anti-IL-5 (TRFK5), and anti-IL-10 (JES5-16E3); BV510-labeled anti-CD4 (RM4-5); and Pacific Blue™-labeled anti-Ly6G (1A8).

To analyze lymphoid and myeloid cell populations, two panels of antibodies were designed. The lymphoid panel was composed of anti-CD8, -CD3, -CD4, and -CD19. The Myeloid panel comprised anti-CD11b, -CD11c, -Siglec-F, -Ly6C, -Ly6G, and -MHC-II. Surface staining of peritoneal and splenic cells was performed in PBS + 0.5% BSA (20min, 4°C) followed by 15 min fixation using 1% PFA. For intracellular staining, splenocytes were cultured for 2 h with PMA/Ionomycin (50/500 ng/mL) and then for 2 h with Brefeldin A (10 μg/mL). Cells were surface stained and then intracellularly after fixation and permeabilization with 1% saponin (all from Sigma) (21). Samples were acquired in a FACSCanto (BD) and analyzed using the FlowJo software v10 (TreeStar, OR, USA).

An initial gate plotting FSC-A versus SSC-A was performed. Afterward, singlets were selected by plotting FSC-A versus FSC-H and the remaining cell populations were resolved. T lymphoid cell populations were defined as $CD3^+/CD4^+$ and $CD3^+/CD8^+$, while B cells were defined as $CD19^+$. Cytokine production by T cells was assessed within $CD3^+/CD4^+$ and $CD3^+/CD8^+$cells. Myeloid cell populations were gated as eosinophils ($Siglec\text{-}F^+/SSC\text{-}H^{int/high}$), neutrophils ($CD11b^{high}/Ly6G^{high}/Siglec\text{-}F^-$), DCs ($CD11c^+/MHC\text{-}II^{int/high}$), and macrophages ($CD11b^+/CD11c^-/Ly6G^-/Siglec\text{-}F^-$).

Determination of Mouse Cytokines by ELISA

Cytokines were quantified, according to the manufacturer's instructions, using the commercial kits: IL-27 ELISA Ready-SET-Go!® (eBiosciences, CA, USA) (detection limit 16 pg/mL); IL-27p28/IL-30 and IL-10 DuoSet ELISA (R&D Systems, MN, USA) (detection limits 15.6 and 31.2 pg/mL, respectively); IL-12p70 and IFN-γ ELISA MAX Deluxe (BioLegend, CA, USA) (detection limit 4 pg/mL for both cytokines).

Statistical Analysis

Results are expressed as mean ± SEM. Statistical differences were analyzed using GraphPad Prism v6.01 (CA, USA). Comparisons between human samples were performed using Mann–Whitney test for unpaired samples and Wilcoxon test for paired data. Mice experimental groups were compared using the unpaired *t*-test unless otherwise stated.

RESULTS

Systemic IL-27 Increases in *L. infantum*-Infected European Patients and BALB/c Mice

To address if the increase of systemic IL-27 is a common fact of VL among different endemic areas (7, 8), we determined this cytokine in the plasma of active *L. infantum* infected individuals from a current outbreak in Spain. Patients with active disease presented higher IL-27 levels than both cured ($p \leq 0.001$) and negative controls ($p \leq 0.001$) (**Figure 1A**). Some patients were re-sampled after cure, which confirmed that IL-27 decreases after successful treatment ($p \leq 0.01$) (**Figure 1A**).

The role of IL-27 during *Leishmania* infection was addressed using mouse models by several authors (10–13, 22). However, whether IL-27 is also increased in the serum of *Leishmania*-infected mice has never been shown. Therefore, we addressed if BALB/c and C57BL/6, two susceptible VL mouse species, displayed a similar systemic increase of IL-27 as observed in *L. infantum*-infected humans. While IL-27 remained unchanged in the serum of infected C57BL/6 mice, infected BALB/c showed an early increase that was significant 4 days after infection ($p \leq 0.05$) and always higher than the IL-27 levels of C57BL/6 mice ($p \leq 0.05$ comparing the day 2 and $p \leq 0.01$ the day 4 after infection) (**Figure 1B**).

Dendritic Cells Are the Main Cellular Source of IL-27 in Infected BALB/c Mice

As the main sources of IL-27 are myeloid cell populations, and macrophages and DCs play critical roles during *Leishmania* infection, we decided to discriminate their contribution to IL-27 response after *L. infantum* infection. For that, the expression of IL-27 subunits in splenic DCs and macrophages sorted from infected BALB/c and C57BL/6 was evaluated. While the expression of EBI3 remained always comparable to basal levels (Figure S1 in Supplementary Material), IL-27p28 expression was significantly upregulated but only in DCs from BALB/c 24 h after infection ($p \leq 0.05$) (**Figure 2A**). The contribution of Kupffer cells, the resident liver macrophages, for the IL-27 response to *L. infantum* was also addressed. The expression of IL-27 subunits was analyzed in Kupffer cells from non-infected and infected BALB/c mice. However, no increase in the RNA levels of IL-27p28 and EBI3 was detected in these cells 24 h after infection (Figure S2 in Supplementary Material), suggesting that DCs, and not macrophages, are the main cell source responsible for the increase of IL-27 in our model.

To confirm our data at protein level, we determined IL-27 and IL-27p28 in supernatants from 24 h *L. infantum*-infected BMMØ and BMDCs. Although after infection the production of IL-27p28 was greater in BMMØ from C57BL/6 than from BALB/c ($p \leq 0.05$), IL-27 concentration was similar in both mouse strains. No difference was found after LPS activation (**Figure 2B**). In line with *ex vivo* results, both IL-27p28 and IL-27 secretion by BMDCs were significantly higher in cells

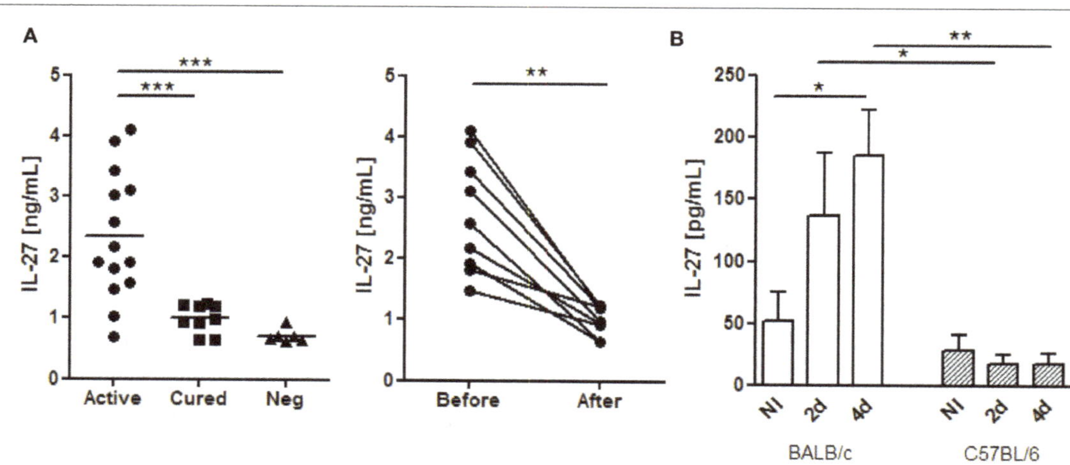

FIGURE 1 | *L. infantum* infection increases systemic IL-27 in European VL patients and in BALB/c mice. (A) Interleukin-27 levels in the plasma of European patients with active VL caused by *L. infantum* (black dots, $n = 14$), cured patients (black squares, $n = 9$), and negative controls (black triangles, $n = 6$). The cytokine was also determined in VL patients before and after treatment ($n = 9$). Each symbol represents one individual; bars represent the mean of the experimental groups. Mann–Whitney test was used to compare clinical groups and Wilcoxon matched pairs test for paired comparisons. **(B)** Interleukin-27 levels in the serum of BALB/c (white columns) and C57BL/6 (patterned columns) mice, infected i.p. with 1×10^8 *L. infantum* promastigotes for 2 and 4 days. Bars represent mean ± SEM of three independent experiments with a minimum of four animals per group and experiment. Unpaired *t*-test was used to assess statistical significances (*$p \leq 0.05$, **$p \leq 0.01$, and ***$p \leq 0.001$).

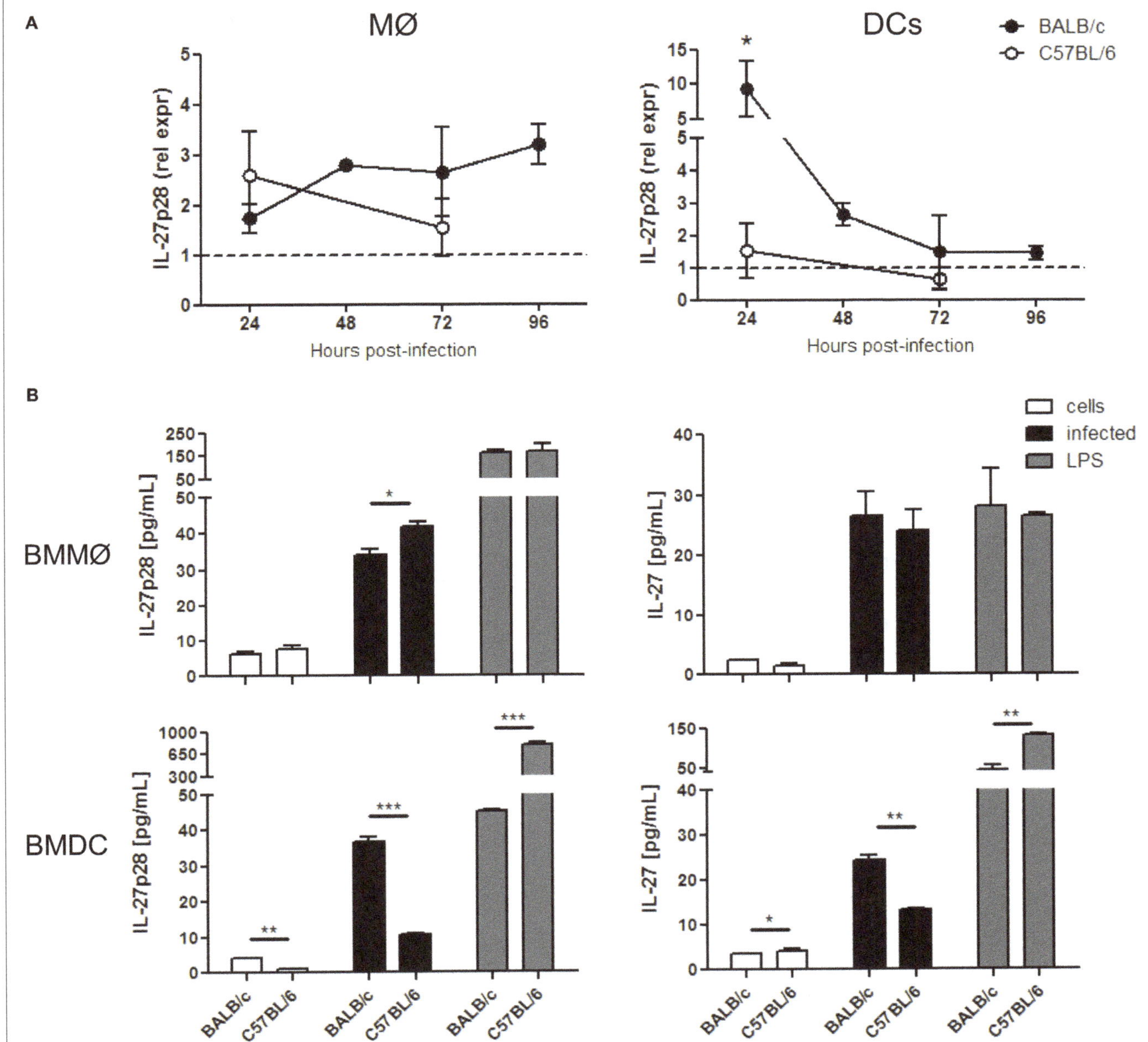

FIGURE 2 | Dendritic cells are the main source of IL-27 after *L. infantum* infection in BALB/c mice. (A) Splenic MØ and DCs were sorted from infected BALB/c (black symbols) and C57BL/6 (open symbols) mice at the indicated time points. The transcription levels of IL-27p28 were quantified by qRT-PCR. Results are relativized to non-infected mice values (=1). Every symbol and bars represent the mean and SEM, respectively, of four different animals per group analyzed in two different independent experiments. Unpaired *t*-test was used to assess statistical significances. **(B)** The secretion of IL-27p28 and IL-27 was quantified by ELISA in 24 h supernatants of BMMØ and BMDC infected with *L. infantum* promastigotes at a 1:10 ratio (black bars). Medium (white bars) and LPS (gray bars) were used as negative and positive controls, respectively. Bars represent the mean ± SEM of two independent experiments, every run in duplicate. Unpaired *t*-test was used to assess statistical significances (*$p \leq 0.05$, **$p \leq 0.01$, and ***$p \leq 0.001$).

from BALB/c when compared to C57BL/6 ($p \leq 0.001$ and $p \leq 0.01$, respectively) (**Figure 2B**). Interestingly, the ability of BMDCs to produce both cytokines after LPS stimulation was higher in C57BL/6 than in BALB/c, indicating that these cells are really capable of producing IL-27, but not in response to *L. infantum* infection. These results suggest that the parasite can actively modulate the secretion of IL-27 and IL-27p28 in BMDCs obtained from BALB/c, but not from C57BL/6 mice.

IL-27 Favors *L. infantum* Infection in Mouse Models

To determine whether IL-27 contribute to the infection outcome, we neutralized IL-27 in BALB/c and administered

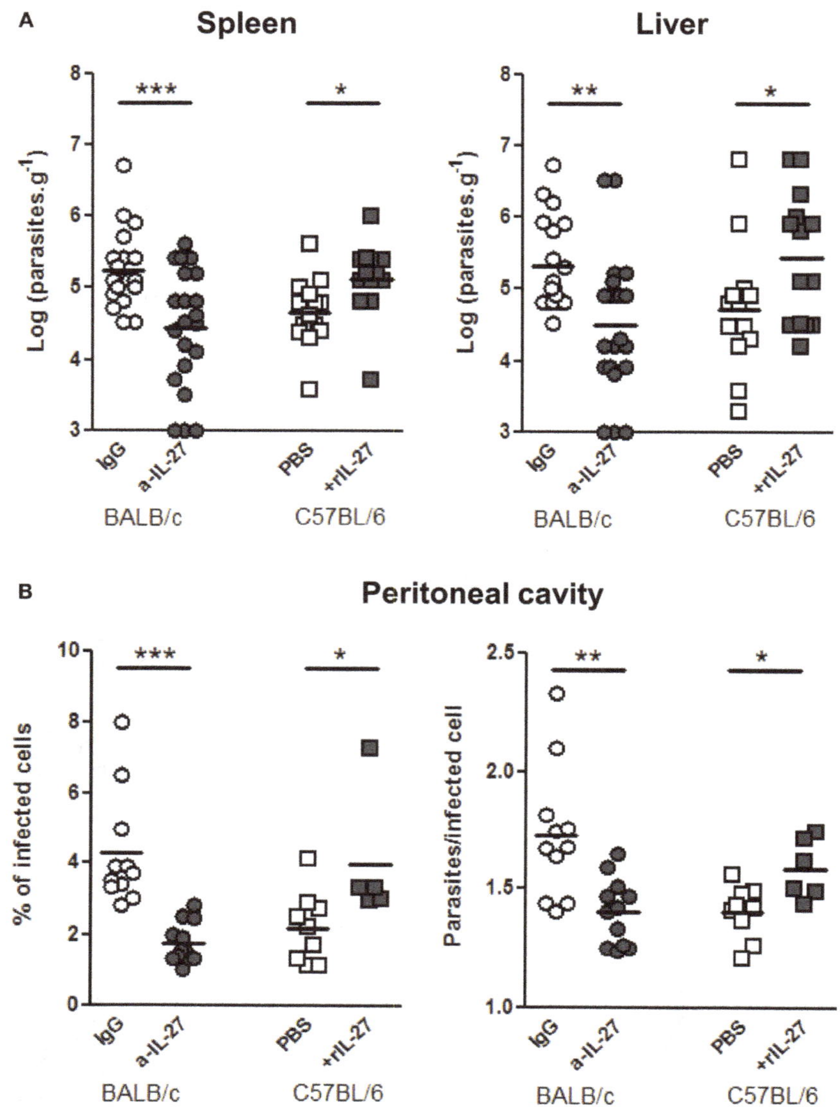

FIGURE 3 | IL-27 favors *L. infantum* infection in mice models. (A) BALB/c (circles) and C57BL/6 (squares) mice were i.p. infected with 1 × 10[8] promastigotes. Twenty-four hours later, BALB/c mice were treated i.p. with 20 μg of a-IL-27 (gray circles) or IgG isotype control (open circles), while C57BL/6 received i.p. 1 μg of mouse rIL-27 (gray squares) or the same volume of PBS (open squares). Three days after treatment, mice were euthanized and the parasite load of spleen and liver determined by limiting dilution. **(B)** In some animals, the peritoneal cavity was washed for collection of recruited cells. Approximately 2 × 10[5] cells from every exudate were cytospined, fixed, and stained with Kaplow modified solution and by the Giemsa method. Finally, slides were observed by optical microscopy at 100x for determination of the percentage of infected cells and the number of parasites/infected cell. All data represent results obtained in three independent experiments. Every symbol represents a mouse and the bars the mean of the group. Unpaired *t*-test was used to assess statistical significances ($^{*}p \leq 0.05$, $^{**}p \leq 0.01$, and $^{***}p \leq 0.001$).

rIL-27 to C57BL/6 mice 24 h after infection, coinciding with the IL-27p28 RNA peak in the spleen and before the IL-27 increase observed in the serum, 2 days after the infection, in BALB/c mice. Seventy-two hours later, these treatments significantly decreased in BALB/c and increased in C57BL/6 splenic and hepatic parasite burdens (**Figure 3A**). We also observed that IL-27 significantly affected the percentage of infected cells and the number of parasites per infected cells in the peritoneal cavity (**Figure 3B**). These results revealed a relation between the levels of IL-27 and the establishment of the infection.

IL-27 Modulates the Cytokine Response in Infected Mice

To elucidate how IL-27 interferes at the early stages of *L. infantum* infection, we performed a kinetic study of the peritoneal and splenic compartments after IL-27 modulation. Interestingly, IL-27 neutralization in infected BALB/c mice transiently decreased IL-10 in the peritoneal cavity ($p \leq 0.01$), and the administration of rIL-27 increased the presence of this cytokine in infected C57BL/6 mice 24 h ($p \leq 0.01$) and 72 h ($p \leq 0.05$) after treatment, always comparing with control infected animals (**Figure 4**). In addition, rIL-27 in C57BL/6 promoted a reduction of IFN-γ ($p \leq 0.05$) and IL-12p70 ($p \leq 0.01$) 24 h after treatment in comparison with infected non-treated animals (**Figure 4**). However, this shift in the cytokine profile determined by IL-27 almost did not alter cell recruitment to the site of infection, as when comparing treated and non-treated animals only the presence of B cells in the peritoneal cavity significantly increased 72 h after IL-27 blockage in BALB/c mice (**Figure 5**). In the spleen, the number of $CD4^+$ T cells increased in BALB/c mice 24 h after IL-27 blockage ($p \leq 0.05$), and the supply of the cytokine decreased the presence of the same cells in C57BL/6 mice after 72 h ($p \leq 0.05$) (**Figure 5**). The administration of rIL-27 also prevented the infiltration of neutrophils in the spleen of C57BL/6 mice ($p \leq 0.01$) (**Figure 6**). Analysis of the cytokine production revealed that IL-27 neutralization increased the numbers of IFN-γ producing $CD4^+$ and $CD8^+$ T cells 24 h post-treatment (**Figure 7**) ($p \leq 0.01$). These differences were not detected at 72 h, likely indicating a reversible effect (**Figure 7**). The potential secretion of other cytokines was also analyzed but no differences between α-IL-27 and IgG receiving mice were observed (Figure S3 in Supplementary Material). In contrast, rIL-27 did not alter the cytokine response of C57BL/6 splenic T cells (**Figure 7**; Figure S3 in Supplementary Material).

DISCUSSION

Interleukin-27 is a cytokine with known immunomodulatory properties involved in the pathogenesis of numerous diseases (5, 6). Several types of infections also course with an increase of IL-27 (23–25). However, whether this fact is a simple host mechanism to control inflammation or a complex pathogen evasion strategy is still unknown. *Leishmania* spp. are expert in modulating immune activity through diverse strategies (4). Previous reports on human leishmaniasis indicate that IL-27 increases when the disease is active in both cutaneous (26–28) and visceral forms (7, 8). Here, for the first time, plasma levels of IL-27 were evaluated in *L. infantum*-infected individuals from Europe. This cytokine was significantly increased in the active phase of our VL patients returning to homeostatic levels after treatment. Interestingly, a relapsing case presented increased circulating IL-27, and positive IL-27 results were obtained even when immunofluorescence antibody test (IFAT) was doubtful (data not shown). Further analysis using a larger cohort of patients will help to better understand the value of IL-27 as a complementary biomarker for human VL diagnosis and even for treatment efficacy monitoring, as has been postulated for this disease (8) and other infections (29).

The role of IL-27 during *Leishmania* infection has been addressed using animal models by several groups (9, 10, 12, 30). The general conclusion was that IL-27 controls inflammation and pathology through limitation of IFN-γ (12) and IL-17 (9) production by $CD4^+$ T cells, resulting in a permissive environment for the infection. However, these results are based on experiments performed on WSX-$1^{-/-}$ or EBI$3^{-/-}$ mice, presenting two main limitations. First, both WSX-1 and EBI3 are subunits shared with the regulatory cytokine IL-35 (31), meaning that the over-inflammation observed in these knockout mice can be a result of the additive loss of the regulatory function of both cytokines. The second issue is that both mice models were generated in the C57BL/6 genetic background. Although both C57BL/6 and BALB/c strains are considered susceptible models for experimental VL (32), here we showed that only BALB/c and not C57BL/6 mice increased IL-27 in the serum early

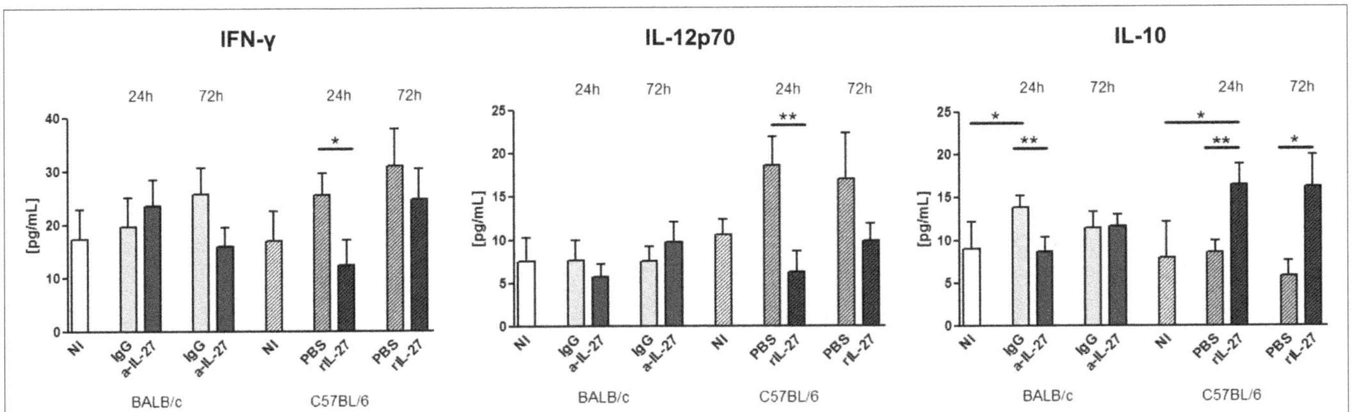

FIGURE 4 | IL-27 influences the cytokine responses in *L. infantum*-infected mice at the infection site. BALB/c and C57BL/6 mice were i.p. infected with 1×10^8 promastigotes. Twenty-four hours later, BALB/c mice were treated i.p. with 20 µg of a-IL-27 (clear dark-gray bars) or IgG isotype control (clear light-gray bars), while C57BL/6 received i.p. 1 µg of mouse rIL-27 (patterned dark-gray bars) or the same volume of PBS (patterned light-gray bars). Twenty-four or 72 h after treatment, mice were euthanized and the peritoneal cavity washed. Non-infected (NI) counterparts were always used as controls (white bars, non-patterned for BALB/c and patterned for C57BL/6 mice). The concentration of IFN-γ, IL-12p70, and IL-10 in the peritoneal exudates was determined by ELISA. Bars represent the mean ± SEM of three independent experiments, a minimum of four animals per condition and experiment was analyzed. Unpaired *t*-test was used to assess statistical significances (*$p \leq 0.05$ and **$p \leq 0.01$).

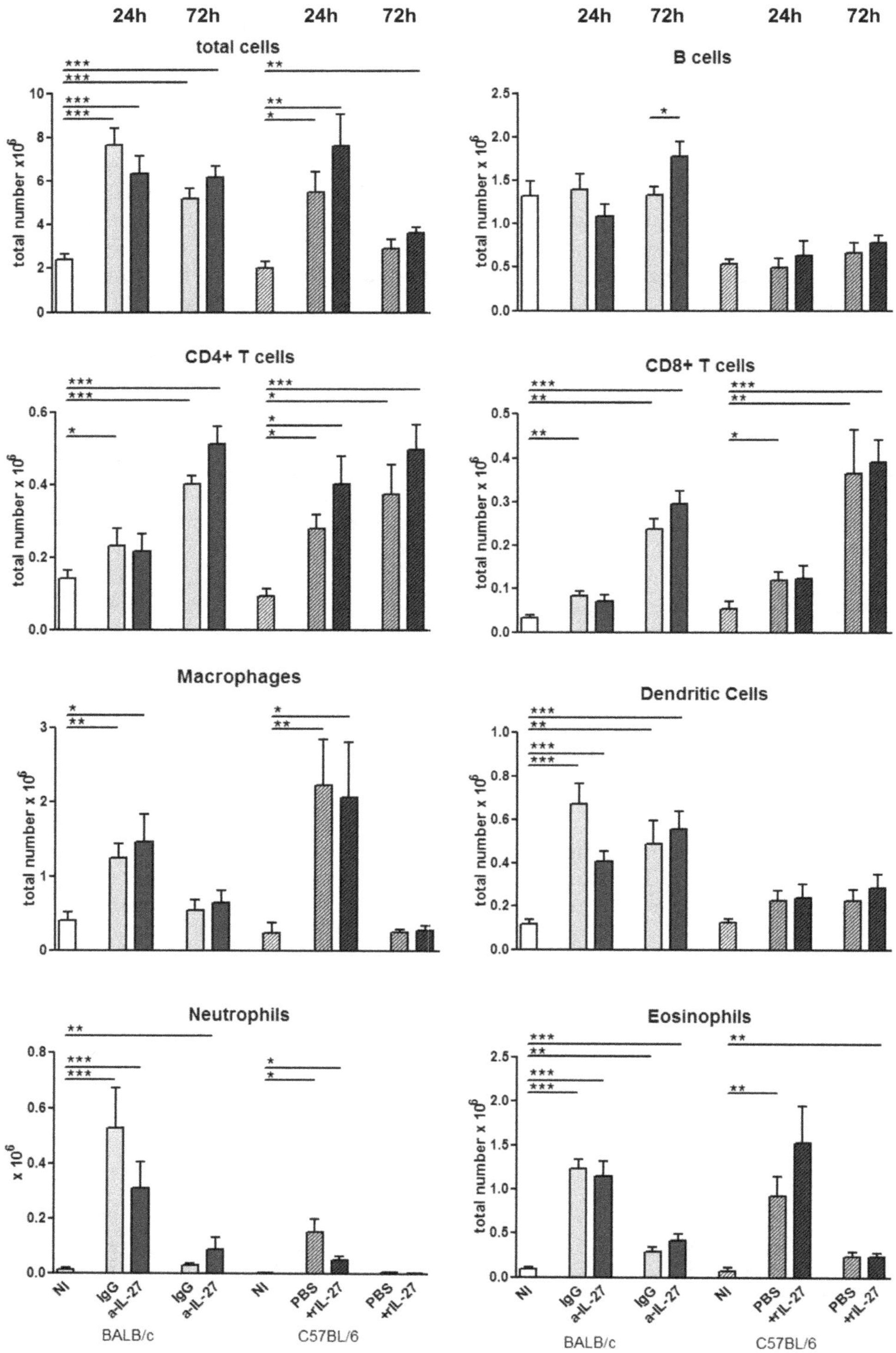

FIGURE 5 | Cell recruitment to the peritoneal cavity in response to *L. infantum* infection after IL-27 modulation. BALB/c and C57BL/6 mice were i.p. infected with 1 × 10^8 promastigotes. Twenty-four hours later, BALB/c mice were treated i.p. with 20 μg of a-IL-27 (clear dark-gray bars) or IgG isotype control (clear light-gray bars), while C57BL/6 received i.p. 1 μg of mouse rIL-27 (patterned dark-gray bars) or the same volume of PBS (patterned light-gray bars). Twenty-four or 72 h after treatment, mice were euthanized and the peritoneal cavity washed. Non-infected (NI) counterparts were always used as controls (white bars, non-patterned for BALB/c and patterned for C57BL/6 mice). Peritoneal cells were then extracellularly stained and acquired by flow cytometry. Bars represent the mean ± SEM of three independent experiments, a minimum of four animals per condition and experiment was analyzed. Unpaired *t*-test was always used to assess statistical significances (*$p \leq 0.05$, **$p \leq 0.01$, and ***$p \leq 0.001$).

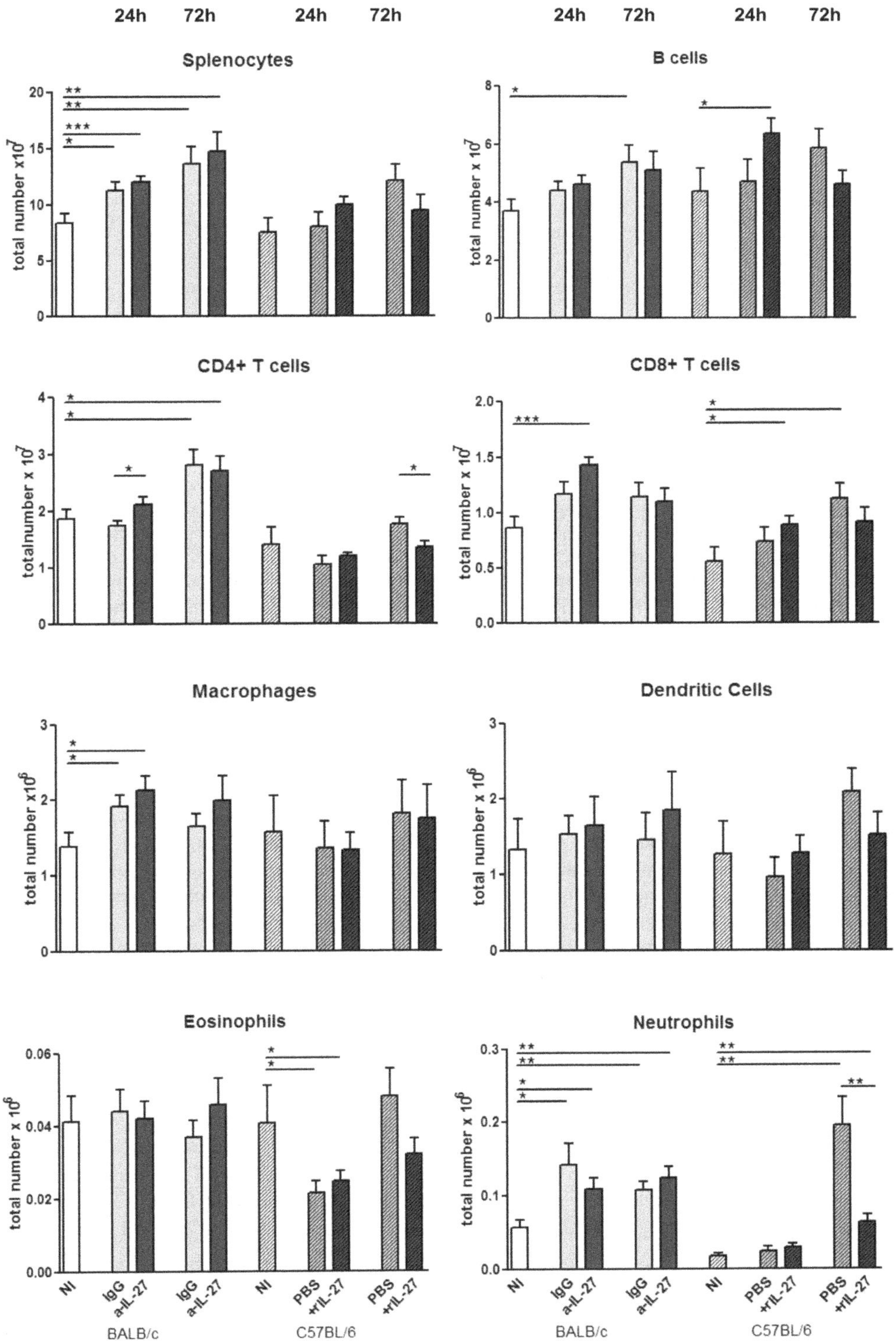

FIGURE 6 | Cellular composition of the spleen from *L. infantum*-infected mice after IL-27 modulation. BALB/c (clear bars) and C57BL/6 (patterned bars) mice were infected i.p. with 1 × 10^8 promastigotes. Twenty-four hours after infection, BALB/c mice were treated i.p. with 20 μg of IL-27 neutralizing antibody (a-IL-27, dark-gray bars) or IgG isotype control (IgG, light-gray bars), while C57BL/6 received i.p. 1 μg of mouse recombinant IL-27 (+rIL-27, dark-gray patterned bars) or the same volume of PBS (PBS, light-gray patterned bars). Non-infected (NI) counterparts were always used as controls (white bars, clear for BALB/c and patterned for C57BL/6 mice). Twenty-four or 72 h after treatment, mice were euthanized and the spleen collected and homogenized. Splenocytes were counted using an automatic cell counter, washed, and phenotyped by flow cytometry. Bars represent the mean and SEM of the three independent experiments, a minimum of four animals was analyzed per condition and experiment. Unpaired *t*-test was used to assess statistical significances (*$p \leq 0.05$, **$p \leq 0.01$, and ***$p \leq 0.001$).

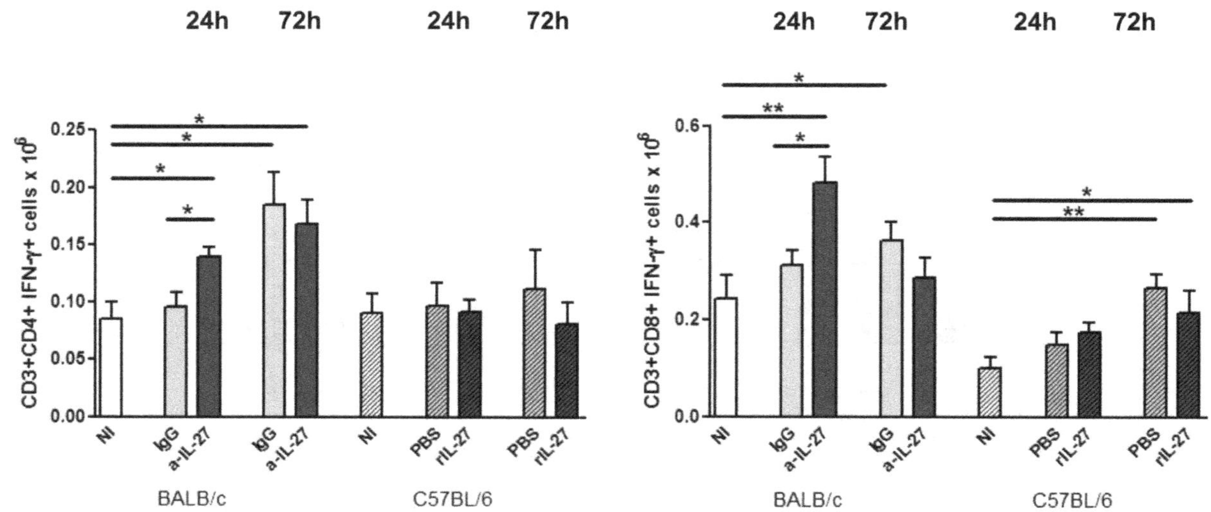

FIGURE 7 | IL-27 neutralization increases the IFN-γ response of splenic T cells in BALB/c mice (clear bars) and C57BL/6 (patterned bars) mice were infected i.p. with 1 × 10⁸ promastigotes. Twenty-four hours after infection, BALB/c mice were treated i.p. with 20 μg of IL-27 neutralizing antibody (a-IL-27, dark-gray bars) or IgG isotype control (IgG, light-gray bars), while C57BL/6 received i.p. 1 μg of mouse recombinant IL-27 (+rIL-27, dark-gray patterned bars) or the same volume of PBS (PBS, light-gray patterned bars). Non-infected (NI) counterparts were always used as controls (white bars, clear for BALB/c and patterned for C57BL/6 mice). Twenty-four or 72 h after treatment, mice were euthanized and the spleen collected and homogenized. Splenocytes were counted with an automatic cell counter, washed, and *in vitro* cultured during 4 h in the presence of PMA + Ionomycin and Brefeldin A. Cells were then extra- and intracellularly stained and acquired by flow cytometry. Bars represent the mean and SEM of the three independent experiments, a minimum of four animals was analyzed per condition and experiment. Unpaired *t*-test was used to assess statistical significances (*$p \leq 0.05$ and **$p \leq 0.01$).

after i.p. infection with *L. infantum*. The difference observed in the IL-27 production between the two mice strains in this study was confirmed at the cellular level, as splenic DCs from BALB/c but not from C57BL/6 mice upregulated the expression of IL-27p28 after infection. Upregulation of IL-27p28 in splenic DCs from BALB/c mice was previously shown after i.v. infection with *Leishmania donovani*, being CD8α$^+$ DCs the major responsible subset (22). The production of IL-27 could restrict the typical Th1 polarization induced by these APCs, known to be essential for parasite limitation (33). In fact, in a conditional IL-27p28 knockout mice model restricted to DCs, CD4$^+$ T cell IFN-γ response was exacerbated (34). Our data suggest that DCs are the main cell source responsible for the increase of IL-27 in BALB/c mice early after *L. infantum* infection probably as a result of active cell function modulation by the parasite. One explanation for the IL-27 divergence observed between the mice strains could be a differential expression of molecules involved in the recognition of parasite structures. An example is TLR-2, more expressed by BALB/c than by C57BL/6 mice (35). It has been demonstrated that TLR-2 signaling induces IL-27 production by respiratory epithelial cells (36). Therefore, this natural high expression of TLR-2 by BALB/c may favor the IL-27 increase early after infection, lowering inflammation, and promoting infection.

We exploited the IL-27 dichotomy in BALB/c and C57BL/6 mice to study the role of this cytokine during the early steps of infection, using an *in vivo* artificial-modulation approach. The resulting data revealed a relation between the levels of IL-27 and infection establishment, as the neutralization or the supply of IL-27 resulted in decreased or increased parasite burdens, respectively. In addition, the administration of rIL-27 significantly increased the production of IL-10 while decreased IFN-γ and IL-12p70 in the peritoneal cavity of C57BL/6 mice. Furthermore, the analysis of the cytokine production by splenic T cells revealed that IL-27 neutralization in BALB/c temporarily increased the numbers of IFN-γ producing CD4$^+$ and CD8$^+$ T cells. These results partially explain the higher parasite burdens quantified in the presence of IL-27. Addition of IL-27 *in vitro* exacerbates the infection of human macrophages by *Leishmania amazonensis via* IL-10 (11) and combined production of IL-27 and IL-10 by *L. donovani*-infected DCs is essential for IL-10 production by Th1 cells, resulting in parasite persistence (13). A recent work in EBI3$^{-/-}$ mice suggested a role for IL-27 in controlling IL-17 production and neutrophil infiltration during the chronic phase of *L. infantum* infection (30). However, whether the absence of the EBI3 subunit has an impact early after infection was not addressed in this work. We can also suggest that the IL-27 produced in response to infection shall not be a product of inflammation as BALB/c mice present higher parasite loads than C57BL/6 during the first days of infection, a difference that is counteracted by the treatments. Probably, the initial immune response of BALB/c is less inflammatory and less capable of limiting infection installation, suggesting again that the parasites directly induce the production of IL-27 for their own benefit. In fact, the absence of IL-27 can also prevent mycobacterial-induced phagosomal maturation arrest, favoring the elimination of the intracellular pathogen by macrophages depending on IFN-γ (37). In addition, IL-27 can impair the protective immunity to *Mycobacterium tuberculosis* in mice, as WSX-1 deficient T cells accumulate more efficiently in the lesions, showing improved capacity to produce IL-2 and reduced expression of cell death markers (25), functions that may also be altered during *Leishmania* infection.

Altogether, our data demonstrate that IL-27 increases after *L. infantum* infection both in humans and in animal models. These results confirm the involvement of IL-27 in mice models of *Leishmania* visceral pathogenesis, limiting inflammation during the initial stages of the infection and favoring parasite persistence, suggesting that the presence of IL-27 early after infection could influence the host immune response and the progression of the disease. Finally, we would like to highlight that IL-27 has the potential to be a useful biomarker for active human VL and for treatment efficacy monitoring, independently of the etiological agent and the geographical region affected.

AUTHOR CONTRIBUTIONS

BP-C, RS, and AC-d-S conceived and designed the experiments; BP-C, PC, AR, and EC performed the experiments; BP-C, PC, RS, EC, JM, JVM, RV, and AC-d-S analyzed the data; JM and AC-d-S contributed with reagents/materials/analysis tools; and BP-C, PC, RV, and AC-d-S wrote the paper.

ACKNOWLEDGMENTS

We thank Dr. Catarina Leitão (Flow cytometry unit, IBMC) and Dr. Sofia Lamas (Animal facilities, IBMC) for all the technical assistance.

FUNDING

This work was supported by Fundação para a Ciência e Tecnologia (FCT)/Ministério da Educação e da Ciência (MEC), co-funded by FEDER under the PT2020 Partnership Agreement through the Research Unit NO. 4293; by European Community's Seventh Framework Programme under grant agreement No. 603182 (Project MuLeVaClin) and by the ISCIII-AES project (project reference PI13/00440). PC and BP-C are supported by fellowships from the European Community's Seventh Framework Programme under grant agreements No. 603182 (Project MuLeVaClin) and No. 603240-2 (Project NMTryPI), respectively.

REFERENCES

1. Institute for Health Metrics and Evaluation (IHME). *Age-Sex Specific All-Cause and Cause-Specific Mortality 1990-2013. Global Burden of Disease Study 2013*. Seattle, WA: GBD Publications (2014).
2. WHO. *Leishmaniasis Fact Sheet N°375*. (2015). Available from: http://www.who.int/mediacentre/factsheets/fs375/en/
3. Gollob KJ, Viana AG, Dutra WO. Immunoregulation in human American leishmaniasis: balancing pathology and protection. *Parasite Immunol* (2014) 36(8):367–76. doi:10.1111/pim.12100
4. Cecilio P, Perez-Cabezas B, Santarem N, Maciel J, Rodrigues V, Cordeiro da Silva A. Deception and manipulation: the arms of *Leishmania*, a successful parasite. *Front Immunol* (2014) 5:480. doi:10.3389/fimmu.2014.00480
5. Aparicio-Siegmund S, Garbers C. The biology of interleukin-27 reveals unique pro- and anti-inflammatory functions in immunity. *Cytokine Growth Factor Rev* (2015) 26(5):579–86. doi:10.1016/j.cytogfr.2015.07.008
6. Yoshida H, Hunter CA. The immunobiology of interleukin-27. *Annu Rev Immunol* (2015) 33:417–43. doi:10.1146/annurev-immunol-032414-112134
7. Ansari NA, Kumar R, Gautam S, Nylen S, Singh OP, Sundar S, et al. IL-27 and IL-21 are associated with T cell IL-10 responses in human visceral leishmaniasis. *J Immunol* (2011) 186(7):3977–85. doi:10.4049/jimmunol.1003588
8. Dos Santos PL, de Oliveira FA, Santos ML, Cunha LC, Lino MT, de Oliveira MF, et al. The severity of visceral leishmaniasis correlates with elevated levels of serum IL-6, IL-27 and sCD14. *PLoS Negl Trop Dis* (2016) 10(1):e0004375. doi:10.1371/journal.pntd.0004375
9. Anderson CF, Stumhofer JS, Hunter CA, Sacks D. IL-27 regulates IL-10 and IL-17 from CD4+ cells in nonhealing *Leishmania major* infection. *J Immunol* (2009) 183(7):4619–27. doi:10.4049/jimmunol.0804024
10. Rosas LE, Satoskar AA, Roth KM, Keiser TL, Barbi J, Hunter C, et al. Interleukin-27R (WSX-1/T-cell cytokine receptor) gene-deficient mice display enhanced resistance to *Leishmania donovani* infection but develop severe liver immunopathology. *Am J Pathol* (2006) 168(1):158–69. doi:10.2353/ajpath.2006.050013
11. Barreto-de-Souza V, Ferreira PL, Vivarini Ade C, Calegari-Silva T, Soares DC, Regis EG, et al. IL-27 enhances *Leishmania amazonensis* infection via ds-RNA dependent kinase (PKR) and IL-10 signaling. *Immunobiology* (2015) 220(4):437–44. doi:10.1016/j.imbio.2014.11.006
12. Artis D, Johnson LM, Joyce K, Saris C, Villarino A, Hunter CA, et al. Cutting edge: early IL-4 production governs the requirement for IL-27-WSX-1 signaling in the development of protective Th1 cytokine responses following *Leishmania major* infection. *J Immunol* (2004) 172(8):4672–5. doi:10.4049/jimmunol.172.8.4672
13. Owens BM, Beattie L, Moore JW, Brown N, Mann JL, Dalton JE, et al. IL-10-producing Th1 cells and disease progression are regulated by distinct CD11c(+) cell populations during visceral leishmaniasis. *PLoS Pathog* (2012) 8(7):e1002827. doi:10.1371/journal.ppat.1002827
14. Smedsrod B, Pertoft H. Preparation of pure hepatocytes and reticuloendothelial cells in high yield from a single rat liver by means of Percoll centrifugation and selective adherence. *J Leukoc Biol* (1985) 38(2):213–30.
15. Neves BM, Silvestre R, Resende M, Ouaissi A, Cunha J, Tavares J, et al. Activation of phosphatidylinositol 3-kinase/Akt and impairment of nuclear factor-kappaB: molecular mechanisms behind the arrested maturation/activation state of *Leishmania infantum*-infected dendritic cells. *Am J Pathol* (2010) 177(6):2898–911. doi:10.2353/ajpath.2010.100367
16. Zal T, Volkmann A, Stockinger B. Mechanisms of tolerance induction in major histocompatibility complex class II-restricted T cells specific for a blood-borne self-antigen. *J Exp Med* (1994) 180(6):2089–99. doi:10.1084/jem.180.6.2089
17. Fujita H, Teng A, Nozawa R, Takamoto-Matsui Y, Katagiri-Matsumura H, Ikezawa Z, et al. Production of both IL-27 and IFN-gamma after the treatment with a ligand for invariant NK T cells is responsible for the suppression of Th2 response and allergic inflammation in a mouse experimental asthma model. *J Immunol* (2009) 183(1):254–60. doi:10.4049/jimmunol.0800520
18. Vasconcellos R, Carter NA, Rosser EC, Mauri C. IL-12p35 subunit contributes to autoimmunity by limiting IL-27-driven regulatory responses. *J Immunol* (2011) 187(6):3402–12. doi:10.4049/jimmunol.1100224
19. Silvestre R, Cordeiro-Da-Silva A, Santarem N, Vergnes B, Sereno D, Ouaissi A. SIR2-deficient *Leishmania infantum* induces a defined IFN-gamma/IL-10 pattern that correlates with protection. *J Immunol* (2007) 179(5):3161–70. doi:10.4049/jimmunol.179.5.3161
20. do Vale A, Afonso A, Silva MT. The professional phagocytes of sea bass (*Dicentrarchus labrax* L.): cytochemical characterisation of neutrophils and

macrophages in the normal and inflamed peritoneal cavity. *Fish Shellfish Immunol* (2002) 13(3):183–98. doi:10.1006/fsim.2001.0394
21. Resende M, Moreira D, Augusto J, Cunha J, Neves B, Cruz MT, et al. *Leishmania*-infected MHC class IIhigh dendritic cells polarize CD4+ T cells toward a nonprotective T-bet+ IFN-gamma+ IL-10+ phenotype. *J Immunol* (2013) 191(1):262–73. doi:10.4049/jimmunol.1203518
22. Maroof A, Kaye PM. Temporal regulation of interleukin-12p70 (IL-12p70) and IL-12-related cytokines in splenic dendritic cell subsets during *Leishmania donovani* infection. *Infect Immun* (2008) 76(1):239–49. doi:10.1128/IAI.00643-07
23. Zhu C, Zhang R, Liu L, Rasool ST, Mu Y, Sun W, et al. Hepatitis B virus enhances interleukin-27 expression both in vivo and in vitro. *Clin Immunol* (2009) 131(1):92–7. doi:10.1016/j.clim.2008.10.011
24. Liu L, Cao Z, Chen J, Li R, Cao Y, Zhu C, et al. Influenza A virus induces interleukin-27 through cyclooxygenase-2 and protein kinase A signaling. *J Biol Chem* (2012) 287(15):11899–910. doi:10.1074/jbc.M111.308064
25. Torrado E, Fountain JJ, Liao M, Tighe M, Reiley WW, Lai RP, et al. Interleukin 27R regulates CD4+ T cell phenotype and impacts protective immunity during *Mycobacterium tuberculosis* infection. *J Exp Med* (2015) 212(9):1449–63. doi:10.1084/jem.20141520
26. Novoa R, Bacellar O, Nascimento M, Cardoso TM, Ramasawmy R, Oliveira WN, et al. IL-17 and regulatory cytokines (IL-10 and IL-27) in *L. braziliensis* infection. *Parasite Immunol* (2011) 33(2):132–6. doi:10.1111/j.1365-3024.2010.01256.x
27. Tolouei S, Ghaedi K, Khamesipour A, Akbari M, Baghaei M, Hasheminia S, et al. IL-23 and IL-27 levels in macrophages collected from peripheral blood of patients with healing vs non-healing form of cutaneous leishmaniasis. *Iran J Parasitol* (2012) 7(1):18–25.
28. Costa DL, Cardoso TM, Queiroz A, Milanezi CM, Bacellar O, Carvalho EM, et al. Tr-1-like CD4+CD25-CD127-/lowFOXP3- cells are the main source of interleukin 10 in patients with cutaneous leishmaniasis due to *Leishmania braziliensis*. *J Infect Dis* (2015) 211(5):708–18. doi:10.1093/infdis/jiu406
29. Sandquist M, Wong HR. Biomarkers of sepsis and their potential value in diagnosis, prognosis and treatment. *Expert Rev Clin Immunol* (2014) 10(10):1349–56. doi:10.1586/1744666X.2014.949675
30. Quirino GF, Nascimento MS, Davoli-Ferreira M, Sacramento LA, Lima MH, Almeida RP, et al. Interleukin-27 mediates susceptibility to visceral leishmaniasis by suppressing the IL-17-neutrophil response. *Infect Immun* (2016) 84(8):2289–98. doi:10.1128/IAI.00283-16
31. Wang RX, Yu CR, Dambuza IM, Mahdi RM, Dolinska MB, Sergeev YV, et al. Interleukin-35 induces regulatory B cells that suppress autoimmune disease. *Nat Med* (2014) 20(6):633–41. doi:10.1038/nm.3554
32. Lipoldova M, Demant P. Genetic susceptibility to infectious disease: lessons from mouse models of leishmaniasis. *Nat Rev Genet* (2006) 7(4):294–305. doi:10.1038/nrg1832
33. Blahoianu MA, Rahimi AAR, Kozlowski M, Angel JB, Kumar A. IFN-γ-induced IL-27 and IL-27p28 expression are differentially regulated through JNK MAPK and PI3K pathways independent of Jak/STAT in human monocytic cells. *Immunobiology* (2014) 219(1):1–8. doi:10.1016/j.imbio.2013.06.001
34. Zhang S, Liang R, Luo W, Liu C, Wu X, Gao Y, et al. High susceptibility to liver injury in IL-27 p28 conditional knockout mice involves intrinsic interferon-γ dysregulation of $CD4^+$ T cells. *Hepatology* (2013) 57(4):1620–31. doi:10.1002/hep.26166
35. Huang L, Hinchman M, Mendez S. Coinjection with TLR2 agonist Pam3CSK4 reduces the pathology of leishmanization in mice. *PLoS Negl Trop Dis* (2015) 9(3):e0003546. doi:10.1371/journal.pntd.0003546
36. Kim HS, Go H, Akira S, Chung DH. TLR2-mediated production of IL-27 and chemokines by respiratory epithelial cells promotes bleomycin-induced pulmonary fibrosis in mice. *J Immunol* (2011) 187(8):4007–17. doi:10.4049/jimmunol.1101654
37. Jung JY, Robinson CM. IL-12 and IL-27 regulate the phagolysosomal pathway in mycobacteria-infected human macrophages. *Cell Commun Signal* (2014) 12:16. doi:10.1186/1478-811X-12-16

4

Human Kinetoplastid Protozoan Infections: Where are we Going Next?

*Alessandra Almeida Filardy[1], Kamila Guimarães-Pinto[1], Marise Pinheiro Nunes[2], Ketiuce Zukeram[1], Lara Fliess[1], Ludimila Pereira[1], Danielle Oliveira Nascimento[1], Luciana Conde[1] and Alexandre Morrot[2,3]**

[1] Department of Immunology, Paulo de Góes Microbiology Institute, Federal University of Rio de Janeiro, Rio de Janeiro, Brazil, [2] Immunoparasitology Laboratory, Oswaldo Cruz Foundation, Oswaldo Cruz Institute, FIOCRUZ, Rio de Janeiro, Brazil, [3] Tuberculosis Research Center, Faculty of Medicine, Federal University of Rio de Janeiro, Rio de Janeiro, Brazil

***Correspondence:**
Alexandre Morrot
alexandre.morrot@ioc.fiocruz.br

Kinetoplastida trypanosomatidae microorganisms are protozoan parasites exhibiting a developmental stage in the gut of insect vectors and tissues of vertebrate hosts. During the vertebrate infective stages, these parasites alter the differential expression of virulence genes, modifying their biological and antigenic properties in order to subvert the host protective immune responses and establish a persistent infection. One of the hallmarks of kinetoplastid parasites is their evasion mechanisms from host immunity, leading to disease chronification. The diseases caused by kinetoplastid parasites are neglected by the global expenditures in research and development, affecting millions of individuals in the low and middle-income countries located mainly in the tropical and subtropical regions. However, investments made by public and private initiatives have over the past decade leveraged important lines of intervention that if well-integrated to health care programs will likely accelerate disease control initiatives. This review summarizes recent advances in public health care principles, including new drug discoveries and their rational use with chemotherapeutic vaccines, and the implementation of control efforts to spatially mapping the kinetoplastid infections through monitoring of infected individuals in epidemic areas. These approaches should bring us the means to track genetic variation of parasites and drug resistance, integrating this knowledge into effective stewardship programs to prevent vector-borne kinetoplastid infections in areas at risk of disease spreading.

Keywords: parasitic infection, kinetoplastid protozoans, *Trypanosoma cruzi*, *Leishmania*, *Trypanosoma brucei*

INTRODUCTION

Protozoan infections are one of the most devastating causes of human death worldwide. These infections are caused by protozoan parasites, microorganisms originally classified in the Kingdom Protozoa, which comprises a diverse group of unicellular eukaryotes (1). Although the majority of the protozoan exists as free-living microorganisms in different aquatic and humid environments, there are many species living in association with host organisms, causing severe human diseases (1, 2). This is the case of Kinetoplastid parasites, a group of flagellated protozoans that parasitize most plant and animal species; and cause human diseases with public health threats and social-economic effects (3).

The kinetoplastids are a monophyletic group related to the euglenids. These microorganisms are distinguished from other protozoan groups mainly by the presence of kinetoplasts, a granule that contains "kDNA," a DNA located in the mitochondria, associated with the base of the flagella (3). Three distinct kinetoplastids cause human disease: *Trypanosoma brucei* [human African trypanosomiasis (HAT) or sleeping sickness], *Trypanosoma cruzi* (Chagas disease), and *Leishmania* spp. (leishmaniasis) (3, 4), which are still recognized as neglected tropical diseases (NTDs) by the World Health Organization. These two genera of parasites are found in the blood and/or tissues of infected humans and are transmitted by arthropod vectors (**Figure 1**) (5).

Although the advances in the development of drug therapies and vector control agents against kinetoplastid diseases (6), new strategies are required for global elimination of epidemies. The main limiting efforts for this accomplishment obviously relies on the global investments in R&D for these NTDs when compared to other diseases with higher levels of financial support, such as malaria, tuberculosis, and HIV, known as "big three" (7). The analysis of the global sums of expenditures for each of these diseases, and their correlations with the social impact indexes on public health indicates a correlation that goes far beyond the political question (8). Such correlation is proportional to the severity of each disease (**Figure 2**), as to the metric of the disability-adjusted

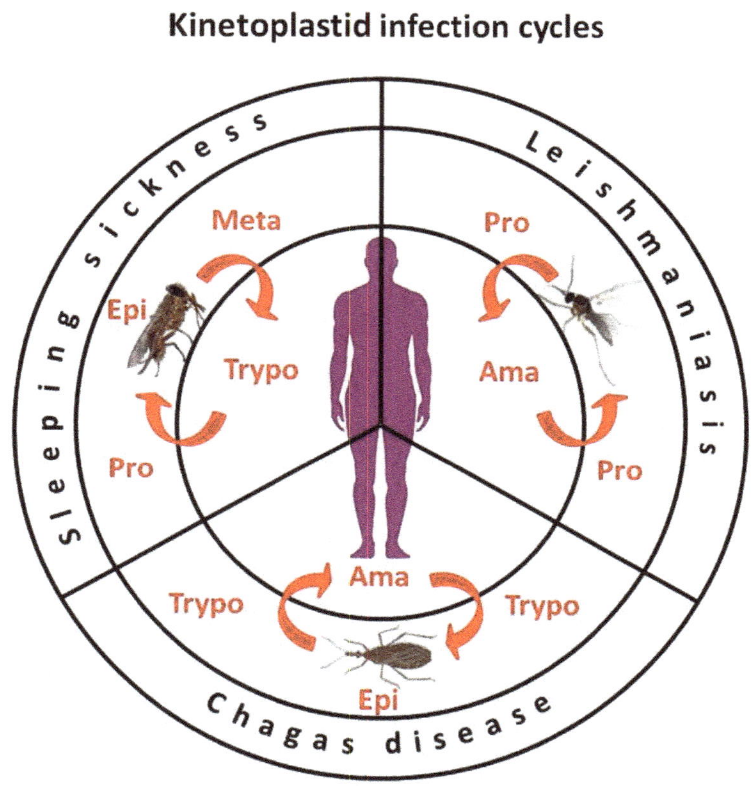

Kinetoplastid	Vector	Invertebrate Stages(IS)/Vertebrate stages(VS)	Disease
Trypanosoma cruzi	Triatomine bugs	Epimastigotes (IS), metacyclic tripomastigotes (IS/IV), trypomastigotes (VS), amastigotes (VS)	Chagas
Trypanosoma brucei	Tsetse flies	Procyclic trypomastigotes (IS), epimastigotes (IS), metacyclic trypomastigotes (IS/VS), trypomastigotes (VS)	African Trypanosomiasis
Leishmania spp	Phlebotomine sandflies	Promastigotes (IV), amastigotes (VS)	Leishmaniasis

FIGURE 1 | Kinetoplastid transmission cycles. The life cycles of kinetoplastid protozoan parasites show development stages in both invertebrate and vertebrate hosts. In leishmaniasis, promastigotes (flagellate and mobile forms) are inoculated into the skin along with the saliva of phlebotomine vectors (Diptera: Psychodidae). In the vertebrate hosts, they are maintained inside phagocytic cells under the proliferative form, amastigotes. When ingested by insect vectors, the amastigote forms are transformed into promastigotes which multiply in the intestinal tissue, then migrate as metacyclic promastigotes into the stomodal valve to be later injected into the skin during blood meal. In Chagas' disease, the etiologic agent *Trypanosoma cruzi* is transmitted to vertebrate hosts as a metacyclic trypomastigote forms by infected triatomine bugs (Triatominae: Reduviidae) during blood feeding. Once in the vertebrate, trypomastigotes differentiate into intracellular amastigote forms. These proliferative stages multiply by binary division, and then differentiate into trypomastigotes, which are released into the bloodstream. When the triatomine bug takes a blood meal from an infected vertebrate host containing circulating parasites, the ingested trypomastigotes forms to differentiate into epimastigotes in the medium intestine of the vector, multiplying by binary division, after which they differentiate into infective metacyclic trypomastigote forms. In sleep sickness or human African trypanosomiasis, the parasite *Trypanosoma brucei* is transmitted by the bite of the tsetse fly (Glossinidae: Glossina). The parasite exists in the saliva of the invertebrate vector and is injected when the insect feeds on human blood. Unlike *Trypanosoma cruzi*, trypomastigotes of *T. brucei* do not invade host cells and, therefore, does not differentiate into intracellular amastigote forms. Instead, *T. brucei* parasites multiply as trypomastigotes in the blood of infected vertebrate host. The parasite cycle continues when a new vector feeds on a contaminated individual. In the invertebrate vector, the parasites differentiate into proliferative epimastigotes forms, invading the insect salivary glands to continue the cycle.

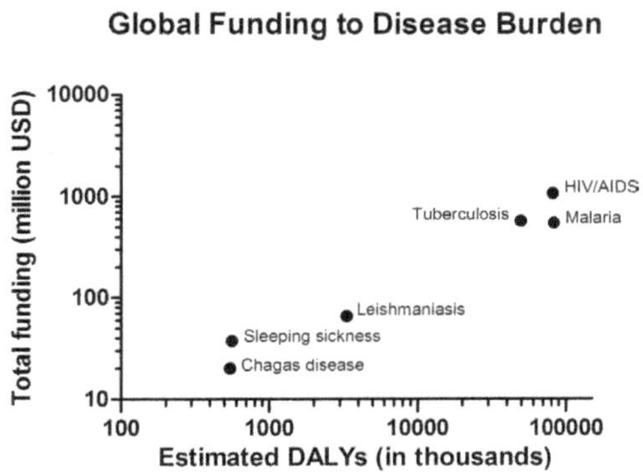

FIGURE 2 | Overall funding for research and development investment correlated with disability-adjusted life years, estimated from the Global Burden of Disease Study.

life year (DALY), an index calculated as the sum of the years of life lost due to premature mortality of patients and the years lost due to disability for people living with the illness (9).

In spite of the low priority of the investments received, studies in the past decades have pointed out the paths for developing effective actions to control human kinetoplastid protozoan infections through a better understanding of the pathogen-vertebrate host interactions during their life cycles, disease pathogenesis in the hosts, and methods that allow the diagnosis, even in the acute phase of the infection (3, 4). This has provided a better opportunity to prospect new therapeutic targets, more effective drug development approaches, and promising vaccines that, together, may combat these diseases more robustly in the near future (5).

TRENDS IN DRUG DEVELOPMENT FOR KINETOPLASTID INFECTIONS

Treatment approaches based on drug therapies in kinetoplastid infections are scarce and have been considered to be highly toxic (10). However, interest in research and exploration of new approaches has given a sign of change. Since kinetoplastid infections lead to chronic persistent diseases, it is critical that drug therapy interventions would be focused on the acute phase, with hopes of achieving complete eradication of disease transmission. To that end, it is necessary to establish technical procedures that allow early diagnosis of acute kinetoplastid infection (5). This intervention approach aims to act at a stage of infection in which pathogen has not yet established itself and is present with a low parasitism burden and few down modulatory mechanisms in place over the host immune responses (1, 11, 12).

In addition, a rapid and efficient intervention during acute phase of the infection, when the host is still under low tissue parasitism, decreases the chances of acquiring drug resistance (13, 14). In Chagas disease, benznidazole and nifurtimox have long been the only clinical treatment options for infection (15). However, progress has been made in the research of new promising drugs against the disease. E1224, a pro-drug of ravuconazole, has shown some efficiency in combating the disease (16). The results of the first phase 2 clinical trial in Bolivia, conducted by drugs for neglected diseases initiative, have shown satisfactory protective results for E1224. This drug was effective in controlling *T. cruzi* parasitism in infected patients. Furthermore, its use in combination with benzanidazole is more effective as compared to monotheraphy-based protocols (16).

To treat HAT, five drugs have been approved: pentamidine, melarsoprol, eflornithine, suramin, and nifurtimox (17). Pentamidine and suramin are used in monotherapies in the early stage of *T.b. gambiense* and *T.b. rhodesiense* infections, whereas melarsoprol is used for the second stage of the disease (18, 19). Nifurtimox has been used since 2009 in combination with eflornithine, mostly in the second stage of *T.b. gambiense* infection. The combination therapy protocols for these two drugs have been improved, although there are still practical restrictions to their potential use in large-scale applications (20). Currently, new drugs designed to improve patient care are being considered to meet current elimination targets. Most of them have been optimized to undergo clinical trials (17).

Fexinidazole and oxaborole SCYX-7158, are already being studied in clinical evaluation as oral therapies in phase IIb/III and phase I trials, respectively (21, 22). Other important R&D studies have focused on the virulence responses of the parasite. The cell surface of African trypanosomes (*T. brucei* spp.) is covered by a dense coat of glycoconjugates that play important roles in the evasion of host immune responses (23). New strategies in drug discovery against HAT aim the development of specific carbohydrate-binding agents capable of inhibiting the action of glycosyltransferases and glycosidases of the parasite, thus altering the nature of the parasite's cell-surface glycans as a treatment target for sleeping sickness (24).

In leishmaniasis, a notable progress in the disease treatment has been made in the preparation of new formulations of amphotericin B, using liposome carriers (25). In addition, new drugs have been extensively studied in clinical trials, although the effects of HIV co-infection in endemic areas contribute to drug unresponsiveness during therapies (26). The use of paromomycin, an aminoglycoside class antibiotic, has also been shown to be efficient at low cost as a first-line drug (27). Alternatively, studies have suggested the effective action of drugs that act on a broad spectrum against *Leishmania* parasites. This is the case of miltefosine, a drug that is also used in the treatment of dogs with leishmaniasis in Brazil (28). The miltefosine has an inhibitory action on several biological pathways of the parasite, such as cytochrome C oxidase, synthesis of phosphatidylcholine, and disruption of parasite Ca^{2+} homeostasis (29–31).

In addition, drug discovery researches for kinetoplastids have benefited from investments made in the field of protozoan genomics. This is clearly seen in the use of data mining, annotation, and analysis of *Leishmania* parasite genome that has lead to the creation of LeishCyc database (32). This systematic approach will allow a complete mapping of *Leishmania* transcriptomics, proteomics, and metabolomics enabling the development of new compounds that can be used in high-throughput screening approaches to search selective drugs against *Leishmania* parasites (32). In fact omics-based analyses have facilitated the broadening of R&D researches in the field of drug development. Lipidomics analyses have yielded the characterization of lipid structures, protein lipidation pathways in post-translational modifications, and their putative functions for kinetoplastid parasites (33, 34). This knowledge will allow the search for new classes of anti-parasitic pharmaceuticals.

RESEARCH AND DEVELOPMENT OF NEW VACCINES AGAINST KINETOPLASTID PARASITES

The major challenge in the preventive control of kinetoplastid infections and other neglected tropic infectious diseases is undoubtedly the implementation of low-cost vaccines for public health programs in affected countries, most of them were low- and middle-income countries (5, 35). This accomplishment would enable to structure intervention actions in health care at the level of mass treatment programs, thus avoiding disease re-emergence. To reach this ideal scenario, there are serious social-political obstacles to overcome in order to ensure the development of clinical tests. The most incisive limitation is unquestionably economic, resulting from a scarce financial incentives and market failures in view of the geopolitical areas where epidemics occur (35). Such constraints are likely to arouse less interest from financial and pharmaceutical institutions in the market development strategies for vaccines against NTDs in general.

There are no licensed vaccines for kinetoplastid infections yet, reinforcing the need for their development, particularly in countries where they are epidemic. Most of the ongoing vaccine studies have been conducted at the level of basic research (5). Particularly, recent advances in the construction of manipulative parasites through genome engineering using CRISPR/Cas9 and Cre recombinase have been dedicated to reprogramming their genome, allowing the identification of regulatory genes associated with the cell fates in the host–parasite interplay (36). These critical virulence genes represent good candidates to be studied as vaccine targets.

Interesting, some kinetoplastid vaccines undergoing clinical trials are promising, since they are cost-effective and show long-term protection against both cutaneous and visceral leishmaniasis. This is the case of vaccines developed by the Infectious Diseases Research Institute, which has included protective *Leishmania* antigen epitopes in its vaccine formulations used in clinical trials (37, 38). Another prominent proposal comes from initiative studies in cooperation with National Institutes of Health. They present a more elaborate vaccine formulation, including protective recombinant *Leishmania* antigens in combination with sand fly salivary gland antigens, capable of inducing a more robust host immune response, considering vector–host interactions in the transmission of *Leishmania* parasites (39).

In the case of Chagas disease, initial studies have pointed out potential antigens in experimental mice models capable of inducing host protective immune responses. They were also effective in reducing cardiac parasite loads and disease pathology, increasing host survival indices. Those studies have proposed the use of Tc24 (calcium binding protein associated with flagellar pocket of *T. cruzi*) and TSA-1 (Trypomastigote surface antigen-1) by a global consortium (40–42). These are the first candidates to be used in vaccine formulations to prevent Chagas disease. Furthermore, the use of vaccines as a therapeutic approach to treat chagasic patients has also been proposed (42).

KEY CHALLENGES TO KINETOPLASTID PARASITE CONTROL: INTEGRATING NEW APPROACHES INTO ERADICATION STRATEGIES

To eradicate kinetoplastid infections in humans, we must gain a better understanding of variants of pathogens and their vectors, the transmission models among their hosts, and efficacious preventive vaccine approaches, to understand and design strategies to intervene in the real dynamics of disease spreading in epidemic areas (43). To achieve that, diagnostic tests capable of detecting infections in the acute phase, and accurate analysis of drug resistance in the parasite spreading are essential to trace a better correlation between variants of pathogens and the clinical spectrum of the disease. Another important step of intervention in the transmission cycles of vector diseases is regarding the application of health care models based on geographic information system (GIS) projects and technologies (44). By using this system, we will be able to follow the infection cycle in terms of spatial data, geographical and geodatabases, which allows us to create mapping models to predict potential areas of risk for transmission of vector-borne diseases (45).

The GIS technology is able to compile multi-analysis related to public health data collected from endemic urban and wild areas, including analyses of disease dispersal, genetic variation of parasites, vector and host habitats, and their relationship with microclimates in affected areas. These metadata analyses can be correlated with geographic positioning system to establish interventions of potential infections, thus allowing for a rational use of medications to prevent the emergence of drug resistance in the context of disease surveillance (44, 45). Nowadays, diverse stochastic models are used as tools for estimating probability distributions of potential outcomes from the understanding of environmental and ecological networks involved in the cycles of vector-borne diseases. These geographic models have allowed disseminating critical information concerning public health surveillance for endemic areas (**Figure 3**).

In kinetoplastid infections, spatial clustering using GIS technology when applied with accurate diagnostic test, analysis of the phylogenetic distribution of *Leishmania* spp. together with surveillance has been demonstrated to be of great value in predicting areas of risk. Epidemiological analysis of the transmission cycles in Europe, and in recent kala-azar outbreaks in Nepal, Kenya, and Brazil, have helped to precisely define that the priority of intervention is in the vector control with the use of insecticides, in order to block the transmission cycle of disease in potential risk areas, identified to be priority to reduce the spread of infection (46–49).

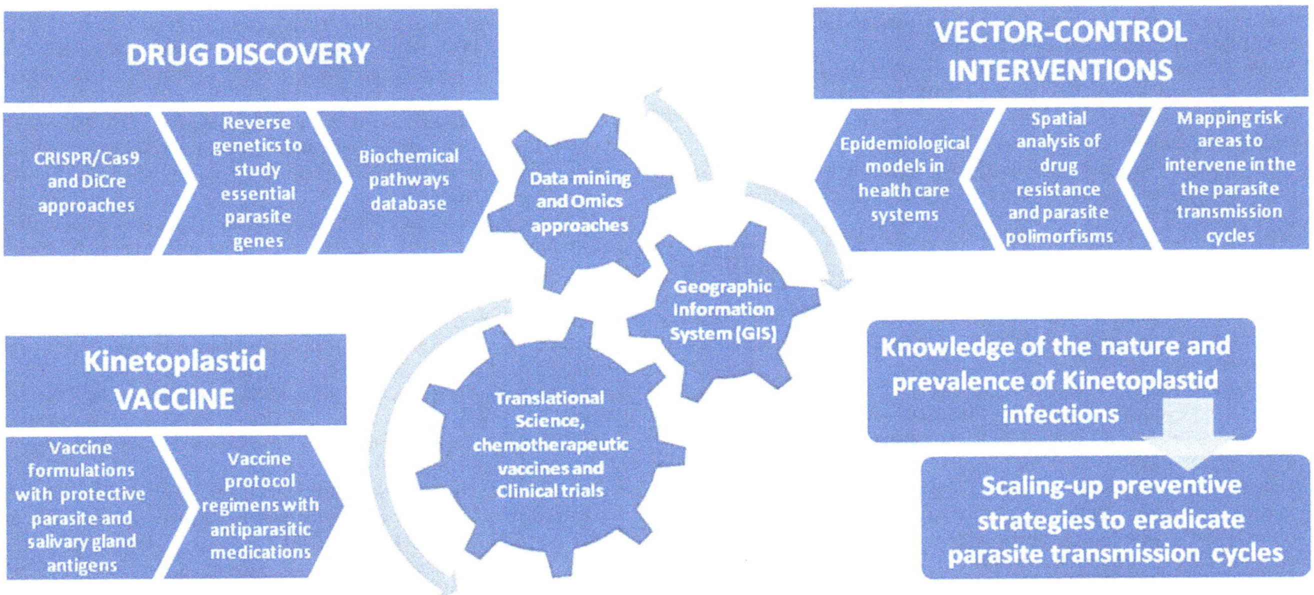

FIGURE 3 | Integrating new approaches into control strategies for kinetoplastid infections. In the past decade, genetic sequencing efforts and manipulation of trypanosomatid genomes have elucidated the characterization of virulence factors and parasite biochemical pathways involved in the pathogenesis disease. These advances allowed the design of new drug targets and therapeutic vaccines capable of reducing the parasitic burden thus controlling the infection and its clinical symptoms. The integration of these tools with epidemiological interventions into public health programs should yield substantial gains in controlling the transmission cycles of these vector-borne diseases. In this line, important studies in the field of vector control interventions have defined a multi-parametric analysis using geographic information system technologies to monitor spatial analysis of drug resistance and parasite polymorphisms to delineate epidemic-prone areas. Those studies have offered a powerful platform for prospecting and development of tools and technologies capable of effectively defining elimination programs in the control and eradication of kinetoplastid diseases.

CONCLUDING REMARKS

Neglected tropical diseases caused by kinetoplastid protozoan parasites are considered endemic in lower-middle-income economies, although in many countries they are in process of epidemiological containment and elimination. However, the eradication of these diseases is a complex issue that must involve health management policies, coordinated among the affected countries, such as the development of public policies to combat parasitic diseases and improvement of social conditions. This will only be possible through the cooperation of local governments in a participatory search for bilateral relations between public and private interests capable of fostering translational studies that guarantee the access of the population to appropriate treatments. The development of accurate diagnosis capable of identifying these diseases in the acute phase of infection, as well as the identification of parasite polymorphisms and variants of drug resistance, together with application of health care models based on GIS technologies will enable both preventive and therapeutic actions based on new generations of drugs and vaccines currently developed for these neglected diseases.

AUTHOR CONTRIBUTIONS

AM conceived the manuscript. AAF and AM wrote the manuscript. AAF, KG-P, MPN, KZ, LF, LP, DON, LC, and AM participated in the preparation of the manuscript.

REFERENCES

1. Sibley LD. Invasion and intracellular survival by protozoan parasites. *Immunol Rev* (2011) 240(1):72–91. doi:10.1111/j.1600-065X.2010.00990.x
2. Kling JC, Körner H. Different regulatory mechanisms in protozoan parasitic infections. *Int J Parasitol* (2013) 43(6):417–25. doi:10.1016/j.ijpara.2013.02.001
3. Jackson AP, Otto TD, Aslett M, Armstrong SD, Bringaud F, Schlacht A, et al. Kinetoplastid phylogenomics reveals the evolutionary innovations associated with the origins of parasitism. *Curr Biol* (2016) 26(2):161–72. doi:10.1016/j.cub.2015.11.055
4. Portman N, Gull K. The paraflagellar rod of kinetoplastid parasites: from structure to components and function. *Int J Parasitol* (2010) 40(2):135–48. doi:10.1016/j.ijpara.2009.10.005
5. Hotez PJ, Pecoul B, Rijal S, Boehme C, Aksoy S, Malecela M, et al. Eliminating the neglected tropical diseases: translational science and new technologies. *PLoS Negl Trop Dis* (2016) 10(3):e0003895. doi:10.1371/journal.pntd.0003895

6. Majumder HK, de Souza W, Chang KP. Target identification and intervention strategies against kinetoplastid protozoan parasites. *Mol Biol Int* (2011) 2011:185413. doi:10.4061/2011/185413
7. Hotez PJ. Blue marble health and "the big three diseases": HIV/AIDS, tuberculosis, and malaria. *Microbes Infect* (2015) 17(8):539–41. doi:10.1016/j.micinf.2015.05.004
8. Pedrique B, Strub-Wourgaft N, Some C, Olliaro P, Trouiller P, Ford N, et al. The drug and vaccine landscape for neglected diseases (2000-11): a systematic assessment. *Lancet Glob Health* (2013) 1(6):e371–9. doi:10.1016/S2214-109X(13)70078-0
9. Horstick O, Tozan Y, Wilder-Smith A. Reviewing dengue: still a neglected tropical disease? *PLoS Negl Trop Dis* (2015) 9(4):e0003632. doi:10.1371/journal.pntd.0003632
10. Gilbert IH. Drug discovery for neglected diseases: molecular target-based and phenotypic approaches. *J Med Chem* (2013) 56(20):7719–26. doi:10.1021/jm400362b
11. Morgan GW, Hall BS, Denny PW, Carrington M, Field MC. The kinetoplastida endocytic apparatus. Part I: a dynamic system for nutrition and evasion of host defences. *Trends Parasitol* (2002) 18(11):491–6. doi:10.1016/S1471-4922(02)02391-7
12. Ouaissi A, Ouaissi M. Molecular basis of *Trypanosoma cruzi* and *Leishmania* interaction with their host(s): exploitation of immune and defense mechanisms by the parasite leading to persistence and chronicity, features reminiscent of immune system evasion strategies in cancer diseases. *Arch Immunol Ther Exp (Warsz)* (2005) 53(2):102–14.
13. Fairlamb AH, Gow NA, Matthews KR, Waters AP. Drug resistance in eukaryotic microorganisms. *Nat Microbiol* (2016) 1(7):16092. doi:10.1038/nmicrobiol.2016.92
14. Alsford S, Kelly JM, Baker N, Horn D. Genetic dissection of drug resistance in trypanosomes. *Parasitology* (2013) 140(12):1478–91. doi:10.1017/S003118201300022X
15. Paucar R, Moreno-Viguri E, Pérez-Silanes S. Challenges in Chagas disease drug discovery: a review. *Curr Med Chem* (2016) 23(28):3154–70. doi:10.2174/0929867323999160625124424
16. Chatelain E. Chagas disease drug discovery: toward a new era. *J Biomol Screen* (2015) 20(1):22–35. doi:10.1177/1087057114550585
17. Cullen DR, Mocerino M. A brief review of drug discovery research for human African trypanosomiasis. *Curr Med Chem* (2017) 24(7):701–17. doi:10.2174/0929867324666170120160034
18. Babokhov P, Sanyaolu AO, Oyibo WA, Fagbenro-Beyioku AF, Iriemenam NC. A current analysis of chemotherapy strategies for the treatment of human African trypanosomiasis. *Pathog Glob Health* (2013) 107(5):242–52. doi:10.1179/2047773213Y.0000000105
19. Kuepfer I, Schmid C, Allan M, Edielu A, Haary EP, Kakembo A, et al. Safety and efficacy of the 10-day melarsoprol schedule for the treatment of second stage Rhodesiense sleeping sickness. *PLoS Negl Trop Dis* (2012) 6(8):e1695. doi:10.1371/journal.pntd.0001695
20. Schmid C, Kuemmerle A, Blum J, Ghabri S, Kande V, Mutombo W, et al. In-hospital safety in field conditions of nifurtimox eflornithine combination therapy (NECT) for *T. b. gambiense* sleeping sickness. *PLoS Negl Trop Dis* (2012) 6(11):e1920. doi:10.1371/journal.pntd.0001920
21. Mesu VKBK, Kalonji WM, Bardonneau C, Mordt OV, Blesson S, Simon F, et al. Oral fexinidazole for late-stage African *Trypanosoma brucei gambiense* trypanosomiasis: a pivotal multicentre, randomised, non-inferiority trial. *Lancet* (2018) 391(10116):144–54. doi:10.1016/S0140-6736(17)32758-7
22. Jacobs RT, Nare B, Wring SA, Orr MD, Chen D, Sligar JM, et al. SCYX-7158, an orally-active benzoxaborole for the treatment of stage 2 human African trypanosomiasis. *PLoS Negl Trop Dis* (2011) 5(6):e1151. doi:10.1371/journal.pntd.0001151
23. Mugnier MR, Stebbins CE, Papavasiliou FN. Masters of disguise: antigenic variation and the VSG coat in *Trypanosoma brucei*. *PLoS Pathog* (2016) 12(9):e1005784. doi:10.1371/journal.ppat.1005784
24. Castillo-Acosta VM, Balzarini J, González-Pacanowska D. Surface: a therapeutic opportunity for diseases. *Trends Parasitol* (2017) 33(10):775–87. doi:10.1016/j.pt.2017.06.009
25. Zaioncz S, Khalil NM, Mainardes RM. Exploring the role of nanoparticles in amphotericin B delivery. *Curr Pharm Des* (2017) 23(3):509–21. doi:10.2174/1381612822666161027103640
26. Jha TK. Drug unresponsiveness & combination therapy for kala-azar. *Indian J Med Res* (2006) 123(3):389–98.
27. Sundar S, Chakravarty J. Paromomycin in the treatment of leishmaniasis. *Expert Opin Investig Drugs* (2008) 17(5):787–94. doi:10.1517/13543784.17.5.787
28. Andrade HM, Toledo VP, Pinheiro MB, Guimarães TM, Oliveira NC, Castro JA, et al. Evaluation of miltefosine naturally infected with *L. infantum* (=L. chagasi) in Brazil. *Vet Parasitol* (2011) 181(2–4):83–90. doi:10.1016/j.vetpar.2011.05.009
29. Luque-Ortega JR, Rivas L. Miltefosine (hexadecylphosphocholine) inhibits cytochrome C oxidase in *Leishmania donovani* promastigotes. *Antimicrob Agents Chemother* (2007) 51(4):1327–32. doi:10.1128/AAC.01415-06
30. Rakotomanga M, Blanc S, Gaudin K, Chaminade P, Loiseau PM. Miltefosine affects lipid metabolism in *Leishmania donovani* promastigotes. *Antimicrob Agents Chemother* (2007) 51(4):1425–30. doi:10.1128/AAC.01123-06
31. Benaim G, García-Marchán Y, Reyes C, Uzcanga G, Figarella K. Identification of a sphingosine-sensitive Ca2+ channel in the plasma membrane of *Leishmania mexicana*. *Biochem Biophys Res Commun* (2013) 430(3):1091–6. doi:10.1016/j.bbrc.2012.12.033
32. Doyle MA, MacRae JI, De Souza DP, Saunders EC, McConville MJ, Likić VA. LeishCyc: a biochemical pathways database for *Leishmania major*. *BMC Syst Biol* (2009) 3:57. doi:10.1186/1752-0509-3-57
33. Biagiotti M, Dominguez S, Yamout N, Zufferey R. Lipidomics and anti-trypanosomatid chemotherapy. *Clin Transl Med* (2017) 6(1):27. doi:10.1186/s40169-017-0160-7
34. Ritzefeld M, Wright MH, Tate EW. New developments in probing and targeting protein acylation in malaria, leishmaniasis and African sleeping sickness. *Parasitology* (2017) 8:1–18.
35. Beaumier CM, Gillespie PM, Hotez PJ, Bottazzi ME. New vaccines for neglected parasitic diseases and dengue. *Transl Res* (2013) 162(3):144–55. doi:10.1016/j.trsl.2013.03.006
36. Duncan SM, Jones NG, Mottram JC. Recent advances in *Leishmania* reverse genetics: manipulating a manipulative parasite. *Mol Biochem Parasitol* (2017) 216:30–8. doi:10.1016/j.molbiopara.2017.06.005
37. Raman VS, Duthie MS, Fox CB, Matlashewski G, Reed SG. Adjuvants for *Leishmania* vaccines: from models to clinical application. *Front Immunol* (2012) 3:144. doi:10.3389/fimmu.2012.00144
38. Alvar J, Croft SL, Kaye P, Khamesipour A, Sundar S, Reed SG. Case study for a vaccine against leishmaniasis. *Vaccine* (2013) 31(Suppl 2):B244–9. doi:10.1016/j.vaccine.2012.11.080
39. Cecílio P, Pérez-Cabezas B, Fernández L, Moreno J, Carrillo E, Requena JM, et al. Pre-clinical antigenicity studies of an innovative multivalent vaccine for human visceral leishmaniasis. *PLoS Negl Trop Dis* (2017) 11(11):e0005951. doi:10.1371/journal.pntd.0005951
40. Dumonteil E, Bottazzi ME, Zhan B, Heffernan MJ, Jones K, Valenzuela JG, et al. Accelerating the development of a therapeutic vaccine for human Chagas disease: rationale and prospects. *Expert Rev Vaccines* (2012) 11(9): 1043–55. doi:10.1586/erv.12.85
41. Seid CA, Jones KM, Pollet J, Keegan B, Hudspeth E, Hammond M, et al. Cysteine mutagenesis improves the production without abrogating antigenicity of a recombinant protein vaccine candidate for human Chagas disease. *Hum Vaccin Immunother* (2017) 13(3):621–33. doi:10.1080/21645515.2016.1242540
42. Konduri V, Halpert MM, Liang D, Levitt JM, Cruz-Chan JV, Zhan B, et al. Genetic adjuvantation of a cell-based therapeutic vaccine for amelioration of chagasic cardiomyopathy. *Infect Immun* (2017) 85(9):e127–117. doi:10.1128/IAI.00127-17
43. DebRoy S, Prosper O, Mishoe A, Mubayi A. Challenges in modeling complexity of neglected tropical diseases: a review of dynamics of visceral leishmaniasis in resource limited settings. *Emerg Themes Epidemiol* (2017) 14:10. doi:10.1186/s12982-017-0065-3
44. Bergquist NR. Vector-borne parasitic diseases: new trends in data collection and risk assessment. *Acta Trop* (2001) 79(1):13–20. doi:10.1016/S0001-706X(01)00099-7
45. Palaniyandi M. The role of remote sensing and GIS for spatial prediction of vector-borne diseases transmission: a systematic review. *J Vector Borne Dis* (2012) 49(4):197–204.

46. Ryan JR, Mbui J, Rashid JR, Wasunna MK, Kirigi G, Magiri C, et al. Spatial clustering and epidemiological aspects of visceral leishmaniasis in two endemic villages, Baringo District, Kenya. *Am J Trop Med Hyg* (2006) 74(2): 308–17.
47. Khanal B, Picado A, Bhattarai NR, Van Der Auwera G, Das ML, Ostyn B, et al. Spatial analysis of *Leishmania donovani* exposure in humans and domestic animals in a recent kala azar focus in Nepal. *Parasitology* (2010) 137(11):1597–603. doi:10.1017/S0031182010000521
48. Tsokana CN, Sokos C, Giannakopoulos A, Mamuris Z, Birtsas P, Papaspyropoulos K, et al. First evidence of *Leishmania* infection in European brown hare (*Lepus europaeus*) in Greece: GIS analysis and phylogenetic position within the *Leishmania* spp. *Parasitol Res* (2016) 115(1):313–21. doi:10.1007/s00436-015-4749-8
49. Sevá AD, Mao L, Galvis-Ovallos F, Tucker Lima JM, Valle D. Risk analysis and prediction of visceral leishmaniasis dispersion in São Paulo State, Brazil. *PLoS Negl Trop Dis* (2017) 11(2):e0005353. doi:10.1371/journal.pntd.0005353

5

Immune Escape Strategies of Malaria Parasites

*Pollyanna S. Gomes[1], Jyoti Bhardwaj[2,3], Juan Rivera-Correa[4], Celio G. Freire-De-Lima[5] and Alexandre Morrot[1]**

[1] Departamento de Microbiologia Geral, Universidade Federal do Rio de Janeiro, Rio de Janeiro, Brazil, [2] Division of Parasitology, Council of Scientific and Industrial Research-Central Drug Research Institute, Lucknow, Uttar Pradesh, India, [3] Academy of Scientific and Innovative Research, Anusandhan Bhawan, New Delhi, India, [4] Division of Parasitology, Department of Microbiology, New York University School of Medicine, New York, NY, USA, [5] Instituto de Biofísica Carlos Chagas Filho, Universidade Federal do Rio de Janeiro, Rio de Janeiro, Brazil

Correspondence:
Alexandre Morrot
morrot@micro.ufrj.br

Malaria is one of the most life-threatening infectious diseases worldwide. Immunity to malaria is slow and short-lived despite the repeated parasite exposure in endemic areas. Malaria parasites have evolved refined machinery to evade the immune system based on a range of genetic changes that include allelic variation, biomolecular exposure of proteins, and intracellular replication. All of these features increase the probability of survival in both mosquitoes and the vertebrate host. *Plasmodium* species escape from the first immunological trap in its invertebrate vector host, the *Anopheles* mosquitoes. The parasites have to pass through various immunological barriers within the mosquito such as anti-microbial molecules and the mosquito microbiota in order to achieve successful transmission to the vertebrate host. Within these hosts, *Plasmodium* species employ various immune evasion strategies during different life cycle stages. Parasite persistence against the vertebrate immune response depends on the balance among virulence factors, pathology, metabolic cost of the host immune response, and the parasites ability to evade the immune response. In this review we discuss the strategies that *Plasmodium* parasites use to avoid the vertebrate host immune system and how they promote successful infection and transmission.

Keywords: plamosdium, evasion strategies, liver stage, blood stage, malaria, microbiology, immulogy

INTRODUCTION

Malaria still remains one of the biggest global health burdens and causes of mortality in the world. Malaria mainly occurs in tropical and subtropical parts of the world, being a serious cause of mortality and morbidity in Sub-Saharan Africa. There are five species of *Plasmodium* that cause disease in humans: *P. ovale, P. malariae, P. vivax, P. falciparum,* and the primate species *P. knowlesi.* In a previous report by the WHO, there were 215 million cases and 438 thousand deaths due to malaria in 2015 (WHO, 2015). Malaria is transmitted by the female *Anopheles* mosquito during a feeding. As the mosquito feeds on its host, sporozoites are released into the blood stream, and they migrate to the liver (Cirimotich et al., 2010). The complete life cycle of *Plasmodium* requires two hosts: the mosquito vector and the vertebrate host (Crompton et al., 2014). In the vertebrate host it undergoes two stages: an asymptomatic pre-erythrocytic stage (liver stage), and a symptomatic erythrocytic stage (blood stage) (Haque and Engwerda, 2014). The journey of sporozoites to the liver is asymptomatic (Zheng et al., 2014), but various reports have described that an initial immune response occurs during this stage. Some of the immunological responses described to occur during the liver stage are: apoptosis of infected cells (Meslin et al., 2007), isolation and targeting of parasites in specific compartments for elimination (Yano and Kurata, 2011), type I IFN production induced by parasite RNA (Liehl et al., 2015) and LC3-mediated autophagy targeting of sporozoites (Risco-Castillo et al., 2015). Nevertheless, several mechanisms such as immune evasion, immune exploitation, and molecular piracy are employed by the parasites to promote their survival in the host (Hisaeda et al., 2005). After the first immunological attack during liver stage, the majority of parasites that survived will replicate within the hepatocytes and amplify their number exponentially leading to the release of hundreds of thousands of merozoites into circulation (Prado et al., 2015). The released merozoites will subsequently initiate the symptomatic blood stage cycle, which is responsible for the clinical features and pathologies associated with malaria (Ocaña-Morgner et al., 2003).

During the blood stage some parasites will differentiate into male and female gametocytes. The gametocytes will be ingested by other feeding mosquitoes where they will further develop inside the mosquito gut (Cirimotich et al., 2010). Within the mosquito, ineffective sporozoites will be kept until the next blood meal, where they will be transmitted to a mammalian host continuing the parasite life cycle (Molina-Cruz et al., 2012). The complexity of the parasite life cycle allows for the use of various immune evasion strategies by *Plasmodium*, which pose a challenge to the development of a malaria vaccine (Hisaeda et al., 2005). In this review, we discuss some of the immune evasion strategies that have been described for *Plasmodium* at both the liver and the blood stages. We also highlight how these immune evasion strategies can promote successful infection, overcoming many of the challenges that human pathogens face with the host immune response.

IMMUNE EVASION DURING THE PRE-ERYTROCYTIC STAGES

Mechanical Strategies to Overcome the First Barrier: the Skin

An infected mosquito bite transmits around 100–200 sporozoites in the human skin and despite innate immune destruction of most of them; some parasites are still able to establish successful infection at very low numbers (Risco-Castillo et al., 2015). The skin is the first barrier that parasites encounter after transmission into the vertebrate host (Cirimotich et al., 2010). Thus, sporozoites have evolved to overcome this barrier by various mechanical strategies such as motility and cell transversal (Tavares et al., 2013). To achieve this, sporozoites are equipped with specialized mechanical proteins that help them achieve successful passage. This has been evidenced by studies that show how the transmission of sporozoites deficient in SPECT-1 (spororozoite microneme protein essential for cell traversal) and SPECT-2 (also called perforin-like protein 1 or PLP1) are blocked in the dermis and are ingested by phagocytes preventing their progression. These proteins were reported to be necessary for cell traversal and for migration to the liver (Patarroyo et al., 2011). The sporozoites can tranverse various kind of cells, wich includes immune cells. The transversal of immune cells can lead to inactivation of immune cell defenses and prevent the clearance of sporozoites (exocytosis) before crossing the barrier (Sinnis and Zavala, 2012). Another protein responsible for motility of sporozoites is TRAP (Thrombospondin-Related Anonymous Protein). This protein is found on the micronemes and the surface of sporozoites. TRAP allows the parasite to interact with surface host molecules that provide gliding motility to exit the dermis. Additionally, TRAP can bind to sulfated glycoconjugate motifs that can aid in recognition and entry to hepatocytes (Müller et al., 1993). Regardless, some of the sporozoites will enter the lymphatic system where they can be recognized and destroyed by immune cells such as dendritic cells (DCs) (Wilson et al., 2016).

Overcoming the Hepatic Immune Defenses to Establish Liver Stage Infection

A successful infection in great part is due to the parasite evading the first attacks of the host immune response, that despite its strength, it is not enough to block the development of the blood stage (Singh et al., 2010). After the sporozoites migrate from the skin, crossing all cellular barriers, they will reach the blood, and consequently the lymphatic system (Crompton et al., 2014). Once inside the circulatory system, sporozoites rapidly reach the sinusoid cavity of the liver. The exoerythrocytic (liver) stage has been described as asymptomatic because the liver is an immunoprivileged organ that is protected against a strong immune response (Liehl et al., 2015). Even though initially the liver stage was considered an unresponsive phase, various reports have showed that the liver immune cells are present and active in different rodent malaria models, suggesting an initial immune response during the liver stage (Liehl et al., 2014). Some reports have described how *Plasmodium* RNA could activate the type I interferon (IFN) pathway via the cytosolic Pattern Recognition Receptor (PRR), MDA5 (Liehl et al., 2014). Type I interferons are potent inflammatory cytokines that are known to inhibit growth of exoerythrocytic forms (Hisaeda et al., 2005). Some of the cells that mediate these anti-parasitic effects include Natural Killer and Natural Killer T cells (NK, NKT), and $\gamma\delta$T cells. These cells mainly inhibit parasite growth through secretion of interferon, including both type I interferons and IFN-γ (Ocaña-Morgner et al., 2003; Risco-Castillo et al., 2015). Other molecules such as hepcidin have been implicated in growth inhibition of exoerytrhrocytic phases (Spottiswoode et al., 2014).

Modulation on of Kupffer Cells

To invade hepatocytes, sporozoites must cross the barrier lined by endothelial cells (ECs) and immune phagocytic cells called Kupffer Cells (KCs) (Tavares et al., 2013). Sporozoites will have to interact with these resident cells in order to establish a successful infection (Meslin et al., 2007).

When the sporozoites reach the liver they are attracted to sulfated molecules that are present in ECs and KCs. This interaction is mainly mediated between the circumsporozoite protein (CSP) and sulfated heparin sulfate proteogycans (HSPGs) in the surface of the host cells. Other molecules that are involved in this process include P39 and CD38 (Cha et al., 2015). Previous studies employing intravital and electron microscopy suggested KCs, but not the ECs are the preferred passage used by sporozoites (Cha et al., 2015). Recent studies proposed that sporozoites exploit multiple paths to cross the sinusoidal barrier. Also, there have been reports that sporozoites pass through gaps between ECs and KCs, not engaging in traversal capacity (Meis et al., 1983). For the sporozoites passing through KCs, it would be interesting to know why the KCs do not degrade parasites even though they efficiently kill other microorganisms that invade hepatocytes (Sinnis and Zavala, 2012). Additionally, it has been described in a mice model that sporozoites can go through KCs and modulate their cytokine profile, leading to the down-regulation of Th1 cytokines (TNF-α, IL-6, and MCP-1) and the upregulation of Th2 cytokines (IL-10) for ensuring safe passage (Klotz and Frevert, 2008). Additionally, CSP can interact with LRP-1 (low-density lipoprotein receptor-related protein) and proteoglycans on the KC surface, which increases the levels of intracellular cAMP/EPAC and prevents the formation of reactive oxygen species (ROS). ROS is a natural byproduct that is produced during environmental stress and can cause cellular damage and it can kill the parasite (Ikarashi et al., 2013). In some cases, the parasite forces the KCs into apoptosis. Lastly, sporozoites can also negatively affect the antigen-presentation capacity of KCs, which display reduced expression of MHC-class I and IL-12 (Steers et al., 2005). Some evidence suggests that sporozoites are able to manipulate the KCs functions and immunosupress the microenvironment for its own advantage.

Modulation of Hepatocytes

After successful penetration of the sinusoidal cell layer, sporozoites enter the hepatocytes and start intra-hepatic development. Sporozoites actively invade the host cells (hepatocytes) employing the cholesterol uptake pathway, which is different from other microorganisms that exploit phagocytic activity of host cells for invasion (Itoe et al., 2014). Additionally, released CSP supports parasite development through the suppression of the NF-κB signaling pathway (Ding et al., 2012) and the up regulation of host heme oxygenase-1 (HO-1), which further promotes the parasite development in the liver by modulating the host inflammatory response (Pamplona et al., 2007). Sporozoite infection of hepatocytes also interferes with the mTOR pathway, which alters the levels of proteins involved in cell survival, proliferation, autophagy, anabolism, and cell growth (Hanson et al., 2013). After invading the final hepatocyte, sporozoites are enclosed in a parasitophorous vacuole (PVM), which physically separates it from the host cytoplasm thereby avoiding degradation by the endocytic/lysosome system. This isolation keeps the parasitophorous vacuole isolated from cell intrinsic defenses such as apoptosis and selective autophagy (Thieleke-Matos et al., 2016). The transition of parasites from liver stage merozoites to initiate blood stage represents another key point of the cycle for immune evasion. In order to start the blood stage, liver stage parasites must exit from the hepatocytes through hepatic spaces where they are exposed to resident phagocytic cells such as KCs and DCs. Merozoites avoid being killed by liver phagocytes by covering themselves in membranes derived from the host known as merosomes (Sturm et al., 2006). The merosomes are derived from infected hepatocytes when they bud off from the cells and manage to avoid recognition by phagocytes to initiate blood stage (Garg et al., 2013). The initiation of blood stage could take days after exiting the liver. Collectively, all of this data demonstrates the long journey that parasites travel to overcome the immune system.

IMMUNE EVASION BY ERYTHROCYTIC PARASITE STAGES

The blood stage is where the clinical symptoms that are characteristic of malaria appear. Blood stage is initiated when merozoites released from hepatocytes invade RBCs to develop into ring shaped, and young and mature trophozoites, undergoing schizogony. In schizogony each one leads to six to 32 daughter clones that will burst out into the bloodstream and reinvade new RBCs (Garg et al., 2013). An effective anti-parasitic immunity has been proven to be complex and involving various elements of the immune system. Antibodies and T-cells have proven to be important components in achieving parasite clearance (Chotivanich et al., 2002). Antibodies can have anti-parasitic activity by binding to infected erythrocytes and mediating their phagocytosis (opsonization) by circulating macrophages (Dups et al., 2014). They can also prevent invasion of red blood cells by binding to extracellular merozoites and marking them for clearance or lysis by complement. T-cells play an essential role by both direct and indirect mechanisms. Direct mechanisms include production of pro-inflammatory cytokines such as IFN-γ and TNF-α that prime macrophages and other components of the anti-parasite immune response (Nasr et al., 2014). They also mediate an indirect mechanism by activating specific B-cell clones that will produce anti-parasite antibodies (Kafuye-Mlwilo et al., 2012). Other innate immune components that have been attributed to play a role include: NK cells, γδT cells (Inoue et al., 2013), host microbiota and natural antibodies (Crompton et al., 2014). Circulating infected blood cells can be targeted for destruction in the spleen but the parasite avoids this by developing several mechanisms to evade the host immune response (Chotivanich et al., 2002). As an example for complement evasion, inhibition of the membrane attack complex (MAC) formation has been described in *P. falciparum*-infected patients and it even correlated with severe malaria cases (Schmidt et al., 2015).

The intracellular survival is the most primitive immune escape mechanism of parasites, which avoid the direct interaction of parasites with the immune cells. Furthermore, RBCs do not express MHC class I molecules on their surface thereby escaping from recognition by $CD8^+$ T cells (Bowen and Walker, 2005). Another feature that parasites use to avoid clearance is the formation of rosettes. Rossettes is a phenomenon where infected erythrocytes cluster with uninfected erythrocytes helping the parasites bind to RBC epitopes and avoid immune recognition. Blood type is one factor correlated with the rosette formation. For example parasites that bind blood type A are more virulent than the ones that bind blood type O because their capacity of forming rosettes is stronger (Moll et al., 2015).

Overall the evasion mechanisms are divided in two fields of strategies. One of them is the expression of variable antigenic proteins at the surface in different life cycle stages of parasites that help camouflage them from the host immune system (Escalante et al., 1998). The evasion of immune clearance is due the highly polymorphic proteins that mediate antigenic variation by changing and adapting to host immune response, promoting long-lasting infections (Wilson et al., 2016). The second is sequestration, which is mediated by genes products of the *PfEMP-1, Var, Rifin* (Mwakalinga et al., 2012), and *Stevor* multigene families (Kraemer and Smith, 2006). These proteins allow iRBC adherence in vascular endothelium hence avoiding clearance, and sequestering them in the microvasculature of various organs. They also exploit host components such as platelets and inflammation that can lead agglutination of uninfected RBCs with iRBCs and promote the appropriate sequestration microenvironment (Helmby et al., 1993).

In the blood stream, merozoites utilize complex set of proteins in order to invade uninfected red blood cells (Helmby et al., 1993). The parasite locates closely its proteins to proteins of the host erythrocytes, mediating reorientation and tight binding allowing them to invade the host RBCs. MSP-1 (merozoite surface proteins) anchors in the host erythrocyte membrane through GPI (glicosilfosfatilinositol) anchors. (Nosjean et al., 1997). MSPs along with other merozoite proteins called erythrocyte binding-like (EBL) proteins exist in several alleles or copies in the genome, showing a high degree of polymorphism (Holder et al., 1999). Several studies about new vaccine candidates against malaria are based in interactions between surface proteins, such as MSPs, GPI and PfEMP-1 (Boyle et al., 2014). The EBL protein family has a sophisticated profile with redundant functions that evolved to promote antigenic variation and immune evasion (Souza-Silva et al., 2014). EBL proteins are proteins that contain a Duffy-binding-like (DBL) which have been shown to mediate host receptor binding, in the case of *P.vivax* infection (VanBuskirk et al., 2004).

All *Plasmodium* species use to the same principle for invasion of the cell through interaction of parasite proteins to host erythrocyte receptor. The most studied invasion mechanisms are the ones used by *P.vivax* and *P.falciparum*. The merozoites of *P.falciparum* have at least five mechanisms of invasion, characterized by its respective receptor in erythrocytes (Baum et al., 2003). *P.vivax* shows great preference to invade immature red blood cell forms, such as reticulocytes. Some studies have reported that people who have the DARC (Duffy antigen receptor chemokines) in erythrocytes are more susceptible to infection by *P. vivax*. Conversely, the lack of this receptor (Souza-Silva et al., 2014) confers resistance to infection by *P. vivax*. However, other studies from west Kenya and Brazil have reported *P.vivax* cases, despite the lack of DARC expression in RBCs, suggesting alternative pathways for *P.vivax* infection (Ryan et al., 2006).

P. falciparum has evolved more adapt ways of immune evasion. One of the most studied strategies is the exposure PfEMP1 on infected red blood cells. The PfEMP-1 expression is a sophisticated apparatus that promotes the ability to bind different host endothelial cells, such as human brain microvascular endothelial cells (HBMEC). This binding helps the parasites avoid clearance by the spleen and it's directly related to complicated falciparum malaria such as cerebral malaria (Abdi et al., 2016).

The alterations in the iRBC membrane created by exposure of these proteins are denominated Knobs. These knobs will mediate cytoadhesion to the endothelium. Some of the targeted endothelium receptors include EPCR, CSA, CD36, and ICAMs (Yipp et al., 2000). Condroitin sulfate A (CSA) is the receptor targeted by the specific variant that leads to placental malaria in pregnant women (Kraemer and Smith, 2006). Each PfEMP variant can promote binding to different receptors in several organs (Hviid and Jensen, 2015). In both iRBC and uninfected RBCs in severe malaria, the erythrocytes become rigid following impediment to their flow through capillaries that have midpoint diameters that are all smaller than the erythrocyte itself (Dondorp et al., 2000). This can block parasite recirculation or recruitment of non-infected RBCs leading to rosettes (Uyoga et al., 2012) and has been associated with severe malaria anemia (Uyoga et al., 2012). Knobs sequestration in post-capillary venules occurs in mature blood stages such trophozoite and schizonts (Sharma, 1991). The presence of the parasite leads to activation of the immune response and production of cytokines, enhancing expression of receptors in endothelial cells targeted by the parasite adhesins (Rowe et al., 2009). This promotes the cyclical fevers associated with malaria while the constant presence of parasite exacerbates the inflammatory immune response (Gazzinelli et al., 2014).

Inadequate Innate and Adaptive Responses against *Plasmodium* Blood Stage Parasites

Even though the parasite has evolved various immune evasion strategies, the host immune response along with its genetic background, are essential for parasite control and prevention of clinical malaria. The human immune system is equipped with both innate and adaptive responses with great anti-parasitic activity. One major component of the innate immune system are Patter Recognition Receptors (PRRs) that recognize Pathogen-associated molecular patterns (PAMPs). In the case of malaria, three PAMPs that have been proposed for Plasmodium parasites are: GPI anchors, Hemozoin and immunostimulatory nucleic acid motifs (Gazzinelli et al., 2014).

Release array of pro and anti-inflammatory can result in either successful parasite control or alternatively an exacerbated immune response leading to pathology (Perkins et al., 2011). Even though mounting a potent immune response is not always completely efficient, it is necessary for controlling parasitemia. An important "bridge" between the innate and adaptive immune response are the dendritic cells (DCs). The DCs have a function of antigen presentation, stimulation of T-cells, and are major mediators of the adaptive immune response (Gowda et al., 2012). During malaria, CD4+ T− helper cells have been implicated for pathogenesis, protection and immune evasion of parasites (Wykes et al., 2014). The role of regulatory T cells (expressing FOXP3 CD4+ CD25+) in immunity has been controversial. For example, lack of T-regs during experimental cerebral malaria mice models renders them more susceptible to disease; while in human cerebral malaria correlates with higher parasitemia (Walther et al., 2005).

The role of CD8+ T cells-mediated immunity in blood stage has been less studied. This is mainly due to the fact that iRBCs don't express MHC class I rendering them resistant to the cytotoxic effect of CD8+ T-cells. Additionally, the high-level of mutations of epitopes in blood stage lead to immune evasion of the cytotoxic T lymphocyte (CTL) response, and hence fail to generate highly effective malaria vaccines (Templeton, 2009). Regardless, experiments using depletion both CD8+ and CD4+ T-cells during blood stage of *P.chabaudi* infections in mice resulted in a delayed clearance of the infection (Podoba and Stevenson, 1991), suggesting a possible role for CD8+ T-cells during blood stage malaria.

B cells have been attributed to an essential protective role during malaria. Antibody responses as immune agents alone can provide sufficient protection to control clinical disease (Wykes et al., 2014). The functions of antibodies can act on limiting the growth of blood stage parasites and the development of clinical symptoms for several mechanisms, like blocking erythrocyte invasion (Blackman et al., 1990), act as opsonins on parasitized erythrocytes (Osier et al., 2014), monocyte-mediated antibody-dependent cellular killing (Bouharoun-Tayoun et al., 1995), and complement-mediated lysis (Boyle et al., 2015), as well as interfering with the adherence of infected erythrocytes to vascular endothelium (Beeson et al., 2004). Unfortunately, the antibody responses to malaria infection from children and adults have been reported to be short-lived and rapidly lost in the absence of continued parasite exposure (Ryg-Cornejo et al., 2016). Collectively, these findings demonstrate that the immune system is efficient at reducing parasite burden but in most cases is not enough to prevent the progress of disease showing the high capacity of immune evasion by the parasite.

CONCLUDING REMARKS

Plasmodium has evolved a range of biomolecular strategies in order to escape the immune response and to guarantee the survival within the host. These parasites have great immune evasion ability across their whole life cycle. From an asymptomatic liver stage to a sophisticated system of proteins (such as PfEMP proteins) that is utilized by the parasite to avoid immune recognition and establish a successful infection. Hence further studies requiring close interactions of biomolecular, genetic, and immune strategies in both host and parasites are needed in order to understand better a protective anti-Plasmodium immunity. Thereby, in this review we summarize some of the important mechanisms that Plasmodium parasites utilize to facilitate evasion of the vertebrate host immune system across its life cycle. The challenges for the development of more effective therapeutics will have to overcome the various parasite immune evasion strategies and as several species cause malaria, several antigenic variations have to be considered. Recently we have a good candidate malaria vaccine in phase III (RST,S - GSK) of implanting, but even with a good initial response, it was also proved to be incomplete in points of recurrence of the disease (Morrison, 2015). Thus, the well-studied avoidance schemes propose an opening of new possibilities for further studies to consolidate the burden that malaria causes to hundreds of thousands of people annually.

AUTHOR CONTRIBUTIONS

PG, JB, JR, CF, and AM wrote the paper. All authors read and approved the final version of the manuscript.

ACKNOWLEDGMENTS

This work was supported by grants from Conselho Nacional de Desenvolvimento Científico e Tecnológico do Brasil (CNPq), Fundação de Amparo à Pesquisa do Estado do Rio de Janeiro (FAPERJ).

REFERENCES

1. Abdi, A. I., Warimwe, G. M., Muthui, M. K., Kivisi, C. A., Kiragu, E. W., Fegan, G. W., et al. (2016). Global selection of *Plasmodium falciparum* virulence antigen expression by host antibodies. *Sci. Rep.* 6:19882. doi: 10.1038/srep19882
2. Baum, J., Pinder, M., and Conway, D. J. (2003). Erythrocyte invasion phenotypes of *Plasmodium falciparum* in The Gambia. *Infect. Immun.* 71, 1856–1863. doi: 10.1128/IAI.71.4.1856-1863.2003
3. Beeson, J. G., Mann, E. J., Elliott, S. R., Lema, V. M., Tadesse, E., Molyneux, M. E., et al. (2004). Antibodies to variant surface antigens of *Plasmodium falciparum*- infected erythrocytes and adhesion inhibitory antibodies are associated with placental malaria and have overlapping and distinct targets. *J. Infect. Dis.* 189, 540–551. doi: 10.1086/381186
4. Blackman, M. J., Heidrich, H. G., Donachie, S., McBride, J. S., and Holder, A. A. (1990). A single fragment of a malaria merozoite surface protein remains on the parasite during red cell invasion and is the target of invasion-inhibiting antibodies. *J. Exp. Med.* 172, 379–382. doi: 10.1084/jem.172.1.379
5. Bouharoun-Tayoun, H., Oeuvray, C., Lunel, F., and Druilhe, P. (1995). Mechanisms underlying the monocyte-mediated antibody-dependent killing of *Plasmodium falciparum* asexual blood stages. *J. Exp. Med.* 182, 409–418. doi: 10.1084/jem.182.2.409
6. Bowen, D. G., and Walker, C. M. (2005). Mutational escape from CD8+ T cell immunity: HCV evolution, from chimpanzees to man. *J. Exp. Med.* 201, 1709–1714. doi: 10.1084/jem.20050808
7. Boyle, M. J., Langer, C., Chan, J., Hodder, A. N., Coppel, R. L., Anders, R. F., et al. (2014). Sequential processing of merozoite surface proteins during and after erythrocyte invasion by *Plasmodium falciparum*. *Infect. Immun.* 82, 924–936. doi: 10.1128/IAI.00866-13
8. Boyle, M. J., Reiling, L., Feng, G., Langer, C., Osier, F. H., Aspeling-Jones, H. et al. (2015). Human antibodies fix complement to inhibit *Plasmodium falciparum* invasion of erythrocytes and are associated with protection against malaria. *Immunity* 42, 580–590. doi: 10.1016/j.immuni.2015.02.012
9. Cha, S. J., Srinivasan, P., Schindler, C. W., van Rooijen, N., van Rooijen, N., Stins, M., et al. (2015). CD68 acts as a major gateway for malaria sporozoite liver infection. *J. Exp. Med.* 212, 1391–1403. doi: 10.1084/jem. 20110575
10. Chotivanich, K., Udomsangpetch, R., McGready, R., Proux, S., Newton, P., Pukrittayakamee, S., et al. (2002). Central role of the spleen in malaria parasite clearance. *J. Infect. Dis.* 185, 1538–1541. doi: 10.1086/340213
11. Cirimotich, C. M., Dong, Y., Garver, L. S., Sim, S., and Dimopoulous, G. (2010). Mosquito immune defenses against Plasmodium infection. *Dev. Comp. Immunol.* 34, 387–395. doi: 10.1016/j.dci.2009.12.005
12. Crompton, P. D., Moebius, J., Portugal, S., Waisberg, M., Hart, G., Garver,

L. S., et al. (2014). Malaria immunity in man and mosquito: insights into unsolved mysteries of a deadly infectious disease. *Annu. Rev. Immunol.* 32, 157–187. doi: 10.1146/annurev-immunol-032713-120220
13. Ding, Y., Huang, X., Liu, T., Fu, Y., Tan, Z., Zheng, H. et al. (2012). The Plasmodium circumsporozoite protein, a novel NF-κB inhibitor, suppresses the growth of SW480. *Pathol. Oncol. Res.* 18, 895–902. doi: 10.1007/s12253-012- 9519-7
14. Dondorp, A. M., Kager, P. A., Vreeken, J., and White, N. J. (2000). Abnormal blood flow and red blood cell deformability in severe malaria. *Parasitol. Today* 16, 228–232. doi: 10.1016/S0169-4758(00)01666-5
15. Dups, J. N., Pepper, M., and Cockburn, I. A. (2014). Antibody and B cell responses to Plasmodium sporozoites. *Front. Microbiol.* 5:625. doi: 10.3389/fmicb.2014. 00625
16. Escalante, A. A., Lal, A. A., and Ayala, F. J. (1998). Genetic polymorphism and natural selection in the malaria parasite *Plasmodium falciparum*. *Genetics* 149, 189–202.
17. Garg, S., Agarwal, S., Kumar, S., Yazdani, S. S., Chitnis, C. E., and Singh, S. (2013). Calcium-dependent permeabilization of erythrocytes by a perforin-like protein during egress of malaria parasites. *Nat. Commun.* 4, 1736. doi: 10.1038/ncomms 2725
18. Gazzinelli, R. T., Kalantari, P., Fitzgerald, K. A., and Golenbock, D. T. (2014). Innate sensing of malaria *parasites. Nat. Rev. Immunol.* 14, 744–757. doi: 10.1038/nri3742
19. Gowda, N. M., Wu, X., and Gowda, D. C. (2012). TLR9 and MyD88 are crucial for the development of protective immunity to malaria. *J. Immunol.* 188, 5073–5085. doi: 10.4049/jimmunol.1102143
20. Hanson, K. K., Ressurreicao, A. S., Buchholz, K., Prudencio, M., Herman-Ornelas, J. D., Rebelo, M., et al. (2013). Torins are potent antimalarials that block replenishment of Plasmodium liver stage parasitophorous vacuole membrane proteins. *Proc. Natl. Acad. Sci. U.S.A.* 110, E2838–E2847. doi: 10.1073/pnas.1306097110
21. Haque, A., and Engwerda, C. (2014). Hepatocytes break the silence during liver- stage malaria. *Nat. Med.* 20, 17–19. doi: 10.1038/nm.3446
22. Helmby, H., Cavelier, L., Pettersson, U., and Wahlgren, M. (1993). Rosetting *Plasmodium falciparum*-infected erythrocytes express unique strain-specific antigens on their surface. *Infect. Immun.* 61, 284–288.
23. Hisaeda, H., Yasutomo, K., and Himeno, K. (2005). Malaria: immune evasion by parasites. *Int. J. Biochem. Cell Biol.* 37, 700–706. doi: 10.1016/j.biocel.2004.10.009
24. Holder, A. A., Guevara Patino, J. A., Uthaipibull, C., Syed, S. E., Ling, I. T., Scott- Finnigan, T., et al. (1999). Merozoite surface protein 1, immune evasion, and vaccines against asexual blood stage malaria. *Parassitologia* 41, 409–414.
25. Hviid, L., and Jensen, A. T. (2015). PfEMP1 - A Parasite Protein Family of Key Importance in *Plasmodium falciparum* malaria immunity and pathogenesis. *Adv. Parasitol.* 88, 51–84. doi: 10.1016/bs.apar.2015.02.004
26. Ikarashi, M., Nakashima, H., Kinoshita, M., Sato, A., Nakashima, M., Miyazaki,
27. H. et al. (2013). Distinct development and functions of resident and recruited liver Kupffer cells/macrophages. *J. Leukoc. Biol.* 94, 1325–1336. doi: 10.1189/jlb.0313144
28. Inoue, S., Niikura, M., Mineo, S., and Kobayashi, F. (2013). Roles of IFN-γ and γδ T Cells in protective immunity against blood-stage malaria. *Front. Immunol.* 4:258. doi: 10.3389/fimmu.2013.00258
29. Itoe, M. A., Sampaio, J. L., Cabal, G. G., Real, E., Zuzarte-Luis, V., March, S. et al. (2014). Host cell phosphatidylcholine is a key mediator of malaria parasite survival during liver stage infection. *Cell Host Microbe* 16, 778–786. doi: 10.1016/j.chom.2014.11.006
30. Kafuye-Mlwilo, M. Y., Mukherjee, P., and Chauhan, V. S. (2012). Kinetics of humoral and memory B cell response induced by the *Plasmodium falciparum* 19-kilodalton merozoite surface protein 1 in mice. *Infect. Immun.* 80, 633–642. doi: 10.1128/IAI.05188-11
31. Klotz, C., and Frevert, U. (2008). Plasmodium yoelii sporozoites modulate cytokine profile and induce apoptosis in murine Kupffer cells. *Int. J. Parasitol.* 38, 1639–1650. doi: 10.1016/j.ijpara.2008.05.018
32. Kraemer, S. M., and Smith, J. D. (2006). A family affair: var genes, PfEMP1 binding, and malaria disease. *Curr. Opin. Microbiol.* 9, 374–380. doi: 10.1016/j.mib.2006.06.006
33. Liehl, P., Meireles, P., Albuquerque, I. S., Pinkevych, M., Baptista, F., Mota, M. M. et al. (2015). Innate immunity induced by Plasmodium liver infection inhibits malaria reinfections. *Infect. Immun.* 83, 1172–1180. doi: 10.1128/IAI.02796-14 Liehl, P., Zuzarte-Luis, V., Chan, J., Zillinger, T., Carapau, D., Carapau, D., et al. (2014). Host-cell sensors for Plasmodium activate innate immunity against liver-stage infection. *Nat. Med.* 20, 47–53. doi: 10.1038/nm.3424
34. Meis, J. F., Verhave, J. P., Jap, P. H., and Meuwissen, J. H. (1983). An ultrastructural study on the role of Kupffer cells in the process of infection by *Plasmodium berghei* sporozoites in rats. *Parasitology* 86(Pt 2), 231–242. doi: 10.1017/S003118200005040X
35. Meslin, B., Barnadas, C., Boni, V., Latour, C., De Monbrison, F., Kaiser, K., et al. (2007). Features of apoptosis in *Plasmodium falciparum* erythrocytic stage through a putative role of PfMCA1 metacaspase-like protein. *J. Infect. Dis.* 195, 1852–1859. doi: 10.1086/518253
36. Molina-Cruz, A., DeJong, R. J., Ortega, C., Haile, A., Abban, E., Rodrigues, J. et al. (2012). Some strains of *Plasmodium falciparum*, a human malaria parasite, evade the complement-like system of *Anopheles gambiae* mosquitoes. *Proc. Natl. Acad. Sci. U.S.A.* 109, E1957–E1962. doi: 10.1073/pnas.1121183109
37. Moll, K., Palmkvist, M., Ch'ng, J., Kiwuwa, M. S., and Wahlgren, M. (2015). Evasion of immunity to *Plasmodium falciparum*: rosettes of blood group a impair recognition of pfemp1. *PLoS ONE* 10:e0145120. doi: 10.1371/journal.pone.0145120
38. Morrison, C. (2015). Landmark green light for Mosquirix malaria vaccine. *Nat Biotechnol.* 33, 1015–1016. doi: 10.1038/nbt1015-1015
39. Müller, H. M., Reckmann, I., Hollingdale, M. R., Bujard, H., Robson, K. J., and Crisanti, A. (1993). Thrombospondin related anonymous protein (TRAP) of *Plasmodium falciparum* binds specifically to sulfated glycoconjugates and to HepG2 hepatoma cells suggesting a role for this molecule in sporozoite invasion of hepatocytes. *EMBO J.* 12, 2881–2889.
40. Mwakalinga, S. B., Wang, C. W., Bengtsson, D. C., Turner, L., Dinko, B., Lusingu, J. P. et al. (2012). Expression of a type B RIFIN in *Plasmodium falciparum* merozoites and gametes. *Malar. J.* 11:429. doi: 10.1186/1475-2875-11-429 Nasr, A., Allam, G., Hamid, O., and Al-Ghamdi, A. (2014). IFN-gamma and TNF associated with severe *falciparum malaria* infection in Saudi pregnant women. *Malar. J.* 13:314. doi: 10.1186/1475-2875-13-314
41. Nosjean, O., Briolay, A., and Roux, B. (1997). Mammalian GPI proteins: sorting, membrane residence and functions. *Biochim. Biophys. Acta* 1331, 153–186. doi: 10.1016/S0304-4157(97)00005-1
42. Ocaña-Morgner, C., Mota, M. M., and Rodriguez, A. (2003). Malaria blood stage suppression of liver stage immunity by dendritic cells. *J. Exp. Med.* 197, 143–151. doi: 10.1084/jem.20021072
43. Osier, F. H., Feng, G., Boyle, M. J., Langer, C., Zhou, J., Richards, J. S. et al. (2014). Opsonic phagocytosis of *Plasmodium falciparum* merozoites: mechanism in human immunity and a correlate of protection against malaria. *BMC Med.* 12:108. doi: 10.1186/1741-7015-12-108
44. Pamplona, A., Ferreira, A., Balla, J., Jeney, V., Balla, G., Epiphanio, S., et al. (2007). Heme oxygenase-1 and carbon monoxide suppress the pathogenesis of experimental cerebral malaria. *Nat. Med.* 13, 703–710. doi: 10.1038/nm1586
45. Patarroyo, M. E., Alba, M. P., and Curtidor, H. (2011). Biological and structural characteristics of the binding peptides from the sporozoite proteins essential for cell traversal (SPECT)-1 and -2. *Peptides* 32, 154–160. doi: 10.1016/j.peptides.2010.09.026
46. Perkins, D. J., Were, T., Davenport, G. C., Kempaiah, P., Hittner, J. B., and Ong'echa, J. M. (2011). Severe malarial anemia: innate immunity and pathogenesis. *Int. J. Biol. Sci.* 7, 1427–1442. doi: 10.7150/ijbs.7.1427
47. Podoba, J. E., and Stevenson, M. M. (1991). CD4+ and CD8+ T lymphocytes both contribute to acquired immunity to blood-stage *Plasmodium chabaudi* AS. *Infect. Immun.* 59, 51–58.
48. Prado, M., Eickel, N., De Niz, M., Heitmann, A., Agop-Nersesian, C., Wacker, R. et al. (2015). Long-term live imaging reveals cytosolic immune responses of host hepatocytes against Plasmodium infection and parasite escape mechanisms. *Autophagy* 11, 1561–1579. doi: 10.1080/15548627.2015.1067361
49. Risco-Castillo, V., Topcu, S., Marinach, C., Manzoni, G., Bigorgne, A. E., Briquet, S., et al. (2015). Malaria sporozoites traverse host cells within transient vacuoles. *Cell Host Microbe* 18, 593–603. doi: 10.1016/j.chom.2015.10.006

50. Rowe, J. A., Claessens, A., Corrigan, R. A., and Arman, M. (2009). Adhesion of *Plasmodium falciparum*-infected erythrocytes to human cells: molecular mechanisms and therapeutic implications. *Expert Rev. Mol. Med.* 11, e16. doi: 10.1017/S1462399409001082
51. Ryan, J. R., Stoute, J. A., Amon, J., Dunton, R. F., Mtalib, R., Koros, J., et al. (2006). Evidence for transmission of Plasmodium vivax among a duffy antigen negative population in Western Kenya. *Am. J. Trop. Med. Hyg.* 75, 575–581.
52. Ryg-Cornejo, V., Ly, A., and Hansen, D. S. (2016). Immunological processes underlying the slow acquisition of humoral immunity to malaria. *Parasitology* 143, 199–207. doi: 10.1017/S0031182015001705
53. Schmidt, C. Q., Kennedy, A. T., and Tham, W. H. (2015). More than just immune evasion: hijacking complement by *Plasmodium falciparum*. *Mol. Immunol.* 67, 71–84. doi: 10.1016/j.molimm.2015.03.006
54. Sharma, Y. D. (1991). Knobs, knob proteins and cytoadherence in falciparum malaria. *Int. J. Biochem.* 23, 775–789. doi: 10.1016/0020-711X(91)90061-Q
55. Singh, S., Alam, M. M., Pal-Bhowmick, I., Brzostowski, J. A., and Chitnis, C. E. (2010). Distinct external signals trigger sequential release of apical organelles during erythrocyte invasion by malaria parasites. *PLoS Pathog.* 6:e1000746. doi: 10.1371/journal.ppat.1000746
56. Sinnis, P., and Zavala, F. (2012). The skin: where malaria infection and the host immune response begin. *Semin. Immunopathol.* 34, 787–792. doi: 10.1007/s00281-012-0345-5
57. Souza-Silva, F. A., Torres, L. M., Santos-Alves, J. R., Tang, M. L., Sanchez, B. A., Sousa, T. N., et al. (2014). Duffy antigen receptor for chemokine (DARC) polymorphisms and its involvement in acquisition of inhibitory anti-duffy binding protein II (DBPII) immunity. *PLoS ONE* 9:e93782. doi: 10.1371/journal.pone.0093782
58. Spottiswoode, N., Duffy, P. E., and Drakesmith, H. (2014). Iron, anemia and hepcidin in malaria. *Front. Pharmacol.* 5:125. doi: 10.3389/fphar.2014.00125
Steers, N., Schwenk, R., Bacon, D. J., Berenzon, D., Williams, J., and Krzych,
59. U. (2005). The immune status of Kupffer cells profoundly influences their responses to infectious *Plasmodium berghei* sporozoites. *Eur. J. Immunol.* 35, 2335–2346. doi: 10.1002/eji.200425680
60. Sturm, A., Amino, R., van de Sand, C., Regen, T., Retzlaff, S., Rennenberg, A., et al. (2006). Manipulation of host hepatocytes by the malaria parasite for delivery into liver sinusoids. *Science* 313, 1287–1290. doi: 10.1126/science.1129720
61. Tavares, J., Formaglio, P., Thiberge, S., Mordelet, E., Van Rooijen, N., Medvinsky, A., et al. (2013). Role of host cell traversal by the malaria sporozoite during liver infection. *J. Exp. Med.* 210, 905–915. doi: 10.1084/jem.20121130
62. Templeton, T. J. (2009). The varieties of gene amplification, diversification and hypervariability in the human malaria parasite, *Plasmodium falciparum*. *Mol. Biochem. Parasitol.* 166, 109–116. doi: 10.1016/j.molbiopara.2009.04.003
63. Thieleke-Matos, C., Lopes da Silva, M., Cabrita-Santos, L., Portal, M. D., Rodrigues, I. P., Zuzarte-Luis, V., et al. (2016). Host cell autophagy contributes to Plasmodium liver development. *Cell. Microbiol.* 18, 437–450. doi: 10.1111/cmi.12524
64. Uyoga, S., Skorokhod, O. A., Opiyo, M., Orori, E. N., Williams, T. N., Arese, P., et al. (2012). Transfer of 4-hydroxynonenal from parasitized to non-parasitized erythrocytes in rosettes. Proposed role in severe malaria anemia. *Br. J. Haematol.* 157, 116–124. doi: 10.1111/j.1365-2141.2011.09015.x
65. VanBuskirk, K. M., Sevova, E., and Adams, J. H. (2004). Conserved residues in the Plasmodium vivax Duffy-binding protein ligand domain are critical for erythrocyte receptor recognition. *Proc. Natl. Acad. Sci. U.S.A.* 101, 15754–15759. doi: 10.1073/pnas.0405421101
66. Walther, M., Tongren, J. E., Andrews, L., Korbel, D., King, E., Fletcher,
67. H. et al. (2005). Upregulation of TGF-beta, FOXP3, and CD4+CD25+ regulatory T cells correlates with more rapid parasite growth in human malaria infection. *Immunity* 23, 287–296. doi: 10.1016/j.immuni.2005.08.006
68. WHO (2015). *World Malaria Report*. Geneva: World Health Organization.
Wilson, K. L., Xiang, S. D., and Plebanski, M. (2016). A model to study the impact of polymorphism driven liver-stage immune evasion by malaria parasites, to help design effective cross-reactive vaccines. *Front. Microbiol.* 7:303. doi: 10.3389/fmicb.2016.00303
69. Wykes, M. N., Horne-Debets, J. M., Leow, C. Y., and Karunarathne, D. S. (2014). Malaria drives T cells *to exhaustion. Front. Microbiol.* 5:249. doi: 10.3389/fmicb.2014.00249
70. Yano, T., and Kurata, S. (2011). Intracellular recognition of pathogens and autophagy as an innate immune host defence. *J. Biochem.* 150, 143–149. doi: 10.1093/jb/mvr083
71. Yipp, B. G., Anand, S., Schollaardt, T., Patel, K. D., Looareesuwan, S., and Ho, M. (2000). Synergism of multiple adhesion molecules in mediating cytoadherence of *Plasmodium falciparum*-infected erythrocytes to microvascular endothelial cells under flow. *Blood* 96, 2292–2298.
72. Zheng, H., Tan, Z., and Xu, W. (2014). Immune evasion strategies of pre-erythrocytic malaria parasites. *Mediators Inflamm.* 2014:362605. doi: 10.1155/2014/362605

6

Vaccination with Altered Peptide Ligands of a *Plasmodium berghei* Circumsporozoite Protein CD8 T-Cell Epitope: A Model to Generate T Cells Resistant to Immune Interference by Polymorphic Epitopes

*Gabriela Minigo[1,2], Katie L. Flanagan[1,3], Robyn M. Slattery[4] and Magdalena Plebanski[1]**

[1] Vaccine and Infectious Diseases Laboratory, Department of Immunology and Pathology, Monash University, Melbourne, VIC, Australia, [2] Global and Tropical Health Division, Menzies School of Health Research, Charles Darwin University, Darwin, NT, Australia, [3] School of Medicine, University of Tasmania, Hobart, TAS, Australia, [4] Diabetes Laboratory, Department of Immunology and Pathology, Monash University, Melbourne, VIC, Australia

***Correspondence:**
Magdalena Plebanski
magdalena.plebanski@monash.edu

Many pathogens, including the malaria parasite *Plasmodium falciparum*, display high levels of polymorphism within T-cell epitope regions of proteins associated with protective immunity. The T-cell epitope variants are often non-cross-reactive. Herein, we show in a murine model, which modifies a protective CD8 T-cell epitope from the circumsporozoite protein (CS) of *Plasmodium berghei* (SYIPSAEKI), that simultaneous or sequential co-stimulation with two of its putative similarly non-cross-reactive altered peptide ligand (APL) epitopes (SYIPSAEDI or SYIPSAEAI) has radically different effects on immunity. Hence, co-immunization or sequential stimulation *in vivo* of SYIPSAEKI with its APL antagonist SYIPSAEDI decreases immunity to both epitopes. By contrast, co-immunization with SYIPSAEAI has no apparent initial effect, but it renders the immune response to SYIPSAEKI resistant to being turned off by subsequent immunization with SYIPSAEDI. These results suggest a novel strategy for vaccines that target polymorphic epitopes potentially capable of mutual immune interference in the field, by initiating an immune response by co-immunization with the desired index epitope, together with a carefully selected "potentiator" APL peptide.

Keywords: cross-reactivity, altered peptide ligand, antagonism, T cell, dendritic cell, vaccine, *Plasmodium*, malaria

INTRODUCTION

Foreign epitopes complexed with host MHC molecules are the target of recognition by cognate antigen-specific T cells. The development of effective preventive vaccines requires the induction of long-lasting immunity in the human population, with the capacity to induce responses to naturally occurring strains of a pathogen bearing different variants of protective epitopes. Pathogens bearing variant epitopes can evade or skew the immune system in a variety of ways leading to loss of protective immunity. A direct form of immune evasion involves the mutation of amino acid residues that are required for peptide binding to MHC. Other more sophisticated forms of polymorphic immune evasion also exist [reviewed in Ref. (1)]. Altered peptide ligand (APL) antagonism involves the concurrent presentation of selected closely related epitope variants. This can inhibit T cell effector functions such as cytokine production, cytotoxicity, or proliferation. The use of APL ligands for immune evasion has been well documented across human immunodeficiency virus (HIV), hepatitis B and C (HBV and HBC), and malaria parasite infections [reviewed in Ref. (1)]. Another form of immune evasion, known as "immune interference," also involves the concurrent or sequential presentation of related epitope variants to T cells. Immune interference results a failure to induce memory T cells from naive precursors. CD8 T-cell epitope variants causing APL antagonism and immune interference have been identified in *Plasmodium falciparum* and are major contributors to the parasite population structure observed in malaria-endemic regions of the world (2, 3).

Variant-specific immunity has been documented for the lead preerythrocytic malaria vaccine, RTS,S, which contains a single polymorphic variant of the circumsporozoite protein (CS) of *P. falciparum* (4). However, vaccines that target individual variants provide limited or short-lasting benefit in protection from malaria. This occurs because the non-targeted parasite variants take over the vacated niches in the vaccine-treated host population [discussed in Ref. (1)]. Attempts to provide more broadly cross-reactive responses against malaria have included mixing polymorphic variants of a single antigenic protein into one vaccine formulation, for example, including both the 3D7 and FC27 variants of merozoite surface protein 2 from *P. falciparum* into a single recombinant erythrocytic-stage vaccine (5); or mixing multiple target proteins into one formulation, for example, including the two key preerythrocytic-stage antigens CS and thrombospondin-related adhesive protein (TRAP) (6). Both attempts yielded disappointing results, with the combination of antigens showing little increase, and in the case of CS and TRAP, even a decrease, in immunity. As an alternative, recent studies have evaluated whether changing the adjuvant used to deliver a protective preerythrocytic *Plasmodium berghei* CD8 T-cell epitope (SYIPSAEKI) in murine models could broaden the pattern of T cell cross-reactivity (7). SYIPSAEKI (KI) is the immunodominant CD8 T-cell epitope of the *P. berghei* circumsporozoite (CS) protein, and the presence of vaccine-induced IFNγ-producing splenic T cells to this epitope correlates with protective efficacy (8). The contact T cell receptor (TCR) amino acid residue has been identified to be position 8, and in recent studies engineered amino acid changes to this position resulted in the generation of useful variants to model how an amino acid change can lead to loss of T cell cross-reactivity, without a decrease in MHC-binding capacity (8). Disappointingly, although both pro-inflammatory (montanide and poly I:C) and non-inflammatory nanoparticle-based vaccines induced comparable and robust peptide-specific responses to KI, they induced limited cross-reactivity to variants SYISAEDI (DI) or SYIPSAEAI (AI) (8). The limited cross-reactivity was also shown not to be due to holes in the naïve T cell repertoire, since vaccines formulated with each APL individually (including KI, AI, or DI) were capable of inducing robust immune responses to the immunizing index APL (7). While neither DI nor AI are natural variants, inclusion of such APLs in malaria vaccines has the potential to induce a broader spectrum of cross-reactive responses different from immunization with the index epitope alone. Conversely, if any of the pooled variants had antagonistic APL properties, such an approach could restrict the spectrum of responses, or turn off preexisting immunity, thus inducing immune interference, as has been described for naturally occurring variants of CS T-cell epitopes (9). Testing the consequences of immunizing with combinations or mixtures of APL variants has not been explored in such previous studies.

Understanding the mechanism by which immune interference promotes parasite survival and influences parasite population dynamics is central to successful vaccine development. In the present study, a murine model was utilized to dissect the complex patterns of immunity induced by well characterized selected APL variants of the *P. berghei* CD8 T-cell epitope KI, DI, and AI. The findings demonstrate a novel vaccination strategy that broadens T cell immunity and is resistant to being "turned off" by immune interference. This new vaccination strategy is likely to be of utility in tackling diverse pathogens beyond malaria that utilizes APLs for immune evasion, such as HIV and hepatitis C [reviewed in Ref. (1)].

ANIMALS AND METHODS

Animals

Female BALB/c (H-2^d) mice, 6–10 weeks of age were sourced from the Walter and Eliza Hall Institute, Melbourne, VIC, Australia, or bred at the Austin Research Institute Biomedical Animal Research Laboratory. The study was approved by Austin Research Institute Animal Care and Use Committee approved all animal procedures.

Peptides

The immunodominant CD8 epitope of *P. berghei* circumsporozoite protein SYIPSAE**K**I, its variants SYIPSAE**D**I and SYIPSAE**A**I, and the influenza CD8 epitope NPKd (TYQRTRALV) were synthesized by to >99% purity by Auspep (Melbourne, VIC, Australia). Peptides were confirmed to be non-toxic at the doses used by incubation of splenocytes overnight and assessment of impairment of ConA responses by ELISPOT.

Immunizations

Bone marrow-derived dendritic cells (DCs) were generated as previously described 10) by culturing bone marrow cells from female BALB/c mice for 6–8 days in RPMI 1640 (Gibco, USA) supplemented with 10% heat inactivated fetal calf serum (CSL, Australia), 20 mM HEPES buffer (JRH, USA), 4 mM L-glutamine, 100 U/mL penicillin, 100 mg/mL streptomycin sulfate, 100 mM β-mercaptoethanol (all Sigma, Australia), 1,000 U/mL granulocyte and macrophage colony stimulating factor (GM-CSF, Pharmingen, USA), and 10 ng/mL of interleukin-4 (IL-4, Pharmingen, USA). Female mice were used to avoid rejection of the transferred DCs. DCs were CD11c+MHCII+ and Gr1− with the majority (>80%) co-expressing CD11b+ indicating an inflammatory DC phenotype (data not shown). Harvested DCs were pulsed with 5 μg/mL peptide at 37°C for 1 h. For co-presentation DCs were pulsed with one peptide for 1 h, followed by the variant peptide for a further 2 h. No phenotypic changes were observed (using markers CD11c, CD11b, Gr1, MHCII, CD40, CD80, or CD86) following the peptide pulse for any of the peptides used, and no changes in inflammatory (IL6, TNF, and IL1) or suppressor cytokines (IL-10) in the supernatant, or changes in DC viability (by trypan blue). 10^6 DCs in 100 µL sterile PBS were injected intradermally into the hind footpads (50 µL per footpad) or into the base of the tail. Experiments involving immunization with one peptide or peptide combination on day 0 followed by booster immunization with another peptide on day 14 included control groups that received the same peptide or peptide combination as single immunization on day 0 only and another group that received a single immunization with the booster peptide on day 14 only. For all sequential immunizations, ELISPOT assays were performed between days 14 and 17 following the last immunization.

Ex Vivo Elispot Assays

ELISPOT assays were carried out in 96 well mixed acetate plates (Millipore, Watford, UK) as previously described (8). MAIPS4510 plates, pretreated with 50 µL/well methanol, were used for IFNγ assays; IL-4 and IL-10 secretion was assessed in MAHAS4510 plates. Plates were coated with 5 µg/mL anti-mouse IFNγ mAb (Mab AN18, Mabtech), 10 µg/mL anti-mouse IL-4 mAb (clone BVD4-1D11, Pharmingen), or 10 µg/mL anti-mouse IL-10 mAb (Pharmingen) and blocked with culture media RPMI 1640 (Gibco, USA) supplemented with 1% heat inactivated mouse serum, 20 mM HEPES buffer (JRH, USA), 4 mM L-glutamine, 100 U/mL penicillin, 100 mg/mL streptomycin sulfate, and 100 mM β-mercaptoethanol (all Sigma, Australia). Around 500,000 freshly isolated splenocytes were cultured in the presence of 10^{-5}–10^{-11} M peptide in triplicate or quadruplicate wells. Plates were incubated at 37°C, 5% CO_2 for 16 h for IFNγ assays, 24 h for IL-4, and 48 h for IL-10 assays. In preliminary assays, cognate responses from splenic T cells from animals immunized with KI, AI, or DI alone were eliminated when splenocytes were depleted of CD8 T cells (Dynabeads, UK) prior to the assay, confirming responses to these minimal CD8 T cell peptide epitopes come from CD8 T cell as expected.

For *In Vitro* Antagonism Assays

Splenocytes were restimulated with a suboptimal concentration of the index peptide KI for 1 h; the altered variant DI was added at different concentrations and incubated for a further 16 h washed, counted, and plated out as per (9).

Plates were incubated with 1 µg/mL biotinylated anti-mouse IFNγ mAb (Mab R4-6A2-Biotin, Mabtech, Sweden), biotinylated anti-mouse IL-4 mAb (clone BVD6-24G2-biotin, Pharmingen, USA), or biotinylated anti-mouse IL-10 mAb (Pharmingen, USA), followed by 1 µg/mL streptavidin–alkaline phosphatase (AP) (Mabtech, Sweden) for IFNγ assay or 0.1 µg/mL extravidin–AP (Sigma, USA) for IL-4 and IL-10 assays and developed using a colorimetric AP Kit (BioRad, Hercules, CA, USA). The number of spot forming units (SFU) per well was scored using the AID ELISPOT reader (Autoimmun Diagnostika GmbH, Germany) with AID ELISpot software version 2.9 (Autoimmun Diagnostika GmbH, Germany).

Statistical Analysis

All statistical analyses were carried out using GraphPad Prism (version 6.01). ELISPOT data were analyzed using two-way ANOVA followed by Tukey's *post hoc* test for comparison of all groups or Dunnett's *post hoc* test for comparison to the index peptide. The significance level used was (α) = 0.05 for all statistical tests.

RESULTS

Co-immunization with Variants KI and DI Impairs the Generation of KI-Specific IFNγ-Secreting CD8 T Cells

To address the question whether co-immunization with epitope variants SYIPSAEKI (KI) and SYIPSAEDI (DI) could broaden the immune response, we immunized BALB/c mice with DCs loaded with both peptides KI and DI. To minimize competition for MHC class I binding clefts, and to ensure KI presentation, DCs were pulsed first with variant KI for 1 h, followed by variant DI for another 2 h at equimolar concentrations (0.5×10^{-6} M). Control mice received DCs pulsed with KI or DI alone or without peptide. No KI-specific IFNγ secreting cells were detected in mice immunized with DI-pulsed DCs, confirming that priming with DI did not induce cross-reactive T cells. DCs pulsed with KI alone induced strong KI-specific IFNγ responses, while DCs co-presenting both KI and DI (KI/DI) induced significantly less KI-specific IFNγ-producing T cells (**Figure 1A**, $p < 0.001$). This significant reduction in KI-specific IFNγ responses was still evident 6 weeks after immunization (**Figure 1B**, $n = 3$, $p < 0.001$). KI-specific IFNγ responses could not be restored to normal level by using more antigen (**Figure 1C**, $n = 3$). To rule out peptide competition for H-2K^d binding, DCs were also pulsed separately with variant KI or DI for 1 h, washed, and then mixed at 1:1 ratio (KI + DI) immediately before injection. Control mice received (i) DCs pulsed with KI + DI, (ii) DCs pulsed with either variant KI or DI alone as positive controls, or (iii) DCs without peptide as a negative control. **Figure 1D** shows that KI-specific IFNγ-secreting cells were reduced irrespective of whether DCs had been loaded with KI and DI together ($p = 0.009$) or separately ($p < 0.001$). No KI-specific IFNγ secretion was observed in DI-immunized mice as observed previously. These data suggest that DI interfered with priming of KI-specific IFNγ secreting T cells *in vivo* when presented together with KI on the same or different APC. Therefore, this interference is unlikely to have been caused by peptide competition for MHC binding. Furthermore, no interference with KI-specific T cell priming was observed with DCs co-presenting KI together with the unrelated H-2K^d-restricted CD8 T-cell epitope NPK^d (TYQRTRALV) from the influenza A virus nucleoprotein (aa 147–155) (11), a peptide with strong binding affinity for H-2k^d (12, 13). The immune interference observed with KI + DI immunization appeared therefore unlikely to be due to the DC-loading protocol but suggests inhibitory effects were mediated specifically by variant DI.

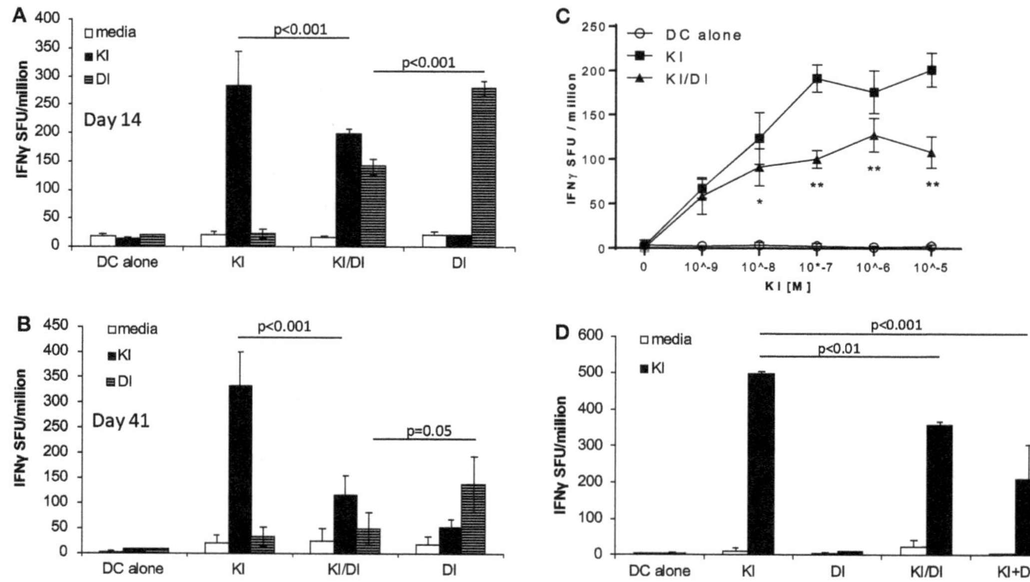

FIGURE 1 | Impaired IFNγ secretion following co-immunization with peptides KI and DI presented on the same or on different DC. BALB/c mice were immunized with dendritic cells (DCs) pulsed with either peptide KI or DI alone or with DCs pulsed with KI for 1 h followed by DI for 2 h. Control mice received DCs without peptide. IFNγ secretion was assessed by *ex vivo* ELISpot assay **(A)** 14 days or **(B)** 41 days after immunization. **(C)** IFNγ secretion upon restimulation with peptide KI at concentrations ranging from 10^{-9} to 10^{-5} M was assessed by *ex vivo* ELISpot assay 13 days after immunization. **(D)** BALB/c mice were immunized with DCs pulsed with either peptide KI or DI alone, with DCs pulsed with KI for 1 h then with DI for 2 h (KI/DI), or with a 1:1 mixture of DCs pulsed separately with KI or DI (KI + DI). IFNγ secretion was assessed by *ex vivo* ELISpot 17 days after immunization. Mean spot forming units ± SD are shown ($n = 3$ mice per group). Two-way ANOVA with Tukey's **(A,B,D)** or Dunnett's **(C)** multiple comparison test was used to test for statistical significance when comparing all groups or when compared to the group immunized with the index peptide KI, respectively.

Co-immunization with Variants KI and AI Does Not Interfere with KI-Specific or AI-Specific T Cell Priming

When we tested the effect of co-immunization of KI with another variant SYIPSAEAI (AI), we observed a different effect. Using the same immunization strategy as above, DCs were pulsed with KI for 1 h followed by AI for 2 h at equimolar concentration (5×10^{6} M) (KI/AI). Control mice were immunized with DCs pulsed with KI and AI alone or without peptide. KI-specific IFNγ responses were assessed by *ex vivo* ELISpot assay. We observed no significant difference in KI-specific IFNγ responses between mice immunized with KI or KI/AI at 2 (**Figure 2A**) or 5 weeks (**Figure 2B**) post-immunization. Titration of peptide KI from 5×10^{-9} to 5×10^{-6} M for *ex vivo* stimulation showed a similar reactivity pattern for KI-immunized mice and KI/AI-immunized mice at all concentrations tested (**Figure 2C**). Together, these data suggest that epitope variant AI does not interfere with KI-specific T cell priming when presented together with KI *in vivo*, indicating a functional difference between the two altered peptide variants AI and DI. To assess whether KI interfered with AI-specific priming, splenocytes from mice immunized with KI/AI or AI alone were assessed for AI-specific IFNγ responses by *ex vivo* ELISpot assay. Titration of peptide AI showed a similar reactivity pattern for AI- or KI/AI-immunized mice at all concentrations tested (**Figure 2D**). These results show that co-presentation of peptides KI and AI does not interfere with T cell priming.

Across experiments, mice immunized with KI-pulsed DC varied in their KI-specific IFNγ responses. **Figure 3A** shows pooled data from 12 experiments. The mean KI-specific IFNγ response in mice immunized with DC pulsed KI/DI (mean 185 ± 146 SFU/million) was significantly lower compared to those immunized with KI alone (mean 330 ± 164 SFU/million; $p < 0.001$). By contrast, KI-specific IFNγ responses in mice co-immunized with KI/AI (mean 285 ± 197 SFU/million) was comparable to those immunized with KI alone (**Figure 3A**).

Variants KI and DI Show Potential Mutual Inhibitory Effects on T Cell Priming

We next tested the effect of KI/DI co-presentation of the priming on DI-specific IFNγ responses after immunization with DCs co-presenting KI and variant DI (KI/DI) or DI alone. Mice immunized with KI/DI had significantly fewer DI-specific IFNγ secreting cells than mice immunized with DI alone (**Figure 1A**, $p < 0.001$), an effect that was less evident at 6 weeks post-immunization (**Figure 1B**, $p = 0.05$). Across experiments KI/DI immunization elicited significantly lower DI-specific IFNγ responses (mean 98 ± 83 SFU/million) compared to mice immunized with DC pulsed with DI alone (mean 164 ± 107 SFU/million; **Figure 3B**; $p < 0.01$). Although we cannot exclude that this effect might have been due to DC being pulsed with KI first followed by DI, this observation suggests that altered peptide variants KI and DI could be mutually antagonistic/immune interfering during T cell priming *in vivo*. KI- or DI-specific IFNγ responses following

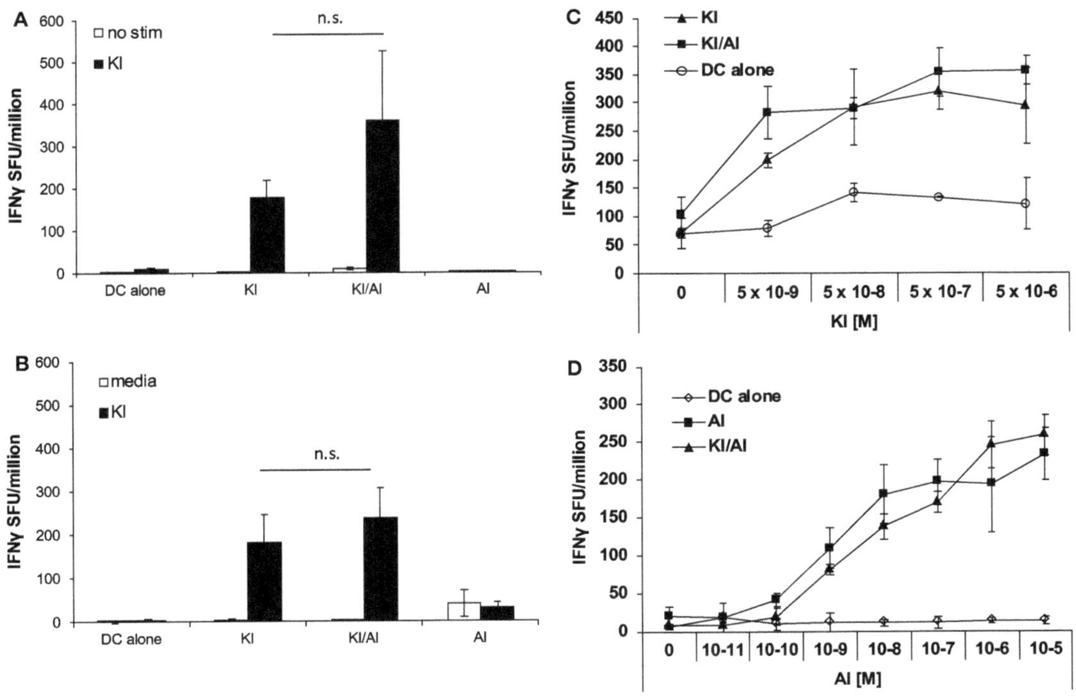

FIGURE 2 | Co-immunization with KI and AI does not interfere with T cell priming. BALB/c mice were immunized with dendritic cells (DCs) pulsed with either peptide KI or AI alone or with DC pulsed with KI for 1 h then with AI for 2 h. Control mice received DCs without peptide. **(A)** 12 days or **(B)** 31 days post-immunization IFNγ secretion was assessed by *ex vivo* ELISpot by restimulation with peptide KI at 0.5 μg/mL. **(C)** BALB/c mice were immunized with DCs pulsed with either peptide KI (triangles) or with DC pulsed with KI for 1 h then with AI for 2 h (squares). Control mice received non-pulsed DCs (open circles). IFNγ secretion was assessed by *ex vivo* ELISpot by restimulation with peptide KI at concentrations ranging from 5×10^{-9} to 5×10^{-6} M 10 days post-immunization. **(D)** BALB/c mice were immunized with DCs pulsed with either peptide AI (triangles) or with DC pulsed with KI for 1 h then with AI for 2 h (squares). Control mice received non-pulsed DCs (open circles). IFNγ secretion was assessed by *ex vivo* ELISpot by restimulation with peptide AI at concentrations ranging from 5×10^{-9} to 5×10^{-6} M 21 days post-immunization. Mean spot forming units ± SD are shown ($n = 3$ mice per group). Two-way ANOVA with Dunnett's multiple comparison test was used to test for statistical significance when compared to the groups immunized with the index peptide KI.

single immunization with the respective peptide displayed a similar response curve with peak responses elicited 2–3 weeks post-immunization (**Figure 3C**). It therefore appears unlikely that the reduced IFNγ responses following co-presentation of both peptides should result from different peptide kinetics. The implication for pathogen immune evasion is that a host exposed to both variants simultaneously might generate impaired IFNγ responses to both epitopes. This potential mutual interference was surprising and led us to investigate what would happen if mice were immunized sequentially with peptides KI and DI.

Variant DI Inhibited KI-Primed Effector T Cells *In Vivo*

To study *in vivo* effects of DI on KI-primed effector T cells, we primed BALB/c mice with the index peptide KI (d0) and 2 weeks later (d14) injected DCs presenting DI. We called this sequential immunization protocol KI–DI. Control mice received KI-pulsed DCs on day 0 (KI) or DI-pulsed DCs on day 14 (DI) or DCs without peptide (DC alone). KI-specific IFNγ responses were measured 14–17 days after the last immunization by *ex vivo* ELISpot assay. Mice primed with the index variant KI that received no further immunizations showed strong KI-specific IFNγ responses detectable 31 days post-immunization (**Figure 4A**). Mice receiving the KI–DI sequential immunizations, however, had significantly reduced numbers of KI-specific IFNγ-secreting cells (**Figure 4A**, black bars; $p < 0.01$). No difference was observed in the numbers of KI-specific IL-4-secreting cells between mice immunized with KI alone or followed by DI 14 days later (**Figure 4B**, black bars), and no KI-specific IL-10 secretion was detected in any of the groups (**Figure 4C**). These results suggest that epitope variant DI has an inhibitory effect on polyclonal KI-primed IFNγ secreting but not IL-4 secreting effector T cells *in vivo*.

DI-specific IFNγ responses were also measured after sequential immunization. Interestingly, there were significantly fewer DI-specific IFNγ-secreting cells detected in mice previously primed with KI compared with mice that were not pre-primed (**Figure 4A**, gray bars, $p < 0.001$). No significant difference in DI-specific IL-4 secretion (**Figure 4B**) and no DI-specific IL-10 secretion (**Figure 4C**) were observed in these mice. These results show that priming with the index peptide KI inhibits subsequent priming with the altered peptide variant DI.

No such interference was observed with AI-specific priming, using the above sequential immunization protocol for KI–AI

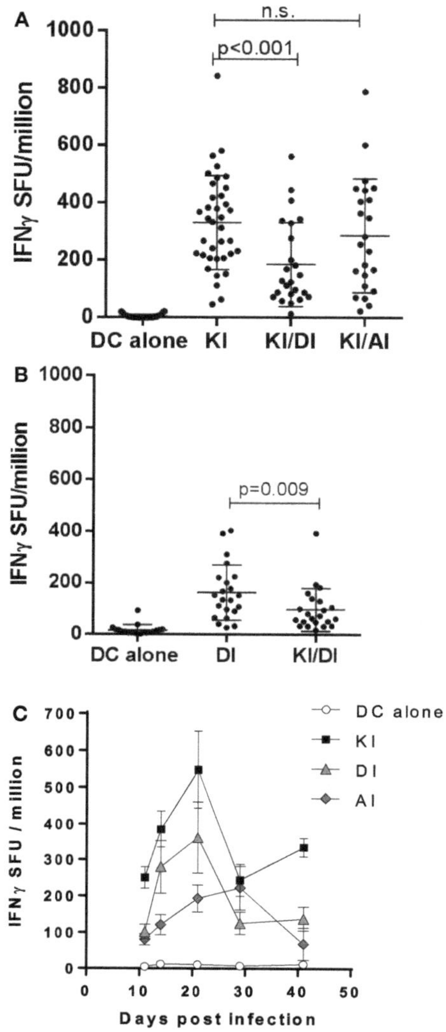

FIGURE 3 | Pooled data. (A) BALB/c mice immunized with dendritic cells (DCs) pulsed with either peptide KI alone (n = 37), with DCs pulsed with KI for 1 h followed by DI for 2 h (n = 24) or with DC pulsed with KI for 1 h then with AI for 2 h (n = 23). Control mice received DCs without peptide (n = 30). KI-specific IFNγ response was assessed by *ex vivo* ELISpot assay. Pooled data from 12 experiments are shown. Dots represent individual mice, and the horizontal line represents the mean ± SD. Data were analyzed using one-way ANOVA followed by Bonferroni's multiple comparison test. **(B)** BALB/c mice were immunized with DCs pulsed with either peptide DI alone or with DCs pulsed with KI for 1 h followed by DI for 2 h. Control mice received DCs without peptide. DI-specific IFNγ response was assessed by *ex vivo* ELISpot assay. Pooled data from eight experiments are shown. Dots represent individual mice, and the horizontal line represents the mean ± SD. Data were analyzed using one-way ANOVA followed by Bonferroni's multiple comparison test. **(C)** Mice were immunized with DCs pulsed with KI (black squares), DI (gray triangles), or AI (gray diamonds) alone and IFNγ responses to their respective peptides measured by *ex vivo* ELISpot assay at different time points. KI response is shown for control mice that received DCs without peptide. Mean spot forming units ± SD are shown (n = 3–9 mice per time point).

immunization. KI-primed mice showed strong KI-specific IFNγ responses irrespective of whether they were later immunized with AI-pulsed DCs or not (**Figure 4D**, black bars) with no statistically significant difference in the frequencies of KI-specific IFNγ-secreting effector T cells between KI- and KI–AI-immunized mice. Variant AI had no inhibitory effect on KI-specific IFNγ effector responses *in vivo*. Similarly, KI-primed mice raised competent AI-specific IFNγ-secreting cells in response KI–AI immunization, similar to AI-immunized mice (**Figure 4D**, gray bars).

KI-Specific IFNγ Responses Were Inhibited in the Presence of Epitope Variant DI *In Vitro*

The effects of antagonistic peptides have been studied on both clonal and polyclonal effector T cell responses (9, 14). Peptide variant DI has previously been shown to partially antagonize KI-specific IFNγ secretion *in vitro* in splenocytes from mice immunized with KI-expressing protein particles derived from a yeast retrotransposon (TyS3) (9). Here, we confirm that peptide DI inhibits KI-specific effector T cell responses *in vitro* using a protocol optimized in previous studies to control for the issue of competition of peptides for binding to MHC (9, 15). For the antagonism assay, splenocytes from KI-immunized mice were incubated with the suboptimal KI concentration of 10^{-8} M (0.01 μg/mL), and after 1 h DI was added at concentrations ranging from 10^{-8} to 10^{-4} M. **Figure 5** shows that addition of the altered variant DI significantly inhibited KI-specific IFNγ secretion from concentrations as low as 10^{-6} M (0.1 μg/mL). The inhibitory effect increased with increasing DI concentration, but inhibition never exceeded 60% of the total IFNγ response to the index peptide KI.

KI/AI-Primed Cells Were Not Susceptible to *In Vivo* Immune Interference by DI

Similar frequencies of KI-specific IFNγ-secreting cells were detected in the spleens from KI-immunized and KI/AI-immunized mice, although mice primed with KI or AI individually showed no cross-reactivity to the other variant (data not shown). In order to determine whether KI-specific CD8 T cells, induced by co-immunization with KI/AI, would have a similar or distinct pattern of cross-reactivity and/or susceptibility to immune interference to those induced with KI alone, mice were immunized with either KI/AI together, or KI alone on DCs (day 0), and 2 weeks later with DI-pulsed DCs (KI/AI–DI and KI–DI, respectively). Control mice received DCs pulsed with KI or without peptide. KI-specific IFNγ responses were measured 2–3 weeks later by *ex vivo* ELISpot assay. Three experiments were performed to assess the effect of variant DI on KI-specific IFNγ responses from KI/AI-primed splenocytes. The responses of mice immunized with KI were as expected susceptible to immune interference by subsequent immunization with DI (**Figure 6**). By contrast, we detected no significant difference in KI-specific IFNγ responses between KI/AI-primed mice that received a subsequent immunization with DI-pulsed DCs on day 14 and those that did not (**Figure 6**). Mice immunized with DCs presenting the variant AI alone on day 0 followed by immunization with DCs pulsed with variant DI on day 14 had no detectable KI-specific IFNγ responses (**Figure 6**), consistent with the previously shown lack

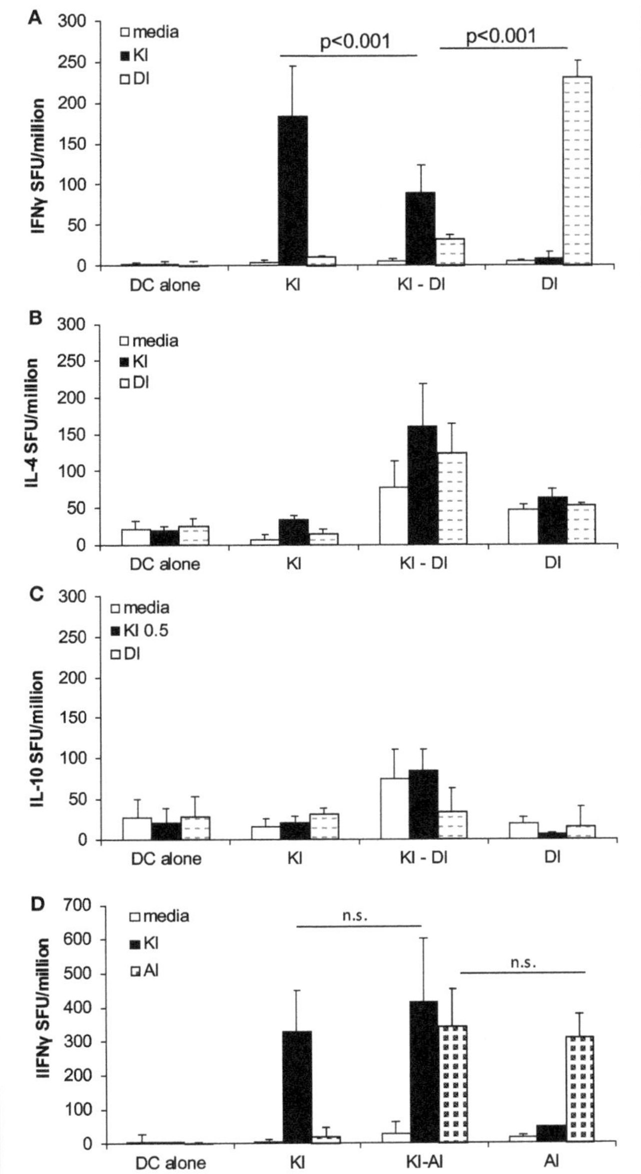

FIGURE 4 | Immunization with variant DI but not variant AI inhibits KI-specific IFNγ-secreting effector T cells *in vivo*. BALB/c mice were immunized with dendritic cells (DCs) pulsed with KI on day 0 (KI), DCs pulsed with DI on day 14 (DI) or with KI-pulsed DCs on day 0 followed by DI-pulsed DCs on day 14 (KI–DI). The negative control group received two immunizations with non-pulsed DCs 14 days apart. Splenocytes were assessed for KI-specific (black bars) and DI-specific (gray bars) **(A)** IFNγ, **(B)** IL-4, and **(C)** IL-10 responses by *ex vivo* ELISpot assay 17 days after the last immunization (day 31). **(D)** BALB/c mice were immunized with DCs pulsed with KI on day 0 (KI), with DCs pulsed with AI on day 14 (AI) or with KI-pulsed DCs on day 0 followed by AI-pulsed DCs on day 14 (KI–AI). The negative control group received two immunizations with non-pulsed DCs 14 days apart. Splenocytes were assessed for KI-specific (black bars) and AI-specific (gray bars) IFNγ responses by *ex vivo* ELISpot assay 14 days after boost immunization (day 28). Mean spot forming units ± SD (n = 3 mice per group). Two-way ANOVA with Tukey's multiple comparison test was used to test for statistical significance when comparing all groups **(A,B,D)**. Two-way ANOVA with Dunnett's multiple comparison test was used to test for statistical significance when comparing to the media control (C).

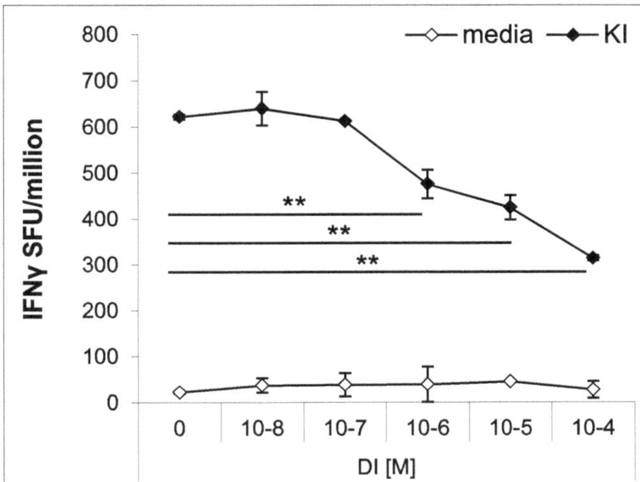

FIGURE 5 | Variant DI antagonizes KI-specific IFNγ secretion *in vitro*. BALB/c mice were immunized with 10^6 dendritic cells (DCs) pulsed with peptide variant KI or with DCs without peptide as negative controls. IFNγ responses were measured 21 days post-immunization by *ex vivo* ELISpot assay. Splenocytes were restimulated with the index peptide KI at 10^{-8} M for 1 h, followed by the altered peptide variant DI at different concentrations (10^{-8}–10^{-4} M). Mean spot forming units ± SD are shown (n = 3 mice per group). Two-way ANOVA with Dunnett's multiple comparison test was used to test for statistical significance when compared to the groups immunized with the index peptide KI.

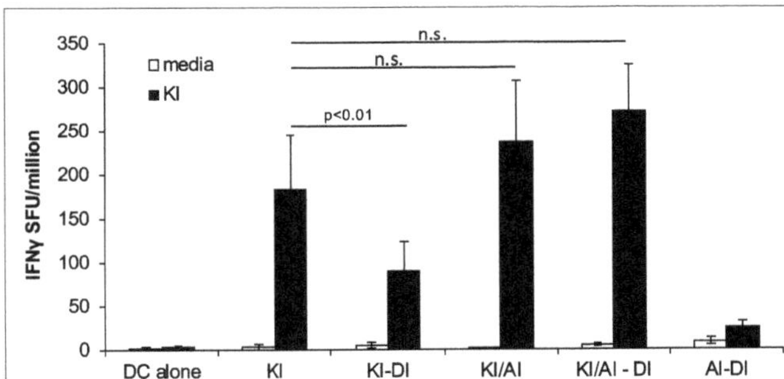

FIGURE 6 | KI/AI-primed cells are resistant to DI-induced immune interference. BALB/c mice were immunized on day 0 with dendritic cells (DCs) pulsed with either KI or AI or with DCs pulsed with KI for 1 h followed by AI for another 2 h. On day 14, three groups received sequential immunization with DI-pulsed DCs (KI–DI, KI/AI–DI, and AI–DI). The negative control group received two immunizations with non-pulsed DCs 14 days apart. Splenocytes were assessed for KI-specific IFNγ responses by *ex vivo* ELISpot assay 17 days after boost immunization (day 31). Mean spot forming units ± SD are shown (n = 3 mice per group). Two-way ANOVA with Dunnett's multiple comparison test was used to test for statistical significance when compared to the groups immunized with the index peptide KI.

of cross-reactivity. Our results show that KI/AI immunization, in contrast to immunization with KI or AI alone, induced T cells that recognize KI and AI, while no longer being susceptible to being turned off by immunization with the antagonistic DI APL, rendering the response therefore resistant to this type of immune interference.

DISCUSSION

The present study shows that immunization with combinations of highly related immunogenic variant peptides (KI, DI, and AI), such as those found naturally in pathogen populations with highly polymorphic T-cell epitopes, can have highly variable, and unpredictable, outcomes, with some combinations capable of decreasing immunity to both immunizing peptides (KI and DI). Moreover, immunizing sequentially with such peptides was shown to be capable of turning off responses, again to both immunizing T-cell epitope variants (KI and DI). The existence of "sequential immune interference" has theoretical consequences for pathogen population structures. It may be that polymorphic variants provide a survival advantage to the pathogen population that allows the species to evade the host immune response. By contrast, co-immunization of KI and AI had apparently little effect on the initial induction of immunity to either epitope, but, unexpectedly, the KI-specific responses generated were no longer susceptible to being turned off by subsequent immunization with DI. This finding offers a new practical strategy to elicit robust immune responses against polymorphic variants (by co-immunizing with an index epitope and a carefully selected "potentiator" epitope), which are then further resistant to being turned off by natural polymorphic variants capable of immune interference. *In vivo* challenge experiments with *P. berghei* sporozoites are needed to quantify the extent to which protective immunity is altered in this model.

Each of the three CD8 T-cell epitopes selected for study (KI, DI, and AI) induced high immune responses to themselves, but not to the other two epitopes, thus at face value they represent simple non-cross-reactive T-cell epitopes. However, co-immunization with DC pre-pulsed with KI and DI together, significantly reduced responses to both epitopes, with this mutual immune interference observed even when KI and DI were injected separately on separately peptide pulsed DC. There was no correlation between the magnitude of induced KI response and the level of interference by DI. Furthermore, the DI peptide was also shown to be capable of turning off effector KI-specific responses in a manner consistent with a classical APL antagonist. However, the fact that immune interference was observed even when presenting the epitopes on separate DC shows that the immune interference observed herein is not acting *via* classical mechanisms used by APL antagonism, such as alterations of the TCR:MHC immune-synaptosome structure (16). Further studies will be required to fully explore the extent to which immune interference by KI and DI is potentially fully reciprocal under a range of co-presentation and sequential immunization combinations.

The activity of some APL antagonist peptides has been shown to depend on a high off-rate in relation to MHC binding, but such mechanisms are unlikely to underlie the observed immune interference described in this study, since we have previously shown similarly high affinity binding to MHC for KI, DI, and AI (1). Temporal separation of stimulation by KI and DI by sequential immunization also resulted in reduced immunity demonstrating that immune interference by DI acts by stimulating KI-specific T cells to change their activity profile. Such switching of an activity profile has been observed *in vitro* for CD4 T-cell epitopes from *P. falciparum*. In this case, stimulation with a variant polymorphic epitope of an index peptide converted IFNγ-producing cells into IL-10 producers; a property demonstrated with human T cell clones to Th2R region variants of CS (2). In our study, immunization with DI did not appear to switch KI-specific responses from IFNγ to IL-10, or convert them into IL-4-producing Th2 cells, which have been noted as previous APL mechanisms capable of down modulating Th1 and cytotoxic immunity. These results do not exclude the hypothesis that stimulation with DI promotes other, less obvious, immunosuppressive cell populations, as well as potentially T cell apoptosis, anergy, or partial activation, related in a number of other studies with low TCR affinity interactions or disturbed TCR stimulating signaling micro-domains [reviewed in Ref. (17, 18)].

By using a combination of the index variant KI together with the "potentiator" peptide AI, we have demonstrated the induction of an immune response that is resistant to immune interference by DI stimulation. This finding lays the experimental foundations for a practical immunization strategy that could induce robust and long-lasting immune responses in the malaria setting. Thus, index epitopes could be paired with potentiator epitopes in a single immunization to induce a robust immune response to a polymorphic epitope, which would be predicted to persist even in vaccinees challenged by repeated pathogen stimulation. This is potentially of great significance for those living in malaria-endemic regions and exposed to persistent reinfection by polymorphic parasites capable of turning off immunity using immune interference (1). Moreover, combinations of engineered and natural variants may offer a new path for vaccines against many different pathogens, to create new modalities of cross-reactive responses.

AUTHOR CONTRIBUTIONS

GM and MP designed the study, interpreted the data, and drafted the manuscript. GM performed experiments and analyzed data. KF and RS critically revised the manuscript.

ACKNOWLEDGMENTS

The authors thank Ms. Jennifer Hanley for technical support.

REFERENCES

1. Flanagan KL, Wilson KL, Plebanski M. Polymorphism in liver-stage malaria vaccine candidate proteins: immune evasion and implications for vaccine design. *Expert Rev Vaccines* (2016) 15(3):389–99. doi:10.1586/14760584.2016.1125785
2. Plebanski M, Flanagan KL, Lee EA, Reece WH, Hart K, Gelder C, et al. Interleukin 10-mediated immunosuppression by a variant CD4 T cell epitope of *Plasmodium falciparum*. *Immunity* (1999) 10(6):651–60. doi:10.1016/S1074-7613(00)80064-3

3. Gilbert SC, Plebanski M, Gupta S, Morris J, Cox M, Aidoo M, et al. Association of malaria parasite population structure, HLA, and immunological antagonism. *Science* (1998) 279(5354):1173–7. doi:10.1126/science.279.5354.1173
4. Neafsey DE, Juraska M, Bedford T, Benkeser D, Valim C, Griggs A, et al. Genetic diversity and protective efficacy of the RTS,S/AS01 malaria vaccine. *N Engl J Med* (2015) 373(21):2025–37. doi:10.1056/NEJMoa1505819
5. Krishnarjuna B, Andrew D, MacRaild CA, Morales RA, Beeson JG, Anders RF, et al. Strain-transcending immune response generated by chimeras of the malaria vaccine candidate merozoite surface protein 2. *Sci Rep* (2016) 6:20613. doi:10.1038/srep20613
6. Kester KE, Gray Heppner D Jr, Moris P, Ofori-Anyinam O, Krzych U, Tornieporth N, et al. Sequential phase 1 and phase 2 randomized, controlled trials of the safety, immunogenicity and efficacy of combined pre-erythrocytic vaccine antigens RTS,S and TRAP formulated with AS02 Adjuvant System in healthy, malaria naive adults. *Vaccine* (2014) 32(49):6683–91. doi:10.1016/j.vaccine.2014.06.033
7. Wilson KL, Xiang SD, Plebanski M. A model to study the impact of polymorphism driven liver-stage immune evasion by malaria parasites, to help design effective cross-reactive vaccines. *Front Microbiol* (2016) 7:303. doi:10.3389/fmicb.2016.00303
8. Plebanski M, Gilbert SC, Schneider J, Hannan CM, Layton G, Blanchard T, et al. Protection from *Plasmodium berghei* infection by priming and boosting T cells to a single class I-restricted epitope with recombinant carriers suitable for human use. *Eur J Immunol* (1998) 28(12):4345–55. doi:10.1002/(SICI)1521-4141(199812)28:12<4345::AID-IMMU4345>3.3.CO;2-G
9. Plebanski M, Lee EA, Hannan CM, Flanagan KL, Gilbert SC, Gravenor MB, et al. Altered peptide ligands narrow the repertoire of cellular immune responses by interfering with T-cell priming. *Nat Med* (1999) 5(5):565–71. doi:10.1038/8444
10. Inaba K, Inaba M, Romani N, Aya H, Deguchi M, Ikehara S, et al. Generation of large numbers of dendritic cells from mouse bone marrow cultures supplemented with granulocyte/macrophage colony-stimulating factor. *J Exp Med* (1992) 176(6):1693–702. doi:10.1038/369403a0
11. Bodmer HC, Pemberton RM, Rothbard JB, Askonas BA. Enhanced recognition of a modified peptide antigen by cytotoxic T cells specific for influenza nucleoprotein. *Cell* (1988) 52(2):253–8. doi:10.1016/0092-8674(88)90514-4
12. Morgan CS, Holton JM, Olafson BD, Bjorkman PJ, Mayo SL. Circular dichroism determination of class I MHC-peptide equilibrium dissociation constants. *Protein Sci* (1997) 6(8):1771–3. doi:10.1002/pro.5560060819
13. Romero P, Corradin G, Luescher IF, Maryanski JL. H-2Kd-restricted antigenic peptides share a simple binding motif. *J Exp Med* (1991) 174(3):603–12. doi:10.1084/jem.174.3.603
14. Klenerman P, Rowland-Jones S, McAdam S, Edwards J, Daenke S, Lalloo D, et al. Cytotoxic T-cell activity antagonized by naturally occurring HIV-1 Gag variants. *Nature* (1994) 369(6479):403–7. doi:10.1038/369403a0
15. Jameson SC, Carbone FR, Bevan MJ. Clone-specific T cell receptor antagonists of major histocompatibility complex class I-restricted cytotoxic T cells. *J Exp Med* (1993) 177(6):1541–50. doi:10.1084/jem.177.6.1541
16. Gascoigne NR, Zal T. Molecular interactions at the T cell-antigen-presenting cell interface. *Curr Opin Immunol* (2004) 16(1):114–9. doi:10.1016/j.coi.2003.11.008
17. Unanue ER. Altered peptide ligands make their entry. *J Immunol* (2011) 186(1):7–8. doi:10.4049/jimmunol.1090118
18. Candia M, Kratzer B, Pickl WF. On peptides and altered peptide ligands: from origin, mode of action and design to clinical application (immunotherapy). *Int Arch Allergy Immunol* (2016) 170(4):211–33. doi:10.1159/000448756

7

Leishmania infantum and *Leishmania braziliensis*: Differences and Similarities to Evade the Innate Immune System

*Sarah de Athayde Couto Falcão[1,2], Tatiana M. G. Jaramillo[1], Luciana G. Ferreira[2], Daniela M. Bernardes[1], Jaime M. Santana[1] and Cecília B. F. Favali[1,2]**

[1] Department of Cell Biology, Biology Institute, University of Brasília, Brasília, Brazil, [2] Núcleo de Medicina Tropical (NMT), University of Brasília, Brasília, Brazil

***Correspondence:**
Cecília B. F. Favali
cfavali@unb.br

Visceral leishmaniasis is a severe form of the disease, caused by *Leishmania infantum* in the New World. Patients present an anergic immune response that favors parasite establishment and spreading through tissues like bone marrow and liver. On the other hand, *Leishmania braziliensis* causes localized cutaneous lesions, which can be self-healing in some individuals. Interactions between host and parasite are essential to understand disease pathogenesis and progression. In this context, dendritic cells (DCs) act as essential bridges that connect innate and adaptive immune responses. In this way, the aim of this study was to compare the effects of these two *Leishmania* species, in some aspects of human DCs' biology for better understanding of the evasion mechanisms of *Leishmania* from host innate immune response. To do so, DCs were obtained from monocytes from whole peripheral blood of healthy volunteer donors and from those infected with *L. infantum* or *L. braziliensis* for 24 h. We observed similar rates of infection (around 40%) as well as parasite burden for both *Leishmania* species. Concerning surface molecules, we observed that both parasites induced CD86 expression when DCs were infected for 24 h. On the other hand, we detected a lower surface expression of CD209 in the presence of both *L. braziliensis* and *L. infantum*, but only the last one promoted the survival of DCs after 24 h. Therefore, DCs infected by both *Leishmania* species showed a higher expression of CD86 and a decrease of CD209 expression, suggesting that both enter DCs through CD209 molecule. However, only *L. infantum* had the ability to inhibit DC apoptotic death, as an evasion mechanism that enables its spreading to organs like bone marrow and liver. Lastly, *L. braziliensis* was more silent parasite, once it did not inhibit DC apoptosis in our *in vitro* model.

Keywords: apoptosis, dendritic cells, *Leishmania infantum*, *Leishmania braziliensis*, CD209

INTRODUCTION

Leishmaniasis is a vector-borne disease that commits millions of people around the world. In 2013, around 215,000 new cases were reported in the world. Of these, around 21,000 were reported in Brazil (1). Around 0.2–0.4 and 0.7–1.2 million visceral leishmaniasis (VL) and cutaneous leishmaniasis (CL), respectively, occur each year. Over 90% of new cases of VL occur in six countries all over the world, including Brazil. About 95% of CL cases occur in the Americas, the Mediterranean basin, and the Middle East and Central Asia (2).

In the sandfly, the flagellated motile forms of *Leishmania* spp. called promastigotes progress through several morphological stages of differentiation, regulating the vector midgut environment (3). Finally, it becomes the non-dividing, infectious metacyclic promastigotes that are transmitted during a sandfly bite, when they are able to infect or be phagocyted by professional phagocytes as macrophages (4) and dendritic cells (DCs) (5). The parasite inside host cells becomes amastigote, a stage without an externalized flagellum that is capable of multiplication in antigen-presenting cells (6). CL is the most common clinical form of leishmaniasis and causes localized skin lesions, especially in arms and legs. In the New World, *Leishmania braziliensis* is able to cause from localized self-limited lesions to tissue destructive mucosal forms (7) that can worsen with age (8). On the other hand, visceral forms are caused by *Leishmania infantum* (9), and the disease, characterized by fever, weight loss, enlargement of the spleen and liver, and anemia, is fatal if left untreated (10).

Host–parasite interactions during innate immune responses determine the fate of adaptive immunity, contributing to healing or parasite persistence in leishmaniasis (11). DCs are professional antigen-presenting cells that interact with pathogens in peripheral tissues and stimulate T lymphocytes after migration to secondary lymphoid organs (12). In the periphery, DCs are in an immature state, with high potential to perform phagocytosis through many receptors that recognize pathogen-associated molecular patterns, as DC-SIGN (CD209) (13–15). Toll-like receptors (TLRs) are also involved in innate response to *Leishmania* parasites. During murine *Leishmania major* infection, data in literature showed that TLR9 was required for the induction of IL-12 in bone marrow-derived DCs (BMDCs) by intact *L. major* parasites or *L. major* DNA. This IL-12 production was essential for early interferon-gamma expression and NK cell activation (16). After pathogen internalization, DC is able to migrate from periphery to secondary tissues, rising MHC expression as well as other co-stimulatory molecules CD86 and CD83. After all these events, DCs are able to properly perform antigen presentation to T cells and determinate the fate of adaptive immune response (17). DCs can also become tolerogenic cells, as observed in the physiologic regulation of apoptosis (18). When *L. braziliensis* were in contact with murine CD11c$^+$ DCs, they were able to produce high levels of IL-12p70 as well as stimulate a significant expression of CD40 and CD83 in the surface of these DCs (19). Another study from the literature, working with mice BMDCs, showed that *L. infantum* could infect and survive inside these cells. Besides, they observed that *L. infantum* promastigotes were not able to upregulate CD40 and CD86 surface expression. The authors also observed that *L. infantum* was able to induce some level of IL-12p40 and IL-10, with no differences in TNF-α levels (20). Another group showed that bystander BMDCs from Balb/c mice increased IL-12p40 and expressed more CD40, CD86, and MHC class II in the cell surface than infected or not exposed cells. These bystander DCs induced a protective CD4$^+$ IFN-γ T cells response, while *L. infantum*-infected DCs polarizing to T-bet+IFN-γ+IL-10+ double producer T cells phenotype (21). On the other hand, human DCs infected with *L. major* showed an increase of HLA-DR, CD86, and CD40. When *L. major*-infected DCs were cocultured with T lymphocytes and treated with anti-CD40 ligand (CD40L), IL-12p70 and IFN-γ production decreased, concluding that IL-12p70 and IFN-γ production are CD40L-dependent (22). When CD86 (B7-2)$^{-/-}$ mice were infected with *L. major*, they presented a resistance, differently CD80 (B7-1)$^{-/-}$, and wild-type Balb/c mice maintained its susceptibility. Moreover, CD86$^{-/-}$ produced more IL-4 than wild-type mice, suggesting that CD86 induced a Th2 response (23). Infection of BALB/c mice by *Leishmania amazonensis* led to higher accumulation of Langerhans cells, and CD4$^+$ and CD8$^+$ T cells were found that produced IL-4 and IL-10. Nevertheless, *L. braziliensis* infection induced dermal DCs accumulation, increased effectors, and activated memory CD4$^+$ T cells and IL-4, IL-10, IFN-γ production by CD4$^+$ and CD8$^+$ T cells (24).

Many pathogens alter DC biology, favoring its persistence in the infected host. Data in literature showed that *L. amazonensis* is able to inhibit human DC differentiation from monocytes (25) and several intracellular signaling pathways (26), altering DC biology and function. Data from murine models of leishmaniasis show that inhibitory pathways are also involved in disease pathogenesis. One example is the OX40L–OX40 pathway that enhances Th2 responses in *L. major*-infected mice (27). Working with *Ox40l*$^{-/-}$ mice, the authors observed that they were very susceptible to *L. major* and *Leishmania mexicana*. Interestingly, only lymphnode cells from *L. major Ox40l*$^{-/-}$ mice produced less IL-4 and IL-10 than *Ox40l*$^{+/+}$. In this way, this pathway is relevant to Th2 development only in the context of *L. major* infection, but it does not alter *L. major* outcome of infection (28, 29). Other surface receptors, the programmed death ligand 1 (PD-L1) and 2 (PD-L2), were studied in susceptible mice infected with *L. mexicana*. PD-L1 knockout mouse demonstrated resistance, decrease of lesion size, as well as parasitic load and IL-4 production after infection. Although PD-L2 knockout mouse showed increase of lesion size, parasitic load, and antibodies production, no difference on IFN-γ and IL-4 production was observed. Both receptors play different roles in response to *L. mexicana* (30).

Another way that pathogens have to adapt to the host is to alter cell death. It is well known that *Mycobacterium tuberculosis* induces cell death through apoptosis, but this event favors antigen presentation (31). Moreover, pathogens as *Leishmania* delay cell death as a way to survive inside host cell. For example, apoptosis of monocyte-derived dendritic cells (moDCs) induced by treatment with camptothecin was downregulated by infection with *L. mexicana* amastigotes, detected by annexin V binding to phosphatidylserine (32).

It is not clear how the regulation of human DC biology is affected in different ways by species of *Leishmania*. In this way, the aim of this study is to analyze the expression of surface molecules relevant to antigen processing and presentation as well as DCs survival after interaction with *L. infantum* or *L. braziliensis*.

MATERIALS AND METHODS

Parasites

Leishmania infantum (MHOM/BR/1974/PP75) and *L. braziliensis* (MHOM/BR/01/BA788) promastigotes were maintained in Schneider's medium (SIGMA) with 20% of calf fetal serum (GIBCO) and gentamicin (50 μm/mL). *Leishmania* stationary-phase promastigotes were quantified in Neubauer chamber. After counting, promastigotes were harvested from culture bottles, washed three times with cold PBS (800 g for 10 min), and adjusted in RPMI medium to be added in DC culture.

Dendritic Cell Culture

Human DCs were differentiated from monocytes. Briefly, venous blood was collected from volunteer healthy donors ($n = 8$), and peripheral blood mononuclear cells (PBMC) were obtained by passage over a Ficoll gradient (GE Healthcare). Cells were harvested, washed, and stained with antibodies, anti-CD14, conjugated with microbeads (Miltenyi Biotec). Stained cells (monocytes) were purified after positive selection in a magnetic field. Monocytes were then counted and cultivated in RPMI 1640 medium supplemented with 2 mM L-glutamine, 100 U/mL penicillin, 100 mg/mL streptomycin (GIBCO), IL-4 (800 IU/mL), and GM-CSF (50 μg/mL) (both from PeproTech) with 10% of fetal serum bovine (GIBCO) in 24-wells plates (5×10^5 cells/wells) for 7 days at 37°C and 5% CO_2. New medium (200 μL) supplemented with cytokines was added on days 3 and 6 of the culture. On day 7, DCs were infected (1 DC:10 parasites), cultivated in 24-wells plates for 24 h at 37°C and 5% CO_2, harvested, and characterized by flow cytometry (FACS Verse BD Biosciences). All experimental conditions and measurements were performed with the same donors.

Flow Cytometry and Antibodies

Dendritic cells were cocultured with *Leishmania* species for 24 h, and control cells were harvested and washed with PBS. Cells were then resuspended in FACS buffer (5×10^6 cells/mL) and incubated at 4°C for 20 min. The cells were stained with CD1a FITC-conjugated (clone HI149), HLA-DR PE-conjugated (clone LN3), CD86 PE-Cy5-conjugated (clone IT2-2), and CD209 PE-conjugated (clone eB-h209) (all eBioscience) and incubated for 30 min at 4°C. Finally, cells were washed, resuspended in FACS buffer, and acquired on a flow cytometer. For cell death experiments, after infection time, the cells were washed and resuspended in 195 μL of binding buffer to each $2–5 \times 10^5$ cells, added 5 μL of annexin V, and incubated for 10 min at room temperature. The cells were washed with PBS 1×, resuspended in 190 μL of binding buffer, added 10 μL propidium iodide (PI) (annexin V and propidium iodide kit, eBioscience), and acquired on a flow cytometer. Stained cells were acquired on a Verse flow cytometer (BD Bioscience) and analyzed using FlowJo Software (Tree Star, Inc.).

Cytokine Assay

Dendritic cells were infected with both *Leishmania* species. After 24 h of infection, supernatant was collected and level of TNF-α was measured by ELISA. TNF-α was quantified (test detection range from 20 to 1000 pg/mL) with purified antihuman TNF-α, antihuman TNF-α biotin, and streptavidin–alkaline phosphatase, according to the instruction of suppliers (Novex, Life Technologies, Invitrogen). Absorbance was measured and analyzed with the program SoftMax Pro (Molecular Devices).

Ethical Statement

Human blood samples were collected after the signature of an informed consent signed by all volunteers, and the project was approved by The Ethical Committee for Human Beings from the Medicine Faculty of University of Brasilia (approval no. 072/2009). Samples were collected by venous puncture by a trained and specialized laboratory technician in the Universidade de Brasília.

Statistical Analysis

The statistical analysis was conducted using GraphPad Prism Software. Samples were tested by Shapiro–Wilk normality test, and the significance of the results was calculated using parametrical paired *t* test, and a p-value of <0.05 was considered significant.

RESULTS

L. braziliensis- or *L. infantum*-Exposed Dendritic Cells Upregulate CD86 and Downregulate CD209 Expression

After 24 h, the parasite load of DCs was accessed by optic microscopy, and we observed 40.67 ± 5.8% *L. infantum* (Li)-infected DCs and 42.13 ± 3.1% *L. braziliensis* (Lb)-infected DCs (**Figure 1A**). The amastigotes number per 100 cells was 249.8 ± 44.23 amastigotes in *L. infantum* (Li)-infected DCs and 185.3 ± 32.73 in

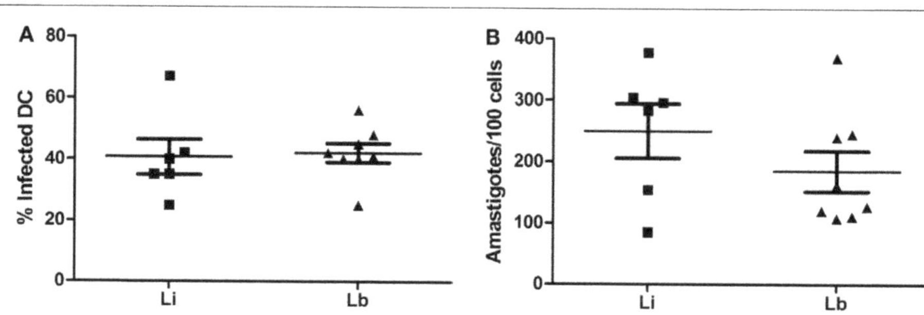

FIGURE 1 | Dendritic cells' infection by *L. infantum* (Li) or *L. braziliensis* (Lb) – immature DCs were infected in a rate of 10 *Leishmania* to 1 DC. Infection after 24 h, in hematoxylin–eosin (HE)-stained slides. Median ± SD. Each point represents one donor. *$p < 0.01$. **(A)** Percentage of infected DCs. **(B)** Amastigotes per 100 cells.

L. braziliensis (Lb)-infected cells (**Figure 1B**). Later, we decided to observe the co-stimulatory and surface molecules expression by DCs after the exposure to *L. infantum* or *L. braziliensis*. Then, we stained the cultured DCs with medium or each parasites species with anti-CD1a, anti-HLA-DR, anti-CD86, and anti-CD209 antibodies. The cells were gated by granularity and size, and the gated cells were further analyzed for expression of CD1a/HLA-DR/CD86/CD209 surface molecules (**Figure 2**). Control DCs, differentiated with media only (M), showed 56.53 ± 8.2% of CD1a expression. This was very similar in DCs exposed to *L. infantum* (60.40 ± 8.1%) as well as exposed to *L. braziliensis* (57.8 ± 8.3%) (**Figure 3A**).

In the same way, we observed a consistent higher expression of HLA-DR in control cells (73.81 ± 5.55%)-, in *L. infantum* (68.27 ± 4.8%)-, and *L. braziliensis* (80.89 ± 2.7%)-exposed DCs, with no significant differences between the groups (**Figure 3B**).

However, both *Leishmania* were able to induce a significant raise in CD86 expression. We observed that CD86 expression was 73.23 ± 5.4% in control cells and increased to 78.16 ± 4.3% in the presence of *L. infantum* and to 92.24 ± 1.9% in the presence of *L. braziliensis* (**Figure 3C**). Moreover, this increase was significantly higher in *L. braziliensis*-infected DCs than in *L. infantum*-infected DCs (**Figure 3C**).

On the other hand, we observed that both *Leishmania* were able to inhibit significantly CD209 expression. Its expression was 80.09 ± 6.8% in control cells, while in the presence of *L. infantum*, it was down modulated to 62.17 ± 9.88%. The presence of *L. braziliensis* also led to a lower CD209 expression (75.36 ± 7.3%) (**Figure 3D**). This decrease was significantly lower in *L. infantum*-infected DCs than *L. braziliensis*-infected DCs (**Figure 3D**).

When we analyzed the mean intensity of fluorescence (MFI) of these molecules, we observed the same effects that we observed in the percentage of expression. The MFI was similar in all experimental conditions for CD1a and HLA-DR (**Figures 4A,B**). On the other hand, we observed a significantly higher CD86 MFI induced by *L. braziliensis* (2060 ± 351.9), but no significant difference was found in the presence of *L. infantum* (1537 ± 169.4) when compared to control cells (1227 ± 152.2) (**Figure 4C**). Also, as we observed in surface expression, the CD209 MFI was significantly lower in the presence of *L. infantum* (856.1 ± 72.8) or *L. braziliensis* (1033 ± 112.6), compared to control cells (1127 ± 116.7) (**Figure 4D**).

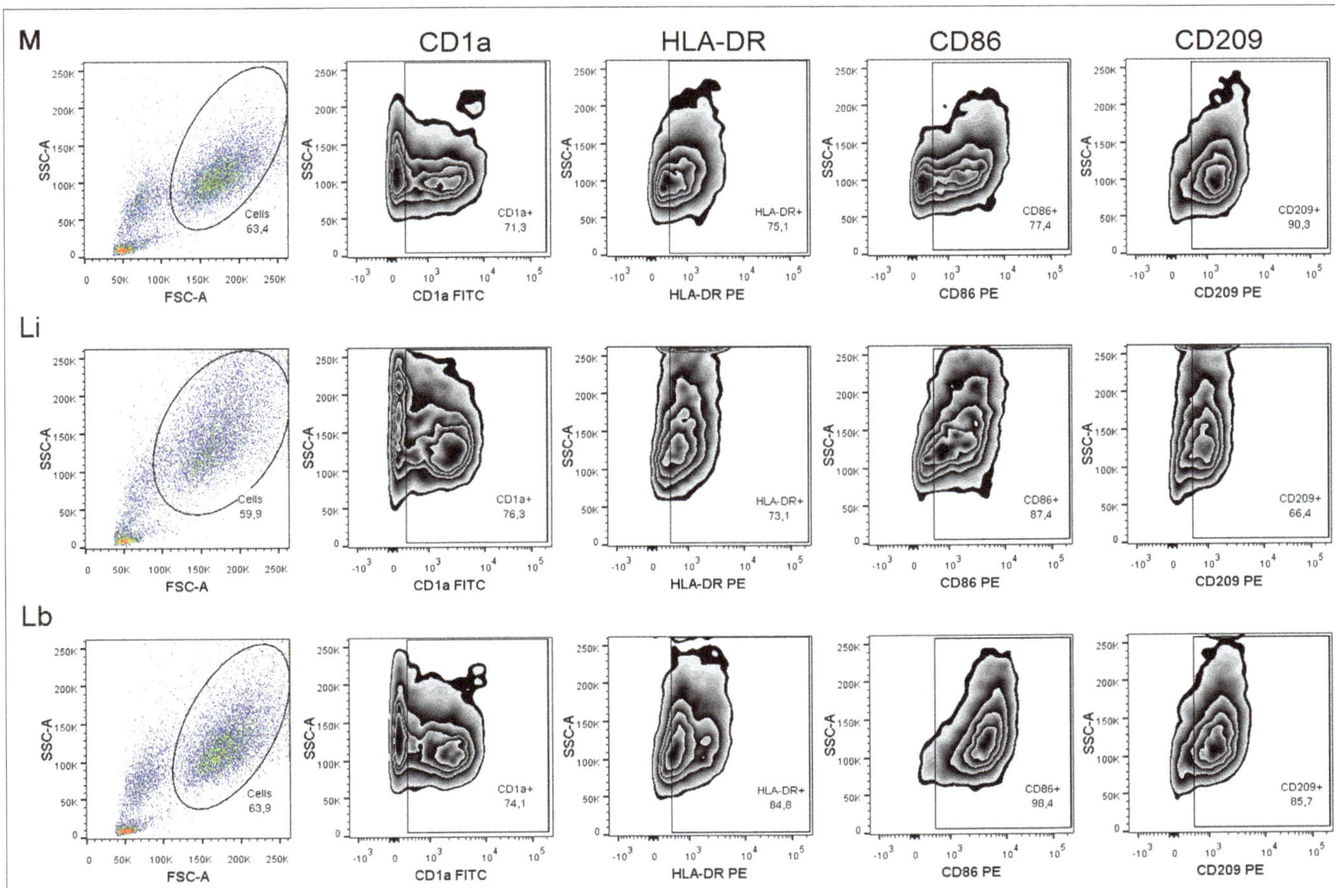

FIGURE 2 | Gating strategy to analyze DCs' regulation by *Leishmania* parasites – DCs in control and infected conditions were gated by granularity and size and further analyzed for expression of CD1a/HLA-DR/CD86/CD209 surface molecules. M, medium, Li, *Leishmania infantum*, Lb, *Leishmania braziliensis*.

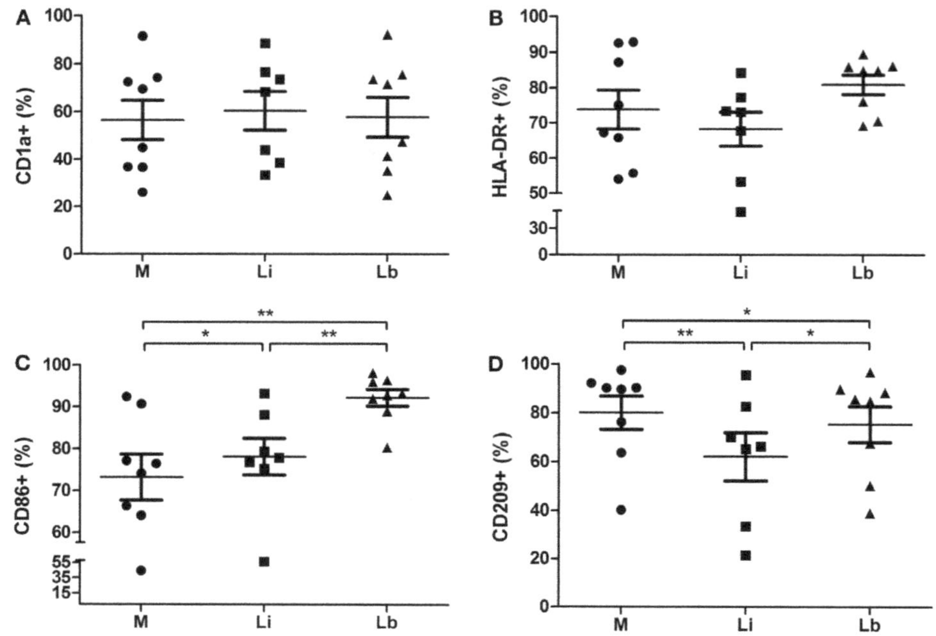

FIGURE 3 | *L. braziliensis*- or *L. infantum*-exposed dendritic cells upregulate CD86 and downregulate CD209 expression – flow cytometry analysis of surface molecule expression in immature DCs differentiated from human monocytes with cytokine-conditioned media (M) or conditioned media in the presence of viable *L. infantum* (Li) or *L. braziliensis* (Lb). CD1a **(A)**, HLA-DR **(B)**, CD86 **(C)**, and CD209 **(D)**. Median ± SD. Each point represents one donor. $^{*}p < 0.05$, $^{**}p < 0.01$.

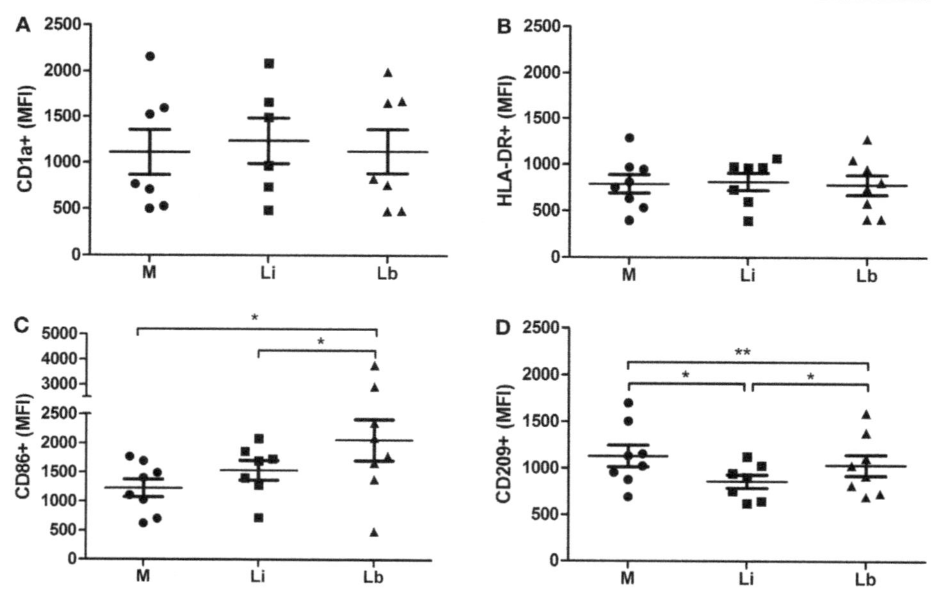

FIGURE 4 | *L. braziliensis*-exposed DCs increase the mean of fluorescence intensity (MFI) of CD86 and decrease CD209 – flow cytometry analyzes of the MFI in immature DCs differentiated from human monocytes with cytokine-conditioned media (M) or conditioned media in the presence of viable *L. infantum* (Li) or *L. braziliensis* (Lb). CD1a **(A)**, HLA-DR **(B)**, CD86 **(C)**, and CD209 **(D)**. Median ± SD. Each point represents one donor. $^{*}p < 0.05$, $^{**}p < 0.01$.

Exposure to *L. infantum* but Not *L. braziliensis* Decreases the Dendritic Cells' Cellular Death

Next, we decided to evaluate if these two *Leishmania* species were able to induce or not cell death of DCs. To do so, after a coculture of the DCs with the two parasite species, we stained the cells with annexin V and PI (**Figure 5A**). We observed no significant differences between DCs only and *L. braziliensis*-exposed DCs in the annexin V+PI− and annexin V+PI+ populations (**Figures 5B,C**, respectively). Nevertheless, the cell population that was annexin V+PI− population significantly decreased in *L. infantum*-exposed DCs, from 5.7 ± 1.0% in control cells to 2.9 ± 0.6%, that is a 50.8% decrease in DC death, showing that the *L. infantum* is able to inhibit cellular death of DCs (**Figure 5B**). However, no significant decrease was observed in the annexin V+PI+ population, 11.36 ± 2% in control cells and 8.3 ± 2.4% in *L. infantum*-exposed DCs (**Figure 5C**).

L. infantum- and *L. braziliensis*-Exposed Dendritic Cells Produced TNF-α

Coculture with *L. infantum* or *L. braziliensis* triggered a significant secretion of TNF-α by DCs. Control cells produced 17.6 ± 4.4 pg/mL, while DCs cocultured with *L. infantum* induced 61.9 ± 10.4 pg/mL, a 3.5-fold significant increase in this cytokine secretion. On the other hand, *L. braziliensis* stimulated significantly even more TNF-α secretion (133.2 ± 43.7 pg/mL), almost an eightfold increase (**Figure 6**).

DISCUSSION

Many data in literature show the relevant role of DCs in diverse pathogen–host interactions, especially in the initial events of innate immunity. These initial events lead the course of adaptive response (33). For a better understanding of *Leishmania* and infected host regulation, we initially cocultured DCs with stationary non-opsonized *L. braziliensis* and *L. infantum* promastigotes for 24 h. The infection rate was similar in our experiments between the two *Leishmania* species (around 40%), and we found no significant difference of internalized parasites number. Concerning infection data, non-opsonized *L. mexicana* promastigotes presented higher phagocytosis than opsonized promastigotes or amastigotes by human moDCs after 3 h. Six hours later, opsonized promastigotes showed higher phagocytosis than non-opsonized promastigotes and amastigotes, but no difference was observed after 24 h of infection (5). Infection of human DCs with *L. amazonensis* showed a similar rate of infection, around 45%, and a parasite burden median of six amastigotes per DC (25).

We observed that both *L. braziliensis* and *L. infantum* were able to induce an increase in CD86 expression and also caused a decrease in CD209 (DC-SIGN) expression in human DCs. A study with *L. amazonensis* showed that the parasite modulates the co-stimulatory molecules expression during the differentiation of human moDCs, affecting the mixed leukocyte reaction and the specific T lymphocytes responses. Similar to our data, *L. amazonensis* also caused an increase in CD86 expression after a 24-h parasite DCs contact (25). On the other hand, murine

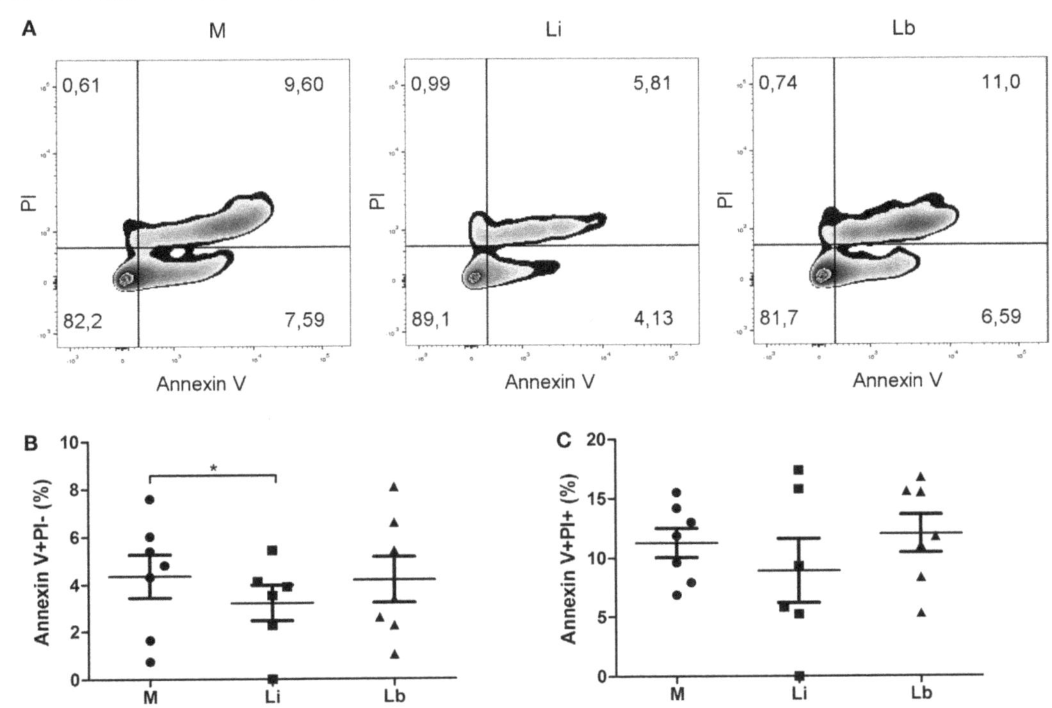

FIGURE 5 | *L. infantum* delayed the cellular death of dendritic cells – flow cytometry gating strategy (A) to perform analyses of annexin V and propidium iodide (PI) staining of control DCs (M) or treated with viable *L. infantum* (Li) or *L. braziliensis* (Lb). Annexin V positive cells **(B)** and annexin V and PI positive cells **(C)**. Median ± SD. Each point represents one donor. *$p < 0.05$, **$p < 0.01$.

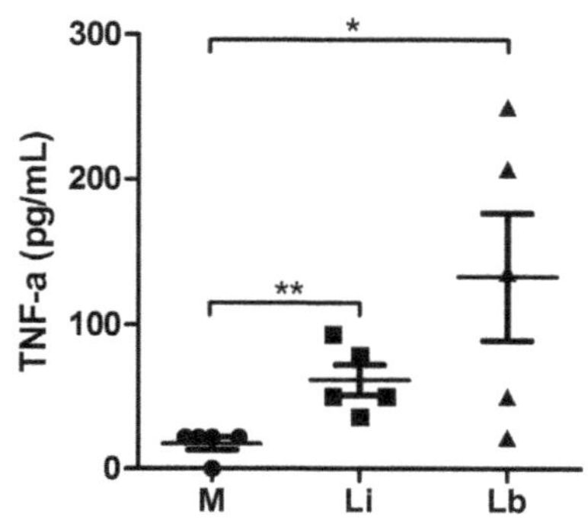

FIGURE 6 | *L. braziliensis* induced TNF-α secretion on immature DCs – cytokine levels measured on culture supernatants after 24 h of infection. Control DCs were cultured in cytokine-conditioned media only or treated with viable *L. infantum* or *L. braziliensis* parasites. Median ± SD. Each point represents one donor. $^*p < 0.05$, $^{**}p < 0.01$.

mature DCs infected with *L. amazonensis* amastigotes presented a decreased antigen presentation, CD40 and CD83 expression, and also a reduced $CD4^+$ T cells priming (34). Contreras et al. (35), showed that *L. mexicana* infection also interfered in the DC maturation process, decreasing co-stimulatory molecules expression and antigen presentation, injuring the presentation to T cells by human DCs. Macrophages cultured with peripheral blood leukocytes (PBL) exhibited CD40 and CD86 expression in the absence of *L. major*, but their expression levels were higher in the presence of the parasite. After blocking CD80, CD86, both, or CD40, macrophages cultured with PBL and *L. major* produced less IFN-γ, IL-5, and IL-12, showing that these co-stimulatory pathways were important to the development of an anti-*Leishmania*-efficient immune response (36). On the other hand, a study performed with VL patients showed that the subset of inflammatory monocytes $CD14^+CD16^+$ remained the same as in the control group. Similarly, the population of $CD54^+HLA\text{-}DR^+$ monocytes was significantly downregulated during active disease. Finally, they observed an increase in CD80 expression level, but a decreased CD86 expression (37). Concerning infection with *L. braziliensis*, data from literature showed that $CD14^+$ monocytes of peripheral blood from CL patients had a decreased expression of CD80 and CD86 following culture with media only or after restimulation with *Leishmania* antigen (38). It seems that monocytes and DCs have different roles in the regulation leishmaniasis. Monocytes seem to have a role in regulating the lesion site during CL pathogenesis, and the authors mentioned before Vieira et al. (38) observed a diminished expression of B7 molecules. In our model, we worked with moDCs from healthy donors' peripheral blood. In this way, it is possible that in these initial interactions, once our experiments were performed after a 24-h infection with *Leishmania* parasites, these DCs regulate CD86 expression positively, being able to activate naive lymphocytes. On the other hand, the effects seem to be opposite for monocytes that migrate to lesion sites, once in patients with CL it is observed a negative regulation of CD86 (38).

Concerning CD209 expression, the decrease of this surface molecule was also observed in *L. major*- and *L. donovani*-infected human DCs (39). It is well established that the receptor CD209 can be used for internalizing microrganisms as parasites (40). In this way, our data are in accordance with data in the literature, suggesting that *L. infantum* and *L. braziliensis* attach to CD209 to access host DCs, which would explain the decrease in CD209 in the surface, as it could be internalized. Nevertheless, CD209 was involved in the phagocytosis of *L. mexicana* promastigotes after 3 h, but not after 6 or 24 h (5). Excreted or secreted recombinant proteins of *L. infantum* interfered in the differentiation of DCs, decreasing the HLA-DR expression but increasing the CD86 expression (41). We observed the same effect concerning CD86, but we observed no significant differences in HLA-DR surface expression caused by *L. infantum* or *L. braziliensis* in our work. Regarding CD86 and CD209 expression, we found a higher expression of CD86 in the presence of *L. braziliensis* than in the presence of *L. infantum*; however, the decrease in CD209 expression was greater in cells infected with *L. infantum* than in *L. braziliensis*-infected ones. Though, the rates of infection as well as the number of internalized amastigotes were similar between both the species of *Leishmania*. This can be explained by the fact that DCs have other recognition receptors that are able to recognize and be involved in *Leishmania* internalization, which were not investigated in this work. We can mention the mannose–fucose receptor, which is present in DCs that can recognize lipophosphoglycan (LPG), GP63, and proteophosphoglicans (PPG) present in the membrane of *Leishmania* species (42, 43). This pathway could explain the DCs' infection rate by *L. braziliensis* and the number of amastigotes to be similar to the *L. infantum*-infection. However, macrophages of B6 mice mannose receptor (MR) knockout showed an increase of parasite load after infection with *L. infantum*. This group showed that MR and Dectin-1 signaling pathways are essential to trigger the oxidative burst in macrophages infected with *L. infantum*, enabling parasite control (44).

Many data in literature showed the relevance of cytokines regulation in leishmaniasis pathogenesis. The presence of *L. amazonensis* during the differentiation of human DC inhibited IL-6 and IL-10 secretion. Besides, these DCs cocultured with *L. amazonensis*, when in contact with autologous lymphocytes, caused a lower secretion of IFN-γ (25). Moreover, amastigotes of *L. amazonensis* suppressed IL-12+p40 and IL-10 production by murine DCs (34). However, we found a higher release of TNF-α after coculture of DCs and *L. braziliensis* or *L. infantum*. The excreted or secreted recombinant proteins of *L. infantum* also induced TNF-α production (41), as we saw for both *Leishmania* species in this work. Studies with fluorescent *L. braziliensis* parasites allowed the observation that the TNF-α production derived from infected DCs, but not from bystander DCs, had contact with *L. braziliensis* in the medium but were not infected. Moreover, soluble parasite products and the TNF-α released by infected DCs provided a more efficient antigen presentation by DCs (45). Data from literature evaluated TNF-α production from PBMC of patients and healthy individuals after stimulation with soluble *L. braziliensis* antigens. The results showed a range in the SD, as expected for human individuals. They showed that healthy donors produced 48.6 ± 77.18 pg/mL of TNF-α (46). Another study that compared PBMC responses from patients with CL and mucosal leishmaniasis (ML), after stimulation with *L. braziliensis* soluble antigen, also detected a wide range of TNF-α levels. In CL, TNF-α levels ranged from 0 to 7440 pg/mL, while in ML patients from 892 to 9173 pg/mL (47). These differences in TNF levels are expected and may exist due to the genetic constitution of the host. On the other hand, data from literature that analyzed immune responses from patients with active VL detected some similarities among VL patients and healthy individuals, concerning cytokines regulation. Analysis *ex vivo* of patient's cells with active VL showed the production of high levels of anti-inflammatory cytokines and lower TNF levels, the last ones very similar to healthy controls (37). Another study with patients with active VL due to *L. infantum* also showed lower TNF-α levels, very similar to healthy controls (48). These observations are similar to our results in which we could not observe the individual variations in healthy donors' DCs infected with *L. infantum*. Another possibility is that even with similar rates of infection and parasites per cell, our results reflect the differences cited before concerning the immunogenicity of *L. braziliensis* and *L. infantum*.

We observed that *L. infantum* caused an inhibition of DC apoptosis. The same phenomenon was not observed for *L. braziliensis*. This demonstrates that possibly only *L. infantum* was able to stimulate the development of an environment adequate for the multiplication inside the cells and that favors a possible spread to other organs as bone marrow and liver. This surviving of DC was also seen in *L. mexicana* infection when apoptosis was induced by camptothecin (49). Indeed, DCs infected with *L. mexicana* amastigotes decreased the phosphorylation of MAP kinase p38 and JNK, causing a decreased DNA fragmentation in the camptothecin stimulated DCs. *L. mexicana* amastigotes activated antiapoptotic pathways, such as PI3K and AKT, allowing the inhibition of infected DCs' cell death (50). The opposite effect was observed with the bacteria *Brucella abortus* that induced apoptosis and necrosis of murine DCs. This apoptosis regulation was performed by caspase-2 in mouse model (51).

A very elegant paper showed that Dectin-1, MR, and DC-SIGN homolog SIGNR3 are able to recognize *L. infantum*, but only DC-SIGN (CD209) and MR triggered pro-IL1 beta processing in a caspase-1-dependent way, being crucial for microbicidal activity of macrophages. On the other hand, signaling through SIGNR3 seems to favor parasite survival because of its modulation of inflammasome activation (44). Once we found a possible correlation of CD209 and cell death, perhaps the internalization of *L. infantum* by CD209 in human DCs could also be interfering in the activation of caspase-1, causing the survival of DCs differently from the data observed on macrophages. On the other hand, *L. braziliensis* seems to not interfere in this pathway of cell death regulation, once we did not observe differences concerning DC survival.

In this way, we can conclude that both *L. infantum* and *L. braziliensis* possibly enter DCs through DC-SIGN, causing a positive regulation on CD86 expression as well as on TNF-α production after this initial interaction. Nevertheless, only *L. infantum* induced a survival in human DCs, probably favoring its establishment and spread in the host, differently from *L. braziliensis* that seems to be more silent in these initial events concerning DC survival. This work shed light in the differences between these two parasites and their interactions with human DCs and opens the field to study the development of intracellular signaling pathways responsible for these phenomena.

AUTHOR CONTRIBUTIONS

SF and CF: conceived and designed the experiments. SF, TJ, LF, DB, and CF: performed the experiments. SF, TJ, and CF: analyzed the data. SF, JS, and CF: contributed reagents/materials/analysis tools. SF and CF: wrote the paper.

REFERENCES

1. WHO. *Accelerating Work to Overcome the Global Impact of Neglected Tropical*. Geneva: WHO (2012).
2. Alvar J, Vélez D, Bern C, Herrero M, Desjeux P, Cano J, et al. Leishmaniasis worldwide and global estimates of its incidence. *PLoS One* (2012) 7:e35671. doi:10.1371/journal.pone.0035671
3. Santos VC, Vale VF, Silva SM, Nascimento AA, Saab NA, Soares RP, et al. Host modulation by a parasite: how *Leishmania infantum* modifies the intestinal environment of *Lutzomyia longipalpis* to favor its development. *PLoS One* (2014) 9:e111241. doi:10.1371/journal.pone.0111241
4. Ramos PK, Brito MV, Silveira FT, Salgado CG, De Souza W, Picanço-Diniz CW, et al. In vitro cytokines profile and ultrastructural changes of microglia and macrophages following interaction with *Leishmania*. *Parasitology* (2014) 141:1052–63. doi:10.1017/S0031182014000274
5. Argueta-Donohué J, Wilkins-Rodríguez AA, Aguirre-García M, Gutiérrez-Kobeh L. Differential phagocytosis of *Leishmania mexicana* promastigotes and amastigotes by monocyte-derived dendritic cells. *Microbiol Immunol* (2015). 60:369–81. doi:10.1111/1348-0421.12325
6. Prina E, Abdi S, Lebastard M, Perret E, Winter N, Antoine J. Dendritic cells as host cells for the promastigote and amastigote stages of *Leishmania amazonensis*: the role of opsonins in parasite uptake and dendritic cell maturation. *J Cell Sci* (2004) 117:315–25. doi:10.1242/jcs.00860
7. Barral A, Barral-Netto M, Almeida R, de Jesus AR, Grimaldi Júnior G, Netto EM, et al. Lymphadenopathy associated with *Leishmania braziliensis* cutaneous infection. *Am J Trop Med Hyg* (1992) 47:587–92.
8. Carvalho AM, Amorim CF, Barbosa JL, Lago AS, Carvalho EM. Age modifies the immunologic response and clinical presentation of American tegumentary leishmaniasis. *Am J Trop Med Hyg* (2015) 92:1173–7. doi:10.4269/ajtmh.14-0631
9. Ready PD. Epidemiology of visceral leishmaniasis. *Clin Epidemiol* (2014) 6:147–54. doi:10.2147/CLEP.S44267
10. Bhattacharya SK, Dash AP. Treatment of visceral leishmaniasis: options and choice. *Lancet Infect Dis* (2016) 16:142–3. doi:10.1016/S1473-3099(15)00528-9
11. Gollob KJ, Viana AG, Dutra WO. Immunoregulation in human American leishmaniasis: balancing pathology and protection. *Parasite Immunol* (2014) 36:367–76. doi:10.1111/pim.12100

12. Cools N, Ponsaerts P, Van Tendeloo VF, Berneman ZN. Balancing between immunity and tolerance: an interplay between dendritic cells, regulatory T cells, and effector T cells. *J Leukoc Biol* (2007) 82:1365–74. doi:10.1189/jlb.0307166
13. Colmenares M, Puig-Kröger A, Pello OM, Corbí AL, Rivas L. Dendritic cell (DC)-specific intercellular adhesion molecule 3 (ICAM-3)-grabbing nonintegrin (DC-SIGN, CD209), a C-type surface lectin in human DCs, is a receptor for *Leishmania amastigotes*. *J Biol Chem* (2002) 277:36766–9. doi:10.1074/jbc.M205270200
14. Vannberg FO, Chapman SJ, Khor CC, Tosh K, Floyd S, Jackson-Sillah D, et al. CD209 genetic polymorphism and tuberculosis disease. *PLoS One* (2008) 3:e1388. doi:10.1371/journal.pone.0001388
15. Jin W, Li C, Du T, Hu K, Huang X, Hu Q. DC-SIGN plays a stronger role than DCIR in mediating HIV-1 capture and transfer. *Virology* (2014) 458-459:83–92. doi:10.1016/j.virol.2014.04.016
16. Liese J, Schleicher U, Bogdan C. TLR9 signaling is essential for the innate NK cell response in murine cutaneous leishmaniasis. *Eur J Immunol* (2007) 37:3424–34. doi:10.1002/eji.200737182
17. Dalod M, Chelbi R, Malissen B, Lawrence T. Dendritic cell maturation: functional specialization through signaling specificity and transcriptional programming. *EMBO J* (2014) 33:1104–16. doi:10.1002/embj.201488027
18. Steinman RM, Turley S, Mellman I, Inaba K. The induction of tolerance by dendritic cells that have captured apoptotic cells. *J Exp Med* (2000) 191:411–6. doi:10.1084/jem.191.3.411
19. Vargas-Inchaustegui DA, Xin L, Soong L. *Leishmania braziliensis* infection induces dendritic cell activation, ISG15 transcription, and the generation of protective immune responses. *J Immunol* (2008) 180:7537–45. doi:10.4049/jimmunol.180.11.7537
20. Neves BM, Silvestre R, Resende M, Ouaissi A, Cunha J, Tavares J, et al. Activation of phosphatidylinositol 3-kinase/Akt and impairment of nuclear factor-kappaB: molecular mechanisms behind the arrested maturation/activation state of *Leishmania infantum*-infected dendritic cells. *Am J Pathol* (2010) 177:2898–911. doi:10.2353/ajpath.2010.100367
21. Resende M, Moreira D, Augusto J, Cunha J, Neves B, Cruz MT, et al. *Leishmania*-infected MHC class II high dendritic cells polarize CD4+ T cells toward a nonprotective T-bet+ IFN-γ+ IL-10+ phenotype. *J Immunol* (2013) 191:262–73. doi:10.4049/jimmunol.1203518
22. Marovich MA, McDowell MA, Thomas EK, Nutman TB. IL-12p70 production by *Leishmania major*-harboring human dendritic cells is a CD40/CD40 ligand-dependent process. *J Immunol* (2000) 164:5858–65. doi:10.4049/jimmunol.164.11.5858
23. Brown JA, Greenwald RJ, Scott S, Schweitzer AN, Satoskar AR, Chung C, et al. T helper differentiation in resistant and susceptible B7-deficient mice infected with *Leishmania major*. *Eur J Immunol* (2002) 32:1764–72. doi:10.1002/1521-4141(200206)32:6<1764::AID-IMMU1764>3.0.CO;2-V
24. Carvalho AK, Carvalho K, Passero LF, Sousa MG, da Matta VL, Gomes CM, et al. Differential recruitment of dendritic cells subsets to lymph nodes correlates with a protective or permissive T-cell response during *Leishmania (Viannia) braziliensis* or *Leishmania* (*Leishmania*) *amazonensis* infection. *Mediators Inflamm* (2016) 2016:7068287. doi:10.1155/2016/7068287
25. Favali C, Tavares N, Clarêncio J, Barral A, Barral-Netto M, Brodskyn C. *Leishmania amazonensis* infection impairs differentiation and function of human dendritic cells. *J Leukoc Biol* (2007) 82:1401–6. doi:10.1189/jlb.0307187
26. Soong L. Modulation of dendritic cell function by *Leishmania* parasites. *J Immunol* (2008) 180:4355–60. doi:10.4049/jimmunol.180.7.4355
27. Ishii N, Ndhlovu LC, Murata K, Sato T, Kamanaka M, Sugamura K. OX40 (CD134) and OX40 ligand interaction plays an adjuvant role during in vivo Th2 responses. *Eur J Immunol* (2003) 33:2372–81. doi:10.1002/eji.200324031
28. Akiba H, Miyahira Y, Atsuta M, Takeda K, Nohara C, Futagawa T, et al. Critical contribution of OX40 ligand to T helper cell type 2 differentiation in experimental leishmaniasis. *J Exp Med* (2000) 191:375–80. doi:10.1084/jem.191.2.375
29. Tuladhar R, Oghumu S, Dong R, Peterson A, Sharpe AH, Satoskar AR. Ox40L-Ox40 pathway plays distinct roles in regulating Th2 responses but does not determine outcome of cutaneous leishmaniasis caused by *Leishmania mexicana* and *Leishmania major*. *Exp Parasitol* (2015) 148:49–55. doi:10.1016/j.exppara.2014.11.002
30. Liang SC, Greenwald RJ, Latchman YE, Rosas L, Satoskar A, Freeman GJ, et al. PD-L1 and PD-L2 have distinct roles in regulating host immunity to cutaneous leishmaniasis. *Eur J Immunol* (2006) 36:58–64. doi:10.1002/eji.200535458
31. Winau F, Weber S, Sad S, de Diego J, Hoops SL, Breiden B, et al. Apoptotic vesicles crossprime CD8 T cells and protect against tuberculosis. *Immunity* (2006) 24:105–17. doi:10.1016/j.immuni.2005.12.001
32. Gutiérrez-Kobeh L, de Oyarzabal E, Argueta J, Wilkins A, Salaiza N, Fernández E, et al. Inhibition of dendritic cell apoptosis by *Leishmania mexicana* amastigotes. *Parasitol Res* (2013) 112:1755–62. doi:10.1007/s00436-013-3334-2
33. Bieber K, Autenrieth SE. Insights how monocytes and dendritic cells contribute and regulate immune defense against microbial pathogens. *Immunobiology* (2015) 220:215–26. doi:10.1016/j.imbio.2014.10.025
34. Xin L, Li K, Soong L. Down-regulation of dendritic cell signaling pathways by *Leishmania amazonensis* amastigotes. *Mol Immunol* (2008) 45:3371–82. doi:10.1016/j.molimm.2008.04.018
35. Contreras I, Estrada JA, Guak H, Martel C, Borjian A, Ralph B, et al. Impact of *Leishmania mexicana* infection on dendritic cell signaling and functions. *PLoS Negl Trop Dis* (2014) 8:e3202. doi:10.1371/journal.pntd.0003202
36. Brodskyn C, Beverley SM, Titus RG. Virulent or avirulent (dhfr-ts-) *Leishmania major* elicit predominantly a type-1 cytokine response by human cells in vitro. *Clin Exp Immunol* (2000) 119:299–304. doi:10.1046/j.1365-2249.2000.01122.x
37. Roy S, Mukhopadhyay D, Mukherjee S, Ghosh S, Kumar S, Sarkar K, et al. A defective oxidative burst and impaired antigen presentation are hallmarks of human visceral leishmaniasis. *J Clin Immunol* (2015) 35:56–67. doi:10.1007/s10875-014-0115-3
38. Vieira ÉL, Keesen TS, Machado PR, Guimarães LH, Carvalho EM, Dutra WO, et al. Immunoregulatory profile of monocytes from cutaneous leishmaniasis patients and association with lesion size. *Parasite Immunol* (2013) 35:65–72. doi:10.1111/pim.12012
39. Revest M, Donaghy L, Cabillic F, Guiguen C, Gangneux JP. Comparison of the immunomodulatory effects of *L. donovani* and *L. major* excreted-secreted antigens, particulate and soluble extracts and viable parasites on human dendritic cells. *Vaccine* (2008) 26:6119–23. doi:10.1016/j.vaccine.2008.09.005
40. Colmenares M, Corbí AL, Turco SJ, Rivas L. The dendritic cell receptor DC-SIGN discriminates among species and life cycle forms of *Leishmania*. *J Immunol* (2004) 172:1186–90. doi:10.4049/jimmunol.172.2.1186
41. Markikou-Ouni W, Drini S, Bahi-Jaber N, Chenik M, Meddeb-Garnaoui A. Immunomodulatory effects of four *Leishmania infantum* potentially excreted/secreted proteins on human dendritic cells differentiation and maturation. *PLoS One* (2015) 10:e0143063. doi:10.1371/journal.pone.0143063
42. Green PJ, Feizi T, Stoll MS, Thiel S, Prescott A, McConville MJ. Recognition of the major cell surface glycoconjugates of *Leishmania* parasites by the human serum mannan-binding protein. *Mol Biochem Parasitol* (1994) 66:319–28. doi:10.1016/0166-6851(94)90158-9
43. Liu D, Uzonna JE. The early interaction of *Leishmania* with macrophages and dendritic cells and its influence on the host immune response. *Front Cell Infect Microbiol* (2012) 2:83. doi:10.3389/fcimb.2012.00083
44. Lefèvre L, Lugo-Villarino G, Meunier E, Valentin A, Olagnier D, Authier H, et al. The C-type lectin receptors dectin-1, MR, and SIGNR3 contribute both positively and negatively to the macrophage response to *Leishmania infantum*. *Immunity* (2013) 38:1038–49. doi:10.1016/j.immuni.2013.04.010
45. Carvalho K, Vallejo M, Camargo Z, Puccia R. Use of recombinant gp43 isoforms expressed in *Pichia pastoris* for diagnosis of paracoccidioidomycosis. *Clin Vaccine Immunol* (2008) 15:622–9. doi:10.1128/CVI.00437-07
46. de Assis Souza M, de Castro MC, de Oliveira AP, de Almeida AF, de Almeida TM, Reis LC, et al. Cytokines and NO in American tegumentary leishmaniasis patients: profiles in active disease, after therapy and in self-healed individuals. *Microb Pathog* (2013) 57:27–32. doi:10.1016/j.micpath.2013.02.004
47. Oliveira WN, Ribeiro LE, Schrieffer A, Machado P, Carvalho EM, Bacellar O. The role of inflammatory and anti-inflammatory cytokines in the pathogenesis of human tegumentary leishmaniasis. *Cytokine* (2014) 66:127–32. doi:10.1016/j.cyto.2013.12.016
48. Nateghi Rostami M, Seyyedan Jasbi E, Khamesipour A, Mohammadi AM. Tumour necrosis factor-alpha (TNF-α) and its soluble receptor type 1 (sTNFR I) in human active and healed leishmaniases. *Parasite Immunol* (2016) 38:255–60. doi:10.1111/pim.12305

49. Valdés-Reyes L, Argueta J, Morán J, Salaiza N, Hernández J, Berzunza M, et al. *Leishmania mexicana*: inhibition of camptothecin-induced apoptosis of monocyte-derived dendritic cells. *Exp Parasitol* (2009) 121:199–207. doi:10.1016/j.exppara.2008.10.020
50. Vázquez-López R, Argueta-Donohué J, Wilkins-Rodríguez A, Escalona-Montaño A, Aguirre-García M, Gutiérrez-Kobeh L. *Leishmania mexicana* amastigotes inhibit p38 and JNK and activate PI3K/AKT: role in the inhibition of apoptosis of dendritic cells. *Parasite Immunol* (2015) 37:579–89. doi:10.1111/pim.12275
51. Li X, He Y. Caspase-2-dependent dendritic cell death, maturation, and priming of T cells in response to *Brucella abortus* infection. *PLoS One* (2012) 7:e43512. doi:10.1371/journal.pone.0043512

8

IL-6 Improves the Nitric Oxide-Induced Cytotoxic CD8+ T Cell Dysfunction in Human Chagas Disease

*Liliana Maria Sanmarco[1], Laura Marina Visconti[2], Natalia Eberhardt[1], Maria Cecilia Ramello[1], Nicolás Eric Ponce[1], Natalia Beatriz Spitale[2], Maria Lola Vozza[2], Germán Andrés Bernardi[2], Susana Gea[1], Angel Ramón Minguez[2] and Maria Pilar Aoki[1]**

[1] Centro de Investigaciones en Bioquímica Clínica e Inmunología CIBICI-CONICET, Facultad de Ciencias Químicas, Universidad Nacional de Córdoba, Córdoba, Argentina, [2] Hospital Nuestra Señora de la Misericordia del Nuevo Siglo, Córdoba, Argentina

***Correspondence:**
Maria Pilar Aoki
paoki@fcq.unc.edu.ar

Reactive oxygen and nitrogen species are important microbicidal agents and are also involved in lymphocyte unresponsiveness during experimental infections. Many of the biological effects attributed to nitric oxide are mediated by peroxynitrites, which induce the nitration of immune cells, among others. Our group has demonstrated that nitric oxide is involved in the suppressive activity of myeloid-derived suppressor cells in *Trypanosoma cruzi*-infected mice, with a higher number of CD8+ T cells suffering surface-nitration compared to uninfected controls. Studying the functional and phenotypic features of peripheral CD8+ T cells from chagasic patients and human cells experimentally infected with *T. cruzi*, we found that different regulatory mechanisms impaired the effector functions of T cytotoxic population from seropositive patients. Peripheral leukocytes from chagasic patients showed increased nitric oxide production concomitant with increased tyrosine nitration of CD8+ T cells. Additionally, this cytotoxic population exhibited increased apoptotic rate, loss of the TCRζ-chain, and lower levels of CD107a, a marker of degranulation. Strikingly, IL-6 stimulation of *in vitro*-infected peripheral blood mononuclear cells obtained from healthy donors, blunted *T. cruzi*-induced nitration of CD3+CD8+ cells, and increased their survival. Furthermore, the treatment of these cultures with an IL-6 neutralizing antibody increased the percentage of *T. cruzi*-induced CD8+ T cell nitration and raised the release of nitric oxide. The results suggest that the under-responsiveness of cytotoxic T cell population observed in the setting of long-term constant activation of the immune system could be reverted by the pleiotropic actions of IL-6, since this cytokine improves its survival and effector functions.

Keywords: tyrosine nitration, peroxynitrite, CD39, CD73, oxidative stress, *Trypanosoma cruzi* infection

INTRODUCTION

CD8+ T cells play a critical role in the immunity against intracellular pathogens, including the protozoan parasite *Trypanosoma cruzi*, the causative agent of Chagas cardiomyopathy (1). Chagas disease is characterized by two distinct phases: the acute phase, which lasts several weeks and is characterized by non-specific symptoms; and the chronic phase, lasting lifelong. The host's ability to control *T. cruzi* infection is substantial, but not fully effective, since most infected individuals tightly limit parasite numbers but fail to completely clear the infection due to diverse and fascinating immune evasion processes (2). Indeed, parasite persistence at low levels into target cells is the hallmark of the indeterminate or asymptomatic chronic phase (3). Up to 40% of infected individuals develop progressive heart disease leading to an end-stage dilated cardiomyopathy.

One key defense mechanism against *T. cruzi* is exerted by nitric oxide (NO), which is produced by inducible NO synthase, among other enzymes, present in monocytes/macrophages and cardiomyocytes (4, 5). The parasite triggers activation of macrophage NADPH oxidase, resulting in a continuous production of superoxide anion $\left(O_2^-\right)$ and also stimulates infected macrophages to produce different amounts of NO. Despite its importance as a microbicidal agent at high levels, persistent low levels of NO have been involved in the establishment and maintenance of lymphocyte unresponsiveness in different experimental models of parasite infections (6–8). These mechanisms illustrate a clear parasite evasion strategy. Moreover, NO induces apoptosis of many different cell types *in vitro* and *in vivo* (9, 10). We found that IL-6 regulates inflammasome activation and, consequently, IL-1β-induced NO production in a murine model of *T. cruzi* infection. The anti-inflammatory action of IL-6 seems to be central for controlling local and systemic oxidative stress, promoting cellular rescue of apoptosis, and protecting infected IL-6-deficient mice against death (unpublished observation). This could be a novel mechanism that regulates NO release in the setting of *T. cruzi* infection.

The presence of low levels of NO rapidly initiates a reaction with the superoxide anion generating peroxynitrites that induce the nitration of surface proteins on T cells (11, 12). It is widely accepted that reactive nitrogen species (NO and peroxynitrites) contribute to the immunosuppressive attitude of myeloid-derived suppressor cells (MDSCs), a heterogeneous cell population associated with tumors, infectious, and inflammatory diseases. Our group has demonstrated that MDSCs during acute *T. cruzi* experimental infection were able to inhibit T cell proliferation *in vitro* (13). Furthermore, we also observed a higher number of splenic CD8+ T cells suffering surface nitration in infected mice compared to uninfected controls.

Chronic exposure to antigens may cause functional defects in pathogen-specific T cells. It has been reported that individuals with more severe clinical disease have a significantly lower frequency of *T. cruzi*-specific CD8+IFNγ+ T cells than subjects in the asymptomatic stage of the infection (14). This impairment in *T. cruzi*-specific CD8+ T cell responses was associated with an increased frequency of fully differentiated memory cells and an increased rate of apoptosis in the total peripheral CD8+ T cell population. The results reveal a progressive exhaustion in the parasite-specific cytotoxic T cell compartment in patients with long-term *T. cruzi* infection. However, during persistent infection, the chronic exposure to an inflammatory microenvironment may also contribute to the impairment of CD8+ T cell responses, resulting in a less efficient control of the pathogen and promoting its persistence.

These findings prompted us to investigate the frequency and functionality of circulating CD8+ T cells from patients with chronic Chagas disease, with particular focus on the molecular mechanisms triggered by IL-6 associated with cytotoxicity and NO-induced cell death. In agreement with previous reports in seropositive patients with Chagas disease, we found a substantial reduction in the total peripheral T cell compartment at the expense of CD8+ T cells (14). Additionally, we observed increased NO-producing leukocytes concomitant with increased nitration of CD8+ T cells and impaired cytotoxic functionality of T cells. Strikingly, IL-6 prevented the nitration of CD8+ T cells and increased their survival when healthy donor peripheral blood mononuclear cells (PBMCs) were infected *in vitro*. In this context, IL-6 led to a decrease in IL-1β levels. The results suggest that the under-responsiveness of the whole cytotoxic T cell population from chagasic patients could be reverted by the pleiotropic actions of IL-6, since this cytokine functions as a survival factor for CD8+ cells and improves the cytotoxic T cell functionality in the setting of long-term constant activation of the immune system.

MATERIALS AND METHODS

Ethics Statement

Subjects were recruited at the "Hospital Nuestra Señora de la Misericordia" (HNSM) from Córdoba-Argentina. All studies were conducted according to the principles expressed in the Declaration of Helsinki. Signed informed consent was obtained from all donors before inclusion in the study. Venous blood was drawn from 46 non-chagasic and chagasic subjects (age 25–60 years) using a protocol that was reviewed and approved by the Comité Institucional de Ética de la Investigación en Salud del Adulto, Ministerio de Salud de la Provincia de Córdoba (Acta number 194/2014, Argentina). *T. cruzi* infection was determined by a combination of indirect hemagglutination (IHA) and enzyme-linked immunosorbent assay (ELISA) performed in the laboratory of HNSM. Subject positive on these two tests were considered infected. Chronic chagasic patients (n = 22) were evaluated clinically and by electrocardiogram and chest X-ray. The uninfected control group (n = 24) consisted of age-matched individuals were serologically negative for *T. cruzi*. All donors with chronic or inflammatory pathology or erythrocyte sedimentation rate >30 mm or white blood cells count <4,000 or >10,000/mm^3 were excluded from the study.

Blood Collection

Approximately 15 mL of blood was drawn from each individual by venipuncture and placed into heparinized tubes (Vacutainer, BD Bioscience). An aliquot of 50 μL of total peripheral blood was stained for FACS analysis and subjected to ACK lysing buffer to remove erythrocytes. PBMCs were isolated through density gradient centrifugation using Ficoll-Hypaque PLUS (GE Healthcare Bioscience) and resuspended in RPMI 1640 (Gibco) supplemented with 10% heat-inactivated FCS (Natocor).

Ex Vivo Flow Cytometry

Peripheral blood was lysed with ACK lysing buffer to remove erythrocytes, and 01 × 10^6 cells were blocked with Fc block and stained with anti-human CD3 Alexa 488 or PerCP, anti-human

CD4 Alexa 647, anti-human CD8 PECy7, anti-human CD39 biotin and streptavidin APC, anti-human CD73 PE (eBioscience and Biolegend), anti-nitrotyrosine (Sigma-Aldrich), and anti-rabbit Alexa 647 or CD20 PECy7 (Biolegend). The intracellular expression of ζ-chain was analyzed with anti-human TCRζ PE antibody (Beckman Coulter). Stained cells were analyzed by flow cytometry (FACS Canto II, Becton Dickinson), with cellular debris being excluded from the analysis. Data were analyzed using the FlowJo software.

Cell Viability Measurement

Leukocytes from peripheral blood were stained with anti-human CD3 Alexa 488, anti-human CD4 Alexa 647, anti-human CD8 PECy7 or APCCy7, anti-human CCR7 Alexa 488, anti-human CD45RA PECy7, and labeled with 5 μL of Annexin VPE (BD Pharmingen) for 15 min on ice. Before acquisition, the cells were stained with 7-AAD (BD Bioscience). A minimum of 300,000 events for each condition were analyzed by flow cytometry. Staining of peripheral blood T cells with antibodies to CD45RA and CCR7 reveals four cells subsets: naïve T cells are CD45RA+CCR7+, central memory cells are CD45RA−CCR7+, effector memory (EM) cells are CD45RA−CCR7−, and terminally differentiated effector memory (EMRA) are CD45RA+CCR7− (15).

To determine Bcl-2 expression, PBMCs stained for CD3 PerCP, CD8, CD4, CCR7, and CD45RA surface expression were permeabilized with FOXP3 staining buffer set (eBioscience) and labeled with anti-Bcl-2 rabbit (Cell Signaling) and then with anti-rabbit Alexa 488 or anti-rabbit Alexa 647. Stained cells were analyzed by flow cytometry.

CD8+ T Cell Functionality

Peripheral blood mononuclear cells were cultured with anti-CD107a PE (Biolegend), monensin, brefeldin A, phorbol 12-myristate 13-acetate (PMA), and ionomycin (Sigma) for 4 h, then stained with anti-IFNγ FITC, anti-TNF APC, and anti-IL-2 APC-Cy7 (Biolegend or eBioscience), and analyzed by flow cytometry.

To evaluate the effect of TCR-dependent activation, PBMCs were cultured with anti-CD3 (1 μg/mL) and anti-CD28 (0.5 mg/mL). After 72 h, PBMCs were cultured with monensin, brefeldin A, and anti-CD107a PE for 6 h and then stained with anti-human CD8 APCCy7, anti-NT rabbit and anti-rabbit Alexa 647, anti-IL-2 PECy7, anti-TNF PerCPCy5.5, or anti-IFNγ PerCPCy5.5.

CD8+ T Cell Exhaustion

Peripheral blood mononuclear cells were cultured with anti-CD3 (1 μg/mL) and anti-CD28 (0.5 mg/mL). After 72 h, the cells were stained with anti-human CD8 APCCy7, anti-Tim3 PerCPCy5.5, anti-PD1 PECy7, anti-CTLA4 PE, anti-CCR7 Alexa 488, and anti-NT rabbit and anti-rabbit Alexa 647.

Measurement of Reactive Oxygen and Nitrogen Species

The nitrite/nitrate content, indicative of NO production, was monitored by the Griess reagent assay (16). In 96-well plates, plasma samples were mixed with 50 μL of Griess reagent, consisting of 1% sulfanilamide in 5% phosphoric acid and 0.1% *N*-(1-napthyl) ethylenediamine dihydrochloride [1:1 ratio (vol/vol)], and incubated for 10 min. The change in absorbance was monitored at 545 nm (standard curve, 0–200 μmol sodium nitrite).

The production of ROS and NO was evaluated using the molecular probes: H_2DCF-DA (10 μM, Invitrogen Inc.) and DAF-FM DA (10 μM, Molecular Probes, Inc.), respectively. All samples were acquired on a FACS Canto II cytometer and then analyzed using the Flow Jo software.

Quantification of Cytokines

Plasma samples were analyzed for TNF, IL-6, IL-10, IFNγ, and IL-4 by using bead-based immunoassays and flow cytometry, according to the manufacturer's instructions (LegendPlex-Biolegend). In cultured supernatant, IL-1β levels were measured by Ready-SET-Go ELISA kit from eBioscience.

Culture of PBMCs and Parasites

Vero cell monolayers were infected with trypomastigote forms of *T. cruzi* Tulahuen strain for 3 h and then washed and maintained in RPMI (Gibco Invitrogen Corporation) at 37°C in a 5% CO_2 atmosphere. After 7 days, the parasites were collected from the supernatant of infected cells and harvested by centrifugation at 4,400 rpm for 5 min.

Peripheral blood mononuclear cells from non-chagasic donors were cultured with *T. cruzi* Tulahuen trypomastigotes (1:1 rate) for 3 h, then the cells were washed and cultured with recombinant bioactive IL-6 (20 ng/mL) or with anti-IL-6 (2 μg/mL) (Biolegend) or anti-IL-6 plus anti-IL-1β (2 μg/mL), or maintained in medium alone for 48 h. Then, culture supernatants were evaluated for IL-1β/NO levels, and the cells were analyzed for NT staining or NO production by flow cytometry. In addition, peripheral blood from chagasic patients and control donors (250 μL) were cultured with 7,500 trypomastigotes with or without IL-6 (20 ng/mL) or maintained in medium for 24 h and then cells were harvested to evaluate NO and ROS production and NT by flow cytometry.

Statistical Analysis

Statistical analysis was performed with GraphPad Prism 5.0 software by using parametric or non-parametric paired *t* test according to data distribution. *p* Values <0.05 were considered significant.

RESULTS

Chagasic Patients Showed a Lower Number of Peripheral Blood CD8+ T Lymphocytes

A total of 46 peripheral blood samples from chagasic and non-chagasic donors of both sexes, collected from people living in Cordoba (Argentina) were analyzed for *T. cruzi*-specific antibodies by ELISA and IHA (**Table 1**). The median value for anti-*T. cruzi* antibody titers detected by IHA was 1/256 (local cutoff titer 1/32). Only one patient showed a complete right-bundle branch block, left anterior hemiblock, and left atrial enlargement, clinical features of chagasic heart disease. Cordoba is considered by the Argentine Ministry of Health to be at high risk for vector transmission, since there is a reemergence of this infection route by an increase in house infestation and a high seroprevalence in vulnerable groups (17).

TABLE 1 | Description of subject groups.

	Non-chagasic donors (n = 24)	Chagasic patients (n = 22)
Age (years old)		
Range	25–60	25–48
Median	30	32
Gender		
Female	$n = 16$	$n = 17$
Male	$n = 8$	$n = 5$
Clinical evaluation		
Electrocardiographic changes	NE	$n = 1$[a]
Echocardiographic changes	NE	$n = 1$[b]
Chest X-rays abnormalities	NE	$n = 0$

[a]*Complete right-bundle branch block and left anterior hemiblock.*
[b]*Left atrial enlargement.*
NE, not evaluated.

TABLE 2 | Peripheral blood lymphocyte subpopulations.

	Non-chagasic donors (n = 15)	Chagasic patients (n = 8)	p-Value
Lymphocyte subsets in peripheral blood			
CD3+ (%)	58.6 ± 3.9	43.2 ± 5.3	$p = 0.03$*
CD3+/μL (absolute number)	1,139 ± 102	754 ± 135	$p = 0.04$*
CD3+CD4+ (%)	58.7 ± 3.7	57.6 ± 2.0	$p = 0.84$
CD3+CD4+/μL (absolute number)	600 ± 72	535 ± 65	$p = 0.59$
CD3+CD8+ (%)	39.9 ± 3.5	30.74 ± 2.2	$p = 0.04$*
CD3+CD8+/μL (absolute number)	381 ± 56	193 ± 32	$p = 0.049$*
CD20+ (%)	14.1 ± 1.5	12.3 ± 1.6	$p = 0.44$
CD20+/μL (absolute number)	305 ± 40	218 ± 32	$p = 0.16$

Values are expressed as mean value ± SE.
**$p < 0.05$, significant.*

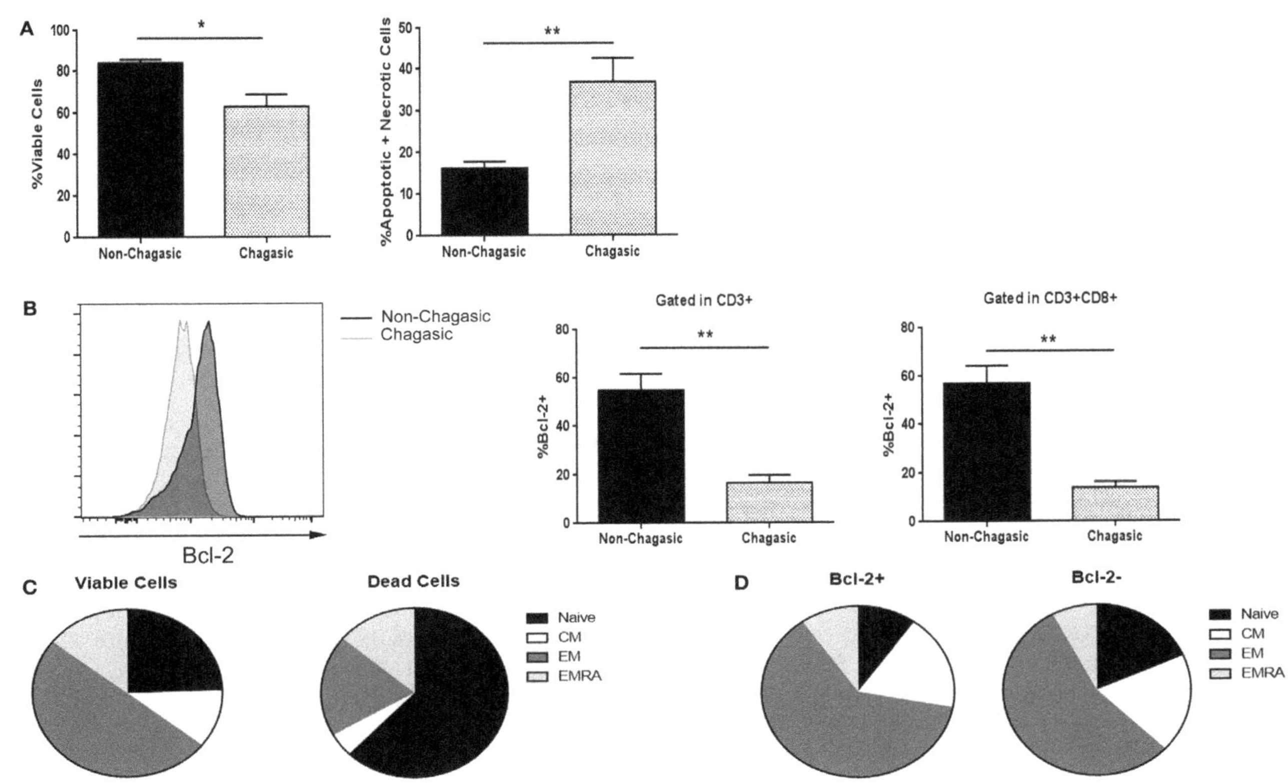

FIGURE 1 | Cytotoxic T lymphocytes from chagasic patients show higher death rate and less Bcl-2 expression. (A) Percentage of viable and apoptotic + necrotic CD3+CD8+ from chagasic patients (n = 5) and non-chagasic donors (n = 5) analyzed by Annexin-V and 7AAD staining. **(B)** Representative histogram of Bcl-2 expression in cytotoxic T cells and percentage of T lymphocytes and CD8+ T cells expressing Bcl-2 in chagasic patients (n = 5) and in non-chagasic donors (n = 5) (*$p < 0.05$ and **$p < 0.01$). **(C)** Frequency of naïve, central memory (CM), effector memory (EM), and effector memory RA (EMRA) gated in viable cells (7AAD−) or dead cells (7AAD+) in CD8+ lymphocytes from seropositive patients (n = 4) (viable naïve vs. dead naïve $p = 0.002$; viable EM vs. dead EM, $p = 0.0002$). **(D)** Frequency of naïve, CM, EM, and EMRA gated in Bcl-2+ or Bcl-2− in CD8+ cells from chagasic patients (n = 4) (naïve Bcl-2+ vs. naïve Bcl-2−, $p = 0.0123$).

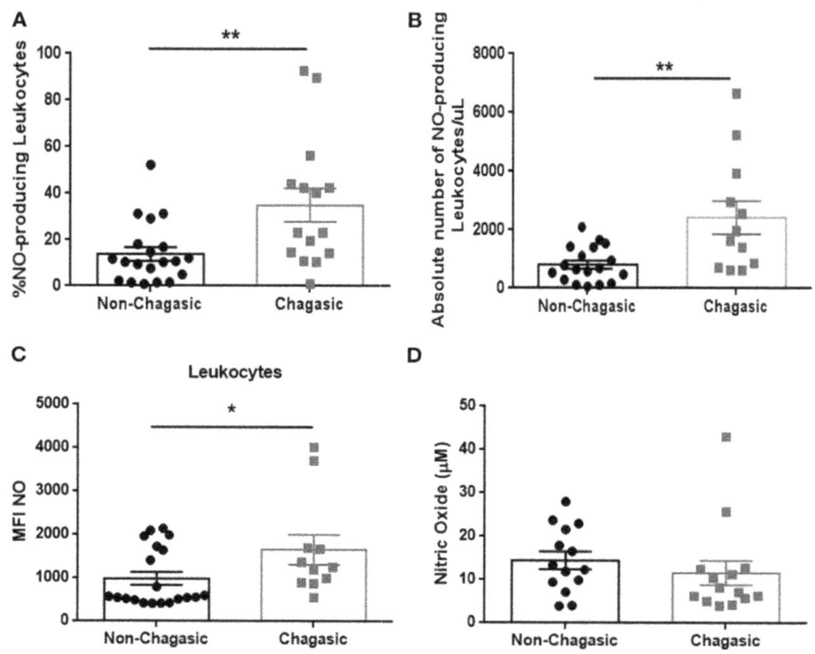

FIGURE 2 | Chagasic patients exhibit a higher number and frequency of nitric oxide-producing leukocytes. **(A)** Percentage and **(B)** absolute number of nitric oxide (NO)-producing leukocytes from chagasic patients ($n = 15$) and non-chagasic donors ($n = 19$). **(C)** Mean fluorescence intensity of NO in leukocytes from chagasic patients ($n = 11$) and non-chagasic donors ($n = 20$). **(D)** Serum nitric oxide levels in seropositive patients ($n = 14$) and seronegative donors ($n = 14$) (* $p < 0.05$ and ** $p < 0.01$).

Seropositive patients with Chagas disease showed a diminished percentage and absolute number of total peripheral T lymphocytes (CD3+) compared to seronegative donors. Although no differences were observed between non-chagasic and chagasic patients in the percentage and absolute number of T helper cells (CD3+CD4+), the percentage and absolute number of cytotoxic T cells (CD3+CD8+) were significantly lower in seropositive than in seronegative patients (**Table 2**).

No differences were observed in the percentage and absolute number of B lymphocytes (CD20+) between the analyzed groups (**Table 2**).

Cytotoxic T Lymphocytes from Chagasic Patients Showed Higher Cell Death and Less Bcl-2 Expression

Through Annexin V and 7-AAD staining, we found that fresh explanted CD8+ T lymphocytes from chagasic patients showed a diminished percentage of viable cells, and concomitantly, a higher rate of apoptotic and necrotic cells compared to non-chagasic donors (**Figure 1A**). In agreement, the expression of the anti-apoptotic protein Bcl-2 was significantly higher in cytotoxic lymphocytes from non-chagasic than from chagasic patients (**Figure 1B**). Among cytotoxic T cells from Chagas patients, naïve CD8 T cells were the phenotype most susceptible to die (viable cells vs. dead cells: 24.53 ± 6.11 vs. 62.48 ± 3.95%). In contrast, EM cytotoxic T cells showed significantly increased survival rate (viable cells vs. dead cells: 49.75 ± 3.06 vs. 19.48 ± 2.45%) (**Figure 1C**). In accordance, the frequency of naïve cells negative for intracellular Bcl-2 expression was significantly lower than naïve cells positive for the expression of this anti-apoptotic protein (Bcl-2+ vs. Bcl-2−: 9.95 ± 0.87 vs. 17.67 ± 2.07) (**Figure 1D**). Furthermore, the percentage of EM CD8 T cells was higher in Chagas subjects in comparison with seronegative donors (Figure S1 in Supplementary Material).

Nitric Oxide-Producing Leukocytes Were Increased in Chagasic Patients

Seropositive patients showed an increased percentage and absolute number of NO-producing leukocytes (**Figures 2A,B**), with higher production of NO per leukocyte (**Figure 2C**), but no significant differences were detected in levels of plasma NO in comparison with seronegative subjects (**Figure 2D**). The infection of peripheral blood from seronegative and seropositive patients with trypomastigotes (Tulahuen strain) significantly increased the percentage of NO- and ROS-producing leukocytes (Figure S2 in Supplementary Material).

CD8+ T Lymphocytes from Chagasic Patients Exhibited High Levels of Nitrated Tyrosine Residues

Non-chagasic individuals exhibited significantly lower tyrosine nitration (NT) of leukocytes, lymphocytes, and T cells than chagasic patients (**Figure 3A**). In particular, chagasic patients showed

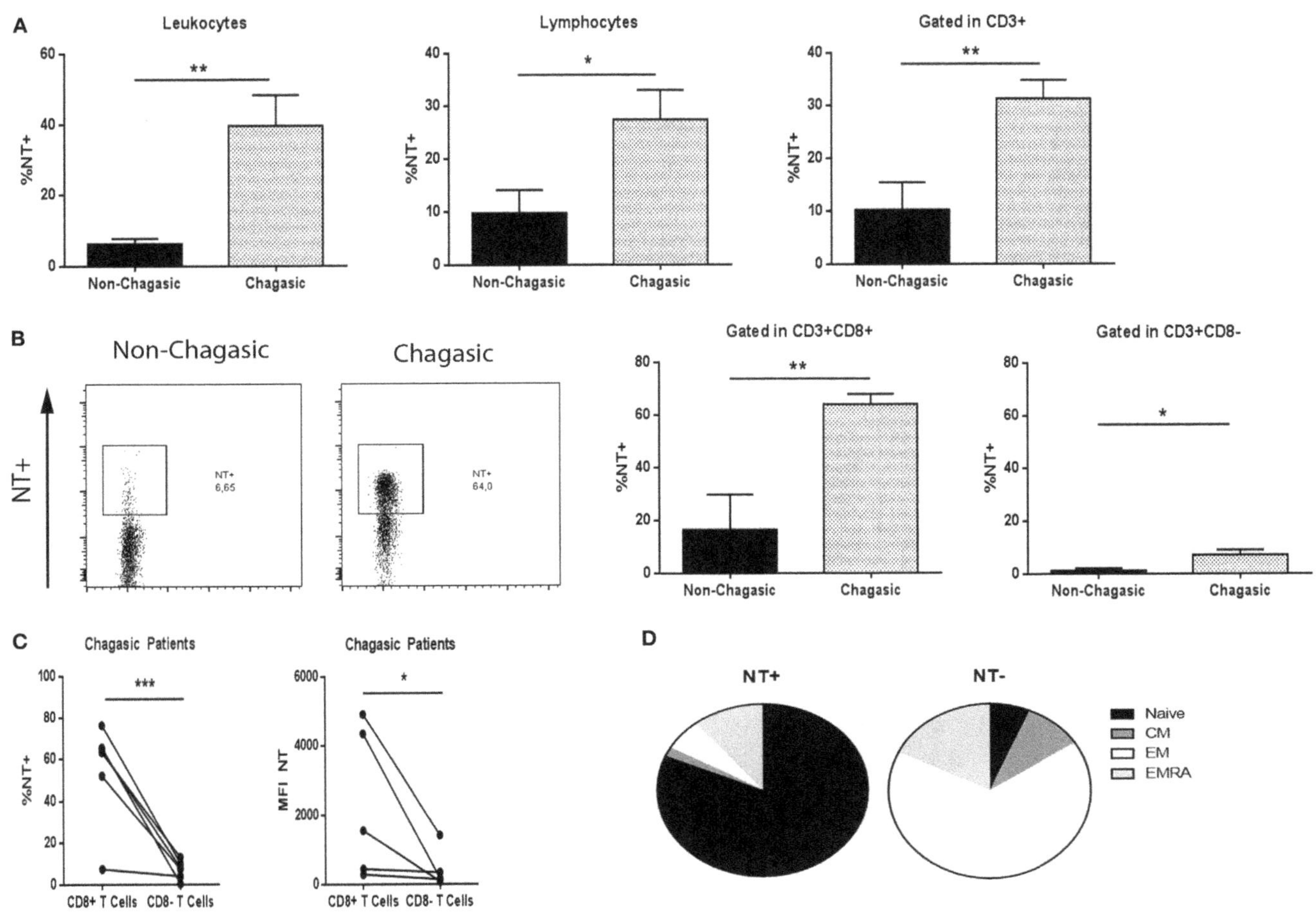

FIGURE 3 | CD8+ T lymphocytes from chagasic patients present high tyrosine nitration. **(A)** Percentage of nitrated (NT) leukocytes, lymphocytes, and T cells from seropositive patients ($n = 6$) and seronegative donors ($n = 6$). **(B)** Representative dot plot of tyrosine nitration on cytotoxic T-cell surface and percentage of NT+CD3+CD8+ and NT+CD3+CD8− lymphocytes from chagasic patients ($n = 6$) and non-chagasic donors ($n = 6$). **(C)** Percentage of NT+CD3+CD8+ and NT+CD3+CD8− and mean fluorescence intensity of NT in CD3+CD8+ and CD3+CD8− cells from chagasic patients ($n = 5$) (*$p < 0.05$, **$p < 0.01$, and ***$p < 0.001$). **(D)** Frequency of naïve, central memory, effector memory (EM), and effector memory RA gated in NT+ or NT− in CD8+ cells from chagasic patients ($n = 4$) (naïve NT+ vs. naïve NT−, $p < 0.0001$; EM NT+ vs. EM NT−, $p < 0.0001$).

more NT+CD8+ T lymphocytes compared to non-chagasic donors (**Figure 3B**). Although nitration also increased in CD8− T cell population from seropositive patients, a main effect was observed in CD8+ T lymphocytes compared to CD8− T cells in this group of patients (**Figure 3C**). Among NT+ cytotoxic cells from Chagas patients, we have identified naïve cells as the main subpopulation that undergoes tyrosine nitration (NT+ vs. NT− 81.45 ± 3.00 vs. 6.50 ± 1.61%). On the contrary, the majority of NT− cells were EM CD8+ T cells (NT+ vs. NT− 5.73 ± 1.22 vs. 66.33 ± 4.46%) (**Figure 3D**).

Cytotoxic T Cells from Chagas Patients Were Less Functional

Even though CD4+ T lymphocytes from seropositive and seronegative individuals showed similar levels of expression of the TCRζ chain, the cytotoxic T cells exhibited a diminished amount of TCRζ in chagasic patients, as compared to non-chagasic donors (**Figure 4A**). In line with these observations, CD8 T cell population from seropositive patients showed lower frequency of CD107a+ cells, as well as IFNγ, TNF, and IL-2-producing cells after stimulation with PMA/Ionomycin (unspecific stimuli) in comparison with the same population from seronegative donors (**Figure 4B**). Furthermore, after anti-CD3/anti-CD28 stimulation (*via* TCR), the percentage of CD8+ T cells from Chagas patients positive for CD107a, IFNγ, TNF, and IL-2 was significantly diminished in NT+ cells compared to NT− cells (**Figure 4C**). The same behavior was observed when we compared the functionality of nitrated vs. no nitrated CD8+ T cells within the EM–EMRA populations (Figure S3 in Supplementary Material). These results indicated that nitrated cytotoxic T cells from chagasic patients were less functional than non-nitrated population. Moreover, chagasic patients showed a decreased percentage of CD39+ and CD73+ lymphocytes compared to control donors (**Figure 4D**). However,

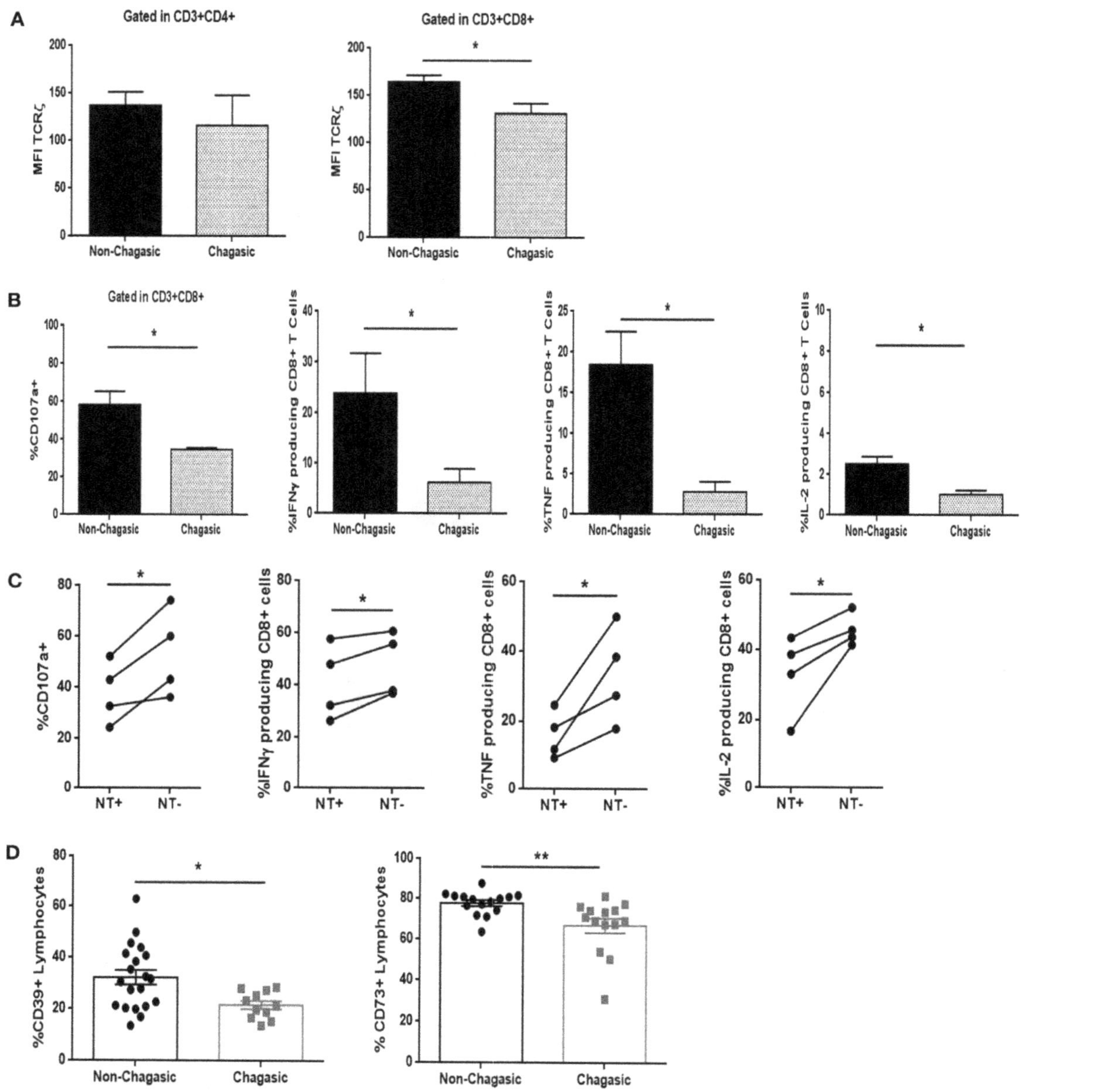

FIGURE 4 | Cytotoxic T cells from chagasic patients are less functional than those from healthy individuals. **(A)** Mean fluorescence intensity of TCRζ-chain in CD3+CD4+ and CD3+CD8+ cells; **(B)** frequency of CD107a+ cells, IFNγ, TNF, and IL-2-producing CD8+ T lymphocytes from chagasic patients ($n = 5$) and seronegative donors ($n = 5$) after PMA/ionomycin stimulation. **(C)** Frequency of CD107a+ cells, IFNγ, TNF, and IL-2-producing NT+ and NT− gated in CD8+ T lymphocytes from chagasic patients ($n = 4$) after anti-CD3+ anti-CD28 stimulation. **(D)** Percentage of CD39+ and CD73+ leukocytes from seropositive ($n = 20$) and seronegative ($n = 14$) individuals (*$p < 0.05$ and **$p < 0.01$).

frequency of CD8+ T cells expressing Tim-3, PD-1, or CTLA-4 was no different between chagasic patients and seronegative donors (Figure S4 in Supplementary Material). The results suggest that although cytotoxic T cells are less functional in seropositive subjects, they appear not to be a classically exhausted population since the expression of inhibitory receptors was not upregulated compared to CD8+ T cells from seronegative subjects.

IL-1β Plasma Levels Were Increased in Seropositive Patients

The cytokine plasma levels were assayed using a panel of capture beads. In seronegative and seropositive individuals, the levels of IL-6, IFNγ, TNF, and IL-4 were similar. However, IL-1β levels were higher, and the amount of IL-10 was lower in plasma from chagasic people compared with control donors (**Figure 5**).

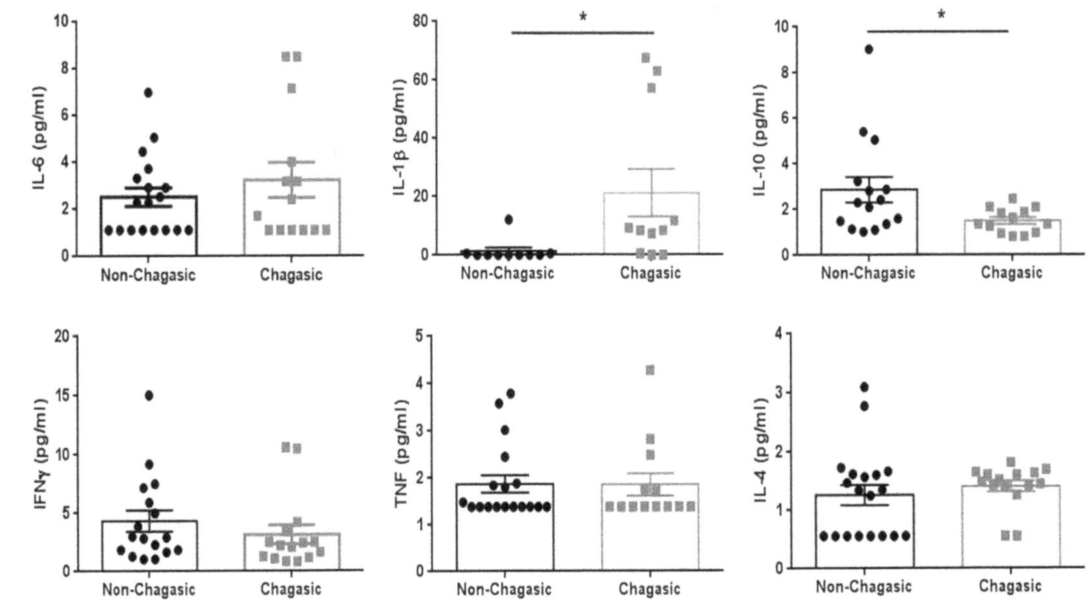

FIGURE 5 | IL-1β plasma levels are higher in seropositive patients than in seronegative donors. Plasma levels of IL-6, IL-10, IFNγ, TNF, and IL-4 (assayed by a panel of capture beads) and IL-1β (evaluated by enzyme-linked immunosorbent assay) in chagasic patients ($n = 18$) and non-chagasic donors ($n = 15$) (*$p < 0.05$).

IL-6 Prevented CD8+ T Cell Nitration and Apoptosis Susceptibility and Decreased IL-1β Production by Infected PBMCs

The IL-6 stimulation of *in vitro*-infected PBMCs obtained from healthy donors blunted *T. cruzi*-induced NT in CD3+CD8+ cells. Conversely, the treatment of these cultures with a neutralizing antibody specific for IL-6 (αIL-6) increased the percentage of *T. cruzi*-induced NT in this subpopulation (**Figure 6A**). Moreover, IL-6 treatment rescued infected CD8+ T cells from apoptosis (**Figure 6B**). Concomitantly, while IL-6 stimulation diminished the levels of IL-1β in culture supernatants from *T-cruzi*-infected PBMCs, αIL-6 treatment increased the release of IL-1β (**Figure 6C**). Furthermore, although IL-6 stimulation did not affect NO production by *T. cruzi*-infected PBMCs, the blockage of IL-6 significantly increased *T. cruzi*-induced NO production (**Figure 6D**). Additionally, IL-6 stimulation diminished NT in infected CD3+CD8+ cells from peripheral blood of chagasic patients (Figure S5 in Supplementary Material). In accordance, we found that blocking IL-6 and IL-1β significantly diminished the percentage of NT+CD8+ T cells from *in vitro*-infected PBMCs in comparison with cultures incubated with anti-IL-6 alone (**Figure 7A**). Moreover, the percentage of NO-producing monocytes significantly diminished when both cytokines were blocked compared with the inhibition of IL-6 alone (**Figure 7B**).

DISCUSSION

Multiple immunological effector mechanisms are critical for resolving *T. cruzi* infection, but considering that this parasite invades and replicates in essentially all types of mammalian cells, T cells and monocytes/macrophages are particularly important for controlling the infection. As with other intracellular parasites, *T. cruzi* antigens are processed and presented on MHC-class I molecules, leading to the recognition of parasite components by CD8+ T cells. In this regard, the study of the induction of CD8+ T cell-mediated protective immunity has become a center of intense research efforts to find control measures and prophylactic tools that could be used to produce effective therapeutic vaccines. This study shows that chronic *T. cruzi* infection leads to a significant nitration of T lymphocytes, mainly of the CD8+ T cell subset. The increased tyrosine nitration was associated with impaired effector functions and a significant fall in the number and percentage of circulating CD8+ T cells in chronic Chagas patients.

Among the reactive oxygen and nitrogen species mediating T-cell suppression is peroxynitrite, one of the most potent oxidants in the body. The hyperproduction of peroxynitrite is associated with nitration of the surface proteins in T cells (11, 12). Regarding CD8+ T cells, nitration of tyrosines within the TCR/CD8 complex disrupts the binding of the specific peptide-MHC dimers to CD8 molecules, which results in the inability of this T cell subset to bind MHC (18, 19). Furthermore, peroxynitrites also inhibit TCR signaling by preventing the association of CD3-ζ with the TCR. Our group has reported that *T. cruzi* induces an increase in splenic NT+CD8+ and NT+CD4+ T cells from infected mice by performing confocal and flow cytometric analysis of immunofluorescence staining (13). In this work, we found that the increased nitration of CD8+ T cells was associated with a lower capacity for activation (TCRζ expression), a

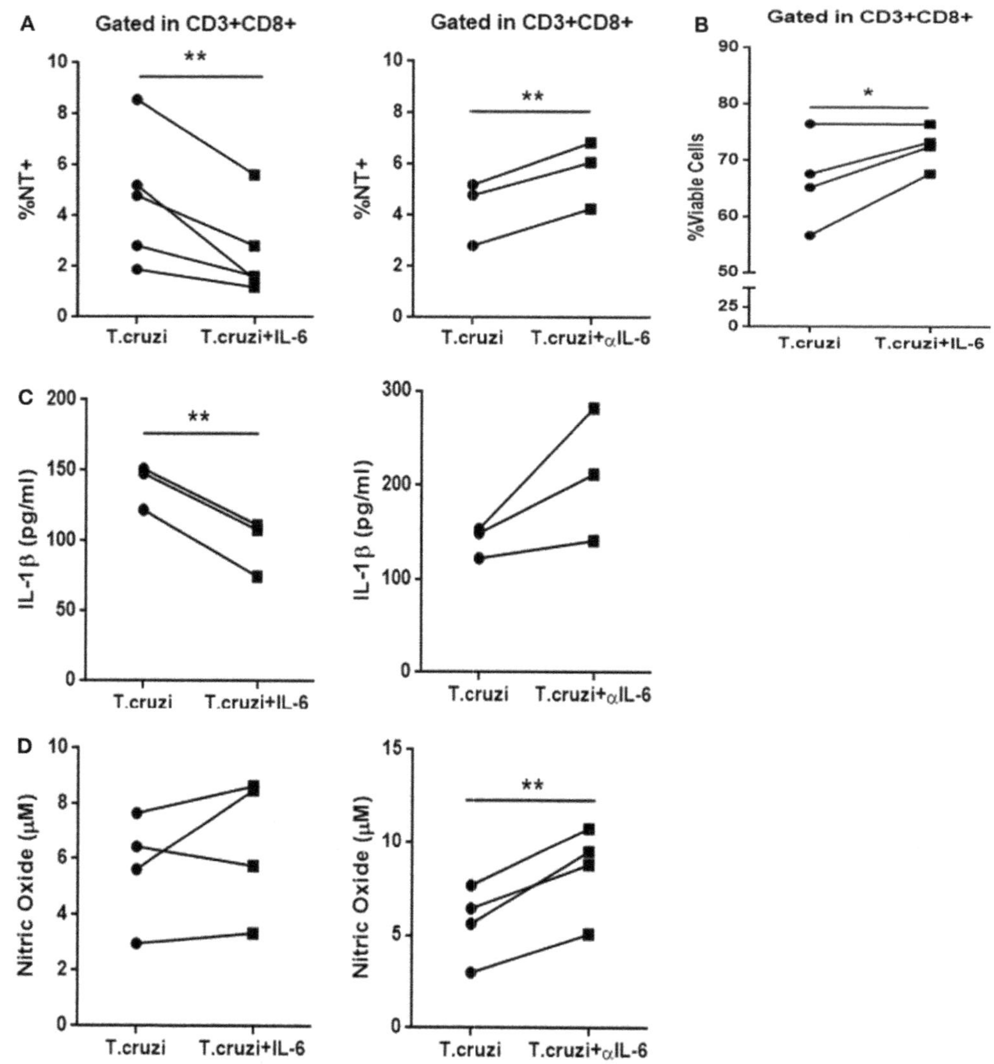

FIGURE 6 | IL-6 prevents nitration, increases survival of CD3+CD8+ cells, and decreases IL-1β levels after infection. (A) Percentage of NT+CD3+CD8+ cells in infected peripheral blood mononuclear cells (PBMCs) from non-chagasic ($n = 5$) donors after 48 h of stimulation with IL-6 (*Trypanosoma cruzi* + IL-6) or αIL-6 (*T. cruzi* + αIL-6) or medium alone (*T. cruzi*). **(B)** Percentage of viable CD3+CD8+ cells infected with *T. cruzi* (*T. cruzi*) or infected and stimulated with IL-6 (*T. cruzi* + IL-6). **(C)** IL-1β levels and **(D)** nitric oxide levels in culture supernatants of infected PBMCs after 48 h of stimulation with IL-6 (*T. cruzi* + IL-6) or αIL-6 (*T. cruzi* + αIL-6) or medium alone (*T. cruzi*) (*$p < 0.05$ and **$p < 0.01$).

diminished production of cytokines (IFNγ, TNF, and IL-2) and deactivation of cytotoxic functions (CD107a expression) in this cell population. Strikingly, cellular nitration seems to be reversible, since the incubation of infected leukocytes from seropositive patients with IL-6 significantly diminished the percentage of NT+ lymphocytes.

Leukocytes from chagasic patients significantly increased the production of NO, which correlated with increased susceptibility of CD8+ T cells to undergo spontaneous apoptosis. NO-mediated suppression of T-cell activation does not seem to be mediated by events triggered by TCR recognition but, instead, with the signaling cascade that is downstream of IL-2 (20). In human T cells, NO affects the stability of IL-2 mRNA and the release of IL-2. In this sense, NO negatively regulates intracellular signaling proteins either directly, by S-nitrosylation of crucial cysteine residues, or indirectly, by activation of cyclic-GMP-dependent protein kinase (21). Furthermore, while NO also sensitizes cells to Fas-L-mediated apoptosis (22), the anti-apoptotic molecule Bcl-2 diminished the susceptibility to NO-induced apoptosis (23). In line with these reports, we found that CD8+ T cells from seropositive individuals showed a significantly decreased expression of Bcl-2 concomitant with the significant diminution in their viability. The increased susceptibility to apoptosis was in accordance with the diminution in the percentage as well as

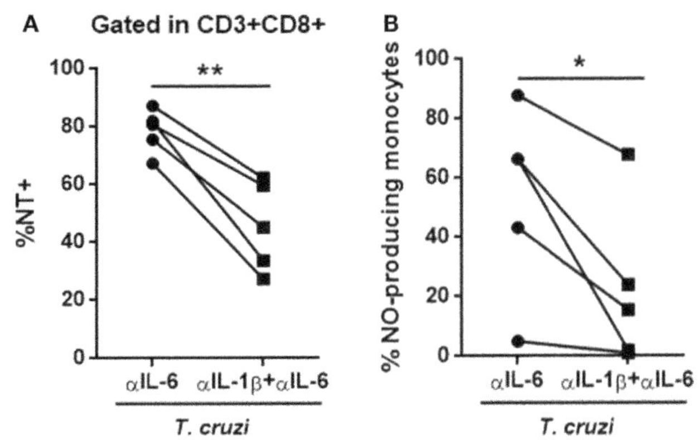

FIGURE 7 | The blockage of IL-6 and IL-1β reverts the phenotype induced by anti-IL-6. **(A)** Percentage of NT+CD8+ T cells and **(B)** NO-producing monocytes (CD14+) in *in vitro*-infected peripheral blood mononuclear cells from seronegative ($n = 5$) subjects after 48 h of stimulation with anti-IL-6 or anti-IL-6 + anti-IL-1β (*$p < 0.05$ and **$p < 0.01$).

absolute number of total T cells at the expense of diminution of CD8+ T cells but not of T helper cells or B cells.

It was reported that NO levels, as measured by Griess reagent assay, were not significantly increased in the plasma of seropositive subjects compared with those in seronegative samples. However, the plasma level of 3-nitrotyrosine (NT), was increased in seropositive subjects (24). The results indicated that seropositive subjects with Chagas disease are exposed to increased nitrosative stress. In total agreement with this report, we observed no significant increase in plasma levels of nitrate/nitrite of seropositive subjects compared with seronegative donors. Nevertheless, the leukocytes from chagasic patients significantly increased the production of NO, suggesting that NO produced by leukocytes, rather than soluble NO, may contribute to increased nitrosative stress in patients with Chagas disease, evidencing the importance of cell-to-cell contact for NO inhibitory effector functions (25, 26). Although tyrosine nitration constitutes one of the mechanisms employed by MDSC to suppress T cell response through cell-to-cell contact, it may also be dependent on the activity of myeloperoxidase, secreted by monocytes and polymorphonuclear neutrophils (27).

In accordance with our recent observations, while IL-1β plasma levels were significantly increased in chagasic patients, the stimulation of *in vitro*-infected PBMCs with IL-6 significantly diminished the production of IL-1β. Moreover, IL-6 diminished the nitration rate and improved the survival of CD8+ T cells. In agreement with this result, we have previously shown that IL-6 acts as a survival factor for infected target cells (28, 29). We have observed that IL-6 regulates IL-1β-induced NO production, and that excessive oxidative stress accounts for the increased mortality of *T. cruzi*-infected IL6KO mice (unpublished results). The anti-inflammatory action of IL-6 appears to be central to controlling cardiac and systemic oxidative stress, promoting cellular rescue against apoptosis, and protecting infected IL-6-deficient mice against death. In this model, this was clearly illustrated by the fact that the percentage of nitrated CD8+ T cells observed after blocking IL-6 was significantly diminished when anti-IL-6 was combined with anti-IL-1β. In accordance, IL-6 stimulation of peripheral blood cells from chagasic patients induced a significant diminution of nitration of CD8+ T cells. Our results strongly suggest that IL-6 could represent a key factor for regulating the nitration of proteins on human cytotoxic T cells.

One potential regulatory system that could have a role in the IL-6-induced anti-inflammatory effects is the extracellular levels of adenosine. *T. cruzi* infection of cardiac tissue induces an influx of immune cells that consume large quantities of oxygen. Ischemic cells rapidly respond to the hypoxic and inflammatory environment by releasing ATP (normally present within cardiomyocytes in millimolar concentrations). Once in the extracellular environment, ATP is converted to AMP and then to adenosine by the CD39 and CD73 ectoenzymes, respectively (30). In pathological conditions, high levels of ATP act as a pro-inflammatory danger signal, activating the inflammasome that processes pro-IL-1β into mature IL-1β (31, 32). In this sense, it has been suggested that CD39 expression may contribute to dampening the ongoing inflammatory processes and/or rescue the cells from ATP-induced apoptosis/necrosis (33). Ultimately, adenosine exerts potent anti-inflammatory effects on different immune cell types. Recently, we reported that purinergic signaling is clue in regulating the immune response to experimental *T. cruzi* infection. The temporal pharmacological inhibition of CD73 during the early acute phase of the infection induces microbicidal mechanisms, with the concomitant reduction in cardiac parasite load, improving the outcome of chronic cardiomyopathy (34). In agreement with a previous report that indicated CD73 expression on T cells is downregulated in chronic HIV infection (35), in this work, we observed lower expression of CD39 and CD73 on fresh explanted lymphocytes from chagasic patients compared to seronegative donor. Thus, it is plausible that the downregulation of ATP catabolic enzymes could be involved in the increased plasma IL-1β levels in chagasic patients.

In summary, the results of this study show that chronic *T. cruzi* infection leads to a decrease in the number and percentage of total circulating CD8+ T cells and that NO produced by leukocytes may contribute to lowering the effector function of these cells, which ultimately may results in an inefficient control of parasite replication. The findings also suggest that IL-6 could be a key factor to improve CD8+ T cell activation and survival.

AUTHOR CONTRIBUTIONS

Conceived and designed the experiments: LS, MR, and MA. Performed the experiments: LS, LV, NE, MR, and NP. Analyzed the data: LS, LV, NE, MR, NP, NS, MV, GB, SG, AM, and MA. Patients handling and human samples: LV, NS, MV, GB, and AM. Wrote the paper: LS and MA.

ACKNOWLEDGMENTS

The authors thank Laura Gatica, Alejandra Romero, Pilar Crespo, and Paula Abadie for their skillful technical assistance. They also thank the staff of the Biochemical Laboratory of Diagnosis of the HNSM for their kind collaboration. MA and SG are members of the scientific career from the Consejo Nacional de Investigaciones Científicas y Técnicas de la República Argentina (CONICET). LS, MR, and NP thank CONICET for the fellowships granted; LV and NE thank fellowship granted from Fundación Florencio Fiorini and ANPCyT-FONCyT, respectively.

FUNDING

This work was supported by Secretaría de Ciencia y Tecnología, Universidad Nacional de Córdoba (Grant number 05/C642), Agencia Nacional de Promoción Científica y Tecnológica (ANPCyT), Fondo para la Investigación Científica y Tecnológica (PICT 2013-2885), Consejo Nacional de Investigaciones Científicas y Técnicas (CONICET) (PIP 11220120100620), and by Ministerio de Ciencia y Tecnología, Gobierno de la Provincia de Córdoba (1143/10).

REFERENCES

1. Tarleton RL. CD8+ T cells in *Trypanosoma cruzi* infection. *Semin Immunopathol* (2015) 37(3):233–8. doi:10.1007/s00281-015-0481-9
2. Savino W, Villa-Verde DM, Mendes-da-Cruz DA, Silva-Monteiro E, Perez AR, Aoki Mdel P, et al. Cytokines and cell adhesion receptors in the regulation of immunity to *Trypanosoma cruzi*. *Cytokine Growth Factor Rev* (2007) 18(1–2):107–24. doi:10.1016/j.cytogfr.2007.01.010
3. Burgos JM, Diez M, Vigliano C, Bisio M, Risso M, Duffy T, et al. Molecular identification of *Trypanosoma cruzi* discrete typing units in end-stage chronic Chagas heart disease and reactivation after heart transplantation. *Clin Infect Dis* (2010) 51(5):485–95. doi:10.1086/655680
4. Aoki MP, Guinazu NL, Pellegrini AV, Gotoh T, Masih DT, Gea S. Cruzipain, a major *Trypanosoma cruzi* antigen, promotes arginase-2 expression and survival of neonatal mouse cardiomyocytes. *Am J Physiol Cell Physiol* (2004) 286(2):C206–12. doi:10.1152/ajpcell.00282.2003
5. Aoki MP, Carrera-Silva EA, Cuervo H, Fresno M, Girones N, Gea S. Nonimmune cells contribute to crosstalk between immune cells and inflammatory mediators in the innate response to *Trypanosoma cruzi* infection. *J Parasitol Res* (2012) 2012:13. doi:10.1155/2012/737324
6. Mabbott NA, Sutherland IA, Sternberg JM. Suppressor macrophages in *Trypanosoma brucei* infection: nitric oxide is related to both suppressive activity and lifespan in vivo. *Parasite Immunol* (1995) 17(3):143–50. doi:10.1111/j.1365-3024.1995.tb01016.x
7. Jenson JS, O'Connor R, Osborne J, Devaney E. Infection with *Brugia microfilariae* induces apoptosis of CD4(+) T lymphocytes: a mechanism of immune unresponsiveness in filariasis. *Eur J Immunol* (2002) 32(3):858–67. doi:10.1002/1521-4141(200203)32:3<858::AID-IMMU858>3.0.CO;2-E
8. Rockett KA, Awburn MM, Rockett EJ, Cowden WB, Clark IA. Possible role of nitric oxide in malarial immunosuppression. *Parasite Immunol* (1994) 16(5):243–9. doi:10.1111/j.1365-3024.1994.tb00346.x
9. Saio M, Radoja S, Marino M, Frey AB. Tumor-infiltrating macrophages induce apoptosis in activated CD8(+) T cells by a mechanism requiring cell contact and mediated by both the cell-associated form of TNF and nitric oxide. *J Immunol* (2001) 167(10):5583–93. doi:10.4049/jimmunol.167.10.5583
10. Hirst DG, Robson T. Nitrosative stress as a mediator of apoptosis: implications for cancer therapy. *Curr Pharm Des* (2010) 16(1):45–55. doi:10.2174/138161210789941838
11. Sawa T, Akaike T, Maeda H. Tyrosine nitration by peroxynitrite formed from nitric oxide and superoxide generated by xanthine oxidase. *J Biol Chem* (2000) 275(42):32467–74. doi:10.1074/jbc.M910169199
12. Gunaydin H, Houk KN. Mechanisms of peroxynitrite-mediated nitration of tyrosine. *Chem Res Toxicol* (2009) 22(5):894–8. doi:10.1021/tx800463y
13. Arocena AR, Onofrio LI, Pellegrini AV, Carrera-Silva AE, Paroli A, Cano RC, et al. Myeloid-derived suppressor cells are key players in the resolution of inflammation during a model of acute infection. *Eur J Immunol* (2014) 44(1):184–94. doi:10.1002/eji.201343606
14. Albareda MC, Laucella SA, Alvarez MG, Armenti AH, Bertochi G, Tarleton RL, et al. *Trypanosoma cruzi* modulates the profile of memory CD8+ T cells in chronic Chagas' disease patients. *Int Immunol* (2006) 18(3):465–71. doi:10.1093/intimm/dxh387
15. Sallusto F, Geginat J, Lanzavecchia A. Central memory and effector memory T cell subsets: function, generation, and maintenance. *Annu Rev Immunol* (2004) 22:745–63. doi:10.1146/annurev.immunol.22.012703.104702
16. Ding AH, Nathan CF, Stuehr DJ. Release of reactive nitrogen intermediates and reactive oxygen intermediates from mouse peritoneal macrophages. Comparison of activating cytokines and evidence for independent production. *J Immunol* (1988) 141:2407–12.
17. Plan.Nacional.de.Chagas. *Plan Nacional de Chagas 2011–2015*. Boletín Oficial Junio – Res 867/2012. Argentina: Official Bulletin of National Ministry of Health (2012).
18. Nagaraj S, Gupta K, Pisarev V, Kinarsky L, Sherman S, Kang L, et al. Altered recognition of antigen is a mechanism of CD8+ T cell tolerance in cancer. *Nat Med* (2007) 13(7):828–35. doi:10.1038/nm1609
19. Nagaraj S, Schrum AG, Cho HI, Celis E, Gabrilovich DI. Mechanism of T cell tolerance induced by myeloid-derived suppressor cells. *J Immunol* (2010) 184(6):3106–16. doi:10.4049/jimmunol.0902661
20. Mazzoni A, Bronte V, Visintin A, Spitzer JH, Apolloni E, Serafini P, et al. Myeloid suppressor lines inhibit T cell responses by an NO-dependent mechanism. *J Immunol* (2002) 168(2):689–95. doi:10.4049/jimmunol.168.2.689
21. Bronte V, Zanovello P. Regulation of immune responses by L-arginine metabolism. *Nat Rev Immunol* (2005) 5(8):641–54. doi:10.1038/nri1668
22. Bonavida B, Garban H. Nitric oxide-mediated sensitization of resistant tumor cells to apoptosis by chemo-immunotherapeutics. *Redox Biol* (2015) 6:486–94. doi:10.1016/j.redox.2015.08.013
23. Messmer UK, Reed UK, Brune B. Bcl-2 protects macrophages from nitric oxide-induced apoptosis. *J Biol Chem* (1996) 271(33):20192–7. doi:10.1074/jbc.271.33.20192
24. Dhiman M, Estrada-Franco JG, Pando JM, Ramirez-Aguilar FJ, Spratt H, Vazquez-Corzo S, et al. Increased myeloperoxidase activity and protein nitration are indicators of inflammation in patients with Chagas' disease. *Clin Vaccine Immunol* (2009) 16(5):660–6. doi:10.1128/CVI.00019-09
25. Gabrilovich DI, Nagaraj S. Myeloid-derived suppressor cells as regulators of the immune system. *Nat Rev Immunol* (2009) 9(3):162–74. doi:10.1038/nri2506
26. Lu T, Gabrilovich DI. Molecular pathways: tumor-infiltrating myeloid cells and reactive oxygen species in regulation of tumor microenvironment. *Clin Cancer Res* (2012) 18(18):4877–82. doi:10.1158/1078-0432.CCR-11-2939
27. Predonzani A, Cali B, Agnellini AH, Molon B. Spotlights on immunological effects of reactive nitrogen species: when inflammation says nitric oxide. *World J Exp Med* (2015) 5(2):64–76. doi:10.5493/wjem.v5.i2.64
28. Ponce NE, Cano RC, Carrera-Silva EA, Lima AP, Gea S, Aoki MP. Toll-like receptor-2 and interleukin-6 mediate cardiomyocyte protection from apoptosis during *Trypanosoma cruzi* murine infection. *Med Microbiol Immunol* (2012) 201(2):145–55. doi:10.1007/s00430-011-0216-z
29. Ponce NE, Carrera-Silva EA, Pellegrini AV, Cazorla SI, Malchiodi EL, Lima AP, et al. *Trypanosoma cruzi*, the causative agent of Chagas disease, modulates interleukin-6-induced STAT3 phosphorylation via gp130 cleavage in different host cells. *Biochim Biophys Acta* (2013) 1832(3):485–94. doi:10.1016/j.bbadis.2012.12.003
30. Antonioli L, Pacher P, Vizi ES, Hasko G. CD39 and CD73 in immunity and inflammation. *Trends Mol Med* (2013) 19(6):355–67. doi:10.1016/j.molmed.2013.03.005

31. Lamkanfi M, Dixit VM. Mechanisms and functions of inflammasomes. *Cell* (2014) 157(5):1013–22. doi:10.1016/j.cell.2014.04.007
32. Garg NJ. Inflammasomes in cardiovascular diseases. *Am J Cardiovasc Dis* (2011) 1(3):244–54.
33. Zhou Q, Yan J, Putheti P, Wu Y, Sun X, Toxavidis V, et al. Isolated CD39 expression on CD4+ T cells denotes both regulatory and memory populations. *Am J Transplant* (2009) 9(10):2303–11. doi:10.1111/j.1600-6143.2009.02777.x
34. Ponce NE, Sanmarco LM, Eberhardt N, Garcia MC, Rivarola HW, Cano RC, et al. CD73 inhibition shifts cardiac macrophage polarization toward a microbicidal phenotype and ameliorates the outcome of experimental Chagas cardiomyopathy. *J Immunol* (2016) 197(3):814–23. doi:10.4049/jimmunol.1600371
35. Toth I, Le AQ, Hartjen P, Thomssen A, Matzat V, Lehmann C, et al. Decreased frequency of CD73+CD8+ T cells of HIV-infected patients correlates with immune activation and T cell exhaustion. *J Leukoc Biol* (2013) 94(4):551–61. doi:10.1189/jlb.0113018

9

Dendritic Cells: A Double-Edged Sword in Immune Responses during Chagas Disease

*Natalia Gil-Jaramillo[1], Flávia N. Motta[1,2], Cecília B. F. Favali[3], Izabela M. D. Bastos[1] and Jaime M. Santana[1]**

[1] Laboratório de Interação Patógeno-Hospedeiro, Instituto de Biologia, Universidade de Brasília, Brasília, Brazil, [2] Faculdade de Ceilândia, Universidade de Brasília, Brasília, Brazil, [3] Laboratório de Biologia do Gene, Instituto de Biologia, Universidade de Brasília, Brasília, Brazil

***Correspondence:**
Jaime M. Santana
jsantana@unb.br

Dendritic cells (DCs) are the most important member of the antigen presenting cells group due to their ability to recognize antigen at the infection site and their high specialized antigen internalization capacity. These cells have central role in connecting the innate and adaptive immune responses against *Trypanosoma cruzi*, the causative agent of Chagas disease. These first line defense cells modulate host immune response depending on type, maturation level, cytokine milieu and DC receptor involved in the interactions with *T. cruzi*, influencing the development of the disease clinic forms. Here, we present a review of DCs–*T. cruzi* interactions both in human and murine models, pointing out the parasite ability to manipulate DCs activity for the purpose of evading innate immune response and assuring its own survival and persistence.

Keywords: chagas disease, *Trypanosoma cruzi*, dendritic cell, immunoregulation, evasion strategy

INTRODUCTION

More than a century has passed since Carlos Chagas discovered the pathogen *Trypanosoma cruzi* and the natural way of its transmission to humans and animals, and elucidated the corresponding human disease it causes (Kropf and Sá, 2009). Chagas disease is also transmitted through blood transfusions or organ transplants, vertically from mother to child through the placenta, and through contaminated food (Andrade et al., 2014). This neglected disease affects predominantly deprived people and induces social and economic impacts by decreasing patient's productivity and earning capacity (Hotez et al., 2007).

With 28,000 new cases per year and 8,000 newborns infected during gestation, Chagas disease affects about 8 million people, beyond 65 million live in areas of exposure and are at risk of contracting the disease (World Health Organization, 2015). Despite the efforts to reduce Chagas disease and the number of infections over the last two decades, it is still endemic in Latin America (Rassi et al., 2010; Strasen et al., 2013) and, as result of global migration, the number of people infected with *T. cruzi* is increasing in North America, Europe, Japan and Oceania (non-endemic areas) (Schmunis, 2007). Since Chagas disease crosses boundaries and spreads, it becomes not only a burden for the endemic countries but a worldwide health concern (Andrade et al., 2014).

Treatment of Chagas disease is one of the greatest therapeutic challenges in tropical medicine since the only drugs approved for human treatment – Nifurtimox and Benznidazole – date from the early 1970s and have carcinogenic properties conferred to nitrofuran and nitroimidazole, their active chemical groups, respectively (Bern, 2011; Wilkinson et al., 2011). Nevertheless, both medicines share similar features: necessity of prolonged administration, effectiveness related to the acute phase and different susceptibility among *T. cruzi* strains (Bermudez et al., 2015). Aditionally, Nifurtimox prescription has been abolished in Brazil, Argentina, Uruguay, Chile and US due to its toxic effects over central nervous system, genotoxicity, and reduced efficacy (Wilkinson et al., 2011).

The natural disease progression consists of an acute phase that can be followed by an asymptomatic indeterminate phase, which represents most of the cases and, one-third of infected population progress to the chronic phase that may lead to death (Machado et al., 2013). Early clinical manifestations include headache, fever, and cough, which are non-specific signs; consequently most of infected individuals are neither notified nor treated. Symptomatic chronic stage of the disease usually occurs from 10 to 25 years after infection and typical manifestations are mild to severe cardiomyopathy and/or dilated digestive tract (megaoesophagus and megacolon) (Steverding, 2014). The mechanisms responsible for patient progression from the indeterminate to the symptomatic chronic phase are not completely understood, although the immunological events initiated during the acute phase undoubtedly drive the organism toward the development of a protective or deleterious immune response (Andrade et al., 2014).

It is unanimity that during the acute phase, dendritic cells (DC), along with macrophages, and natural killer (NK) cells, guarantee the host first line of defense against the parasite (Watanabe Costa et al., 2016). Guide by this context, our purpose is to present a review about DC–*T. cruzi* interaction pointing out the parasite ability to evade innate immune response to assure its own survival and persistence.

Trypanosoma cruzi

Trypanosoma cruzi is an obligate intracellular protozoan of the Kinetoplastea Class, characterized by the presence of one flagellum and a single mitochondrion comprising the kinetoplast, a specialized DNA-containing structure. The Order Trypanosomatida comprises other parasites responsible for severe diseases in humans and other species, for instance *Leishmania* sp. (leishmaniasis), *Trypanosoma brucei* (African trypanosomiasis), *Phytomonas* sp. (plant diseases), and *Crithidia* sp. (arthropods diseases) (Stevens, 2008), that show adaptability toward their hosts with numerous sophisticated immune evasion strategies (D'Avila-Levy et al., 2015).

Trypanosoma cruzi strains present diversity in morphology, infection capacity, cell surface predominant antigens and other biological and biochemical features (de Lana et al., 2010). In 2009, *the Second Satellite Meeting* held in Buzios, Brazil suggested six Discrete Typing Units (DTUs) for classifying the several *T. cruzi* strains, named TcI to TcVI (Zingales et al., 2009). A DTU is a population set that is more genetically related among themselves than to any other population, showing common genetic, immunological and molecular markers (Tibayrenc, 1998). These DTUs subsets have different distribution among the American continent due to parasite adaptations to different vectors and reservoirs (Zingales et al., 2012), and, although, some characteristics are shared within the same DTU, differences in many aspects can be found among strains. *T. cruzi* Colombian and G strains, belonging to TcI group, are a clear example of this intra-DTU diversity. Colombian strain, isolated from humans, is highly infective (Ramírez et al., 2010), but no human infections were reported from G strain, which was isolated from anal gland secretions of an opossum (Deane et al., 1984). *T.* cruzi G strain has gp35/50 as predominant surface glycoprotein that appears to be related to its poor internalization by humans cells (Yoshida, 2006).

T. cruzi life cycle alternates between reduviid bug vectors and mammal hosts. Domestic and wild animals like opossum, bats, armadillo, and monkey may also act as reservoir host (Coura et al., 2002). The parasite presents different forms during its life cycle – epimastigotes remains in the insect gut; non-divinding and infective metacyclic trypomastigotes (MT) find in the insect feces and/or urine; bloodstream trypomastigotes that can circulate in the mammalian blood and, finally, the intracellular, proliferative and rounded amastigote form. A triatomine insect picks up the parasite trypomastigote forms by feeding on the blood of an infected mammal (Teixeira et al., 2009) and, once inside the vector, those forms differentiate into epimastigotes and multiply in midgut (Manchola et al., 2015). After migration to the bug's hindgut, epimastigotes attach to the waxy gut cuticle by their flagella and differentiate into infectious MT, which will be deposited along with feces/urine on the skin of the victim (Muñoz-Saravia et al., 2012). The parasite penetrates the new host through lesions caused by its bite or a variety of mucosal membranes. MTs invade host cells entering a parasitophorous vacuole (Romano et al., 2012), which fuses to lysosomes. Once free in the cytoplasm, the parasite differentiates into amastigotes that undergo binary fission multiplication and transform back to trypomastigotes, which are released upon rupture of the host cell membrane and infect neighboring cells or enter the bloodstream (Stecconi-Silva et al., 2003; Tonelli et al., 2004). Bloodstream trypomastigotes may begin another infection cycle when they are taken in the blood feeding of the vector (Bern, 2015). Humans and animals can be infected orally through the ingestion of food and drink contaminated by crushed infected insect vectors or their feces (Nóbrega et al., 2009; Bastos et al., 2010).

Immune evasion strategies developed by *T. cruzi* are essential to the establishment of a long-life infection. Complement inactivation, escape from phagolysosome, antibodies with no *T-cruzi* specificity and delayed immune response are some examples of those strategies (Reviewed by Nardy et al., 2015; Cardoso et al., 2016). Another mechanism involved in parasite persistence is the manipulation of DC functions, which impairs an adequate host immune defense.

DENDRITIC CELLS

Dendritic cells are bone-marrow-derived cells that belong to the antigen presenting cells (APC) group, being considered the most important member due to their high capacity to recognize and internalize antigens at the infection site (Haniffa et al., 2009; Collin et al., 2013). They link innate and adaptive immune responses by capturing, processing and expressing antigens in the cell surface membrane (Planelles et al., 2003; Steinman, 2007). Immature DCs have a wide range of innate receptors that enables the recognition of pathogens via pattern recognition receptors (PRRs), which activate DCs through signaling pathways eliciting their maturation (Pearce and Everts, 2015). Toll-like receptors (TLRs), abundant in APC, are one of the best-characterized PPRs and efficiently detect pathogen-associated molecular patterns (PAMPs) that are located on the cell surface or in the lumen of endosomes. The presence of TLRs on the cell surface or in the lumen of endosomes enables efficient pathogen recognition and the development of an adequate innate immune response; i.e., TLR2, located in DCs plasma membrane, senses various components of pathogens and its stimulation induces the production of various proinflammatory cytokines. TLR9, located in DCs endolysosome, is involved in virus, bacteria, protozoa nucleic acid recognition and its activation also leads to the production of proinflammatory cytokines (Takeuchi and Akira, 2010). After antigen recognition, DCs can travel along the body from peripheral tissues to lymphoid organs/tissues where they present the processed antigens through their major histocompatibility complexes (MHC) to T cells (Lipscomb and Masten, 2002). Maturation process comprises differentiation from antigen-capturing specialized cells to presenting and stimulating specialized cells. Mature DCs can be identified by morphological aspects like cytoplasmic extensions and abundant intracellular structures (lysosomes, endosomes, granules, etc.) related to antigen processing and by modulation of molecular markers such as up-regulation of CD83, of co-stimulatory molecules like CD80 (or B7-1) and CD86 (or B7-2) and MHC (O'Neill et al., 2004).

Dendritic cells present antigens to lymphocytes $CD8^+$ and $CD4^+$ T by MHC class I and MHC class II, respectively (Blum et al., 2013). For MHC class I molecules, these antigens originate from intracellular sources; for MHC class II, from exogenous sources. Some DCs have an atypical ability, called cross-presentation that allows to load peptides from exogenous antigens onto MHC class I molecules (Vyas et al., 2008; Neefjes et al., 2011; Segura and Amigorena, 2015). MHC class I molecules are expressed by all nucleated cells and their antigen presentation pathway consists in a series of reactions: (1) intracellular proteins are degraded by the proteasome; (2) the peptides are delivered to the endoplasmic reticulum by the transporter associated with antigen processing complex; (3) antigens are loaded onto MHC class I molecules; (4) peptide–MHC class I complexes are transported via the Golgi to cell surface for presentation to $CD8^+$ T cells (Vyas et al., 2008; Neefjes et al., 2011). Recently it was demonstrated that infection of HeLa cells with *T. cruzi* Y strain promotes a down-regulation of the immunoproteasome subunits biosynthesis as well as the MHC class I molecule expression, which could be considered a mechanism of parasite persistence inside the cell (Camargo et al., 2014). Unlike MHC class I expression, MHC class II are mainly expressed by APCs such as DCs, macrophages and B cells (Vyas et al., 2008; Neefjes et al., 2011). Extracellular antigens are taken up by APCs and placed into the phagosome. This compartment fuses with lysosomes to form phagolysosomes, where MHC class II molecules interact with the antigens. Peptide-loaded MHC class II molecules are then transported to the cell surface where they engage antigen-specific $CD4^+$ T cells (Vyas et al., 2008; Neefjes et al., 2011). Curiously, MHC II molecules are in constant recycle and degradation process in immature DCs, but mature DCs exhibits a stable and prolonged antigen presentation (den Haan et al., 2014). It is worth mentioning that DCs antigen presentation is not enough for T lymphocytes activation and proliferation. Co-stimulatory molecules expression and cytokine production are also required and they are efficiently provided by mature DCs (den Haan et al., 2014). Following activation via TLRs, DCs may produce acute innate cytokines involved in local and systemic responses such as IL-1β, IL-6, IL-8, IL-12, and TNF-α (Verhasselt et al., 1997; Holdsworth and Can, 2015), however, DCs, under specific conditions, are also able to produce IL-10 and TGF-β for directing a regulatory response (**Table 1**).

Different DC subsets and maturation levels can produce distinct kinds of cytokines or co-stimulatory molecules that can lead either to an inflammatory or a regulatory response. Among DC subsets, myeloid (mDC or classical DC), plasmocytoid (pDC), Langerhans cells (LCs), and derived from monocytes (monocyte DC) are some well-known examples. In murines, mDCs are composed of two main groups: resident and migratory, which are further divided into two subsets: Batf3-dependent and IRF4-dependent DCs (Reviewed by Segura, 2016). mDC Batf3-dependent/migratory expresses CD11c, Clec9A, XCR1, CD103, and CD207; the resident one expresses CD11c, Clec9A, XCR1, and CD8. On the other hand, mDC IRF4-dependent/resident expresses CD11c, CD11b, CD172a; the same markers are found in the migratory subsets along with CD206. The major markers for pDC are CD11c, Ly6c, B220 and SiglecH. For monocyte DC, they are CD11c, CD11b, CD64, FcεRI, CD206, CD14, CD172a, and Ly6c (Reviewed by Segura, 2016). Finally, LCs is a special DC population present in epidermis and other stratified squamous epithelia, such as oral and genital mucous membranes and bronchus. Despite of being associated with these tissues, LCs may differentiate into migratory cells for antigen presentation; their principal markers are CD11c, CD207, EpCAM, and E-cadherin. Human mDCs classical markers are $CD1c^+$, Dectin 1 (CLEC 7A), and Dectin 2 (CLEC6A). Regarding pDCs, CD303 (CLEC4C), CD304 (neuropilin), and CD123 (IL-3R) are human usual markers. Monocyte DCs may express CD14, CD209 (DC-SIGN), CD16, and CD1c (Reviewed by Collin et al., 2013). Lewis and Reizis (2012) have proposed the existence of two more kinds of DCs within these subsets: "receptors", cells more specialized in capturing antigens and producing cytokines and "presenters", cells that benefit from these cytokines and travel to lymph nodes for presenting the antigens. It represents another level of specialization among DCs, stating their diversity and their capacity to guide polarity, magnitude and specificity of immune responses (Lewis and Reizis, 2012).

Some studies have demonstrated that acute and chronic phases of Chagas disease require different polarizations of

TABLE 1 | Study conditions in murine models.

DC source	Markers	*T. cruzi* strain	Study conditions	Disease phase	Result	Reference
Spleen	CD11c	Tehuantepec	Tehuantepec *in vivo* infection	Acute	↓CD86; ↓ migration capacity	Chaussabel et al., 2003
Bone-marrow	CD11b; CD11c	RA	RA *in vitro* infection	Acute	↓Cytokine production; ↓endocytic capacity	Poncini et al., 2008
Spleen	CD11c	RA	RA *in vivo* infection	Acute	↓Cytokine production; ↓MHC II expression	Alba Soto et al., 2003
Spleen	CD11c	K98	K98 *in vivo* infection	Acute	↑Co-stimulatory molecules expression; ↑MHC II expresion	Alba Soto et al., 2003
Bone-marrow	CD11b; CD11c	AQ1.7, MUTUM (TcI); 1849, 2369 (TcII)	*In vitro* infections	Acute	↑Anti-inflammatory cytokine production; ↑ TLR2 expression	da Costa et al., 2014
Spleen	CD11c	Y	*In vivo* infection using different mouse lineages	Acute	↓Co-stimulatory molecules expression; ↓MHC II expression	Planelles et al., 2003
Bone-marrow	CD11c	Queretaro	*In vivo* infection using MIF-deficient mice	Acute	IL-12 role in protection	Terrazas et al., 2011
Bone-marrow	CD11b; CD11c	RA	IL-10-deficient DCs were injetec along RA strain in mice	From acute to chronic	↓Cytokine production; ↓MHC II expression	Alba Soto et al., 2010
Bone-marrow	CD11b; CD11c	RA	*In vitro* infections	Acute	↑Anti-inflammatory cytokine production; ↓T cell induction	Poncini et al., 2010
Bone-marrow DCs and NK cells	CD11c	RA	Study of NK cells and DCs interaction in mice	Acute	Unbalanced DC population	Batalla et al., 2013
Spleen	CD11b; CD11c	Colombian	300, 3000, and 30000 initial inocula in mice	From acute to chronic	Less favorable host response in medium inocula	Borges et al., 2012
Bone-marrow		CL Brener	*In vitro* assay using CpG islands	Acute	Recognition by TLR9; ↑IL-12 and IFN-γ production	Bartholomeu et al., 2008
Spleen	CD11c	Y	*In vivo* infection studying TLR9 expression	Acute	↑Recognition by TLR9; ↑inflammatory cytokine production	Gravina et al., 2013
Bone-marrow		Tulahuen	*In vivo* and *in vitro* infection using MyD88/TRIF-deficient mice	Acute	No IFN-β production and no parasite clearance	Koga et al., 2006
Spleen	CD11c	CL Brener	*In vivo* infection using UNC93B1deficient mice	Acute	No correct TLR activation; ↓IL-12p40 and IFN-γ	Caetano et al., 2011
Spleen	CD11c	Dm28c	*In vitro* infections using B2R-deficient DCs	Acute	No IL-12 production	Monteiro et al., 2007
Spleen	CD11c	Dm28c	*In vitro* infections using C5a antagonist	Acute	No IL-12p40/70 and IFN-γ production	Schmitz et al., 2014
Spleen	CD11c	RA	*In vitro* infections using Gal-1-deficient DCs	Acute	Regulatory T Cell induction	Poncini et al., 2015
Spleen	CD11c	Tehuantepec	*In vivo* infections studying Gal-3 expression	Acute	↑Gal-3 expression;↓Migration capacity	Vray et al., 2004
Bone-marrow	CD11c	Tulahuen	*In vitro* infections blocking Siglec-E	Acute	↓Inflammatory cytokine production; ↓T cell induction	Erdmann et al., 2009
Bone-marrow	CD11c	Tehuantepec	*In vitro* infections blocking Siglec-E	Acute	Parasite clearance	Erdmann et al., 2009
Spleen	CD11b; CD11c	Y	*In vitro* infectionn using Slamf1-deficient splenic DCs	From acute to chronic	↓IFN-γ production; no intracellular *T. cruzi* replication	Calderón et al., 2012

immune response: Th1 profile is protective in an acute state and regulatory responses are important in preventing the chronic phase (Andrade et al., 2014; Dutra et al., 2015). For this reason, DCs are a key group of cells in Chagas disease: they could modulate response depending on type, maturation level, cytokine milieu and DC receptor involved, having a fundamental role in the development of the disease clinic forms including the undetermined stage.

DENDRITIC CELL–*T. cruzi* INTERACTION: MURINE MODELS

Studies on acute Chagas disease in humans are limited due to lack of unique symptoms that characterize this disease state. Nonetheless, extending our knowledge about the acute phase is important because immunological events that take place in this stage have a great influence on the possible development of the chronic phase (Andrade et al., 2014). In this context, experimental murine infection may mimic the human disease, giving us a similar view on what happens at the beginning of *T. cruzi* infection.

Unlikely the habitual DCs response during an infection, the expression of important surface molecules like MHC, CD80 or CD86 can be reduced when DCs recognize *T. cruzi* antigens in a strain dependent manner, limiting DC maturation and antigen presenting capacity. During acute phase, splenic DCs infected by *T. cruzi* Tehuantepec strain shows low expression of CD86 molecules and are not able to migrate toward lymphoid organs/tissues (Chaussabel et al., 2003). *T. cruzi* high virulent RA strain (TcVI) induces bone-marrow DCs downregulation of cytokine production and of endocytic capacity added to a suppression of MHC class II, compared to non-infected cells (Poncini et al., 2008). These data are in concordance with the regulation studied by Alba Soto and coworkers, where they also detected a diminished MHC II expression in infected splenic DCs by the same *T. cruzi* strain. Additionally, they showed that the DC manipulated behavior induced by RA strain is not repeated for non-virulent K98 *T. cruzi* strain (TcI) (**Figure 1**; Alba Soto et al., 2003). Another comparative infection study, using mDCs, was performed using TcI (AQ1.7 and MUTUM) and TcII strains (1849 and 2369). The results demonstrated that both *T. cruzi* DTUs may modulate DCs to different extents and this modulation varied more between strains than between DTUs themselves. In general, both DTUs induced the production and expression of anti-inflammatory molecules, such as IL-10, production and PD-L1 and TLR2 expression. Regarding TLR2 expression, it seems that *T. cruzi* has molecules that bind this receptor promoting the production of anti-inflammatory cytokines such as IL-10. Oppositely, proinflammatory molecules did not present a pattern, varying depending on the strain. Finally, they also demonstrated that DC expression of differentiation and activation molecules was not polarized, which suggests that each strain of *T. cruzi* has possibly evolved specific evasion strategies (da Costa et al., 2014). Interestingly, when two mice lineages were infected by high virulent *T. cruzi* Y strain (TcII), the susceptible one showed splenic DCs with reduced capacity of antigen presentation and lower expression of CD40 and CD86 molecules compared with resistant lineages (Planelles et al., 2003). It is well known that the deficiency of co-stimulatory signals during cross-presentation may reduce T cell stimulation or lead to an anergic state (Boussiotis et al., 1996). Thus, it seems that impaired function by DC maybe helps parasite to evade the host immune system.

Cytokine production is another important aspect during DCs–*T. cruzi* interaction, particularly the production of IL-12, considered a protective molecule during the acute infection once it drives a polarized Th1 adaptive response that enables the host to adequately control parasite growth through IFN-γ (Andrade et al., 2014). In concordance, DCs from *T. cruzi*-resistant mouse lineages overexpressed IL-12 and TNF-α while the susceptible lineages produced the Th2 cytokine IL-4 (Planelles et al., 2003). IL-4 is known to mediate host susceptibility to *T. cruzi* but is also required for preventing immune hyperactivity and organ immunopathology (Abrahamsohn and Coffman, 1996; Laucella et al., 1996). Terrazas et al. (2011) demonstrated the protective role of IL-12 through *T. cruzi* Queretaro (TcI) strain infection of MIF (macrophage migration inhibitory factor)-deficient mice. MIF is a pleiotropic cytokine produced by multiple different cell types, including DCs that modulates the expression of several proinflammatory molecules (Cooke et al., 2009). It seems that it favors DC maturation through IL-12 secretion and activation of p38 MAPK protein, a kinase already known to be involved in DC maturation. On the other hand, MIF-deficient mice showed lower levels of IL-12 production and immature bone-marrow DCs, leading to a susceptibility of *T. cruzi* Queretaro (TcI) strain infection (Terrazas et al., 2011). The regulatory IL-10 cytokine is also associated with host susceptibility during acute stage of Chagas disease by limiting DCs induction of antimicrobial effector mechanism such as suppressing DC trafficking to draining lymph nodes (Corinti et al., 2001; Demangel et al., 2002; Alba Soto et al., 2010). A single intravenous injection of IL-10-deficient DCs that were pulsed with parasite antigens conferred an effective control against a lethal challenge with *T. cruzi* RA strain in mice. IL-10 deficient DCs were high Th1 cytokines producers and inducers of antigen-specific T lymphocytes after immunization (Alba Soto et al., 2010). On the other hand, Poncini et al. (2010) have showed that interaction of DCs with *T. cruzi* trypomastigotes was not able to activate the DCs, and these cells became TGF-β and IL-10 producers and were not efficient as lymphocyte stimulators, being classified as regulatory DCs. Furthermore, mature DCs have the capacity to induce NK cells activation and proliferation. NK cells play a significant role in innate immune response and surveillance as a result of their cytokine production and cytolysis of infected cells. Moreover, NK cells secrete IFN-γ, TNF-α, and GM-CSF, which promote DC maturation and activation of T-cell (Gerosa et al., 2002; Piccioli et al., 2002). Batalla et al. (2013) used RA and K98 *T. cruzi* strains to demonstrate the role of NK cells in regulating the maturation level of DCs. During both infections, NK cell was functionally activated and produced IFN-γ but also IL-10; NK cells from mice infected with *T. cruzi* RA strain (high virulence) exhibit reduced ability to lyse and fail to induce maturation

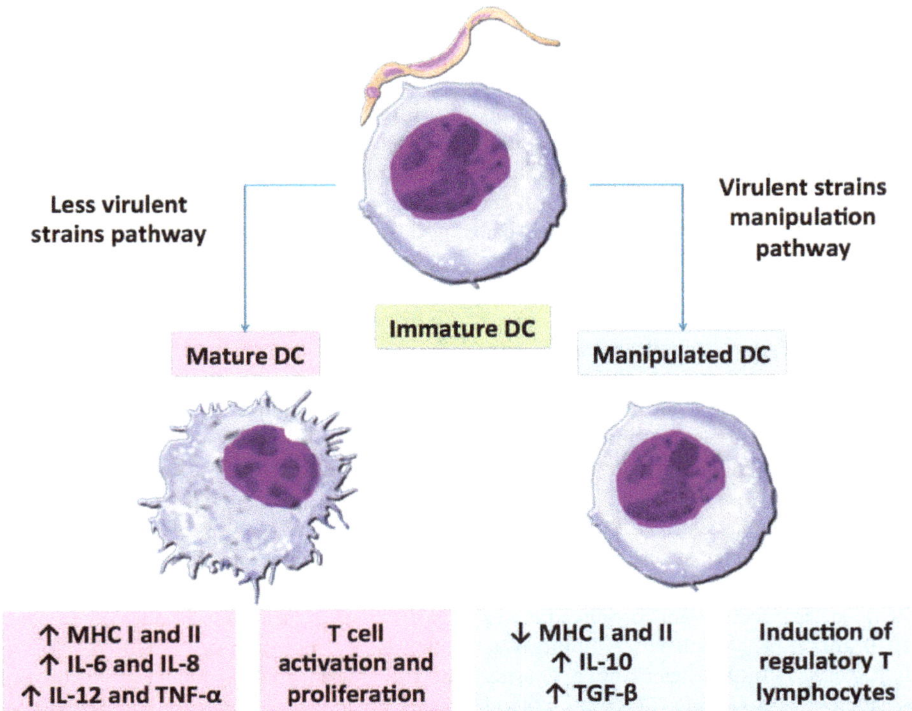

FIGURE 1 | Possible scenarios after dendritic cells (DCs)–*Trypanosoma cruzi* interaction. DCs may maturate, up-regulating major histocompatibility complexes (MHC) molecule expression and proinflammatory cytokine production, which may stimulate antigen-specific T lymphocyte activation and proliferation to control parasitemia (magenta); or DCs may be manipulated and the resultant low MHC expression together with high regulatory cytokine production may lead to a weak T cell activation, helping parasite establishment (blue). DC deviant behavior pathway could represent a potent immune evasion strategy of virulent *T. cruzi* strains to successfully set host infection. On the other hand, less virulent *T. cruzi* strains lack DC modulation capacity, which enables host immune response and parasite control.

of bone marrow-derived immature DCs. This unbalanced DC population could difficult T cell stimulation for an adequate response. Finally, that IL-10 production observed by NK cells after infection with *T. cruzi* RA strain might lead to parasite persistence but can also limit the induction of a vigorous tissue-damaging T-cell response (Batalla et al., 2013). Cytokine production may also be modulated by parasite initial inocula. Three different inocula of *T. cruzi* Colombian strain were used to infect mice, resulting in differential expression of IFN-γ, IL-17, TNF-α, IL-4, and IL-23 by immune cells in heart infiltrates. Curiously, the medium inoculum showed the less favorable host response, which may indicate the existence of an ideal initial inoculum to help parasite evade host immune response (Borges et al., 2012).

It also has been shown the important role of TLRs in *T. cruzi* recognition by first line of defense cells, including DCs. Campos et al. (2004) demonstrated that *T. cruzi* employs a myeloid differentiation factor 88 (MyD88)-, a key adaptor for most TLRs, dependent pathway to elicit cytokine production by the host cells. Intraperitoneal macrophages lacking MyD88 produced less IFN-γ, IL-12, TNF-α and reactive nitrogen intermediates, they also presented higher parasitemia and mortality (Campos et al., 2004). The role of TLRs in the establishment of critical effector mechanisms mediated by $CD8^+$ T cells during *T. cruzi* infection was also investigated (Oliveira et al., 2010). The analysis of induction of IFN-γ and cytotoxic activity *in vivo* in TLR2-, TLR4-, TLR9-, or MyD88-deficient mice during infection showed that neither the absence of TLR2, TLR4, or TLR9 individually, nor the ablation of all MyD88-mediated pathways affect the development of cytotoxic and IFN-γ-producing $CD8^+$ T cells. Nonetheless, TLR4 deficient macrophages presented a reduced production of TNF-α and nitric oxide (NO), pointing to an important role of the TLR4 pathway and NO production to the innate immune response against *T. cruzi* infection (Oliveira et al., 2010). With regard specifically to DCs, infection with *T. cruzi* parasites promotes recruitment of TLR9 to the DC endolysosome compartment, promoting their interaction during initial phagocytosis. Stimulatory motifs containing CpG islands of *T. cruzi* CL Brener, particularly those formed by genes coding for mucin like proteins, also led TLR9 into lysosomes of bone-marrow DCs and the induction of IL-12 as well as IFN-γ synthesis (Bartholomeu et al., 2008). Such potent proinflammatory activity and, consequently, control of parasite replication could lead to host resistance to infection or avoiding host lethality and maintenance of parasite life cycle long-term parasite persistence. The second hypothesis suggests another adaptation of *T. cruzi* to the host cell-mediated immunity (Bartholomeu et al., 2008). Gravina et al. (2013) stated that DC population constitutes the main source of IL-12/IL-23p40 production in a TLR9-dependent manner in *T. cruzi* Y strain infection. Moreover, when DCs were unable to produce IL-12/IL-23p40, macrophages recovered their capacity to respond to TLR9 agonist, which may represent a compensatory response. Therefore, modulation of TLR9 is important to control the inflammatory response in the different cell populations but TLR9 acts fundamentally on DC inflammatory activity in *T. cruzi* infection (Gravina et al., 2013). Synergy among TLRs in parasite infected DC has also been studied. When MyD88/TRIF (Toll/IL-1R domain-containing adaptor-inducing IFN-β) deficient mice (i.e., with no functional activation of TLRs) were infected with *T. cruzi* Tulahuen strain (TcVI), parasite clearance was impaired mainly by absence of IFN-β production (Koga et al., 2006). In the same work, it was proposed that proinflammatory cytokine production is a MyD88-dependent induction and the expression of IFN-β is a TRIF-dependent. In any case, both TLR adaptors contribute to innate immune responses against *T. cruzi* infection (Koga et al., 2006). UNC93B1, a protein that interacts with TLR3, TLR7, and TLR9, seems to play an essential role in host protection against *T. cruzi* infection (Caetano et al., 2011). UNC93B1 mice deficient were more susceptible to *T. cruzi* infection and produced lower concentration of IL-12p40 and IFN-γ. Such susceptibility was also achieved during TLR3/TLR7/TLR9-deficient mice *T. cruzi* infection, showing that nucleic acid-sensing TLRs are critical determinants of host resistance to primary infection with *T. cruzi* (Caetano et al., 2011).

Other receptors also have been proposed to play an important role during the acute phase of Chagas disease. G-protein-coupled bradykinin (BK) B2 receptors (B_2R)-deficient mice were more susceptible to *T. cruzi* Dm28c strain (TcI) infection than WT animals (Monteiro et al., 2007). B_2Rs recognize *T. cruzi* released kinins, mediators related to bradykinin that activate immature DCs (Monteiro et al., 2006). Splenic DCs without B_2R receptor do not produce IL-12, appointing a critical role for the kinin signaling pathway in the development of type-1 effector T cells (Monteiro et al., 2007). In a recent study, the same group demonstrated that blockage of B_2R along with C5a receptor resulted in splenic DCs unable to produce IL-12p40/70 and IFN-γ (Schmitz et al., 2014). C5a is an anaphylatoxin derived from proteolysis of C5 complex of complement system, whose biological function is to activate cells from myeloid lineage (Klos et al., 2009). Yet, they showed that, as for kinins, C5a molecules seems to be produced through *T. cruzi* cruzipain activity during infection and can promote DC activation and a Th1 protective response (Schmitz et al., 2014). Galectins, a lectin receptor, can also act as pathogen recognition receptors and as modulators of innate and adaptive response (Vasta, 2009). It has been shown that those receptors are widely expressed in B cell, macrophages and DCs during *T. cruzi* infection (Vray et al., 2004; Zúñiga et al., 2001a,b). Concerning DCs, Galectin-1 seems to be a negative immune regulator that limits the host protective response by driving tolerogenic circuits in DCs. Those tolerogenic DCs induce regulatory T cells activation, which would favor parasite persistence in host tissues or limit collateral tissue damage through suppression of inflammatory responses (Poncini et al., 2015). Galectin-3 (Gal-3) and its specific ligands were over-expressed in splenic DCs after infection by *T. cruzi* Tehuantepec strain, which lead to DC increased adhesiveness and reduced migration (Vray et al., 2004). Therefore, *T. cruzi* modulates Gal-3 and its ligands functionality to improve infection, another immunomodulatory property of *T. cruzi* (Vray et al., 2004). Another lectin-like receptor expressed by immune system cells, Siglec-E (sialic acid-binding Ig-like lectin-E), has also been implicated in *T. cruzi* infection. It is well known that transference of sialic acid by *T. cruzi trans*-sialidase (TS) from host cell to parasite surface mucin-like molecules confers resistance to human complement, contributing to infection (Tomlinson et al., 1994). In this context, pathogenic *T. cruzi* Tulahuen strain (high TS activity) interacted more to Siglec-E than non-pathogenic *T. cruzi* Tehuantepec strain (reduced TS activity). This interaction led to an inhibitory effect on DCs modulation, suppressing the production of cytokine IL-12 and subsequent T-cell activation. In contrast, *T. cruzi* Tehuantepec strain could not install an important parasitemia (Erdmann et al., 2009). Together, those findings suggest that *T. cruzi* (or parasite products) may lead to immunosuppression through its interaction with DC lectin receptors (Terrazas et al., 2010). Slamf1 (self-ligand adhesion molecule - CD150) is a co-stimulatory molecule present in myeloid lineage and required at the interface of antigen presenting cells and T cells (van Driel et al., 2016). *In vitro* and *in vivo* experiments revealed that Slamf1-deficient myeloid cells showed altered production of cytokines and reduced parasite replication. For instance, much lower IFN-γ production was detected in the heart of Slamf1 deficient mice than in the heart of WT mice. Additionally, Slamf1 deficient mice presented reduced cardiac damage despite of the comparable number of infiltrating DCs, macrophages, CD4 and CD8 T lymphocytes to that of WT animals. Therefore, *T. cruzi* requires Slamf1 to replicate in DCs and its absence leads to less production of myeloid cell specific factors by DCs, which are key compounds to host immune response and infection outcomes (Calderón et al., 2012).

Currently, there is an enormous amount of data that states a direct association between mouse DC functional specializations (antigen presentation or pathogen sensing) and their subsets. However, after our meticulous review of literature in the field, it is not unrealistic to conclude that the role of DC subsets in innate immune response against *T. cruzi* needs to be more properly addressed by researches since most cited works emphasize only one surface phenotype as if all DCs are equally functional. The same statement is valid for *T. cruzi* strains, a missing pattern respect to DCs subsets and their level of activation and to *T. cruzi* strains, which hampers an association concerning published data. **Table 1** summarizes the limited actual data in the murine DC-*T. cruzi* system.

HUMAN DC—*T. cruzi* INTERACTION: *IN VITRO* STUDIES

The first experiment that confirmed the ability of *T. cruzi* to infect and reproduce inside a human DC was performed in 1999 (Van Overtvelt et al., 1999), a biological process that had already been known for *Leishmania* (Moll et al., 1995). The authors also demonstrated that DCs, derived from monocytes and infected with *T. cruzi* Tehuantepec strain, significantly reduced HLA-DR and CD40 expression. In addition, these infected DCs were neither IL-12 nor TNF-α producers (Van Overtvelt et al., 1999). In a different study, using the same *T. cruzi* strain, Van Overtvelt and co-workers showed that *T. cruzi* soluble factor(s) released by the parasite itself into the DC culture medium inhibits LPS induced MHC class I up-regulation on the surface of human DC. Such inhibition may decrease the protective effect of specific $CD8^+$ T since infected DCs had a weaker capacity of cross-presentation. This reduction of DC function may influence the *in vivo* host's ability to competently combat *T. cruzi* infection (Van Overtvelt et al., 2002). It is well known that a small family of type 1 glycoinositolphospholipids (GIPLs) is abundant in *T. cruzi* cell surface and, therefore, such molecules seem to have immunoregulatory activities (Brodskyn et al., 2002; Medeiros et al., 2007). GIPLs isolated from *T. cruzi* G (TcI) and Y (TcII) strains were incubated along with LPS to stimulate DCs derived from monocytes. The results showed that *T. cruzi* GIPL antigens direct the down-regulation of both proinflammatory cytokines, such as TNF-α and IL-12 and anti-inflammatory, such IL-10, in DCs. The parasite GIPL also inhibited the expression of co-stimulatory molecules HLA-DR, CD83, CD86, CD80, and CD40 on DC surface. Similar results were achieved when the ceramide portion of GIPL molecule alone was used to stimulate DC, suggesting that fragments from the parasite glycoproteins could represent an evasion strategy of *T. cruzi*. Altogether, GIPL seems to contribute to parasite protection from the innate responses, allowing the beginning of infection and also acts in an inhibitory way on DC maturation, postponing an adequate immune response against *T. cruzi* (Brodskyn et al., 2002). Otherwise, a parasite released protein belonging to thiol-disulfide oxidoreductase family (Tc52) binds to and induces human and murine DC maturation by TLR2 activation. DCs derived from monocytes treated with Tc52 showed higher expression of CD83, CD86, CD54 and HLA-DR and an elevated production of IL-8, MCP-1, MIP-1α. These *in vitro* data suggest that Tc52 may provide local recruitment and activation of leukocyte and then DC migration to the lymph node, where they can trigger B and T cell immune responses (Ouaissi et al., 2002).

Yet, *T. cruzi* Tulahuen strain parasites enhance expression of CD40 and CD80 on cord blood mDCs in a higher level compared to mDCs from adult donors. $CD8^+$ T cells proliferation was also stimulated by those cord blood mDCs. In early life, immune responses are considered of partial effectiveness, owing to the relative immaturity of the human immune system therefore it is possible that maternally transmitted IgGs might contribute to overcome some deficiency of fetal/neonatal DCs and to protect the fetus/newborn against pathogens that have already come into contact with the mother (Rodriguez et al., 2012a). Another study, performed by the same group, showed that *T. cruzi* can induce maturation of this DC type without infecting them. Rodriguez and coworkers found that blood cord and adult mDCs that had contact with parasite but were not yet infected also expressed high levels of CD80 and CD83. In addition, they demonstrated that either infected mDCs or *T. cruzi* lysates co-incubated mDCs have a similar expression pattern of their surface molecules. The authors also showed that infection rate in mDCs is lower than in monocytes and granulocytes, maybe due to their enhanced capacity of phagocytosis when compared to mature DCs (Rodriguez et al., 2012b). Consistent with the results shown in murine model, modulation of DCs function varies according to *T. cruzi* strain. In a comparative study, Magalhães and colleagues demonstrated that *T. cruzi* Col cl1.7 (TcI) but not Y (TcII) strain induces higher CD80 and CD86 expression, while *T. cruzi* Y strain induces up-regulation of IL-10, TNF-α and granzyme A production. Also, $CD8^+$ T lymphocytes activated by Col cl1.7 strain produced higher level of IL-17. Then, TcI strain were capable of a higher monocyte activation, while the profile induced by TcII was more inflammatory (Magalhães et al., 2015). **Figure 2** summarizes DC receptors referred to in this review.

The present knowledge about the interaction between human DCs and *T. cruzi* is restricted to *in vitro* models where expression of some cytokines and surface molecules were analyzed, but the specific functions of human DC subsets are only beginning to be unraveled. Contradictory studies have been published concerning DC–*T. cruzi* interactions, both in human and mouse models. However it seems that *T. cruzi* virulent strains probably take advantage of susceptible DCs to overcome host immune response and successfully install the infection. Remarkably, those modulated DCs will conduct a weak adaptive response with low expression of MHC class I and II molecules and proinflammatory cytokines, which are fundamental for controlling parasite survival (Poncini et al., 2008, 2010; Alba Soto et al., 2010; da Costa et al., 2014).

FUTURE: NEEDS AND EXPECTATIONS

Dendritic cells are crucial decision-making cells of the immunological system as they direct tolerance, anergy, and initiation/regulation of the adaptive immune responses (Banchereau and Steinman, 1998). For these reasons, DC has been proposed as targets for immunotherapy in diseases related to autoimmunity and exacerbated immune responses, such as autoimmune encephalomyelitis (Menges et al., 2002), thyroiditis (Verginis et al., 2005), and arthritis (Jaen et al., 2009) or to improve unsatisfactory immune responses toward tumor or pathogens (Dubsky et al., 2005). Targeting these cells with recombinant antibodies conjugated to autoantigens or pathogen antigens could direct a less exacerbated response against certain disease (Lutz, 2012).

ASP-2, an amastigote protein from *T. cruzi* Y strain, was conjugated with αDEC205 antibody, DEC205 is a C-type lectin endocytic receptor expressed in some DC populations and is widely used for targeting DCs. Recombinant ASP-2/DEC205 antibody was injected in mice, resulting in higher IFN-γ production by splenocytes and high proliferation of antigen-specific $CD4^+$ T cells (Rampazo et al., 2015). Thus, targeted regulatory DCs could be used as an immunotherapy strategy during disease undetermined form to prevent evolution to

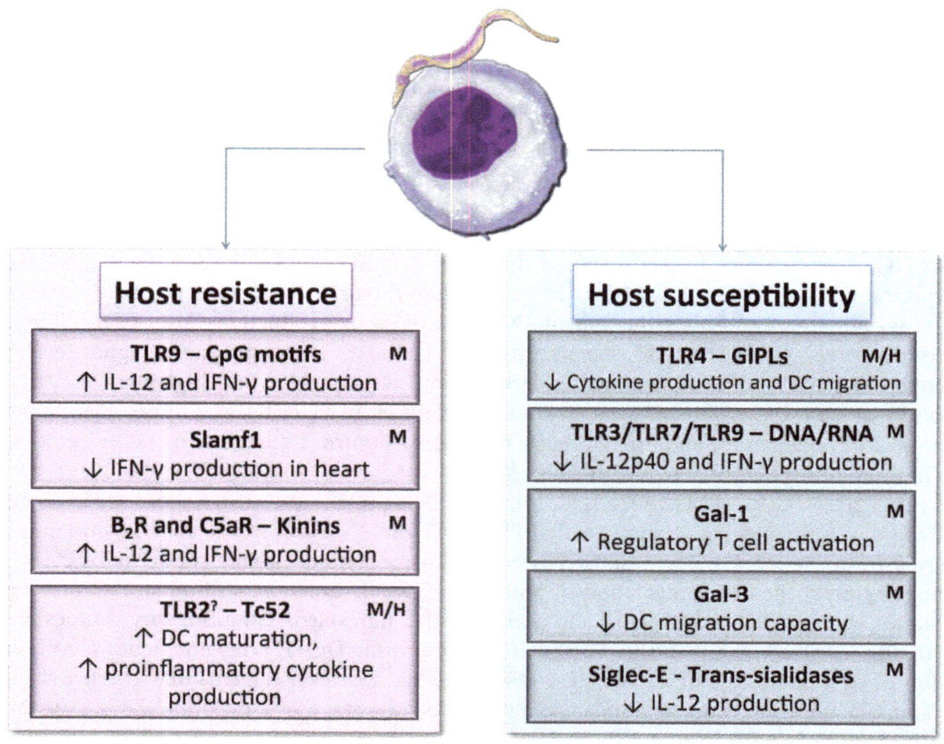

FIGURE 2 | Dendritic cell receptor–*T. cruzi* antigen interactions may induce host resistance or susceptibility to parasite by activating different DCs signaling pathways. DCs maturation, cytokine production, and migration capacity could be up or down-regulated depending on the signaling pathways triggered during the initial contact between DCs and the parasite. **H**: DC receptors already known to interact with parasite in human model. **M**: DC receptors already known to interact with parasite in murine model. **?**: May act as a maturation inducer or as regulatory cytokines activator.

the chronic phase. Nevertheless, host receptor and parasite antigen should be carefully elected because they could influence maturation signals received by DCs for orchestration of the immune response (Cohn and Delamarre, 2014). Furthermore, trypomastigote lysate -pulsed IL-10-deficient DC conferred protection against *T. cruzi* infection to recipient mice by secreting increased amounts of IFN-γ, enhancing antigen-specific production and inducing endogenous DC activation. This DC-based vaccination against *T. cruzi* also demonstrated that IL-10 produced by sensitizing DC has a key role in inhibiting the protection response (Alba Soto et al., 2010). DC-based vaccine has also been successfully tested in *Leishmania*. Freshly isolated pDC from mice pulsed with *Leishmania* antigen and reinjected into host resulted in a protective effect, presenting mixed Th1/Th2 response with secretion of IFN-γ, IL-4 and IL-10 (Remer et al., 2007).

Unfortunately, DC immunizations have an elevated cost, which turns up this approach less attractive added to relative efficiency of the current treatment for Chagas disease during acute phase (Rassi et al., 2010; Cohn and Delamarre, 2014). Nonetheless, this neglected disease remains with no vaccines or antiparasitic drugs proven efficient in chronically infected adults, when most patients are diagnosed. Thus, future DCs immunization researches could be directed toward treatment for the undetermined stage targeting tolerogenic DCs.

CONCLUSION

Although efforts have been devoted to deciphering DCs—*T. cruzi* interaction, there is still much to be investigated before the complete understanding of DC role in the induction of immunity against *T. cruzi*. Moreover, our knowledge about that interaction is mostly based on the regulation, differentiation and function of the DC lineage from mouse. A challenge that needs to be overcome is the difficulty in isolating subsets of DCs from human tissue; only then we might be able to improve the understanding of human DCs in a molecular level and perhaps develop vaccines for the prevention or treatment of Chagas disease. Our review reiterates that *T. cruzi* capacity to modulate host DCs is an indispensable strategy to escape from innate immune response with the purpose of its own survival. Nevertheless, DCs present an efficient machinery to capture, process, and present antigens to T cells and to activate B cells therefore their immunotherapeutic potential may not be disregarded.

AUTHOR CONTRIBUTIONS

NG-J: participated in design and manuscript writing. FM: participated in design and manuscript writing. CF: participated in design and manuscript writing. IB: participated in design, coordination, and manuscript writing. JS: participated in design, coordination, and manuscript writing.

ACKNOWLEDGMENT

We thank Julian E. Palacio Hernández for image editions.

REFERENCES

1. Abrahamsohn, I. A., and Coffman, R. L. (1996). *Trypanosoma cruzi*: IL-10, TNF, IFN-gamma, and IL-12 regulate innate and acquired immunity to infection. *Exp. Parasitol.* 84, 231–244. doi: 10.1006/expr.1996.0109
2. Alba Soto, C. D., Mirkin, G. A., Solana, M. E., and González Cappa, S. M. (2003). *Trypanosoma cruzi* infection modulates in vivo expression of major histocompatibility complex class II molecules on antigen-presenting cells and T-cell stimulatory activity of dendritic cells in a strain-dependent manner. *Infect. Immun.* 71, 1194–1199. doi: 10.1128/IAI.71.3.1194
3. Alba Soto, C. D., Solana, M. E., Poncini, C. V., Pino-Martinez, A. M., Tekiel, V., and González-Cappa, S. M. (2010). Dendritic cells devoid of IL-10 induce protective immunity against the protozoan parasite *Trypanosoma cruzi*. *Vaccine* 28, 7407–7413. doi: 10.1016/j.vaccine.2010.08.105
4. Andrade, D. V., Gollob, K. J., and Dutra, W. O. (2014). Acute chagas disease: new global challenges for an old neglected disease. *PLoS Negl. Trop. Dis.* 8:e3010. doi: 10.1371/journal.pntd.0003010
5. Banchereau, J., and Steinman, R. M. (1998). Dendritic cells and the control of immunity. *Nature* 392, 245–252. doi: 10.1038/32588
6. Bartholomeu, D. C., Ropert, C., Melo, M. B., Parroche, P., Junqueira, C. F., Teixeira, S. M. R., et al. (2008). Recruitment and endo-lysosomal activation of TLR9 in dendritic cells infected with *Trypanosoma cruzi*. *J. Immunol.* 181, 1333–1344. doi: 10.4049/jimmunol.181.2.1333
7. Bastos, C. J. C., Aras, R., Mota, G., Reis, F., Dias, J. P., de Jesus, R. S., et al. (2010). Clinical outcomes of thirteen patients with acute chagas disease acquired through oral transmission from two urban outbreaks in Northeastern Brazil. *PLoS Negl. Trop. Dis.* 4:e711. doi: 10.1371/journal.pntd.0000711
8. Batalla, E. I., Pino Martínez, A. M., Poncini, C. V., Duffy, T., Schijman, A. G., González Cappa, S. M., et al. (2013). Impairment in natural killer cells editing of immature dendritic cells by infection with a virulent *Trypanosoma cruzi* population. *J. Innate Immun.* 5, 494–504. doi: 10.1159/000350242
9. Bermudez, J., Davies, C., Simonazzi, A., Real, J. P., and Palma, S. (2015). Current drug therapy and pharmaceutical challenges for Chagas disease. *Acta Trop.* 156, 1–16. doi: 10.1016/j.actatropica.2015.12.017
10. Bern, C. (2011). Antitrypanosomal therapy for chronic Chagas' disease. *N. Engl. J. Med.* 364, 2527–2534. doi: 10.1056/NEJMct1014204
11. Bern, C. (2015). Chagas' Disease. *N. Engl. J. Med.* 373, 456–466. doi: 10.1056/NEJMra1410150
12. Blum, J. S., Wearsch, P. A., and Cresswell, P. (2013). Pathways of antigen processing. *Annu. Rev. Immunol.* 31, 443–473. doi: 10.1146/annurev-immunol- 032712-095910
13. Borges, D. C., Araújo, N. M., Cardoso, C. R., and Lazo Chica, J. E. (2012). Different parasite inocula determine the modulation of the immune response and outcome of experimental *Trypanosoma cruzi* infection. *Immunology* 138, 145–156. doi: 10.1111/imm.12022
14. Boussiotis, V. A., Freeman, G. J., Gribben, J., and Nadler, L. (1996). The role of B7-1/B7-2:CD28/CTLA-4 pathways in the prevention of anergy, induction of productive immunity and down-regulation of the immune response. *Immunol. Rev.* 153, 5–26. doi: 10.1111/j.1600-065X.1996.tb00918.x
15. Brodskyn, C., Patricio, J., Oliveira, R., Lobo, L., Arnholdt, A., Mendonça-previato, L., et al. (2002). Glycoinositolphospholipids from *Trypanosoma cruzi* interfere with macrophages and dendritic cell responses. *Infect. Immun.* 70, 3736–3743. doi: 10.1128/IAI.70.7.3736-3743.2002
16. Caetano, B. C., Carmo, B. B., Melo, M. B., Cerny, A., dos Santos, S. L., Bartholomeu, D. C., et al. (2011). Requirement of UNC93B1 reveals a critical role for Toll- Like Receptor 7 in host resistance to primary infection with *Trypanosoma cruzi*. *J. Immunol.* 187, 1903–1911. doi: 10.4049/jimmunol.1003911
17. Calderón, J., Maganto-Garcia, E., Punzón, C., Carrión, J., Terhorst, C., and Fresno, M. (2012). The receptor Slamf1 on the surface of myeloid lineage cells controls susceptibility to infection by *Trypanosoma cruzi*. *PLoS Pathog.* 8:e1002799. doi: 10.1371/journal.ppat.1002799
18. Camargo, R., Faria, L. O., Kloss, A., Favali, C. B. F., Kuckelkorn, U., Kloetzel, P. M., et al. (2014). *Trypanosoma cruzi* infection down-modulates the immunoproteasome biosynthesis and the MHC class I cell surface expression in HeLa cells. *PLoS ONE* 9:e95977. doi: 10.1371/journal.pone.0095977
19. Campos, M. A., Closel, M., Valente, E. P., Cardoso, J. E., Akira, S., Alvarez- leite, J. I., et al. (2004). Impaired production os proinflammatory cytokines and host resistance to acute infection with *Trypanosoma cruzi* in mice lacking functional myeliod differentation factor 88. *J. Immunol.* 172, 1711–1718. doi: 10.4049/jimmunol.172.3.1711
20. Cardoso, M. S., Reis-cunha, J. L., Bartholomeu, D. C., Fernandez, M. M., and Bartholomeu, D. C. (2016). Evasion of the Immune Response by *Trypanosoma cruzi* during Acute Infection. *Front. Immunol.* 6:659. doi: 10.3389/fimmu.2015.00659
21. Chaussabel, D., Pajak, B., Vercruysse, V., Bisseyé, C., Garzé, V., Habib, M., et al. (2003). Alteration of migration and maturation of dendritic cells and T-Cell depletion in the course of experimental *Trypanosoma cruzi* infection. *Lab. Investig.* 83, 1373–1382. doi: 10.1097/01.LAB.0000087587.93781.6F
22. Cohn, L., and Delamarre, L. (2014). Dendritic cell-targeted vaccines. *Front. Immunol.* 5:255. doi: 10.3389/fimmu.2014.00255
23. Collin, M., Mcgovern, N., and Haniffa, M. (2013). Human dendritic cell subsets. *Immunology* 140, 22–30. doi: 10.1111/imm.12117
24. Cooke, G., Armstrong, M. E., and Donnelly, S. C. (2009). Macrophage migration inhibitory factor (MIF), enzymatic activity and the inflammatory response. *Biofactors* 35, 165–168. doi: 10.1002/biof.27
25. Corinti, S., Albanesi, C., la Sala, A., Pastore, S., and Girolomoni, G. (2001). Regulatory activity of autocrine IL-10 on dendritic cell functions. *J. Immunol.* 166, 4312–4318. doi: 10.4049/jimmunol.166.7.4312
26. Coura, J. R., Dias, J. C. P., Frasch, A. C. C., Guhl, F., Lazzari, J. O., Lorca, M., et al. (2002). Control of Chagas disease. *Adv. Parasitol.* 61, 129–165. doi: 10.1016/S0065-308X(05)61004-4.
27. da Costa, T. A., Silva, M. V., Mendes, M. T., Carvalho-Costa, T. M., Batista, L. R., Lages-Silva, E., et al. (2014). Immunomodulation by *Trypanosoma cruzi*: toward understanding the association of dendritic cells with infecting TcI and TcII populations. *J. Immunol. Res.* 2014, 1–12. doi: 10.1155/2014/962047
28. D'Avila-Levy, C. M., Boucinha, C., Kostygov, A., Santos, H. L. C., Morelli, K. A., Grybchuk-Ieremenko, A., et al. (2015). Exploring the environmental diversity of kinetoplastid flagellates in the high-throughput DNA sequencing era. *Mem. Inst. Oswaldo Cruz* 110, 956–965. doi: 10.1590/0074-02760150253
29. de Lana, M., Marques, E., and Machado, D. M. (2010). *Biology of "Trypanosoma cruzi" and Biological Diversity*, 1st Edn. Amsterdam: Elsevier Inc.
30. Deane, M. P., Lenzi, H. L., and Jansen, A. (1984). *Trypanosoma cruzi*: vertebrate and invertebrate cycles in the same mammal host, the opossum *Didelphis marsupialis*. *Mem. Inst. Oswaldo Cruz* 79, 513–515. doi: 10.1590/S0074- 02761984000400021

31. Demangel, C., Bertolino, P., and Britton, W. J. (2002). Autocrine IL-10 impairs dendritic cell (DC)-derived immune responses to mycobacterial infection by suppressing DC trafficking to draining lymph nodes and local IL-12 production. *Eur. J. Immunol.* 32, 994–1002. doi: 10.1002/1521-4141(200204)32:4<994::AID-IMMU994>3.3.CO;2-Y
32. den Haan, J. M. M., Arens, R., and van Zelm, M. C. (2014). The activation of the adaptive immune system: cross-talk between antigen-presenting cells, T cells and B cells. *Immunol. Lett.* 162, 103–112. doi: 10.1016/j.imlet.2014. 10.011
33. Dubsky, P., Ueno, H., Piqueras, B., Connolly, J., Banchereau, J., and Palucka, A. K. (2005). Human dendritic cell subsets for vaccination. *J. Clin. Immunol.* 25, 551–572. doi: 10.1007/s10875-005-8216-7
34. Dutra, W. O., Menezes, C. A. S., Magalhães, L. M. D., and Gollob, K. J. (2015). Immunoregulatory networks in human Chagas disease. *Parasite Immunol.* 36, 377–387. doi: 10.1111/pim.12107
35. Erdmann, H., Steeg, C., Koch-nolte, F., Fleischer, B., and Jacobs, T. (2009). Sialylated ligands on pathogenic *Trypanosoma cruzi* interact with Siglec-E (sialic acid-binding Ig-like lectin-E). *Cell. Microbiol.* 11, 1600–1611. doi: 10.1111/j.1462-5822.2009.01350.x
36. Gerosa, F., Baldani-Guerra, B., Nisii, C., Marchesini, V., Carra, G., and Trinchieri, G. (2002). Reciprocal activating interaction between natural killer cells and dendritic cells. *J. Exp. Med.* 195, 327–333. doi: 10.1084/jem.20010938 Gravina, H. D., Antonelli, L., Gazzinelli, R. T., and Ropert, C. (2013). Differential Use of TLR2 and TLR9 in the regulation of immune responses during the infection with *Trypanosoma cruzi. PLoS ONE* 8:e63100. doi: 10.1371/journal.pone.0063100
37. Haniffa, M., Ginhoux, F., Wang, X.-N., Bigley, V., Abel, M., Dimmick, I., et al. (2009). Differential rates of replacement of human dermal dendritic cells and macrophages during hematopoietic stem cell transplantation. *J. Exp. Med.* 206, 371–385. doi: 10.1084/jem.20081633
38. Holdsworth, S. R., and Can, P. Y. (2015). Cytokines: names and numbers you should care about. *Clin. J. Am. Soc. Nephrol.* 10, 2243–2254. doi: 10.2215/CJN.07590714
39. Hotez, P. J., Molyneux, D. H., Fenwick, A., Kumaresan, J., Sachs, S. E., Sachs,
40. J. D., et al. (2007). Control of neglected tropical diseases. *N. Engl. J. Med.* 357, 1018–1027. doi: 10.1056/NEJMra064142
41. Jaen, O., Rullé, S., Bessis, N., Zago, A., Boissier, M. C., and Falgarone, G. (2009). Dendritic cells modulated by innate immunity improve collagen-induced arthritis and induce regulatory T cells in vivo. *Immunology* 126, 35–44. doi: 10.1111/j.1365-2567.2008.02875.x
42. Klos, A., Tenner, A. J., Johswich, K. O., Ager, R. R., Reis, E. S., and Köhl, J. (2009). The role of the anaphylatoxins in health and disease. *Mol. Immunol.* 46, 2753–2766. doi: 10.1016/j.molimm.2009.04.027
43. Koga, R., Hamano, S., Kuwata, H., Atarashi, K., Ogawa, M., Hisaeda, H., et al. (2006). TLR-dependent induction of IFN- β mediates host defense against *Trypanosoma cruzi. J. Immunol.* 177, 7059–7066. doi: 10.4049/jimmunol.177.10.7059
44. Kropf, S. P., and Sá, M. R. (2009). The discovery of *Trypanosoma cruzi* and Chagas disease (1908-1909): tropical medicine in Brazil. *Hist. Cienc. Saude Manguinhos.* 16(Suppl. 1), 13–34. doi: 10.1590/S0104-59702009000500002
45. Laucella, S. A., Rottenberg, M. E., and de Titto, E. H. (1996). Role of cytokines in resistance and pathology in *Trypanosoma cruzi* infection. *Rev. Argent Microbiol.* 28, 99–109.
46. Lewis, K. L., and Reizis, B. (2012). Dendritic cells: arbiters of immunity and immunological tolerance. *Cold Spring Harb. Perspect. Biol.* 4:a007401. doi: 10.1101/cshperspect.a007401
47. Lipscomb, M. F., and Masten, B. J. (2002). Dendritic cells: immune regulators in health and disease. *Physiol. Rev.* 82, 97–130. doi: 10.1152/physrev.00023.2001 Lutz, M. B. (2012). Therapeutic potential of semi-mature dendritic cells for tolerance induction. *Front. Immunol.* 3:123. doi: 10.3389/fimmu.2012.00123 Machado, F. S., Dutra, W. O., Esper, L., Gollob, K., Teixeira, M., Factor, S. M., et al.
48. (2013). Current understanding of immunity to *Trypanosoma cruzi* infection and pathogenesis os Chagas disease. *Semin. Immunopathol.* 34, 753–770. doi: 10.1007/s00281-012-0351-7
49. Magalhães, L. M. D., Viana, A., Chiari, E., Galvão, L. M. C., Gollob, K. J., and Dutra, O. (2015). Differential activation of human monocytes and lymphocytes by distinct strains of *Trypanosoma cruzi. PLoS Negl. Trop. Dis.* 9:e0003816. doi: 10.1371/journal.pntd.0003816
50. Manchola, N. C., Rapado, L. N., Barison, M. J., and Silber, A. M. (2015). Biochemical characterization of branched chain amino acids uptake in *Trypanosoma cruzi. J. Eukaryot. Microbiol.* 63, 299–308. doi: 10.1111/jeu.12278 Medeiros, M. M., Peixoto, J. R., Oliveira, A.-C., Cardilo-Reis, L., Koatz, L. G., Van Kaer, L., et al. (2007). Toll-like receptor 4 (TLR4)- dependent proinflammatory and immunomodulatory properties of the glycoinositolphospholipid (GIPL) from *Trypanosoma cruzi. J. Leukoc. Biol.* 82, 488–496. doi: 10.1189/jlb.0706478
51. Menges, M., RöBner, S., Voigtländer, C., Schindler, H., Kukutsch, N. A., Bogdan, C., et al. (2002). Repetitive injections of dendritic cells matured with tumor necrosis factor alpha induce antigen-specific protection of mice from autoimmunity. *J. Exp. Med.* 195, 15–21. doi: 10.1084/jem.20011341
52. Moll, H., Flohé, S., and Röllinghoff, M. (1995). Dendritic cells in *Leishmania major*- immune mice harbor persistent parasites and mediate an antigen-specific T cell immune response. *Eur. J. Immunol.* 25, 693–699. doi: 10.1002/eji.1830250310
53. Monteiro, A. C., Schmitz, V., Morrot, A., de Arruda, L. B., Nagajyothi, F., Granato, A., et al. (2007). Bradykinin B 2 receptors of dendritic cells, acting as sensors of kinins proteolytically released by *Trypanosoma cruzi*, are critical for the development of protective Type-1 responses. *PLOS Pathog.* 3:e185. doi: 10.1371/journal.ppat.0030185
54. Monteiro, A. C., Schmitz, V., Svensjo, E., Gazzinelli, R. T., Almeida, I. C., Todorov, A., et al. (2006). Cooperative activation of TLR2 and bradykinin B2 receptor is required for induction of type 1 immunity in a mouse model of subcutaneous infection by *Trypanosoma cruzi. J. Immunol.* 177, 6325–6335. doi: 10.4049/jimmunol.177.9.6325
55. Muñoz-Saravia, S. G., Haberland, A., Wallukat, G., and Schimke, I. (2012). Chronic Chagas' heart disease: a disease on its way to becoming a worldwide health problem: epidemiology, etiopathology, treatment, pathogenesis and laboratory medicine. *Heart Fail. Rev.* 17, 45–64. doi: 10.1007/s10741-010-9211-5
56. Nardy, A. F., Freire-de-Lima, C. G., and Morrot, A. (2015). Immune evasion strategies of *Trypanosoma cruzi. J. Immunol. Res.* 2015:7. doi: 10.1155/2015/178947
57. Neefjes, J., Jongsma, M. L., Paul, P., and Bakke, O. (2011). Towards a systems understanding of MHC class I and MHC class II antigen presentation. *Nat. Rev. Immunol.* 11, 823–836. doi: 10.1038/nri3084
58. Nóbrega, A. A., Garcia, M. H., Tatto, E., Obara, M. T., Costa, E., Sobel, J., et al. (2009). Oral transmission of chagas disease by consumption of Açaí palm fruit, Brazil. *Emerg. Infect. Dis.* 15, 653–655. doi: 10.3201/eid1504.081450
59. Oliveira, A., Alencar, B. C., De Tzelepis, F., Klezewsky, W., Raquel, N., Neves, F. S., et al. (2010). Impaired innate immunity in Tlr4 2 / 2 mice but preserved CD8 + T cell responses against *Trypanosoma cruzi* in Tlr4-, Tlr2-, Tlr9- or myd88- deficient mice. *PLoS Pathog.* 6:e1000870. doi: 10.1371/journal.ppat.1000870
60. O'Neill, D. W., Adams, S., and Bhardwaj, N. (2004). Manipulating dendritic cell biology for the active immunotherapy of cancer. *Blood J.* 104, 2235–2246. doi: 10.1182/blood-2003-12-4392
61. Ouaissi, A., Guilvard, E., Delneste, Y., Caron, G., Magistrelli, G., Herbault, N., et al. (2002). The *Trypanosoma cruzi* Tc52-released protein induces human dendritic cell maturation, signals via toll-like receptor 2, and confers protection against lethal infection. *J. Immunol.* 168, 6366–6374. doi: 10.4049/jimmunol.168.12.6366
62. Pearce, E. J., and Everts, B. (2015). Dendritic cell metabolism. *Nat. Rev. Immunol.* 15, 18–29. doi: 10.1038/nri3771
63. Piccioli, D., Sbrana, S., Melandri, E., and Valiante, N. M. (2002). Contact-dependent stimulation and inhibition of dendritic cells by natural killer cells. *J. Exp. Med.* 195, 335–341. doi: 10.1084/jem.20010934
64. Planelles, L., Thomas, M. C., Marañón, C., Morell, M., and López, M. C. (2003). Differential CD86 and CD40 co-stimulatory molecules and cytokine expression pattern induced by *Trypanosoma cruzi* in APCs from resistant or susceptible mice. *Clin. Exp. Immunol.* 131, 41–47. doi: 10.1046/j.1365-2249.2003.02022.x
65. Poncini, C. V., Giménez, G., Pontillo, C. A., Alba-Soto, C. D., de Isola, E. L. D., Piazzón, I., et al. (2010). Central role of extracellular signal-regulated kinase and Toll-like receptor 4 in IL-10 production in regulatory dendritic cells induced by *Trypanosoma cruzi. Mol. Immunol.* 47, 1981–1988. doi: 10.1016/j.molimm.2010.04.016

66. Poncini, C. V., Ilarregui, J. M., Batalla, E. I., Engels, S., Cerliani, J. P., Cucher, M. A., et al. (2015). *Trypanosoma cruzi* infection imparts a regulatory program in dendritic cells and T cells via galectin-1-dependent mechanisms. *J. Immunol.* 195, 3311–3324. doi: 10.4049/jimmunol.1403019
67. Poncini, C. V., Soto, C. D. A., Batalla, E., Solana, M. E., and Gonzalez Cappa, S. M. (2008). *Trypanosoma cruzi* induces regulatory dendritic cells in vitro. *Infect. Immun.* 76, 2633–2641. doi: 10.1128/IAI.01298-07
68. Ramírez, J. D., Guhl, F., Rendón, L. M., Rosas, F., Marin-Neto, J. A., and Morillo, C. A. (2010). Chagas cardiomyopathy manifestations and *Trypanosoma cruzi* genotypes circulating in chronic chagasic patients. *PLoS Negl. Trop. Dis.* 4:e899. doi: 10.1371/journal.pntd.0000899
69. Rampazo, E. V., Amorim, K. N. S., and Yamamoto, M. M. (2015). Antigen targeting to dendritic cells allows the identification of a CD4 T-Cell epitope within an immunodominant *Trypanosoma cruzi* antigen. *PLoS ONE* 10:e0117778. doi: 10.1371/journal.pone.0117778
70. Rassi, A., Rassi, A., and Marin-Neto, J. A. (2010). Chagas disease. *Lancet* 375, 1388–1402. doi: 10.1016/S0140-6736(10)60061-X
71. Remer, K. A., Apetrei, C., Schwarz, T., Linden, C., and Moll, H. (2007). Vaccination with plasmacytoid dendritic cells induces protection against infection with *Leishmania major* in mice. *Eur. J. Immunol.* 37, 2463–2473. doi: 10.1002/eji.200636780
72. Rodriguez, P., Carlier, Y., and Truyens, C. (2012a). Activation of cord blood myeloid dendritic cells by *Trypanosoma cruzi* and parasite-specific antibodies, proliferation of CD8 + T cells, and production of IFN-gamma. *Med. Microbiol. Immunol.* 201, 157–169. doi: 10.1007/s00430-011-0217-y
73. Rodriguez, P., Carlier, Y., and Truyens, C. (2012b). *Trypanosoma cruzi* activates cord blood myeloid dendritic cells independently of cell infection. *Med. Microbiol. Immunol.* 201, 287–296. doi: 10.1007/s00430-012- 0230-9
74. Romano, P. S., Cueto, J. A., Casassa, A. F., Vanrell, M. C., Gottlieb, R. A., and Colombo, M. I. (2012). Molecular and cellular mechanisms involved in the *Trypanosoma cruzi*/host cell interplay. *IUBMB Life* 64, 387–396. doi: 10.1002/iub.1019
75. Schmitz, V., Almeida, L. N., Svensjö, E., Monteiro, A. C., Köhl, J., and Scharfstein, J. (2014). C5a and bradykinin receptor cross-talk regulates innate and adaptive immunity in *Trypanosoma cruzi* infection. *J. Immunol.* 193, 3613–3623. doi: 10.4049/jimmunol.1302417
76. Schmunis, G. A. (2007). Epidemiology of Chagas disease in non-endemic countries: the role of international migration. *Mem. Inst. Oswaldo Cruz* 102, 75–85. doi: 10.1590/S0074-02762007005000093
77. Segura, E. (2016). "Review of mouse and human dendritic cell subsets," in *Dendritic Cell Protocols*, eds E. Segura and N. Onai (New York, NY: Springer Science+Business Media), 3–15. doi: 10.1007/978-1-4939-3606-9_1
78. Segura, E., and Amigorena, S. (2015). *Cross-Presentation in Mouse and Human Dendritic Cells*, 1st Edn. Amsterdam: Elsevier Inc.
79. Stecconi-Silva, R. B., Andreoli, W. K., and Mortara, R. A. (2003). Parameters affecting cellular invasion and escape from the parasitophorous vacuole by different infective forms of *Trypanosoma cruzi*. *Mem. Inst. Oswaldo Cruz* 98, 953–958. doi: 10.1590/S0074-02762003000700016
80. Steinman, R. M. (2007). Dendritic cells: versatile controllers of the immune system. *Nat. Med.* 13, 1155–1159. doi: 10.1038/nm1643
81. Stevens, J. R. (2008). Kinetoplastid phylogenetics, with special reference to the evolution of parasitic trypanosomes. *Parasite* 15, 226–232. doi: 10.1051/parasite/2008153226
82. Steverding, D. (2014). The history of chagas disease. *Parasit Vectors* 7, 1–8. doi: 10.1186/1756-3305-7-317
83. Strasen, J., Williams, T., Ertl, G., Zoller, T., Stich, A., and Ritter, O. (2013). Epidemiology of chagas disease in Europe: many calculations, little knowledge. *Clin. Res. Cardiol.* 103, 1–10. doi: 10.1007/s00392-013-0613-y
84. Takeuchi, O., and Akira, S. (2010). Pattern recognition receptors and inflammation. *Cell* 140, 805–820. doi: 10.1016/j.cell.2010.01.022
85. Teixeira, A., Vinaud, M., and Castro, A. M. (2009). *Emerging Chagas Disease*. Brasília: Bentham.
86. Terrazas, C. A., Huitron, E., Vazquez, A., Juarez, I., Camacho, G. M., Calleja, E. A., et al. (2011). MIF synergizes with *Trypanosoma cruzi* antigens to promote efficient dendritic cell maturation and IL-12 production via p38 MAPK. *Int. J. Biol. Sci.* 7, 1298–1310. doi: 10.7150/ijbs.7.1298
87. Terrazas, C. A., Terrazas, L. I., and Gómez-García, L. (2010). Modulation of dendritic cell responses by parasites: a common strategy to survive. *J. Biomed. Biotechnol.* 2010:357106. doi: 10.1155/2010/357106
88. Tibayrenc, M. (1998). Genetic epidemiology of parasitic protozoa and other infectious agents: the need for an integrated approach. *Int. J. Parasitol.* 28, 85–104. doi: 10.1016/S0020-7519(97)00180-X
89. Tomlinson, S., Pontes de Carvalho, L. C., Vandekerckhove, F., and Nussenzweig, V. (1994). Role of sialic acid in the resistance of *Trypanosoma cruzi* trypomastigotes to complement. *J. Immunol.* 153, 3141–3147.
90. Tonelli, R. R., Silber, A. M., Almeida-de-Faria, M., Hirata, I. Y., Colli, W., and Alves, J. M. (2004). L-proline is essential for the intracellular differentiation of *Trypanosoma cruzi*. *Cell. Microbiol.* 6, 733–741. doi: 10.1111/j.1462- 5822.2004.00397.x
91. van Driel, B. J., Liao, G., Engel, P., and Terhorst, C. (2016). Responses to microbial challenges by SLAMF receptors. *Front. Immunol.* 7:4. doi: 10.3389/fimmu.2016.00004
92. Van Overtvelt, L., Andrieu, M., Verhasselt, V., Connan, F., Choppin, J., Vercruysse, V., et al. (2002). *Trypanosoma cruzi* down-regulates lipopolysaccharide-induced MHC class I on human dendritic cells and impairs antigen presentation to specific CD8 + T lymphocytes. *Int. Immunol.* 14, 1135–1144. doi: 10.1093/intimm/dxf077
93. Van Overtvelt, L., Vanderheyde, N., Verhasselt, V., Ismaili, J., De Vos, L., Goldman, M., et al. (1999). *Trypanosoma cruzi* infects human dendritic cells and prevents their maturation: inhibition of cytokines, HLA-DR, and costimulatory molecules. *Infect. Immun.* 67, 4033–4040.
94. Vasta, G. R. (2009). Roles of galectins in infection. *Nat. Rev. Microbiol.* 7, 424–438. doi: 10.1038/nrmicro2146
95. Verginis, P., Li, H. S., and Carayanniotis, G. (2005). Tolerogenic semimature dendritic cells suppress experimental autoimmune thyroiditis by activation of thyroglobulin-specific CD4+CD25+ T cells. *J. Immunol.* 174, 7433–7439. doi: 10.4049/jimmunol.174.11.7433
96. Verhasselt, V., Buelens, C., Willems, F., De Groote, D., Haeffner-Cavaillon, N., and Goldman, M. (1997). Bacterial lipopolysaccharide stimulates the production of cytokines and the expression of costimulatory molecules by human peripheral blood dendritic cells: evidence for a soluble CD14-dependent pathway. *J. Immunol.* 158, 2919–2925.
97. Vray, B., Camby, I., Vercruysse, V., Mijatovic, T., Bovin, N. V., Ricciardi-Castagnoli, P., et al. (2004). Up-regulation of galectin-3 and its ligands by *Trypanosoma cruzi* infection with modulation of adhesion and migration of murine dendritic cells. *Glycobiology* 14, 647–657. doi: 10.1093/glycob/cwh068
98. Vyas, J. M., Van der Veen, A. G., and Ploegh, H. L. (2008). The known unknowns of antigen processing and presentation. *Nat. Rev. Immunol.* 8, 607–618. doi: 10.1038/nri2368
99. Watanabe Costa, R., da Silveira, J. F., and Bahia, D. (2016). Interactions between *Trypanosoma cruzi* secreted proteins and host cell signaling pathways. *Front. Microbiol.* 7:388. doi: 10.3389/fmicb.2016.00388
100. Wilkinson, S. R., Bot, C., Kelly, J. M., and Hall, B. S. (2011). Trypanocidal activity of nitroaromatic prodrugs: current treatments and future perspectives. *Curr. Top. Med. Chem.* 11, 2072–2084. doi: 10.2174/156802611796575894
101. World Health Organization (2015). *World Health Organization: Chagas Disease.* Available at: http://www.who.int/mediacentre/factsheets/fs340/en/ Yoshida, N. (2006). Molecular basis of mammalian cell invasion by *Trypanosoma cruzi*. *An. Acad. Bras. Cienc.* 78, 87–111. doi: 10.1590/S0001-37652006000100010
102. Zingales, B., Andrade, S. G., Briones, M. R. S., Campbell, D. A., Chiari, E., Fernandes, O., et al. (2009). A new consensus for *Trypanosoma cruzi* intraspecific nomenclature: second revision meeting recommends TcI to TcVI. *Mem. Inst. Oswaldo Cruz* 104, 1051–1054. doi: 10.1590/S0074-02762009000700021
103. Zingales, B., Miles, M. A., Campbell, D. A., Tibayrenc, M., Macedo, A. M., Teixeira, M. M. G., et al. (2012). The revised *Trypanosoma cruzi* subspecific nomenclature: rationale, epidemiological relevance and research applications. *Infect. Genet. Evol.* 12, 240–253. doi: 10.1016/j.meegid.2011.12.009
104. Zúñiga, E., Gruppi, A., Hirabayashi, J., Kasai, K. I., and Rabinovich, G. A. (2001a). Regulated expression and effect of galectin-1 on *Trypanosoma cruzi*-infected macrophages: modulation of microbicidal activity and survival. *Infect. Immun.* 69, 6804–6812. doi: 10.1128/IAI.69.11.6804-6812.2001
105. Zúñiga, E., Rabinovich, G. A., Iglesias, M. M., and Gruppi, A. (2001b). Regulated expression of galectin-1 during B-cell activation and implications for T-cell apoptosis. *J. Leukoc. Biol.* 70, 73–79.

10

Is the Antitumor Property of *Trypanosoma cruzi* Infection Mediated by its Calreticulin?

Galia Ramírez-Toloza[1]*, Paula Abello[2] and Arturo Ferreira[2]*

[1] *Faculty of Veterinary Medicine and Livestock Sciences, University of Chile, Santiago, Chile,* [2] *Program of Immunology, Faculty of Medicine, Institute of Biomedical Sciences (ICBM), University of Chile, Santiago, Chile*

***Correspondence:**
Galia Ramírez-Toloza
galiaram@uchile.cl;
Arturo Ferreira
aferreir@med.uchile.cl

Eight to 10 million people in 21 endemic countries are infected with *Trypanosoma cruzi*. However, only 30% of those infected develop symptoms of Chagas' disease, a chronic, neglected tropical disease worldwide. Similar to other pathogens, *T. cruzi* has evolved to resist the host immune response. Studies, performed 80 years ago in the Soviet Union, proposed that *T. cruzi* infects tumor cells with similar capacity to that displayed for target tissues such as cardiac, aortic, or digestive. An antagonistic relationship between *T. cruzi* infection and cancer development was also proposed, but the molecular mechanisms involved have remained largely unknown. Probably, a variety of *T. cruzi* molecules is involved. This review focuses on how *T. cruzi* calreticulin (TcCRT), exteriorized from the endoplasmic reticulum, targets the first classical complement component C1 and negatively regulates the classical complement activation cascade, promoting parasite infectivity. We propose that this C1-dependent TcCRT-mediated virulence is critical to explain, at least an important part, of the parasite capacity to inhibit tumor development. We will discuss how TcCRT, by directly interacting with venous and arterial endothelial cells, inhibits angiogenesis and tumor growth. Thus, these TcCRT functions not only illustrate *T. cruzi* interactions with the host immune defensive strategies, but also illustrate a possible co-evolutionary adaptation to privilege a prolonged interaction with its host.

Keywords: calreticulin, *Trypanosoma cruzi*, trypomastigotes, complement system, C1q, cC1qR, tumor growth, immune response

INTRODUCTION

Trypanosoma cruzi (the protozoan agent of Chagas' disease) cell infection is preceded by a variety of molecular interactions (1). Of relevance is the generation of a synapsis involving parasite endoplasmic reticulum (ER)-resident *T. cruzi* calreticulin (TcCRT) that, after translocation, interacts with complement component C1. C1 is then inactivated and recognized by cC1qR (a membrane form of mammalian CRT). The complement system, an important arm of innate and adaptive immune responses, is thus inhibited and parasite infectivity increased.

A significant decrease in experimental tumor growth is observed in experimental animals treated with recombinant TcCRT (rTcCRT) or infected with *T. cruzi*. A unifying molecular basis for these apparently unrelated phenomena is proposed herein. These molecular interactions do provide benefits for both the host and the parasite.

Through evolution, microbial agents have developed different mechanisms to resist the host immune response. In apparently unrelated strategies, some infectious agents elicit antitumor immune responses, leading to inhibition of cancer progression (2). Although these antitumor effects have been reported for several decades now, for a variety of infections, information on pathogen molecules involved is scarce (3).

Eight to 10 million people in 21 endemic countries are infected with *T. cruzi*. In about 30% of those infected, manifests, Chagas' disease, a worldwide neglected tropical chronic illness (4, 5). The disease, originally endemic in Latin America, is now global, mainly because of migrations to USA, Canada, Europe, Oceania, and Asia (6), where transmission is mainly through blood transfusions, organ transplants, or congenital (7).

Eighty years ago, it was proposed that *T. cruzi* possesses an anticancer activity. Several *T. cruzi* strains displayed growth inhibitory effects over multiple transplanted or spontaneous tumors, in animal experimental models and humans (8, 9). This property was attributed to a "toxic substance" secreted by the parasite (10, 11). This "toxin" reduced pain, tumor growth, bleeding, and local inflammation in humans affected by a variety of tumors (12).

Chronically infected rats are more resistant to a carcinoma induced by 1,2-dimethylhidrazyne (9), and *T. cruzi* has a tropism for tumor cells, suggesting an antagonistic relationship between Chagas' disease and cancer development (8). Elemental Darwinian reasoning allows us to propose that, if host survival is favored, chances for improved parasite persistence are evident.

Some authors have proposed that tumor and parasites compete for nutrients with consequent inhibition of tumor growth (13). However, this hypothesis is not entirely satisfactory since tumor growth is a multistep and complex process involving development of new blood vessels (angiogenesis) that provide the tumor with the necessary nutrients, oxygen, and means for waste removal (14). Other investigators have demonstrated, using a recombinant non-pathogenic *T. cruzi* clone as vector of a testis tumor antigen, the activation of T cell-mediated immunity. This specific cell immunity could delay tumor development in infected mice (15). In this work, it would have been important to define whether the non-pathogenic *T. cruzi* clone used translocates-externalizes its CRT. Non-infective epimastigotes are strongly impaired in their capacity to translocate this chaperone (16). Moreover, hemiallelic *TcCRT* KO, wild type, and transgenic parasites, respectively carrying one, two, and three *TcCRT* gene copies, express increased levels of the protein, *in vitro* resistance to human complement, and higher infectivity (16, 17).

Most likely, multiple parasite molecules and mechanisms are involved in the tumor resistance mediated by *T. cruzi* infection. Understanding these mechanisms may contribute to identify new therapeutic targets against cancer and Chagas' disease.

Our laboratory has been working for more than 20 years now with TcCRT, a multifunctional ER-resident protein that the parasite translocates to the external milieu (as depicted in **Figures 1A,B**). TcCRT is involved in a multiplicity of

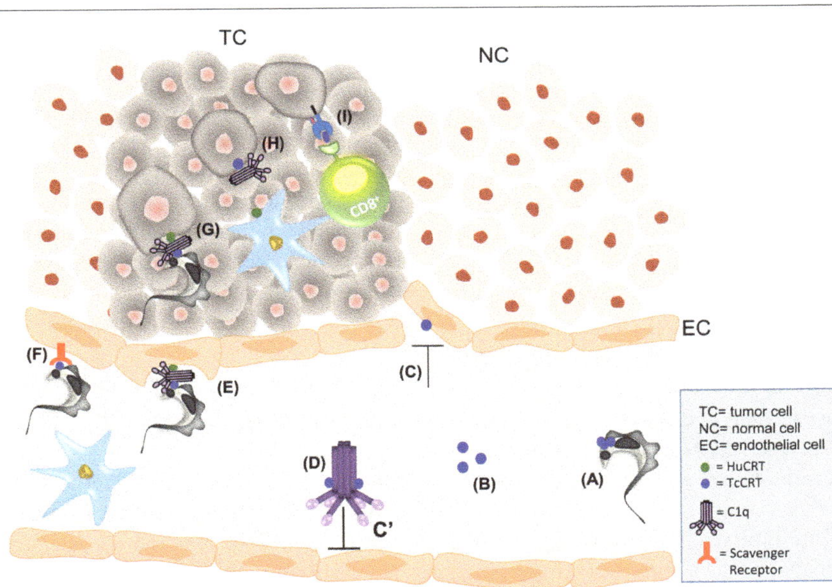

FIGURE 1 | The antitumor effect of *T. cruzi* infection may be explained by TcCRT. TcCRT is exposed on the parasite surface **(A)** and secreted **(B)**. TcCRT inhibits angiogenesis **(C)** and the activation of the classical pathway of the complement system through C1 inactivation **(D)**. TcCRT, present on the parasite surface, recruits C1. On the EC membrane, a trimolecular synapse is formed by HuCRT/C1q/TcCRT. This interaction increases the infectivity process **(E)**. TcCRT is also recognized by SRs on ECs, promoting infectivity **(F)**. The HuCRT/C1q/TcCRT interaction can also promote *T. cruzi* infectivity in TCs **(G)**. Moreover, TcCRT could mediate induction of an anamnestic antitumor immune response. Parasite could translocate TcCRT bound to the tumor cell with subsequent capture of host C1 **(H)**. This C1 will be recognized by HuCRT present on an antigen-presenting cell (APC), followed by internalization of this complex. Among many other possibilities, APCs will cross-process TcCRT, and specific peptides from this parasite protein will be loaded onto MHC I molecules. APCs will enter the regional lymph node and present these nTcCRT-specific peptides to cytotoxic T lymphocytes, thus leading to their activation. These CD8+ cytotoxic T lymphocytes will leave the lymph node and kill tumor cells that also present TcCRT-derived peptides **(I)**.

host–pathogen interactions. Thus, TcCRT is a potent virulence factor that inhibits the angiogenesis and a likely responsible, for at least in important part, of the antitumor effects of *T. cruzi* infection.

IN EUKARYOTES, CALRETICULIN, AN ER-RESIDENT CHAPERONE PROTEIN, MEDIATES ANTITUMOR PROPERTIES

Calreticulin (CRT) is a 45 kDa protein, mainly residing in the ER (18). CRT participates in a variety of physiological and pathological processes in different cellular types (19). Thus, CRT contributes in multiple physiological processes such as control of glycoprotein folding quality system and binding to monoglucosylated high mannose glycans (20). Moreover, CRT is involved in quality control process during protein synthesis, including integrins, surface receptors, and transporters (21), and it is considered as an intracellular Ca^{2+} regulator (22).

Calreticulin is also found in the cytosol, nucleus, secretory granules, on the plasma membrane, and free in the extracellular milieu (18), accelerating cutaneous wound healing (23–25) and regulating cell adhesion by interacting with the cytosolic tail of the integrin alpha subunit (18); nuclear export of some steroid hormone receptors (26–28) and the stability or translation of a variety of RNAs (29–33). CRT is an mRNA binding protein that regulates mRNA stability (19).

Calreticulin also participates in the immune response against apoptotic cancer cells (34–38), and surface exposure of CRT participates as an "eat me" signal required for phagocytosis on dying tumor cells (39). Tumor tissues express significant higher levels of CRT compared to normal tissues (40). Indeed, its expression is related to the clinical stage and lymph node metastasis in several types of cancer (41, 42).

Over 40 functions have been described for human CRT (HuCRT) (43). These functions reside in three different domains: globular N-terminal (N), proline-rich (P), and acidic C-terminus (18). HuCRT and its N-terminal fragment bind laminin (44) with antiangiogenic properties *in vitro* and *in vivo* (45, 46) and inhibit the growth in several tumor models (47–49).

Vasostatin, a CRT 180 amino acid N-terminal fragment, is an endogenous inhibitor of angiogenesis and suppressor of tumor growth. It inhibits vascular endothelial growth factor (VEGF)-induced endothelial cell (EC) proliferation and tube formation in Matrigel and induces cell apoptosis under oxygen deprivation (50).

Calreticulin is present in humans (51), insects (52, 53), nematodes (54–57), protozoans (58–61), and plants (62). A high identity is shared among CRTs from different species. Thus, *Onchocerca volvulus*, *Schistosoma mansoni*, and *Leishmania donovani* share 50% of the identity in amino acid sequence with HuCRT.

Examples of important evasive strategies performed by CRTs from different parasite species are *Amblyomma americanum* [secretes CRT during the feeding process (63)] and *Schistosoma cercariae* [uses CRT in the penetration of gland cells or skin and parasite migration (54)].

HOW DOES *T. CRUZI* CALRETICULIN PARTICIPATE IN THE HOST–PARASITE INTERPLAY?

Given the important pleiotropic HuCRT behavior, the CRT model opens interesting research opportunities on how this protein, alone or interacting with others, intervenes in the host–parasite interactions.

For 25 years now, our laboratory has worked with TcCRT. This protein is coded by only one gene with a variable number of copies whose involvement in TcCRT expression will depend on the *T. cruzi* clone and strain studied (unpublished data). A TcCRT gene was cloned, sequenced, and expressed in our laboratory in 1991 (58). We identified variable low plasma levels of anti-native TcCRT antibodies in *T. cruzi*-infected humans (64), thus revealing the immunogenic capacity of the native protein.

Trypanosoma cruzi calreticulin also binds monoglucosylated glycans (60) and participates in the maturation of cruzipain, a lysosomal protease (65) present in *T. cruzi*. Although TcCRT locates mainly in the ER, it is also found in the Golgi complex, reservosomes, flagellar pocket, cell surface, cytosol, nucleus, and kinetoplast (66, 67). However, the mechanisms involved in these diverse TcCRT localizations are unknown. Thus, TcCRT, in spite of its KEDL-ER retention sequence [KDEL in mammal CRTs (18)], translocates from the ER to the extracellular environment (**Figures 1A,B**) where, besides inhibiting complement (66) and acting as a virulence factor (68), it mediates antitumor effects.

In spite of the long evolutionary distance, TcCRT still shares 50% of overall sequence homology with HuCRT, reaching up to 80% in critical functional domains. Moreover, the general globular N-domain, responsible of antiangiogenic properties and the structural features of the extended arm P-domain also share structure homologies, thus announcing the possibility of functional similarities (69).

Two important TcCRT functions may explain the relationship between *T. cruzi* infection and cancer. First, TcCRT is an important complement inhibitor (**Figure 1D**) and virulence factor (**Figure 1E**). Second, TcCRT inhibits angiogenesis (**Figure 1C**). Both functions are central to inhibit tumor growth.

TcCRT IS AN IMPORTANT VIRULENCE FACTOR IN *T. CRUZI*

Similar to HuCRT (70, 71), TcCRT inhibits the complement system by interacting with C1 (**Figure 1D**), the first component of its classical pathway (66, 72–74). TcCRT is translocated from the ER to the area of flagellum emergence (**Figure 1A**) (66), where C1 is recruited by parasite-bound TcCRT and inhibited at the earliest complement activation step (C4b generation) (**Figure 1D**). TcCRT also affects the ability of C1s to activate C4, in a calcium-independent manner (74). Inhibition of C1 is a significant complement evasion strategy, with consequences in the host–parasite relationships. Although HuCRT and TcCRT prevent binding of the serine proteases to C1q, they do not displace the serine proteases from the preformed stabilized C1 (C1q, r_2, and s_2) complex (74). TcCRT also binds to MBL and

Ficolins (75). C1, MBL, and Ficolins are three complement "danger signal" recognition macromolecular modules present in plasma. These molecular complexes are genetically, structurally, and functionally related, but they differ in the nature of the recognized danger signals (76). More recently, we have proposed that L-Ficolin binds TcCRT, inhibiting the lectin pathway. This inhibition may represent other *T. cruzi* strategy to inhibit the host immune response (75). In agreement with these findings, TcCRT is present on the parasite surface co-localizing with C1q (66).

Human CRT is also a membrane receptor for C1q [cC1qR (77)], and it may bridge TcCRT on the parasite surface with HuCRT present on the host cell (**Figure 1E**) (78). The TcCRT/C1q/HuCRT synapsis represents the culmination of an important molecular mimicry strategy. Apoptotic cells to be phagocytized use a similar mechanism (34, 36, 37). The CRT/C1q complex is recognized as an "eat me" signal by cC1qR on phagocytes. This signal is also used by *T. cruzi* as an "apoptotic mimicry" strategy (i.e., by capturing C1 in the area of flagellum emergence), thus facilitating the invasion/infectivity of host cells (79). This TcCRT-C1q-mediated parasite infectivity correlates with significant increases in TcCRT mRNA levels during early (cell contact and penetration) infection stages (36, 66, 68, 69, 72, 79). The TcCRT–C1q interaction can be prevented with anti-TcCRT $F(ab')_2$ fragments (devoid of the C1-binding Fc domains) (80). Indeed, passive immunization of mice with these fragments decreases infectivity (68). Congenital transmission is an important *T. cruzi* transmission pathway. Human pregnancy is a condition of elevated circulating CRT (81, 82). Moreover, human placenta expresses high CRT levels (83). We have recently proposed that the TcCRT/C1q/HuCRT interaction is very important in an *ex vivo* model of infection of human placenta (84), indicating a possible mechanism to explain the congenital transmission.

TcCRT PARTICIPATES IN THE INHIBITION OF TUMOR GROWTH

Cancer is omnipresent in human history, and it also affects most of the living animal species, as a natural phenomenon of sporadic cellular dysfunction. Mammary, prostate, lung, cervix/uterine are just a few examples of cancer that, taken together, have epidemic proportions.

Interestingly, in patients infected with *T. cruzi*, cancer is rare (10, 12). About 80 years ago, Roskin, Ekzempliarskaia, and Klyuyeva, researchers from the former Soviet Union, postulated an experimental anticancer toxic activity derived from this infection. When they inoculated *T. cruzi* extracts, directly in a peritumoral area, in different tumors, both in experimental animals and in humans, similar results related to reduction of tumor size were obtained (10–13, 85, 86). More recently, the parasite capacity to infect preferentially tumor cells, as compared to normal host cells, was described (8). Although, in general, these data suggest an antagonism between *T. cruzi* infection and tumor growth (8), and research progress in these areas was seriously hampered by the intense international political problems of those years (i.e., the Cold War) (11). Although several publications on these issues have appeared during the last decades, the molecular basis of this phenomenon has remained elusive.

We propose that TcCRT is an important mediator of the antitumor effects of *T. cruzi* infection. Similar to HuCRT, TcCRT is antiangiogenic in *in vitro*, *ex vivo*, and *in vivo* models (**Figure 1C**) (3, 87, 88). Moreover, TcCRT inhibits the growth of a mammary adenocarcinoma and a melanoma in different experimental animal models (3, 87–89). The inhibition of tumor angiogenesis was proposed as a cancer therapy almost 40 years ago (90). For this reason, molecules or drugs with capacity to inhibit angiogenesis are currently applicable to a wide variety of tumors, often as a complement to other therapies (91).

Trypanosoma cruzi calreticulin and its N-terminal domain (N-TcCRT) were studied in different experimental set ups in mammals, *Homo sapiens* included (3). Thus, rTcCRT and its N-TcCRT inhibit capillary growth *ex vivo* in *Rattus rattus* aortic rings, morphogenesis, proliferation, and chemotaxis in human umbilical cord endothelial cells (HUVECs) (3) and *in vivo* angiogenesis in the *Gallus gallus* chorioallantoid membrane (CAM) assay (87). TcCRT was overall more effective, in molar terms, than HuCRT (3). Interestingly, in the CAM assay, the antiangiogenic TcCRT effect was fully reverted by polyclonal antibodies against rTcCRT (88).

In agreement with the previously described facts, the *in vivo* antitumor capacity of *T. cruzi* infection is paralleled by the inoculation of rTcCRT, with inhibits by 60–70% the time-course development of a murine mammary methotrexate multiresistant adenocarcinoma (TA3-MTX-R) (7).

T. CRUZI INFECTS NEOPLASTIC CELLS AND PROMOTES AN IMMUNE RESPONSE

Native TcCRT (nTcCRT) on the parasite contacts ECs, mediating internalization of *T. cruzi* and inhibition of tumor growth. This nTcCRT/EC contact may be indirect, mediated by C1q (**Figure 1E**) or by direct binding to scavenger receptors (SRs) (**Figure 1F**). TcCRT has affinity for collagenous structures, a possible explanation for its binding to human C1 and to SRs (66, 68). Fluid-phase Fucoidan, bearing extensive collagen-like sequences, inhibits the binding of CRT to SR-A present on both phagocytic cells (92) and the internalization of TcCRT by ECs (3).

IS NATIVE TcCRT RESPONSIBLE FOR THE ANTITUMOR EFFECT OF *T. CRUZI* INFECTION?

Recombinant TcCRT has important *in vivo* antiangiogenic and antitumor activities (3, 88). The antitumor effect of *T. cruzi* extract has been recently reproduced in a rat model. Experimental animals showed a strong cytotoxic response against tumor, with activation of $CD4^+$ and $CD8^+$ T cells and splenocytes. Moreover, a humoral adaptive immune response is generated. These anti-*T. cruzi* antibodies cross-reacted with tumor cells, inducing an antibody-dependent cellular toxicity *in vitro* (93). In a mouse model, we have reverted the antitumor effect of a *T. cruzi* epimastigote extract with specific antibodies against rTcCRT. Moreover, anti-rTcCRT F(ab′)$_2$ antibodies (devoid of their capacity to interact with C1) neutralize the antitumor activity of *T. cruzi* infection, thus identifying nTcCRT as a mediator of this effect (unpublished data).

HOW DOES TcCRT INHIBIT TUMOR GROWTH IN INDIVIDUALS INFECTED WITH *T. CRUZI*?

We propose that, during *T. cruzi* infection, nTcCRT mediates key alterations in the tumor cell microenvironment leading to an adaptive immune response, with significant antitumor effects. Once in the circulation, *T. cruzi* must swiftly invade ECs (**Figures 1E,F**). Translocated-exteriorized TcCRT (**Figures 1A,B**) (92) will recruit and inactivate plasma complement C1 (**Figure 1D**) and inhibits angiogenesis (**Figure 1C**). This will allow the parasite to contact ECs *via* cC1qR (**Figure 1E**) (77, 94). Otherwise, the chaperone protein could interact directly with SR-A1 on ECs (**Figure 1F**) (95–97). Both pathways may lead to antiangiogenesis and generate a stressful environment where tumor cells will externalize their CRT, as previously shown with other stressing agents, such as Antracyclins (37). C1 recruitment and increased tumor cell phagocytosis by dendritic cells will follow (**Figure 1H**).

On the other hand, an adaptive immune response may be invoked by inoculated TcCRT or by its native counterpart timely externalized by infecting trypomastigotes (66) or present in epimastigote extracts (75). The chaperone protein should reach the surface of tumor cells (or ECs), thus generating a site for C1 binding (**Figure 1G**), followed by phagocytosis of these complexes by dendritic cells (**Figure 1H**). Targeting these activities on tumor cells should be favored by the parasite tropism for these tissues. The relevant novelty of parasite TcCRT is its difference in amino acidic sequence with the mammal (murine, in this case) counterpart. This difference may reach 50%, while mammal CRTs differ among them by no more than 10% (73). Upon arrival to the regional lymph nodes, these dendritic cells will present antigenic peptides derived from TcCRT, thus activating cytotoxic T lymphocytes, among other possibilities. Whether tumor cells can cross-present peptides derived from endocytosed TcCRT to cytotoxic T cells (**Figure 1I**) is a matter of current research in our laboratory. Activated cytotoxic T cells should then return to the tumor site and act against neoplastic tumor cells. Activation of CD4$^+$ T cells *via* MHC II presentation, with stimulation of B cells and resulting ADCC against tumor cells, is a possibility that should also be entertained.

In our murine models, these antitumor effects are better performed by TcCRT, as compared to HuCRT. Among mammals, CRTs are at least 95% homologous in amino acidic differences. CRT immunogenicity across mammal species is thus restricted. On the other hand, because of extensive evolutionary distances, TcCRT amino acidic sequence differs by 50% with its mammal counterparts. Thus, TcCRT is more capable of generating immunogenic epitopes on the surface of mammal tumors. Recently, the expression of CRT has been correlated with a favorable prognosis of cancer. The high expression of CRT on tumor cells has been associated with a high density of infiltrating mature dendritic cells and effector memory T-cell subsets, suggesting that CRT triggers the activation of an adaptive immune response in the tumor microenvironment (98). Thus, TcCRT expressed and secreted by the parasite may be also important in this regard.

CONCLUDING REMARKS

Infection with *T. cruzi* correlates with increased resistant to tumors. Since, during infection, nTcCRT is translocated to the parasite exterior and experimental parenteral administration of rTcCRT mimics the antitumor effects of the infection, nTcCRT is the most likely responsible molecule for these effects. Moreover, the antitumor effects of parasite infection can be specifically reverted by anti-rTcCRT antibodies. Since, in a large set of experimental animals treated with rTcCRT, no clinical deleterious effects have been detected by standard clinical veterinary criteria, we can now propose that rTcCRT or derived domains are interesting immunological tools to be considered in more advanced preclinical trials (e.g., rTcCRT capacity to bind to human mammary tumor cell lines *in vitro*, to subsequently incorporate C1, with increased capacity to induce phagocytosis).

AUTHOR CONTRIBUTIONS

GR-T, PA, and AF designed experiments. GR-T and PA performed experiments. GR-T, PA, and AF interpreted the data. GR-T, PA, and AF generated key reagents. GR-T, PA, and AF wrote, revised, and edited the manuscript. GR-T, PA, and AF approved the manuscript.

REFERENCES

1. Yoshida N. Molecular basis of mammalian cell invasion by *Trypanosoma cruzi*. *An Acad Bras Cienc* (2006) 78:87–111. doi:10.1590/S0001-37652006000100010
2. Oikonomopoulou K, Brinc D, Hadjisavvas A, Christofi G, Kyriacou K, Diamandis EP. The bifacial role of helminths in cancer: involvement of immune and non-immune mechanisms. *Crit Rev Clin Lab Sci* (2014) 51:138–48. doi:10.3109/10408363.2014.886180
3. Lopez NC, Valck C, Ramirez G, Rodriguez M, Ribeiro C, Orellana J, et al. Antiangiogenic and antitumor effects of *Trypanosoma cruzi* Calreticulin. *PLoS Negl Trop Dis* (2010) 4:e730. doi:10.1371/journal.pntd.0000730
4. Coura JR, Vinas PA. Chagas disease: a new worldwide challenge. *Nature* (2010) 465:S6–7. doi:10.1038/nature09221
5. Perez-Molina JA, Perez AM, Norman FF, Monge-Maillo B, Lopez-Velez R. Old and new challenges in Chagas disease. *Lancet Infect Dis* (2015) 15:1347–56. doi:10.1016/S1473-3099(15)00243-1
6. Tanowitz HB, Weiss LM, Montgomery SP. Chagas disease has now gone global. *PLoS Negl Trop Dis* (2011) 5:e1136. doi:10.1371/journal.pntd.0001136
7. Ramirez-Toloza G, Aguilar-Guzman L, Valck C, Abello P, Ferreira A. Is it all that bad when living with an intracellular protozoan? The role of *Trypanosoma cruzi* calreticulin in angiogenesis and tumor growth. *Front Oncol* (2014) 4:382. doi: 10.3389/fonc.2014.00382

8. Kallinikova VD, Matekin PV, Ogloblina TA, Leikina MI, Kononenko AF, Sokolova NM, et al. [Anticancer properties of flagellate protozoan *Trypanosoma cruzi* Chagas, 1909]. *Izv Akad Nauk Ser Biol* (2001) 3:299–311.
9. Oliveira EC, Leite MS, Miranda JA, Andrade AL, Garcia SB, Luquetti AO, et al. Chronic *Trypanosoma cruzi* infection associated with low incidence of 1,2-dimethylhydrazine-induced colon cancer in rats. *Carcinogenesis* (2001) 22:737–40. doi:10.1093/carcin/22.5.737
10. Klyuyeva NG, Roskin GI. *Biotherapy of Malignant Tumours*. New York: Pergamon Press (1963). 315 p.
11. Krementsov NL. *The Cure: A Story of Cancer and Politics from the Annals of the Cold War*. Chicago: University of Chicago Press (2002). 261 p.
12. Roskin G. Toxin therapy of experimental cancer; the influence of protozoan infections upon transplanted cancer. *Cancer Res* (1946) 6:363–5.
13. Hauschka TS, Goodwin MB. *Trypanosoma cruzi* Endotoxin (KR) in the treatment of malignant mouse tumors. *Science* (1948) 107:600–2. doi:10.1126/science.107.2788.600
14. Folkman J. Fundamental concepts of the angiogenic process. *Curr Mol Med* (2003) 3:643–51. doi:10.2174/1566524033479465
15. Junqueira C, Santos LI, Galvao-Filho B, Teixeira SM, Rodrigues FG, DaRocha WD, et al. *Trypanosoma cruzi* as an effective cancer antigen delivery vector. *Proc Natl Acad Sci U S A* (2011) 108:19695–700. doi:10.1073/pnas.1110030108
16. Sanchez Valdez FJ, Perez Brandan C, Zago MP, Labriola C, Ferreira A, Basombrio MA. *Trypanosoma cruzi* carrying a monoallelic deletion of the calreticulin (TcCRT) gene are susceptible to complement mediated killing and defective in their metacyclogenesis. *Mol Immunol* (2013) 53:198–205. doi:10.1016/j.molimm.2012.08.001
17. Sanchez-Valdez FJ, Perez Brandan C, Ramirez G, Uncos AD, Zago MP, Cimino RO, et al. A monoallelic deletion of the TcCRT gene increases the attenuation of a cultured *Trypanosoma cruzi* strain, protecting against an in vivo virulent challenge. *PLoS Negl Trop Dis* (2014) 8:e2696. doi:10.1371/journal.pntd.0002696
18. Michalak M, Groenendyk J, Szabo E, Gold LI, Opas M. Calreticulin, a multi-process calcium-buffering chaperone of the endoplasmic reticulum. *Biochem J* (2009) 417:651–66. doi:10.1042/BJ20081847
19. Lu YC, Weng WC, Lee H. Functional roles of calreticulin in cancer biology. *Biomed Res Int* (2015) 2015:526524. doi:10.1155/2015/526524
20. Michalak M, Milner RE, Burns K, Opas M. Calreticulin. *Biochem J* (1992) 285(Pt 3):681–92. doi:10.1042/bj2850681
21. Michalak M, Corbett EF, Mesaeli N, Nakamura K, Opas M. Calreticulin: one protein, one gene, many functions. *Biochem J* (1999) 344(Pt 2):281–92. doi:10.1042/0264-6021:3440281
22. Baksh S, Michalak M. Expression of calreticulin in *Escherichia coli* and identification of its Ca2+ binding domains. *J Biol Chem* (1991) 266:21458–65.
23. Arias I, Sepulveda C, Bravo P, Hamilton-West C, Maldonado I, Ferreira A. Comparative effect of human and *Trypanosoma cruzi* calreticulin in wound healing. *J Tissue Eng Regen Med* (2012) 9(1):41–54. doi:10.1002/term.1613
24. Gold LI, Rahman M, Blechman KM, Greives MR, Churgin S, Michaels J, et al. Overview of the role for calreticulin in the enhancement of wound healing through multiple biological effects. *J Investig Dermatol Symp Proc* (2006) 11:57–65. doi:10.1038/sj.jidsymp.5650011
25. Nanney LB, Woodrell CD, Greives MR, Cardwell NL, Pollins AC, Bancroft TA, et al. Calreticulin enhances porcine wound repair by diverse biological effects. *Am J Pathol* (2008) 173:610–30. doi:10.2353/ajpath.2008.071027
26. Burns K, Duggan B, Atkinson EA, Famulski KS, Nemer M, Bleackley RC, et al. Modulation of gene expression by calreticulin binding to the glucocorticoid receptor. *Nature* (1994) 367:476–80. doi:10.1038/367476a0
27. Dedhar S, Rennie PS, Shago M, Hagesteijn CY, Yang H, Filmus J, et al. Inhibition of nuclear hormone receptor activity by calreticulin. *Nature* (1994) 367:480–3. doi:10.1038/367480a0
28. Holaska JM, Black BE, Love DC, Hanover JA, Leszyk J, Paschal BM. Calreticulin is a receptor for nuclear export. *J Cell Biol* (2001) 152:127–40. doi:10.1083/jcb.152.1.127
29. Iakova P, Wang GL, Timchenko L, Michalak M, Pereira-Smith OM, Smith JR, et al. Competition of CUGBP1 and calreticulin for the regulation of p21 translation determines cell fate. *EMBO J* (2004) 23:406–17. doi:10.1038/sj.emboj.7600052
30. Nickenig G, Michaelsen F, Muller C, Berger A, Vogel T, Sachinidis A, et al. Destabilization of AT(1) receptor mRNA by calreticulin. *Circ Res* (2002) 90:53–8. doi:10.1161/hh0102.102503
31. Singh NK, Atreya CD, Nakhasi HL. Identification of calreticulin as a rubella virus RNA binding protein. *Proc Natl Acad Sci U S A* (1994) 91:12770–4. doi:10.1073/pnas.91.26.12770
32. Timchenko LT, Iakova P, Welm AL, Cai ZJ, Timchenko NA. Calreticulin interacts with C/EBPalpha and C/EBPbeta mRNAs and represses translation of C/EBP proteins. *Mol Cell Biol* (2002) 22:7242–57. doi:10.1128/MCB.22.20.7242-7257.2002
33. Totary-Jain H, Naveh-Many T, Riahi Y, Kaiser N, Eckel J, Sasson S. Calreticulin destabilizes glucose transporter-1 mRNA in vascular endothelial and smooth muscle cells under high-glucose conditions. *Circ Res* (2005) 97:1001–8. doi:10.1161/01.RES.0000189260.46084.e5
34. Obeid M, Panaretakis T, Joza N, Tufi R, Tesniere A, van Endert P, et al. Calreticulin exposure is required for the immunogenicity of gamma-irradiation and UVC light-induced apoptosis. *Cell Death Differ* (2007) 14:1848–50. doi:10.1038/sj.cdd.4402201
35. Obeid M, Panaretakis T, Tesniere A, Joza N, Tufi R, Apetoh L, et al. Leveraging the immune system during chemotherapy: moving calreticulin to the cell surface converts apoptotic death from "silent" to immunogenic. *Cancer Res* (2007) 67:7941–4. doi:10.1158/0008-5472.CAN-07-1622
36. Obeid M, Tesniere A, Ghiringhelli F, Fimia GM, Apetoh L, Perfettini JL, et al. Calreticulin exposure dictates the immunogenicity of cancer cell death. *Nat Med* (2007) 13:54–61. doi:10.1038/nm1523
37. Obeid M, Tesniere A, Panaretakis T, Tufi R, Joza N, van Endert P, et al. Ecto-calreticulin in immunogenic chemotherapy. *Immunol Rev* (2007) 220:22–34. doi:10.1111/j.1600-065X.2007.00567.x
38. Tesniere A, Apetoh L, Ghiringhelli F, Joza N, Panaretakis T, Kepp O, et al. Immunogenic cancer cell death: a key-lock paradigm. *Curr Opin Immunol* (2008) 20:504–11. doi:10.1016/j.coi.2008.05.007
39. Gardai SJ, McPhillips KA, Frasch SC, Janssen WJ, Starefeldt A, Murphy-Ullrich JE, et al. Cell-surface calreticulin initiates clearance of viable or apoptotic cells through trans-activation of LRP on the phagocyte. *Cell* (2005) 123:321–34. doi:10.1016/j.cell.2005.08.032
40. Zamanian M, Veerakumarasivam A, Abdullah S, Rosli R. Calreticulin and cancer. *Pathol Oncol Res* (2013) 19:149–54. doi:10.1007/s12253-012-9600-2
41. Chen CN, Chang CC, Su TE, Hsu WM, Jeng YM, Ho MC, et al. Identification of calreticulin as a prognosis marker and angiogenic regulator in human gastric cancer. *Ann Surg Oncol* (2009) 16:524–33. doi:10.1245/s10434-008-0243-1
42. Lwin ZM, Guo C, Salim A, Yip GW, Chew FT, Nan J, et al. Clinicopathological significance of calreticulin in breast invasive ductal carcinoma. *Mod Pathol* (2010) 23:1559–66. doi:10.1038/modpathol.2010.173
43. Eggleton P, Bremer E, Dudek E, Michalak M. Calreticulin, a therapeutic target? *Expert Opin Ther Targets* (2016) 25:1–11. doi:10.1517/14728222.2016.1164695
44. Yao L, Pike SE, Tosato G. Laminin binding to the calreticulin fragment vasostatin regulates endothelial cell function. *J Leukoc Biol* (2002) 71:47–53.
45. Pike SE, Yao L, Jones KD, Cherney B, Appella E, Sakaguchi K, et al. Vasostatin, a calreticulin fragment, inhibits angiogenesis and suppresses tumor growth. *J Exp Med* (1998) 188:2349–56. doi:10.1084/jem.188.12.2349
46. Pike SE, Yao L, Setsuda J, Jones KD, Cherney B, Appella E, et al. Calreticulin and calreticulin fragments are endothelial cell inhibitors that suppress tumor growth. *Blood* (1999) 94:2461–8.
47. Cai KX, Tse LY, Leung C, Tam PK, Xu R, Sham MH. Suppression of lung tumor growth and metastasis in mice by adeno-associated virus-mediated expression of vasostatin. *Clin Cancer Res* (2008) 14:939–49. doi:10.1158/1078-0432.CCR-07-1930
48. Jazowiecka-Rakus J, Jarosz M, Kozlowska D, Sochanik A, Szala S. Combination of vasostatin and cyclophosphamide in the therapy of murine melanoma tumors. *Acta Biochim Pol* (2007) 54:125–33.
49. Yao L, Pike SE, Pittaluga S, Cherney B, Gupta G, Jaffe ES, et al. Anti-tumor activities of the angiogenesis inhibitors interferon-inducible protein-10 and the calreticulin fragment vasostatin. *Cancer Immunol Immunother* (2002) 51:358–66. doi:10.1007/s00262-002-0294-2
50. Shu Q, Li W, Li H, Sun G. Vasostatin inhibits VEGF-induced endothelial cell proliferation, tube formation and induces cell apoptosis under oxygen deprivation. *Int J Mol Sci* (2014) 15:6019–30. doi:10.3390/ijms15046019
51. McCauliffe DP, Zappi E, Lieu TS, Michalak M, Sontheimer RD, Capra JD. A human Ro/SS-A autoantigen is the homologue of calreticulin and is highly homologous with onchocercal RAL-1 antigen and an aplysia "memory molecule". *J Clin Invest* (1990) 86:332–5. doi:10.1172/JCI114704

52. Ferreira CA, Da Silva Vaz I, da Silva SS, Haag KL, Valenzuela JG, Masuda A. Cloning and partial characterization of a Boophilus microplus (Acari: Ixodidae) calreticulin. *Exp Parasitol* (2002) 101:25–34. doi:10.1016/S0014-4894(02)00032-2
53. Smith MJ. Nucleotide sequence of a *drosophila melanogaster* gene encoding a calreticulin homologue. *DNA Seq* (1992) 3:247–50. doi:10.3109/10425179209034025
54. Kasper G, Brown A, Eberl M, Vallar L, Kieffer N, Berry C, et al. A calreticulin-like molecule from the human hookworm *Necator americanus* interacts with C1q and the cytoplasmic signalling domains of some integrins. *Parasite Immunol* (2001) 23:141–52. doi:10.1046/j.1365-3024.2001.00366.x
55. Khalife J, Pierce RJ, Godin C, Capron A. Cloning and sequencing of the gene encoding *Schistosoma mansoni* calreticulin. *Mol Biochem Parasitol* (1993) 62:313–5. doi:10.1016/0166-6851(93)90120-M
56. Rokeach LA, Zimmerman PA, Unnasch TR. Epitopes of the *Onchocerca volvulus* RAL1 antigen, a member of the calreticulin family of proteins, recognized by sera from patients with onchocerciasis. *Infect Immun* (1994) 62:3696–704.
57. Smith MJ. A C. elegans gene encodes a protein homologous to mammalian calreticulin. *DNA Seq* (1992) 2:235–40. doi:10.3109/10425179209020808
58. Aguillon JC, Ferreira L, Perez C, Colombo A, Molina MC, Wallace A, et al. Tc45, a dimorphic *Trypanosoma cruzi* immunogen with variable chromosomal localization, is calreticulin. *Am J Trop Med Hyg* (2000) 63:306–12.
59. Joshi M, Pogue GP, Duncan RC, Lee NS, Singh NK, Atreya CD, et al. Isolation and characterization of *Leishmania donovani* calreticulin gene and its conservation of the RNA binding activity. *Mol Biochem Parasitol* (1996) 81:53–64. doi:10.1016/0166-6851(96)02676-X
60. Labriola C, Cazzulo JJ, Parodi AJ. *Trypanosoma cruzi* calreticulin is a lectin that binds monoglucosylated oligosaccharides but not protein moieties of glycoproteins. *Mol Biol Cell* (1999) 10:1381–94. doi:10.1091/mbc.10.5.1381
61. Oladiran A, Belosevic M. *Trypanosoma carassii* calreticulin binds host complement component C1q and inhibits classical complement pathway-mediated lysis. *Dev Comp Immunol* (2010) 34:396–405. doi:10.1016/j.dci.2009.11.005
62. Denecke J, Carlsson LE, Vidal S, Hoglund AS, Ek B, van Zeijl MJ, et al. The tobacco homolog of mammalian calreticulin is present in protein complexes in vivo. *Plant Cell* (1995) 7:391–406. doi:10.1105/tpc.7.4.391
63. Jaworski DC, Higgins JA, Radulovic S, Vaughan JA, Azad AF. Presence of calreticulin in vector fleas (Siphonaptera). *J Med Entomol* (1996) 33:482–9. doi:10.1093/jmedent/33.3.482
64. Marcelain K, Colombo A, Molina MC, Ferreira L, Lorca M, Aguillon JC, et al. Development of an immunoenzymatic assay for the detection of human antibodies against *Trypanosoma cruzi* calreticulin, an immunodominant antigen. *Acta Trop* (2000) 75:291–300. doi:10.1016/S0001-706X(00)00062-0
65. Conte I, Labriola C, Cazzulo JJ, Docampo R, Parodi AJ. The interplay between folding-facilitating mechanisms in *Trypanosoma cruzi* endoplasmic reticulum. *Mol Biol Cell* (2003) 14:3529–40. doi:10.1091/mbc.E03-04-0228
66. Ferreira V, Valck C, Sanchez G, Gingras A, Tzima S, Molina MC, et al. The classical activation pathway of the human complement system is specifically inhibited by calreticulin from *Trypanosoma cruzi*. *J Immunol* (2004) 172:3042–50. doi:10.4049/jimmunol.172.5.3042
67. Souto-Padron T, Labriola CA, de Souza W. Immunocytochemical localisation of calreticulin in *Trypanosoma cruzi*. *Histochem Cell Biol* (2004) 122:563–9. doi:10.1007/s00418-004-0724-7
68. Ramirez G, Valck C, Molina MC, Ribeiro CH, Lopez N, Sanchez G, et al. *Trypanosoma cruzi* calreticulin: a novel virulence factor that binds complement C1 on the parasite surface and promotes infectivity. *Immunobiology* (2011) 216:265–73. doi:10.1016/j.imbio.2010.04.001
69. Ramirez G, Valck C, Ferreira VP, Lopez N, Ferreira A. Extracellular *Trypanosoma cruzi* calreticulin in the host-parasite interplay. *Trends Parasitol* (2011) 27:115–22. doi:10.1016/j.pt.2010.12.007
70. Stuart GR, Lynch NJ, Day AJ, Schwaeble WJ, Sim RB. The C1q and collectin binding site within C1q receptor (cell surface calreticulin). *Immunopharmacology* (1997) 38:73–80. doi:10.1016/S0162-3109(97)00076-3
71. Stuart GR, Lynch NJ, Lu J, Geick A, Moffatt BE, Sim RB, et al. Localisation of the C1q binding site within C1q receptor/calreticulin. *FEBS Lett* (1996) 397:245–9. doi:10.1016/S0014-5793(96)01156-8
72. Ferreira V, Molina MC, Schwaeble W, Lemus D, Ferreira A. Does *Trypanosoma cruzi* calreticulin modulate the complement system and angiogenesis? *Trends Parasitol* (2005) 21:169–74. doi:10.1016/j.pt.2005.02.005
73. Ferreira V, Molina MC, Valck C, Rojas A, Aguilar L, Ramirez G, et al. Role of calreticulin from parasites in its interaction with vertebrate hosts. *Mol Immunol* (2004) 40:1279–91. doi:10.1016/j.molimm.2003.11.018
74. Valck C, Ramirez G, Lopez N, Ribeiro CH, Maldonado I, Sanchez G, et al. Molecular mechanisms involved in the inactivation of the first component of human complement by *Trypanosoma cruzi* calreticulin. *Mol Immunol* (2010) 47:1516–21. doi:10.1016/j.molimm.2010.01.019
75. Sosoniuk E, Vallejos G, Kenawy H, Gaboriaud C, Thielens N, Fujita T, et al. *Trypanosoma cruzi* calreticulin inhibits the complement lectin pathway activation by direct interaction with L-Ficolin. *Mol Immunol* (2014) 60:80–5. doi:10.1016/j.molimm.2014.03.014
76. Ramirez G, Valck C, Aguilar L, Kemmerling U, Lopez-Munoz R, Cabrera G, et al. Roles of *Trypanosoma cruzi* calreticulin in parasite-host interactions and in tumor growth. *Mol Immunol* (2012) 52:133–40. doi:10.1016/j.molimm.2012.05.006
77. Eggleton P, Tenner AJ, Reid KB. C1q receptors. *Clin Exp Immunol* (2000) 120:406–12. doi:10.1046/j.1365-2249.2000.01218.x
78. Malhotra R. Collectin receptor (C1q receptor): structure and function. *Behring Inst Mitt* (1993) (93):254–61.
79. Rimoldi MT, Tenner AJ, Bobak DA, Joiner KA. Complement component C1q enhances invasion of human mononuclear phagocytes and fibroblasts by *Trypanosoma cruzi* trypomastigotes. *J Clin Invest* (1989) 84:1982–9. doi:10.1172/JCI114388
80. Aguilar L, Ramirez G, Valck C, Molina MC, Rojas A, Schwaeble W, et al. F(ab')2 antibody fragments against *Trypanosoma cruzi* calreticulin inhibit its interaction with the first component of human complement. *Biol Res* (2005) 38:187–95. doi:10.4067/S0716-97602005000200008
81. Crawford KE, Kalionis B, Stevenson JL, Brennecke SP, Gude NM. Calreticulin has opposing effects on the migration of human trophoblast and myometrial endothelial cells. *Placenta* (2012) 33:416–23. doi:10.1016/j.placenta.2012.02.003
82. Gu VY, Wong MH, Stevenson JL, Crawford KE, Brennecke SP, Gude NM. Calreticulin in human pregnancy and pre-eclampsia. *Mol Hum Reprod* (2008) 14:309–15. doi:10.1093/molehr/gan017
83. Houen G, Koch C. Human placental calreticulin: purification, characterization and association with other proteins. *Acta Chem Scand* (1994) 48:905–11. doi:10.3891/acta.chem.scand.48-0905
84. Castillo C, Ramirez G, Valck C, Aguilar L, Maldonado I, Rosas C, et al. The interaction of classical complement component C1 with parasite and host calreticulin mediates *Trypanosoma cruzi* infection of human placenta. *PLoS Negl Trop Dis* (2013) 7:e2376. doi:10.1371/journal.pntd.0002376
85. Hauschka T, Sake L, Rlair M. *Trypanosoma cruzi* in treatment of mouse tumours. *J Natl Cancer Inst* (1947) 7:189.
86. Malisoff WM. The action of the endotoxin of *Trypanosoma cruzi* (KR) on malignant mouse tumors. *Science* (1947) 106(2763):591–4. doi:10.1126/science.106.2763.591-a
87. Molina MC, Ferreira V, Valck C, Aguilar L, Orellana J, Rojas A, et al. An in vivo role for *Trypanosoma cruzi* calreticulin in antiangiogenesis. *Mol Biochem Parasitol* (2005) 140:133–40. doi:10.1016/j.molbiopara.2004.12.014
88. Toledo V, Ramirez G, Valck C, Lopez N, Ribeiro CH, Maldonado I, et al. Comparative in vivo antiangiogenic effects of calreticulin from *Trypanosoma cruzi* and Homo sapiens sapiens. *Biol Res* (2010) 43:287–9. doi:10.4067/S0716-97602010000300004
89. Aguilar-Guzman L, Lobos-Gonzalez L, Rosas C, Vallejos G, Falcon C, Sosoniuk E, et al. Human survivin and *Trypanosoma cruzi* calreticulin act in synergy against a murine melanoma in vivo. *PLoS One* (2014) 9:e95457. doi:10.1371/journal.pone.0095457
90. Baillie CT, Winslet MC, Bradley NJ. Tumour vasculature – a potential therapeutic target. *Br J Cancer* (1995) 72:257–67. doi:10.1038/bjc.1995.323
91. Griffioen AW, Molema G. Angiogenesis: potentials for pharmacologic intervention in the treatment of cancer, cardiovascular diseases, and chronic inflammation. *Pharmacol Rev* (2000) 52:237–68.
92. Berwin B, Hart JP, Rice S, Gass C, Pizzo SV, Post SR, et al. Scavenger receptor-A mediates gp96/GRP94 and calreticulin internalization by antigen-presenting cells. *EMBO J* (2003) 22:6127–36. doi:10.1093/emboj/cdg572
93. Ubillos L, Freire T, Berriel E, Chiribao ML, Chiale C, Festari MF, et al. *Trypanosoma cruzi* extracts elicit protective immune response against chemically induced colon and mammary cancers. *Int J Cancer* (2016) 138:1719–31. doi:10.1002/ijc.29910

94. van den Berg RH, Faber-Krol MC, Sim RB, Daha MR. The first subcomponent of complement, C1q, triggers the production of IL-8, IL-6, and monocyte chemoattractant peptide-1 by human umbilical vein endothelial cells. *J Immunol* (1998) 161:6924–30.
95. Adachi H, Tsujimoto M, Arai H, Inoue K. Expression cloning of a novel scavenger receptor from human endothelial cells. *J Biol Chem* (1997) 272:31217–20. doi:10.1074/jbc.272.50.31217
96. Canton J, Neculai D, Grinstein S. Scavenger receptors in homeostasis and immunity. *Nat Rev Immunol* (2013) 13:621–34. doi:10.1038/nri3515
97. Zani IA, Stephen SL, Mughal NA, Russell D, Homer-Vanniasinkam S, Wheatcroft SB, et al. Scavenger receptor structure and function in health and disease. *Cells* (2015) 4:178–201. doi:10.3390/cells4020178
98. Fucikova J, Becht E, Iribarren K, Goc J, Remark R, Damotte D, et al. Calreticulin expression in human non-small cell lung cancers correlates with increased accumulation of antitumor immune cells and favorable prognosis. *Cancer Res* (2016) 76:1746–56. doi: 10.1158/0008-5472.CAN-15-1142

11

Comparative Genomics of *Glossina palpalis gambiensis* and *G. morsitans morsitans* to Reveal Gene Orthologs Involved in Infection by *Trypanosoma brucei gambiense*

*Illiassou Hamidou Soumana[1], Bernadette Tchicaya[1], Stéphanie Rialle[2, 3, 4, 5], Hugues Parrinello[2, 3, 4, 5] and Anne Geiger[1]**

[1] *UMR 177, Institut de Recherche pour le Développement-CIRAD, CIRAD TA A-17/G, Montpellier, France,* [2] *Centre National de la Recherche Scientifique Unité Mixte de Recherche 5203, Institut de Génomique Fonctionnelle, Montpellier, France,* [3] *Institut National de la Santé Et de la Recherche Médicale U661, Montpellier, France,* [4] *Universités de Montpellier 1 and 2, UMR 5203, Montpellier, France,* [5] *Montpellier GenomiX, c/o Institut de Génomique Fonctionnelle, Montpellier, France*

Correspondence:
Anne Geiger
anne.geiger@ird.fr

Blood-feeding *Glossina palpalis gambiense* (Gpg) fly transmits the single-celled eukaryotic parasite *Trypanosoma brucei gambiense* (Tbg), the second *Glossina* fly African trypanosome pair being *Glossina morsitans/T.*brucei rhodesiense. Whatever the *T. brucei* subspecies, whereas the onset of their developmental program in the zoo-anthropophilic blood feeding flies does unfold in the fly midgut, its completion is taking place in the fly salivary gland where does emerge a low size metacyclic trypomastigote population displaying features that account for its establishment in mammals-human individuals included. Considering that the two *Glossina—T. brucei* pairs introduced above share similarity with respect to the developmental program of this African parasite, we were curious to map on the *Glossina morsitans morsitans* (Gmm), the Differentially Expressed Genes (DEGs) we listed in a previous study. Briefly, using the gut samples collected at days 3, 10, and 20 from Gpg that were fed or not at day 0 on Tbg—hosting mice, these DGE lists were obtained from RNA seq—based approaches. Here, post the mapping on the quality controlled DEGs on the Gmm genome, the identified ortholog genes were further annotated, the resulting datasets being compared. Around 50% of the Gpg DEGs were shown to have orthologs in the Gmm genome. Under one of the three *Glossina* midgut sampling conditions, the number of DEGs was even higher when mapping on the Gmm genome than initially recorded. Many Gmm genes annotated as "Hypothetical" were mapped and annotated on many distinct databases allowing some of them to be properly identified. We identify *Glossina* fly candidate genes encoding (a) a broad panel of proteases as well as (b) chitin—binding proteins, (c) antimicrobial peptide production—Pro3 protein, transferrin, mucin, atttacin, cecropin, etc—to further select in functional studies, the objectives being to probe and validated fly genome manipulation that prevents the onset of the developmental program of one or the other *T. brucei* spp. stumpy form sampled by one of the other bloodfeeding *Glossina* subspecies.

Keywords: human African Trypanosomiasis, *Glossina palpalis gambiensis*, *Glossina morsitans morsitans*, *Trypanosoma brucei gambiense*, differentially expressed genes, heterologous genes

INTRODUCTION

Trypanosomes causing either Human African Trypanosomiasis (HAT, i.e., sleeping sickness) or Animal African Trypanosomiasis (AAT, i.e., Nagana) are transmitted by *Glossina* spp. (tsetse flies). These hematophagous flies acquire their parasite during a blood meal on an infected host, and transmit the mature form of the parasite to another host during a subsequent blood meal. Two forms of HAT have been reported: a chronic and an acute form (Hoare, 1972; Aksoy et al., 2014; Beschin et al., 2014). The chronic form, spread throughout 24 sub-Saharan countries of West Africa, is caused by *Trypanosoma brucei gambiense* (Tbg) and is transmitted by *Glossina palpalis*; this form represents over 90% of all sleeping sickness cases (Welburn et al., 2009). The acute form, endemic to 12 East African countries, is caused by *Trypanosoma brucei rhodesiense* (Tbr), and is transmitted by *Glossina morsitans morsitans* (Gmm). Currently the disease persists in sub-Saharan countries (Louis et al., 2002), where more than 60 million people are exposed to the trypanosomiasis risk. Progress in deciphering the mechanisms of host-parasite interactions involves identifying the genes encoding the factors that govern tsetse fly vector competence (Vickerman et al., 1988; Maudlin and Welburn, 1994; Van den Abbeele et al., 1999), which may promote the development of anti-vector strategies that are alternative or complementary to current strategies.

Using a microarray approach, we recently investigated the effect of trypanosome ingestion by *G. palpalis gambiensis* (Gpg) flies on the transcriptome signatures of *Sodalis glossinidius* (Farikou et al., 2010; Hamidou Soumana et al., 2014a) and *Wigglesworthia glossinidia* (Hamidou Soumana et al., 2014b), two symbionts of tsetse flies (Aksoy et al., 2014). The aim of this previous work was to identify the genes that are differentially expressed in trypanosome infected vs. non-infected or self-cured (refractory) flies and that, consequently, can be suspected to positively or negatively control fly infection. Similarly, using the RNA-seq *de novo* assembly approach, we investigated the differential expression of *G. p. gambiensis* genes in flies challenged or not with trypanosomes (Hamidou Soumana et al., 2015). Furthermore, transcriptome profiling of *T. b. brucei* development in Gmm has recently been reported (Savage et al., 2016).

Since the acute form of HAT is caused by the Gmm/Tbr vector/parasite "couple," the identification of molecular targets common to both Gpg and Gmm (i.e., orthologous genes) deserves further consideration. Indeed, identification of these targets would allow the development of common approaches to fight both forms of HAT. As Gpg and Gmm are two separate *Glossina* species, their genomes should display some differences between each other. Furthermore, the Gmm genome and the sequences of the Gpg RNA-seq *de novo* assembled genes have been annotated with reference to two distinct database sets: the first set comprises *Drosophila melanogaster*, *Aedes aegypti*, *Anopheles gambiae*, *Culex quinquefasciatus*, and *Phlebotomus papatasi* (International Glossina Genome Initiative, 2014), whereas the second set comprises *Ceratitis capitata*, *Drosophila melanogaster*, *D. willistoni*, *D. virilis*, *D. mojavensis*, *Acyrthosiphon pisum*, *Hydra magnipapillata*, *Anopheles* sp., *Bombyx* sp., *Aedes* sp., and *Glossina morsitans* (data that were available before the publication of the whole genome sequence; Hamidou Soumana et al., 2015). This indicates that only the *D. melanogaster* database was common to the two database sets used to annotate the differentially expressed Gpg genes and the Gmm genome, respectively. Thus, for the present study, it was necessary to map the sequences of the Gpg RNA-seq *de novo* assembled genes on the Gmm genome and annotate them on the corresponding database. This has been achieved, and the Gpg genes that were previously shown to be differentially expressed (i.e., stimulated vs. non-stimulated flies, and infected vs. non-infected flies; Hamidou Soumana et al., 2015) were annotated on the Gmm database. Finally, the data resulting from the best hits annotation, which provide a translation product for each gene (and thus its potential biological function and physiological role), were compared with data resulting from the previous annotation of the same genes on the set of above-mentioned databases. The overall results provide a data platform that can be applied for further identification of candidate genes involved in the vector competence of both fly species. Importantly, these data could represent promising targets in the development of new anti-vector strategies in the fight against the chronic or acute forms of sleeping sickness.

MATERIALS AND METHODS

Ethical Statement

All animal experiments in this report were conducted according to internationally recognized guidelines. The experimental protocols were approved by the Ethics Committee on Animal Experiments and the Veterinary Department of the Centre International de Recherche Agronomique pour le Développement (CIRAD; Montpellier, France).

Sample Processing, RNA-Seq Library Preparation, and Sequencing

Samples for this study were previously used to identify the differentially expressed genes (DEGs) in Gpg. The different steps are described in the corresponding report (Hamidou Soumana et al., 2015), as well as *pro parte* in reports related to the differential expression of *S. glossinidius* and *W. glossinidia* genes (Hamidou Soumana et al., 2014a,b). Sample processing is summarized in **Figure 1**.

Preparation and Sequencing of the RNA-Seq Libraries

The sequential steps consisted of: RNA extraction from the pooled midguts of each biological replicate, resuspension of RNA pellets in nuclease-free water, concentration, RNA quantification, and quality control (to confirm the absence of any DNA contamination).

Generation of RNA-Seq Libraries

RNA-seq libraries were generated using the Illumina TruSeq™ RNA Sample Preparation Kit (Illumina; San Diego, USA). The sequential steps consisted of: mRNA purification from 4 μg total RNA using poly-T oligo-linked magnetic beads; fragmentation of RNA using divalent cations under elevated temperature (Illumina fragmentation buffer); first-strand cDNA

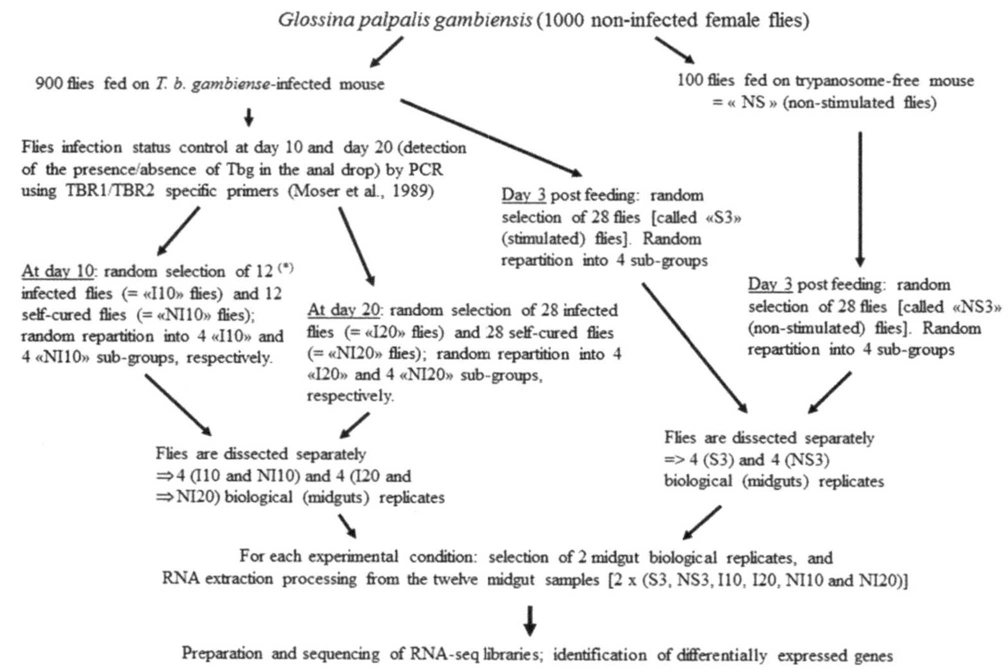

FIGURE 1 | Samples processing. (*) at day 10 the rate of infected flies was law, thus only 12 infected flies ("I10") could be sampled (instead of 28 at day 20). Self-cured flies are flies that have ingested trypanosomes (while they have taken a blood meal on an infected mouse), but the anal drops of which were trypanosome negative.

synthesis using random oligonucleotides and SuperScript II; second-strand cDNA synthesis using DNA Polymerase I and RNase H; conversion of remaining overhangs into blunt ends via exonuclease/polymerase activities and enzyme removal; and adenylation of 3′ ends of cDNA fragments, with ligation of Illumina PE adapter oligonucleotides for further hybridization. Finally, cDNA fragments were selected (preferably 200 bp in length) in which fragments with ligated adaptor molecules on both ends were selectively enriched using Illumina PCR Primer Cocktail, and the products were purified and quantified using the Agilent DNA assay on the Agilent Bioanalyzer 2100 system.

Brief Summary of the Pipeline for Generating Quality-Controlled Reads

A total of 12 RNA-seq libraries were prepared, sequenced, and compared, including two biological replicates for each of the NS3, S3, I10, NI10, I20, and I20 samples. Clustering of the index-coded samples was performed on a cBot Cluster Generation System using TruSeq PE Cluster Kit-cBot-HS (Illumina). After cluster generation, the library preparations were sequenced on an Illumina Hiseq 2000 platform, and 100-bp paired-end reads were generated. Image analyses and base calling were performed using the Illumina HiSeq Control Software and Real-Time Analysis component. Demultiplexing was performed using CASAVA 1.8.2. The quality of the raw data was assessed using FastQC (Babraham Institute) and the Illumina software SAV (Sequencing Analysis Viewer). Raw sequencing reads from this study were exported in the FASTQ format and were deposited at the NCBI Short Read Archive (SRA) with the accession number SRP046074; aligned BAM files are available on request.

Identification of DEGs Once the Reads Generated from the 12 Gpg Fly Gut RNA Seq Libraries Were Mapped and Annotated on a Panel of Non-insect and Insect Genome Databases, One of Them Being Gmm

The RNA-seq reads that satisfied the quality control (i.e., removal of ambiguous nucleotides, low-quality sequences with quality scores <20, and sequences <15 bp in length) were mapped on the *G. m. morsitans* genome (13,807 scaffolds; International Glossina Genome Initiative, 2014) from VectorBase (www.vectorbase.org) and GenBank (accession no. CCAG010000000). This was achieved via the splice junction mapper TopHat 2.0.13 (Kim et al., 2013) using Bowtie 2.1.0 (Langmead and Salzberg, 2012), to align RNA-seq reads to the *Glossina morsitans* genome (GmorY1 assembly, release date: January 2014). Final read alignments with more than 12 mismatches were discarded.

Gene counting (number of reads aligned on each gene) was performed before statistical analysis, using HTSeq count 0.5.3p9 (union mode; Anders et al., 2014). Genes with <10 reads (cumulating all analyzed samples) were filtered and removed. We used the Bioconductor (Gentleman et al., 2004) software package EdgeR (Robinson et al., 2010) 3.6.7. to identify genes displaying a modified expression profile as a result of fly infection by trypanosomes. Data were normalized using the upper quartile normalization factors, using the quartiles method (Bullard et al., 2010). Genes with an adjusted $p < 5\%$ according to the False Discovery Rate (FDR) method from Benjamini and Hochberg (1995) were declared differentially expressed.

Bio Informatics-Based Approaches Aimed to Identify Molecular DEGs in Both Gmm and Gpg Once the Latter are Subverted as T. brucei spp Hosts *Per se*

Tsetse fly gene orthologs were tentatively identified using BLAST searches (Mount, 2007) with annotation against the NCBI non-redundant (Nr) sequence database, using an *E*-value cut-off of 10^{-5} ($E < 0.00001$), according to the best hits against known sequences. This was performed to retrieve orthologous genes with the highest sequence similarity to the given unigenes along with putative functional annotations. The official gene symbols of tsetse fly gene orthologs were used for functional annotation. Along with Nr annotations, the "Database for Annotation, Visualization and Integrated Discovery" (DAVID; Dennis et al., 2003) was used to obtain GO annotations of unigenes. The KEGG pathway annotations of tsetse fly gene orthologs were performed using the BLASTX software against the KEGG database (Wixon and Kell, 2000).

Analyzing the two annotation processes of the Gpg DEGs consisted in comparing the list of the "best hits" resulting from the Gpg DEG annotation on the Gmm database with the list resulting from the Gpg DEG annotation previously performed on a set of other databases (*Ceratitis capitata*, *Drosophila melanogaster*, *D. willistoni*, *D. virilis*, *D. mojavensis*, *Acyrthosiphon pisum*, *Hydra magnipapillata*, *Anopheles* sp., *Bombyx* sp., *Aedes* sp., and *Glossina morsitans*; Hamidou Soumana et al., 2015). The first step consisted in mixing the DEGs identified at the three experimental times (3, 10, and 20 days) and removing the duplicates, so as to take into account all recorded DEGs except for one of each. The second step consisted in removing the DEGs in which the annotation (best hit) resulted in "hypothetical" or "uncharacterized" proteins, as well as those identified with a numerical identifier, in order to only consider identified and named proteins. Finally, the names of the proteins (best hits) were standardized and alphabetically classified. This process was performed separately for the DEGs annotated with reference to the Gmm database, as well as those previously annotated on the above-characterized set of other databases. The two final listings were then combined (Microsoft Excel software), and their content was arranged according to the alphabetical order of protein names. This procedure facilitated the detection of the best hits that are common to both annotation processes and their corresponding genes.

RESULTS

Mapping of PolyA+ mRNA

A total of 459,555,846 clusters were generated from the 12 RNA-seq libraries. Quality controls were performed to ensure the reliability of the libraries after removal of ambiguous nucleotides, low-quality sequences (quality scores < 20), and sequences <15 bp in length. Finally, 436,979,101 clean clusters were obtained (**Table 1**). Clean reads had Phred-like quality scores at the Q20 level (i.e., a sequencing error probability of 0.01). These clean sequenced reads with no strand-specificity were mapped to the Gmm reference genome using TopHat (with Bowtie 2) software in order to identify exon-exon splice junctions and to ensure enough sensitivity in mapping reads with polymorphisms.

Filtering and removing any genes with <10 mapped reads allowed mapping 8,286 (stimulated vs. non-stimulated flies; 3 days), 8,032 (infected vs. refractory flies; 10 days) and 8,101 Gpg genes (infected vs. refractory flies; 20 days) on the Gmm reference genome (International Glossina Genome Initiative, 2014). Further, analyses to reveal differential expression (DE) were performed using the bioinformatics tools HTseq and EdgeR from Bioconductor (http://www.bioconductor.org/), which use the R statistical programming language and are widely accepted for modeling the inherent variation between biological replicates. **Figure 2** presents the $\log_2$ fold-change (stimulated vs. non-stimulated flies at day-3 post-infected blood meal) against the $\log_2$ of the reads concentration (log-counts-per-million) for each gene after normalization. The generated cloud shows a log fold-change centered on 0 (ordinate axis), signifying that the libraries are properly normalized. Genes that are differentially expressed between the S and NS samples ($p < 0.05$) are represented in red. Similar results were obtained for the other experimental conditions.

Identification of DEGs and Functional Annotation

The EdgeR method identified a total of 284, 139, and 59 Gmm genes corresponding respectively to the Gpg DEG samples S3

TABLE 1 | Assembly quality of Gpg libraries at the three different sampling times.

Samples	Number of crude clusters (CC)	Number of clusters after filtering (CAF)	% CAF/CC
NS 3-day sample[a]	36,002,596	34,386,734	95.51
NS 3-day sample[b]	41,153,580	39,330,015	95.57
S 3-day sample	32,726,727	31,257,269	95.51
S 3-day sample	33,386,646	31,848,385	95.39
NI 10-day sample	33,159,650	31,593,962	95.28
NI 10-day sample	30,632,671	29,185,036	95.27
I 10-day sample	42,223,049	40,108,756	94.99
I 10-day sample	43,418,918	41,279,341	95.07
NI 20-day sample	41,882,170	39,688,764	94.76
NI 20-day sample	38,192,692	36,205,087	94.80
I 20-day sample	40,587,354	38,401,915	94.62
I 20-day sample	46,189,793	43,693,837	94.60
Total	459,555,846	436,979,101	–
Mean	38,296,320	36,414,925	95.08

The superscipts [a] and [b] are two replicates of the "non-stimulated samples" at day 3. Idem for the other sampling conditions. S, stimulated; NS, non-stimulated; NI, non-infected; I, infected.

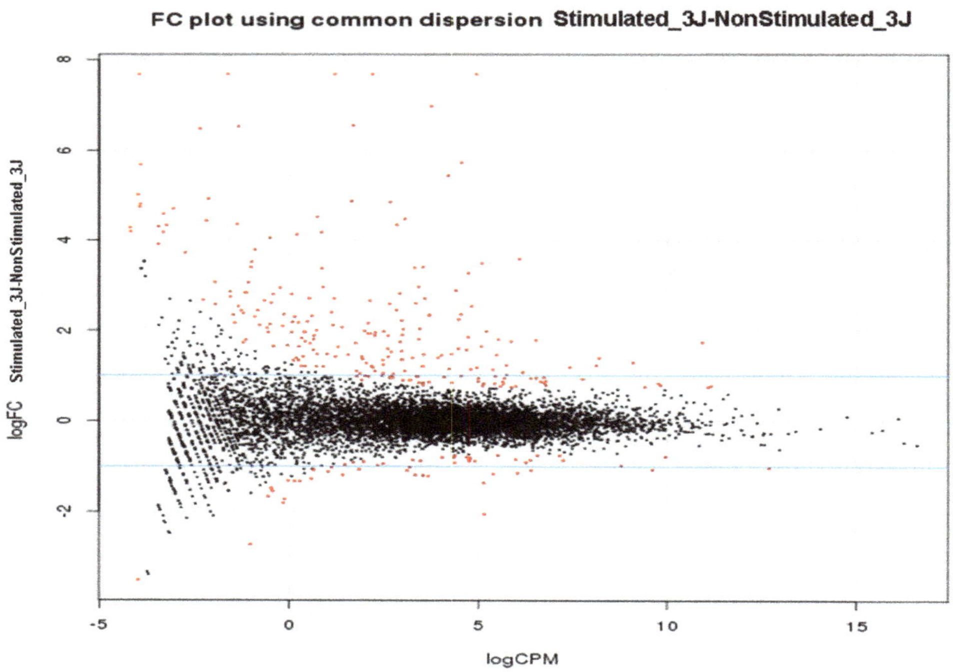

FIGURE 2 | Smear plot of libraries. Samples are from trypanosome stimulated-/-non-stimulated tsetse fly midguts sampled 3 days post-infected blood meal, after normalization using the upper quartile method.

TABLE 2 | Number of differentially expressed genes in Gpg.

Experimental conditions	Number of identified genes	Significantly differentially expressed genes			
		Overall	Overexpressed	Fold-change	
				2 < $\log_2$ FC or $\log_2$ FC < −2	3 < $\log_2$ FC or $\log_2$ FC < −3
S vs. NS (3 days)	8,286	284	229 (80.6%)	97 (34.1%)	44 (15.5%)
I vs. NI (10 days)	8,032	139	119 (85.6%)	60 (43.1%)	35 (25.2%)
I vs. NI (20 days)	8,101	59	37 (62.7%)	19 (32.2%)	6 (10.2%)

S, stimulated; NS, non-stimulated; NI, non-infected; I: infected.

vs. NS3 (Supplementary Table S1), I10 vs. NI10 (Supplementary Table S2), and I20 vs. NI20 (Supplementary Table S3), at a $p < 0.05$. Most of these genes were overexpressed regardless of the experimental condition. Specifically, there were 229 out of 284 genes (80.6%) in the day-3 samples (S3 vs. NS3), 119 out of 139 genes (85.6%) in I-10 vs. NI-10 samples, and 37 out of 59 genes (62.7%) in I20 vs. NI20. Furthermore, the number of DEGs were highly differentially overexpressed ($\log_2$ FC > 2) or underexpressed ($\log_2$ FC < −2). Specifically, there were 97 out of 284 DEGs (34%; S3 vs. NS3), 60 out of 139 DEGs (43%; I10 vs. NI10), and 19 out of 59 DEGs (32%; I20 vs. NI20). These data are summarized in **Table 2**. Genes exhibiting a highly differential overexpression or underexpression under the different experimental conditions (i.e., S vs. NS, I10 vs. NI10, and I20 vs. NI20) are grouped together in **Table 3**. Most DEGs encode a wide range of proteases, although 91 DEGs presented in Supplementary Tables S1–S3 could not be properly annotated (i.e., best hit description = "hypothetical"), signifying that the panel of databases used for the annotation process should be enlarged or that the genes may be specific to the Gmm genome. In addition, several of the DEGs were very highly overexpressed. For example the $\log_2$ FC of GMOY009756, which encodes a trypsin, had a fold-change of 7.14 in S3 vs. NS3 samples, and GMOY002278, which encodes the proteinase inhibitor I2, had a fold-change of 9.47 in I10 vs. NI10. In contrast, some DEGs were underexpressed: the $\log_2$ FC of GMOY005345, which encodes an aspartic peptidase, had a fold-change of −6.51 in I20 vs. NI20 samples. **Table 3** is presented so as to facilitate comparison of differential expression levels for a given gene along the three sampling times. For instance, the levels (in $\log_2$ FC) of GMOY005345, which encodes an aspartic peptidase, are 3.39 (S3 vs. NS3), 2.70 (I10 vs. NI10), and −6.51 (I20 vs. NI20).

Table 3 also provides the functional annotation data for each gene at each sampling time. To obtain an overview of the

TABLE 3 | Annotation on the *Glossina morsitans morsitans* genome of Gpg genes differentially expressed in response to Tbg infection.

Genes	Fold-change log_2 FC	Encoded proteins (best hits)	Gene Ontology (GO)		
			Biological process	Molecular function	Cellular component
PROTEASES AND PROTEASE INHIBITORS					
GMOY005345	3.39	Aspartic peptidase	GO:0006508 proteolysis	GO:0004190 aspartic-type endopeptidase activity	No terms assigned
GMOY005345	2.70	Aspartic peptidase	GO:0006508 proteolysis	GO:0004190 aspartic-type endopeptidase activity	No terms assigned
GMOY005345	−6.51	Aspartic peptidase	GO:0006508 proteolysis	GO:0004190 aspartic-type endopeptidase activity	No terms assigned
GMOY007305	2.09	Destabilase	No terms assigned	GO:0003796 lysozyme activity	No terms assigned
GMOY007305	3.00	Destabilase	No terms assigned	GO:0003796 lysozyme activity	No terms assigned
GMOY000103	2.64	Fat body c-type lysozyme	No terms assigned	No terms assigned	No terms assigned
GMOY000103	2.74	Fat body c-type lysozyme	No terms assigned	No terms assigned	No terms assigned
GMOY002036	−2.75	Peptidase S1A, chymotrypsin-type	GO:0006508 proteolysis	GO:0004252 serine-type endopeptidase activity	No terms assigned
GMOY003273	2.30	Peptidase S1A, chymotrypsin-type	GO:0006508 proteolysis	GO:0004252 serine-type endopeptidase activity	No terms assigned
GMOY003994	4.19	Peptidase S1A, chymotrypsin-type	GO:0006508 proteolysis	GO:0004252 serine-type endopeptidase activity	No terms assigned
GMOY006266	3.72	Peptidase S1A, chymotrypsin-type	GO:0006508 proteolysis	GO:0004252 serine-type endopeptidase activity	No terms assigned
GMOY008964	3.32	Peptidase S1A, chymotrypsin-type	GO:0006508 proteolysis	GO:0004252 serine-type endopeptidase activity	No terms assigned
GMOY008965	3.52	Peptidase S1A, chymotrypsin-type	GO:0006508 proteolysis	GO:0004252 serine-type endopeptidase activity	No terms assigned
GMOY008966	3.35	Peptidase S1A, chymotrypsin-type	GO:0006508 proteolysis	GO:0004252 serine-type endopeptidase activity	No terms assigned
GMOY008966	4.41	Peptidase S1A, chymotrypsin-type	GO:0006508 proteolysis	GO:0004252 serine-type endopeptidase activity	No terms assigned
GMOY009436	2.11	Peptidase S1A, chymotrypsin-type	GO:0006508 proteolysis	GO:0004252 serine-type endopeptidase activity	No terms assigned
GMOY009757	2.76	Peptidase S1A, chymotrypsin-type	GO:0006508 proteolysis	GO:0004252 serine-type endopeptidase activity	No terms assigned
GMOY010768	2.73	Peptidase S1A, chymotrypsin-type	GO:0006508 proteolysis	GO:0004252 serine-type endopeptidase activity	No terms assigned
GMOY010768	2.06	Peptidase S1	GO:0006508 proteolysis	GO:0004252 serine-type endopeptidase activity	No terms assigned
GMOY002729	3.01	Serine protease 1	GO:0006508 proteolysis	GO:0004252 serine-type endopeptidase activity	No terms assigned
GMOY000672	6.95	Serine protease 6	GO:0006508 proteolysis	GO:0004252 serine-type endopeptidase activity	No terms assigned
GMOY000672	6.78	Serine protease 6	GO:0006508 proteolysis	GO:0004252 serine-type endopeptidase activity	No terms assigned
GMOY009756	7.14	Trypsin	GO:0006508 proteolysis	GO:0004252 serine-type endopeptidase activity	No terms assigned
GMOY009756	3.48	Trypsin	GO:0006508 proteolysis	GO:0004252 serine-type endopeptidase activity	No terms assigned
GMOY008967	2.55	Trypsin	GO:0006508 proteolysis	GO:0004252 serine-type endopeptidase activity	No terms assigned
GMOY008967	3.37	Trypsin-like cysteine/serine peptid. domain	No terms assigned	GO:0003824 catalytic activity	No terms assigned
GMOY010488	6.83	Imune reactive putative protease inhibitor	No terms assigned	No terms assigned	No terms assigned
GMOY010488	4.69	Immune reactive putative protease inhibitor	No terms assigned	No terms assigned	No terms assigned

(Continued)

TABLE 3 | Continued

Genes	Fold-change $\log_2$ FC	Encoded proteins (best hits)	Gene Ontology (GO)		
			Biological process	Molecular function	Cellular component
GMOY002277	2.31	Proteinase inhibitor I2, Kunitz metazoa	No terms assigned	GO:0004867 serine-type endopeptidase inhibit. Activ.	No terms assigned
GMOY002277	4.10	Proteinase inhibitor I2, Kunitz metazoa	No terms assigned	GO:0004867 serine-type endopeptidase inhibit. Activ.	No terms assigned
GMOY002278	6.54	Proteinase inhibitor I2, Kunitz metazoa	No terms assigned	GO:0004867 serine-type endopeptidase inhibit. Activ.	No terms assigned
GMOY002278	9.47	Proteinase inhibitor I2, Kunitz metazoa	No terms assigned	GO:0004867 serine-type endopeptidase inhibit. Activ.	No terms assigned
GMOY008344	2.94	Trypsin Inhibitor-like	No terms assigned	No terms assigned	No terms assigned
GMOY008344	4.38	Trypsin Inhibitor-like	No terms assigned	No terms assigned	No terms assigned
ESTERASES—HYDROLASES					
GMOY000067	3.35	Alkaline phosphatase	GO:0008152 metabolic process	GO:0016791 phosphatase activity	No terms assigned
GMOY000067	3.60	Alkaline phosphatase	GO:0008152 metabolic process	GO:0003824 catalytic activity	No terms assigned
GMOY004731	2.06	Alkaline phosphatase-like, alpha/beta/alpha	GO:0008152 metabolic process	GO:0003824 catalytic activity	No terms assigned
GMOY006875	–2.02	Alkaline phosphatase-like, alpha/beta/alpha	GO:0008152 metabolic process	GO:0003824 catalytic activity	No terms assigned
GMOY004236	2.36	Acylphosphatase-like	No terms assigned	GO:0003998 acylphosphatase activity	No terms assigned
GMOY006958	2.60	Carboxylesterase	No terms assigned	No terms assigned	No terms assigned
GMOY011249	2.83	Carboxylesterase	No terms assigned	No terms assigned	No terms assigned
GMOY012368	2.53	Exonuclease	No terms assigned	No terms assigned	No terms assigned
GMOY007402	3.85	Extracellular Endonuclease, subunit A	No terms assigned	GO:0016787 hydrolase activity	No terms assigned
GMOY012360	–2.93	Extracellular Endonuclease, subunit A	No terms assigned	GO:0016787 hydrolase activity	No terms assigned
GMOY009375	7.56	Glycoside hydrolase	GO:0005975 carbohyd. metabolic process	GO:0003824 catalytic activity	No terms assigned
GMOY012361	–2.55	Tsal2 protein precursor	No terms assigned	GO:0016787 hydrolase activity	No terms assigned
GMOY004309	2.44	Thiolase-like	GO:0008152 metabolic process	GO:0003824 catalytic activity	No terms assigned
GMOY007148	2.10	Thiolase-like	GO:0008152 metabolic process	GO:0003824 catalytic activity	No terms assigned
BINDING					
GMOY010194	4.12	Araucan	No terms assigned	GO:0003677 DNA binding	No terms assigned
GMOY009525	7.53	Armadillo-type fold	No terms assigned	GO:0005488 binding	No terms assigned
GMOY009611	2.60	Barrier- to-autointegration factor, BAF	No terms assigned	GO:0003677 DNA binding	No terms assigned
GMOY009394	–5.56	Basic-leucine zipper domain	GO:0006355 regulation of transcription	GO:0003700 sequence-specific	No terms assigned
GMOY010195	5.99	Caupolican	GO:0006355 regul. of transcrip,DNA-templated	GO:0003677 DNA binding	GO:0005634 nucleus
GMOY002708	7.89	Chitin binding	GO:0006030 chitin metabolic process	GO:0008061 chitin binding	GO:0005576 extracel
GMOY005278	2.93	Chitin binding domain	GO:0006030 chitin metabolic process	GO:0008061 chitin binding	GO:0005576 extracel
GMOY003840	4.12	Chitin binding domain	GO:0006030 chitin metabolic process	GO:0008061 chitin binding	GO:0005576 extracel
GMOY011054	6.08	Chitin binding domain	GO:0006030 chitin metabolic process	GO:0008061 chitin binding	GO:0005576 extracel
GMOY011810	6.55	Chitin binding domain	GO:0006030 chitin metabolic process	GO:0008061 chitin binding	GO:0005576 extracel

(Continued)

TABLE 3 | Continued

Genes	Fold-change log_2 FC	Encoded proteins (best hits)	Gene Ontology (GO)		
			Biological process	Molecular function	Cellular component
GMOY011809	8.08	Pro1 (Chitin related)	GO:0006030 chitin metabolic process	GO:0008061 chitin binding	GO:0005576 extracel
GMOY004647	4.24	Cupredoxin	No terms assigned	GO:0005507 copper ion binding	No terms assigned
GMOY004364	2.90	Haemolymph juvenile hormone binding	No terms assigned	No terms assigned	No terms assigned
GMOY005487	3.48	Lim3	No terms assigned	GO:0008270 zinc ion binding	No terms assigned
GMOY007084	2.39	NAD(P)-binding domain	No terms assigned	No terms assigned	No terms assigned
GMOY002356	2.31	Nucleotide-binding	No terms assigned	GO:0000166 nucleotide binding	No terms assigned
GMOY002825	4.47	Odorant binding protein 2	No terms assigned	GO:0005549 odorant binding	No terms assigned
GMOY002825	2.03	Odorant binding protein 2	No terms assigned	No terms assigned	No terms assigned
GMOY005548	2.99	Odorant binding protein 7	No terms assigned	No terms assigned	No terms assigned
GMOY001476	2.20	Odorant binding protein 22	No terms assigned	GO:0005549 odorant binding	No terms assigned
GMOY008769	4.95	Small GTPase	GO:0007165 signal transduction	GO:0005525 GTP binding	GO:0016020 membrane
GMOY004228	5.44	Transferrin family	GO:0006879 cellular iron ion homeostasis	GO:0008199 ferric iron binding	GO:0005576 extracel
GMOY004228	2.63	Transferrin family, iron binding site	GO:0006879 cellular iron ion homeostasis	GO:0008199 ferric iron binding	GO:0005576 extracel
GMOY008315	2.05	Winged helix-turn-helix DNA-binding domain	GO:0006355 regul. of transcrip,DNA-templated	GO:0043565 sequence-specific DNA binding Transcription Factor Activity	No terms assigned
TRANSPORT/TRANSFERASE ACTIVITY					
GMOY004684	−2.39	Cellul. retinaldehyde binding/a-tocopherol transport	GO:0006810 transport	GO:0005215 transporter activity	GO:0005622 intracel
GMOY008601	2.58	Fatty acid synthase 3	GO:0008152 metabolic process	GO:0016740 transferase activity	No terms assigned
GMOY008601	4.11	Fatty acid synthase 3	GO:0008152 metabolic process	GO:0016740 transferase activity	No terms assigned
GMOY008602	2.02	Fatty acid synthase 4	GO:0008152 metabolic process	GO:0016740 transferase activity	No terms assigned
GMOY008602	−2.55	Fatty acid synthase 4	GO:0008152 metabolic process	GO:0016740 transferase activity	No terms assigned
GMOY005442	2.35	Lipid transport protein	GO:0006869 lipid transport	GO:0005319 lipid transporter activity	No terms assigned
GMOY005442	2.40	Lipid transport protein	GO:0006869 lipid transport	GO:0005319 lipid transporter activity	No terms assigned
GMOY003490	4.50	Major Facilitator Superfamily transporter	GO:0055085 transmembrane transport	No terms assigned	GO:0016021 integral
GMOY003491	3.97	Major Facilitator Superfamily transporter	GO:0055085 transmembrane transport	No terms assigned	GO:0016021 integral
GMOY005103	2.77	Major Facilitator Superfamily transporter	GO:0055085 transmembrane transport	No terms assigned	GO:0016021 integral
GMOY007627	2.09	Major Facilitator Superfamily transporter	GO:0055085 transmembrane transport	No terms assigned	GO:0016021 integral
GMOY005102	6.28	N-acetylgalactosaminyltransferase	GO:0008152 metabolic process	No terms assigned	No terms assigned
GMOY011877	2.37	Na+ channel, amiloride-sensitive	GO:0006814 sodium ion transport	GO:0005272 sodium channel activity	GO:0016020 membrane
GMOY009903	2.75	Neurotransmitter-gated ion-channel	GO:0006811 ion transport	No terms assigned	GO:0016021 integral
GMOY005934	2.72	Pyridoxal phosphate-dependent transferase	No terms assigned	GO:0003824 catalytic activity	No terms assigned

(Continued)

TABLE 3 | Continued

Genes	Fold-change log_2 FC	Encoded proteins (best hits)	Gene Ontology (GO)		
			Biological process	Molecular function	Cellular component
GMOY009343	8.14	Sodium:neurotransmitter symporter	GO:0006836 neurotransmitter transport	GO:0005328 neurotransmitter:Na symporter act	GO:0016021 integral
GMOY009343	6.43	Sodium:neurotransmitter symporter	GO:0006836 neurotransmitter transport	GO:0005328 neurotransmitter:Na symporter act	GO:0016021 integral
GMOY009386	2.44	Sodium:neurotransmitter symporter	GO:0006836 neurotransmitter transport	GO:0005328 neurotransmitter:Na symporter act	GO:0016021 integral
GMOY002486	2.59	Two pore domain K channel, TASK family	GO:0071805 K ion transmemb, transport	GO:0005267 potassium channel activity	GO:0016020 membrane
GMOY012088	4.05	Tyrosine aminotransferase	GO:0009072 aromatic amino acid family metabolic process	GO:0004838 L-tyrosine:2-oxoglutarate aminotransferase Activity	No terms assigned
OXIDO-REDUCTION PROCESS					
GMOY001939	2.50	Cytochrome P450-4g1	GO:0055114 oxidation-reduction process	GO:0016705 oxidoreductase activity	No terms assigned
GMOY002598	2.15	Cytochrome P450	GO:0055114 oxidation-reduction process	GO:0016705 oxidoreductase activity	No terms assigned
GMOY006475	2.28	Cytochrome P450-4g1	GO:0055114 oxidation-reduction process	GO:0016705 oxidoreductase activity	No terms assigned
GMOY006761	2.42	Cytochrome P450-4g1	GO:0055114 oxidation-reduction process	GO:0016705 oxidoreductase activity	No terms assigned
GMOY006761	−2.08	Cytochrome P450-4g1	GO:0055114 oxidation-reduction process	GO:0016705 oxidoreductase activity	No terms assigned
GMOY007181	3.49	Cytochrome P450	GO:0055114 oxidation-reduction process	GO:0016705 oxidoreductase activity	No terms assigned
GMOY007652	3.43	Cytochrome P450	GO:0055114 oxidation-reduction process	GO:0016705 oxidoreductase activity	No terms assigned
GMOY009767	3.96	Cytochrome P450	GO:0055114 oxidation-reduction process	GO:0016705 oxidoreductase activity	No terms assigned
GMOY009909	3.35	Cytochrome P450	GO:0055114 oxidation-reduction process	GO:0016705 oxidoreductase activity	No terms assigned
GMOY007529	4.49	Dehydrogenase/reductase	GO:0008152 metabolic process	GO:0016491 oxidoreductase activity	No terms assigned
GMOY004332	2.12	Fatty acyl-CoA reductase	No terms assigned	GO:0080019 fatty-acyl-CoA reductase activity	No terms assigned
GMOY007497	6.25	NADH-cytochrome b-5 reductase 2	GO:0055114 oxidation-reduction process	GO:0016491 oxidoreductase activity	No terms assigned
GMOY010446	2.40	2-oxoglutarate dioxygenase	GO:0055114 oxidation-reduction process	GO:0050353 trimethyllysine dioxygenase activity	No terms assigned
HYPOTHETICAL					
GMOY000215	4.17	Hypothetical	No terms assigned	No terms assigned	No terms assigned
GMOY000215	5.24	Hypothetical	No terms assigned	No terms assigned	No terms assigned
GMOY000257	2.90	Hypothetical	No terms assigned	No terms assigned	No terms assigned

(Continued)

TABLE 3 | Continued

Genes	Fold-change log_2 FC	Encoded proteins (best hits)	Gene Ontology (GO)		
			Biological process	Molecular function	Cellular component
GMOY001239	2.53	Hypothetical	No terms assigned	No terms assigned	No terms assigned
GMOY002434	3.22	Hypothetical	No terms assigned	No terms assigned	No terms assigned
GMOY002933	2.07	Hypothetical	No terms assigned	No terms assigned	No terms assigned
GMOY002986	2.69	Hypothetical	No terms assigned	No terms assigned	No terms assigned
GMOY003011	2.30	Hypothetical	No terms assigned	No terms assigned	No terms assigned
GMOY003030	4.38	Hypothetical	No terms assigned	No terms assigned	No terms assigned
GMOY003034	–2.10	Hypothetical	No terms assigned	No terms assigned	No terms assigned
GMOY003158	2.70	Hypothetical	No terms assigned	No terms assigned	No terms assigned
GMOY003197	2.04	Hypothetical	No terms assigned	No terms assigned	No terms assigned
GMOY003830	2.75	Hypothetical	No terms assigned	No terms assigned	No terms assigned
GMOY003830	3.68	Hypothetical	No terms assigned	No terms assigned	No terms assigned
GMOY003974	2.28	Hypothetical	No terms assigned	No terms assigned	No terms assigned
GMOY003976	3.89	Hypothetical	No terms assigned	No terms assigned	No terms assigned
GMOY004022	–2.06	Hypothetical	No terms assigned	No terms assigned	No terms assigned
GMOY004337	5.80	Hypothetical	No terms assigned	No terms assigned	No terms assigned
GMOY004337	6.61	Hypothetical	No terms assigned	No terms assigned	No terms assigned
GMOY005055	6.08	Hypothetical	No terms assigned	No terms assigned	No terms assigned
GMOY005606	6.32	Hypothetical	No terms assigned	No terms assigned	No terms assigned
GMOY005797	6.60	Hypothetical	No terms assigned	No terms assigned	No terms assigned
GMOY005797	6.49	Hypothetical	No terms assigned	No terms assigned	No terms assigned
GMOY005798	3.98	Hypothetical	No terms assigned	No terms assigned	No terms assigned
GMOY005798	6.25	Hypothetical	No terms assigned	No terms assigned	No terms assigned
GMOY005799	2.24	Hypothetical	No terms assigned	No terms assigned	No terms assigned
GMOY006671	4.00	Hypothetical	No terms assigned	No terms assigned	No terms assigned
GMOY006276	2.33	Hypothetical	No terms assigned	No terms assigned	No terms assigned
GMOY007187	3.59	Hypothetical	No terms assigned	No terms assigned	No terms assigned
GMOY007637	4.06	Hypothetical	No terms assigned	No terms assigned	No terms assigned
GMOY008016	4.65	Hypothetical	No terms assigned	No terms assigned	No terms assigned
GMOY008016	6.67	Hypothetical	No terms assigned	No terms assigned	No terms assigned
GMOY008627	3.64	Hypothetical	No terms assigned	No terms assigned	No terms assigned
GMOY009539	2.28	Hypothetical	No terms assigned	No terms assigned	No terms assigned
GMOY009540	2.19	Hypothetical	No terms assigned	No terms assigned	No terms assigned
GMOY009541	2.40	Hypothetical	No terms assigned	No terms assigned	No terms assigned
GMOY009951	3.11	Hypothetical	No terms assigned	No terms assigned	No terms assigned
GMOY010224	6.87	Hypothetical	No terms assigned	No terms assigned	No terms assigned
GMOY010224	3.57	Hypothetical	No terms assigned	No terms assigned	No terms assigned
GMOY010232	–2.44	Hypothetical	No terms assigned	No terms assigned	No terms assigned
xGMOY012069	9.07	Hypothetical	No terms assigned	No terms assigned	No terms assigned
GMOY012069	5.33	Hypothetical	No terms assigned	No terms assigned	No terms assigned
GMOY008956	2.90	hypothetical conserved protein	No terms assigned	No terms assigned	No terms assigned
MISCELLANEOUS					
GMOY008458	5.74	Actin-related protein	No terms assigned	No terms assigned	No terms assigned
GMOY008368	2.22	Adipokinetic hormone recept isoform A	No terms assigned	No terms assigned	No terms assigned
GMOY004147	4.32	Apolipophorin-III superfamily	No terms assigned	No terms assigned	No terms assigned
GMOY011562	2.29	Cecropin	No terms assigned	No terms assigned	GO:0005576 extracel
GMOY011562	2.36	Cecropin	No terms assigned	No terms assigned	GO:0005576 extracel
GMOY011563	2.77	Cecropin	No terms assigned	No terms assigned	GO:0005576 extracel
GMOY010882	3.02	Chemosensory protein 3	No terms assigned	No terms assigned	No terms assigned
GMOY007457	2.47	Cytochrome b561/ferric reduct transmembrane	No terms assigned	No terms assigned	GO:0016021 integral

(Continued)

TABLE 3 | Continued

Genes	Fold-change $\log_2$ FC	Encoded proteins (best hits)	Gene Ontology (GO)		
			Biological process	Molecular function	Cellular component
GMOY003354	2.48	Elongase 9	No terms assigned	No terms assigned	GO:0016021 integral
GMOY003354	6.25	Elongase 9	No terms assigned	No terms assigned	GO:0016021 integral
GMOY008821	3.10	Elongase 4	No terms assigned	No terms assigned	GO:0016021 integral
GMOY009277	3.72	Insect cuticle protein	No terms assigned	GO:0042302 structural constituent of cuticle	No terms assigned
GMOY003876	2.08	Insect cuticle protein	No terms assigned	GO:0042302 structural constituent of cuticle	No terms assigned
GMOY011216	2.40	Insect cuticle protein	No terms assigned	GO:0042302 structural constituent of cuticle	No terms assigned
GMOY002258	2.03	Insulin-like	No terms assigned	GO:0005179 hormone activity	GO:0005576 extracel
GMOY003944	9.22	LIM and senesc, cell antigen-like-protein 1	GO:0009987 cellular process	GO:0005198 structural molecule activity	GO:0043226 organelle
GMOY011997	3.02	Mammalian NeuroPept, Y like receptor	No terms assigned	No terms assigned	GO:0016021 integral
GMOY012052	3.40	Mammalian NeuroPept, Y like receptor	No terms assigned	No terms assigned	GO:0016021 integral
GMOY009745	2.02	Milk gland protein 1	No terms assigned	No terms assigned	No terms assigned
GMOY001342	−2.40	Milk gland protein 2	No terms assigned	No terms assigned	No terms assigned
GMOY001342	2.14	Milk gland protein 2	No terms assigned	No terms assigned	No terms assigned
GMOY012125	3.57	Milk gland protein 3	No terms assigned	No terms assigned	No terms assigned
GMOY001343	2.50	Milk gland protein 6	No terms assigned	No terms assigned	No terms assigned
GMOY012016	−4.00	Milk gland protein 8	No terms assigned	No terms assigned	No terms assigned
GMOY012016	2.36	Milk gland protein 8	No terms assigned	No terms assigned	No terms assigned
GMOY012369	2.24	Milk gland protein 10	No terms assigned	No terms assigned	No terms assigned
GMOY010160	2.78	Mpv17/PMP22	No terms assigned	No terms assigned	GO:0016021 integral membrane
GMOY009494	−3.95	Rhodanese-like domain	No terms assigned	No terms assigned	No terms assigned
GMOY010675	2.12	Single domain Von Willebrand factor type C	No terms assigned	No terms assigned	No terms assigned
GMOY007078	2.52	Single domain Von Willebrand factor type C	No terms assigned	No terms assigned	No terms assigned

Gpg genes that were previously shown to be differentially expressed (DEGs) 3, 10, and 20 days after being challenged with Tbg were mapped on the Gmm genome and annotated on this reference genome. The table presents Gmm genes that are heterologs of the Gpg DEGs, in addition to the annotation results and the gene ontology. Only highly differential expressed genes ($\log_2FC < -2$ or $\log_2FC > 2$) have been considered. ***Black*** *fonts: genes that are differentially expressed in stimulated vs. non-stimulated flies (at day 3 after fly challenge).* ***Blue*** *and* ***Red*** *fonts: genes differentially expressed at day 10 and day 20 after fly challenge, respectively.*

functional groups and categories, we used the GO assignment to classify the functions of the unigenes. According to this process the genes expressed at high levels were classified into three GO groups (**Figure 3**) and further subdivided into categories: biological process (14 categories), molecular functions (22 categories), and cellular component (6 categories). The category "No terms assigned" was predominant across all GO groups at any investigated time.

Comparing Gpg Gene Annotation on the Gmm Genome and on a Previously Used Panel of Genomes

The global and detailed results of this comparative approach are presented in Supplementary Table S4. **Table 4**, which is a refined list of Supplementary Table S4, focuses on the expression of Gmm genes that are similar to Gpg genes previously identified as differentially expressed in response to Tbg infection. The results indicate that a high number of Gpg DEGs have orthologs in the Gmm genome. Furthermore, a large number of Gpg (22) and Gmm genes (23) encoding serine proteases were idenetified. Similarly, nine Gpg and nine Gmm genes were identified as encoding chitin binding proteins. Finally, whereas 14 Gmm genes encoding a "Major Facilitator Superfamily transporter" were identified, only one such gene was characterized in Gpg.

Homologies between Identified Gmm Genes That Are Heterologous to Gpg DEGs with Genes from Other Organisms

In order to identify genes previously annotated as "uncharacterized" or "hypothetical," we used the BLASTx program to identify heterologous genes among various organisms listed in the NCBI databases. Homologies with a

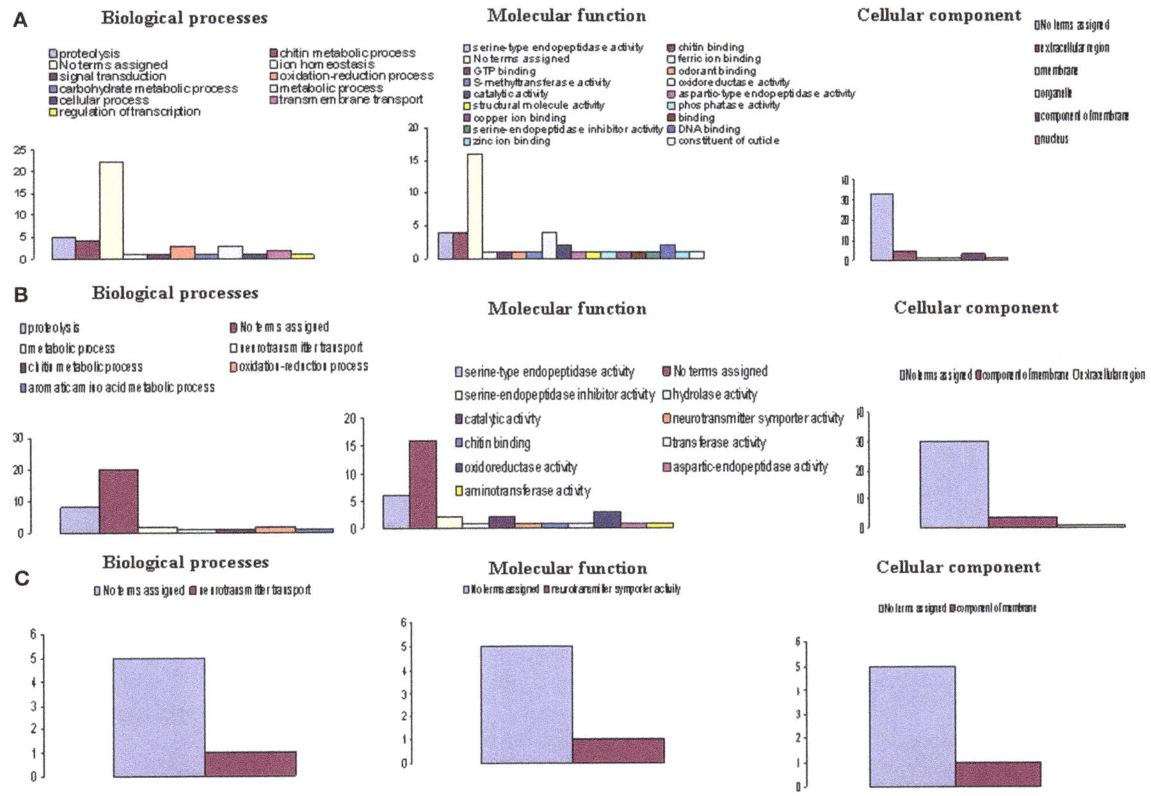

FIGURE 3 | Functional classes of Gmm genes heterologous to highly differentially expressed Gpg genes. Highly differentially expressed genes ($\log_2$ FC > +3 or $\log_2$ FC < −3) were observed in **(A)**. Tbg stimulated vs. non-stimulated Gpg flies (day-3 sampling); **(B)** Tbg infected vs. non-infected Gpg flies (day-10 sampling); and **(C)** Tbg infected vs. non-infected Gpg flies (day-20 sampling). The X-axis designates the Gene Ontology (GO) category, while the Y-axis provides the number of genes in each GO category.

cut-off $E < 10^{-5}$ and-/-or displaying the highest hits score were selected; the minimum accepted homology level was 60%. **Table 5** presents the results of the recorded annotation, and **Figure 4** presents the species from which genomes the genes to be annotated displayed the best match.

Among the 284 Gmm genes heterologous to the day-3 Gpg DEGs samples, 54 genes showed significant matches with other organisms in the investigated databases. The top homology matches were *Drosophila* sp. (11.1%), *Ceratitis capitata* (13%), and *Musca domestica* (68.5%). The remaining 7.4% of genes matched with either *Homo sapiens* (1.8%), *Lucilia sericata* (3.5%), or *Volvox carteri* (2.1%). Similarly, among the 139 Gmm genes heterologous to the day-10 Gpg DEGs samples, 33 genes showed significant matches with other organisms. The top homology matches were *Drosophila* (18.2%), *Ceratitis capitata* (21.3%), and *Musca domestica* (51.5%). The remaining 9% of genes matched with either *Loxodonta africana* (2.9%) or *Volvox carteri* (6.1%). Finally, among the 59 DEGs from day-20 samples, 12 DEGs displayed significant matches with *Musca domestica* (58.7%), *Ceratitis capitata* (8.3%), or *Drosophila* sp (33%).

Several trends appear when comparing results from the annotation reported in **Table 5** with those reported in Supplementary Tables S1–S3 (or in **Table 3**, regarding the genes in which the differential expression level was $-2 < \log_2$ FC or $\log_2$ FC > 2). First, many genes were not annotated; second, for genes that were annotated, the fold-change was identical; and finally, several genes that were annotated as "Hypothetical" when mapped on the Gmm genome could be identified when mapped on other databases. This was the case regarding the genes GMOY003830 (i.e., => Pherophorin-dz1 protein, when annotated on *Volvox carteri*), GMOY004337 (i.e., => Bardet –Biedl syndrome 4 protein homolog, when annotated on *D. willistoni* or *Ceratitis capitata*), GMOY005606 (i.e., => leucine-rich repeat-containing protein 15-like, when annotated on *Musca domestica*), GMOY007560 (i.e., => N-acetylgalactosaminyl transferase 2-like, when annotated on *C. capitata*), GMOY007584 (i.e., => Synaptotagmin-1-like, when annotated on *C capitata*), and GMOY008070 (i.e., => Pherophorin-dz1 protein, when annotated on *Volvox carteri*).

DISCUSSION

The chronic and acute forms of sleeping sickness endemic to sub-Saharan Africa are caused by two *Trypanosoma* subspecies, Tbg and Tbr, which are, respectively, transmitted to their

TABLE 4 | Identification of Gmm gene orthologs of Gpg genes on the basis of their expression products.

Glossina palpalis gambiensis genes	Best hit description-/-name of the encoded proteins	*Glossina morsitans morsitans* genes
GLOS_ARP3.1.1	Actin-related protein [*Drosophila melanogaster*]	
	Actin-related protein	GMOY008458
GLOS_DVIR_GJ17549.1.1	Acyltransferase—GJ17549 [*Drosophila virilis*]	
	Acyl-CoA N-acyltransferase	GMOY003123
GLOS_LOC101462532.1.1	Adenylosuccinate lyase-like [*Ceratitis capitata*]	
	Adenylosuccinase	GMOY002461
GLOS_LOC101450467.1.1	Alkaline phosphatase-like—membrane-bound [*Ceratitis capitata*]	
	Alkaline phosphatase	GMOY000067
GLOS_LOC101455841.1.3	Alpha-2-macroglobuline—CD109 antigen-like isoform X5 [*C. capitata*]	
	Alpha-2-macroglobulin	GMOY010996
GLOS_LOC101461571.2.2	Aspartic protease-like (lysosomal) [*Ceratitis capitata*]	
	Aspartic peptidase	GMOY005345; GMOY010103
GLOS_DVIR_GJ18228.1.1; GLOS_FDL.1.2	Beta-hexosaminidase—GJ18228 [*Drosophila virilis/D. melanogaster*]	
	Beta-hexosaminidase domain 2-like	GMOY001794
GLOS_KCC2A.2.2	Ca2+/calmodulin-dependent protein kinase type II	
	Ca2+/calmodulin-dependent protein kinase	GMOY006719
GLOS_CEC.2.2; GLOS_CECC.1.1; GLOS_CG10252.2.2	Cecropin [*G. m. morsitans/D. yakuba/D. melanogaster*]	
	Cecropin (anti-microbial peptide)	GMOY011562; GMOY011563
GLOS_DANA_GF24496.1.1; GLOS_DANA_GF24494.3.12	Chitin binding—GF24496 [*Drosophila ananassae*]	
GLOS_DGRI_GH11353.5.6; GLOS_DGRI_GH14440.1.1	Chitin binding—GH11353 [*Drosophila grimshawi*]	
GLOS_DMOJ_GI10981.2.2; GLOS_DMOJ_GI13574.3.3	Chitin binding—GI10981 [*Drosophila mojavensis*]	
GLOS_DWIL_GK11657.1.1; GLOS_DWIL_GK13541.1.5	Chitin binding—GK11657 [*Drosophila willistoni*]	
GLOS_DPER_GL15114.1.3	Chitin binding—GL15114 [*Drosophila persimilis*]	
	Chitin binding	GMOY002708; GMOY003840; GMOY005251; GMOY005278;
		GMOY009806; GMOY009807; GMOY011054; GMOY011809
		GMOY011810
GLOS_LOC101462140.1.1	Chitinase 3-like [*Ceratitis capitata*]	
	Chitinase-like protein Idgf5	GMOY009161
GLOS_CP305.1.2; GLOS_C4AC3.1.1; GLOS_CP6G1.1.1;	Cytochrome P450 305a1 [*D. melanogaster*]	
GLOS_CP9F2.9.9; GLOS_CP6W1.1.1	Cytochrome P450 9f2 [*D. melanogaster*]	
	cytochrome P450-4g1	GMOY001150; GMOY001939; GMOY006475; GMOY006761
	Cytochrome P450	GMOY002598; GMOY002627; GMOY005461; GMOY007064;
		GMOY007181; GMOY007270; GMOY007652;
		GMOY009767; GMOY009909
GLOS_RN181.1.1	E3 ubiquitin-protein ligase RNF181 homolog	
	E3 ubiquitin-protein ligase SINA like	GMOY002938; GMOY008903
GLOS_ELP2.1.1	Elongator complex protein 2; D. m. GN = Elp2 PE = 1 SV = 1	
	Elongase 4; 9	GMOY008821; GMOY003354
GLOS_LOC101461359.1.1	Endoplasmic reticulum metallopeptidase 1-like isoform X1 [*C. capitata*]	
	Endoplasmic reticulum metallopeptidase 1	GMOY009845; GMOY010241
GLOS_LOC101454791.1.1	Enkurin-like [*Ceratitis capitata*]	
	Enkurin	GMOY009600

(Continued)

TABLE 4 | Continued

Glossina palpalis gambiensis genes	Best hit description-/-name of the encoded proteins	*Glossina morsitans morsitans* genes
GLOS_LOC101459623.1.5	Exonuclease 3′-5′ domain-containing protein 2-like [*C. capitata*]	
	Exonuclease	GMOY012368
GLOS_LOC101459395.1.1	Gamma-glutamyl hydrolase-like [*Ceratitis capitata*]	
	Gamma-glutamyl hydrolase	GMOY000946
GLOS_GSTT1.2.5; GLOS_GST.1.1	Glutathione S-transferase 1-1 [*L. cuprina/Musca domestica*]	
	Glutathione S-transferase	GMOY002000; GMOY009373
GLOS_LOC101449625.1.1	Glyoxalase domain-containing protein 4-like isoform X1 [*C. capitata*]	
	Glyoxylase	GMOY008525
GLOS_DVIR_GJ19325.1.1	G-protein receptor activity—GJ19325 [*Drosophila virilis*]	
	G-protein coupled receptor	GMOY009447
GLOS_DWIL_GK15016.1.2	Haemolynph juvenile hormone binding- GK15016- [*D. willistoni*]	
	Haemolymph juvenile hormone binding	GMOY004364
GLOS_H12.1.1	Histone H1.2 [*Drosophila virilis*]	
	Histone H1	GMOY002746
GLOS_IMDH.2.2	Inosine-5′-monophosphate dehydrogenase [*D. melanogaster*]	
	Inosine-5′-monophosphate dehydrogenase	GMOY006458
GLOS_LECA.10.13	Lectin subunit alpha [*Sarcophaga peregrina*]	
	Lectin-like C-type	GMOY001011; GMOY009274
GLOS_LRRX1.1.4	Leucine-rich repeat-containing protein— [*D. discoideum*]	
	Leucine rich repeat containing protein	GMOY010344
GLOS_LSD1.1.1	Lipid storage droplets surface-binding protein 1	
	lipid storage droplet-1	GMOY007510
GLOS_DWIL_GK13707.1.1	Lipid transporter—GK13707 [*Drosophila willistoni*]	
	Lipid transport protein	GMOY002410; GMOY005442; GMOY005442;
GLOS_LOC101449088.1.1	lysM—peptidoglycan-binding domain-containing protein 1-like [*C. capitata*]	
	LysM domain	GMOY008891
GLOS_DPER_GL12526.1.1	Major Facilitator Superfamily-type transporter / — [*D. persimilis*]	
	Major Facilitator Superfamily transporter	GMOY001742; GMOY003428; GMOY003490; GMOY003491;
		GMOY003839; GMOY004738; GMOY005103; GMOY005106;
		GMOY005109; GMOY005501; GMOY007545; GMOY007627;
		GMOY012075; GMOY012352
GLOS_LOC101462556.1.1	MD-2-related lipid-recognition protein-like [*Ceratitis capitata*]	
	MD-2-related lipid-recognition domain	GMOY006406
GLOS_MYSN.1.1	Myosin heavy chain, non-muscle [*D. melanogaster*]	
	Myosin heavy chain	GMOY007533; GMOY008852
GLOS_DMOJ_GI24301.1.1	Neuropeptide Y receptor—GI24301 [*Drosophila mojavensis*]	
	NeuroPeptide Y like receptor / mammalian (Putative)	GMOY011997; GMOY012052
GLOS_DGRI_GH13991.1.1; GLOS_DVIR_GJ10540.1.1	Odorant binding—GH13991 [*Drosophila grimshawi*]/*Drosophila virilis*	
GLOS_OB99B.1.1	Odorant-binding protein 99b	

(Continued)

TABLE 4 | Continued

Glossina palpalis gambiensis genes	Best hit description-/-name of the encoded proteins	*Glossina morsitans morsitans* genes
	Odorant binding protein 1; 2; 7	GMOY000890; GMOY002825; GMOY005548;
	Odorant binding protein 21; 22	GMOY006418; GMOY001476
GLOS_LOC101453268.1.1	Period circadian protein-like [*Ceratitis capitata*]	
	Period circadian protein	GMOY012110
GLOS_LOC101458811.1.1	Pyridoxal kinase-like [*Ceratitis capitata*]	
	Pyridoxal phosphate-dependent transferase	GMOY005488; GMOY005934
GLOS_DMOJ_GI20119.1.1; GLOS_DMOJ_GI16517.2.2; GLOS_DSEC_GM17695.1.1; GLOS_LOC101456159.4.4; GLOS_DMOJ_GI18413.1.2; GLOS_DANA_GF15448.2.3; GLOS_AAEL_AAEL007969.1.1; GLOS_LOC101461009.2.2; GLOS_EAST.2.2; GLOS_LOC101457953.1.5; GLOS_LOC101462986.1.1; GLOS_DWIL_GK19454.1.1 GLOS_LOC101459895.9.9; GLOS_DWIL_GK24139.1.1; GLOS_LOC101455430.10.10; GLOS_LOC101455604.4.10; GLOS_DMOJ_GI21244.4.5; GLOS_DMOJ_GI24442.1.1; GLOS_DVIR_GJ21497.1.3; GLOS_DVIR_GJ22718.8.10; GLOS_DVIR_GJ21498.1.1; GLOS_DVIR_GJ21499.1.1;	Serine proteases (see details in Supplementary Table S4)	GMOY000672; GMOY002036; GMOY002729; GMOY003271 GMOY003273; GMOY003280; GMOY003693; GMOY003994 GMOY006266; GMOY006369; GMOY006991; GMOY008468 GMOY008469; GMOY008958; GMOY008962; GMOY008964 GMOY008965; GMOY008966; GMOY009418; GMOY009436 GMOY009757; GMOY010502; GMOY010768
GLOS_DMOJ_GI19420.1.1; GLOS_DVIR_GJ17584.1.1	Serine protease inhibitor (Serpin) GI19420 [*D. mojavensis/D. virilis*]	
GLOS_DANA_GF14653.1.2; GLOS_DERE_GG24413.1.1;	Serine-type endopeptidase inhibitor— [*D. ananassae/D. erecta*]	
GLOS_DWIL_GK10999.1.1; GLOS_LOC101459846.1.2	Serine-type endopeptidase inhibitor /Metalloendopeptidase [*D. willistoni*]	
	Serine proteinase inhibitors (Kazal domain)	GMOY010058
GLOS_DWIL_GK15974.5.7; GLOS_DMOJ_GI22128.1.1	Single domain von Willebrand factor type C [*D. willistoni*]	
	Single domain Von Willebrand factor type C	GMOY003774; GMOY005237; GMOY007078; GMOY010675
GLOS_DWIL_GK22031.1.1	Sulfate transmembrane transporter—GK22031 [*Drosophila willistoni*]	
	Sulfate transporter	GMOY000550
GLOS_LOC101448839.1.1; GLOS_LOC101454308.1.2	Timeless-like isoform X1 protein (circadian rhythm regulation) [*C. capitata*]	
	Timeless protein	GMOY006112
GLOS_TRF.1.1	Transferrin [*Sarcophaga peregrina*]	
	Transferrin family, iron binding site	GMOY004228
GLOS_LOC101463325.1.1	Trypsin-like [*Ceratitis capitata*]	
	Trypsin-like cysteine/serine peptidase domain	GMOY002535; GMOY008308
GLOS_DWIL_GK18237.1.1	UDP-glucuronosyl/UDP-glucosyltransferase—GK18237 [*D. willistoni*]	
	UDP-glucuronosyl/UDP-glucosyltransferase	GMOY007046
GLOS_LOC101451574.1.1	WD repeat-containing protein 81-like isoform X1 [*Ceratitis capitata*]	
	WD40/YVTN repeat-like-containing domain	GMOY010092
GLOS_LOC101458997.1.1	Yellow-like protein (protein of the gelly) [*Ceratitis capitata*]	
	yolk protein 3	GMOY006227

The table compares the results of the previous Gpg DEG annotation on a panel of various genomes with the corresponding annotation on the Gmm genome. A comparison is presented between the Gpg and the Gmm genes on the basis of the identified proteins they encode.

TABLE 5 | Gmm gene heterologs of Gpg DEGs matching genes from other organism databases.

Genes	log_2 FC	Homology with other organisms (>60%)
GMOY000550	-0.90	*Musca domestica* sodium-independent sulfate anion transporter-like (LOC101893700), mRNA
GMOY001137	1.09	*Musca domestica* aminomethyltransferase, mitochondrial-like (LOC101895864), mRNA
GMOY001742	-0.9	*Ceratitis capitata* synaptic vesicle glycoprotein 2B-like (LOC101452461), transcript variant X3, mRNA
GMOY002004	-1.78	*Musca domestica* putative fatty acyl-CoA reductase CG5065-like (LOC101898308), mRNA
GMOY002004	1.8	*Musca domestica* putative fatty acyl-CoA reductase CG5065-like (LOC101898308), mRNA
GMOY002024	0.96	*Musca domestica* phosphotriesterase-related protein-like (LOC101890186), mRNA
GMOY002356	2.31	*C. capitata* CUGBP Elav-like family member 2-like (LOC101455154), transcript variant X1 to X3, mRNA
GMOY002461	0.82	*Musca domestica* adenylosuccinate lyase-like (LOC101900029), mRNA
GMOY002486	2.6	*Musca domestica* potassium channel subfamily K member 9-like (LOC101895107), mRNA
GMOY002535	1.5	*Ceratitis capitata* serine protease easter-like (LOC101451852), mRNA
GMOY002729	1.91	*Lucilia sericata* clone LScDNA1 putative salivary trypsin mRNA, complete cds
GMOY002729	3.0	*Musca domestica* serine proteinase stubble-like (LOC101890358), mRNA
GMOY002938	-1.10	*Musca domestica* uncharacterized LOC101893009 (LOC101893009), mRNA
GMOY003158	2.70	*Musca domestica* uncharacterized LOC101895341 (LOC101895341), mRNA
GMOY003161	1.44	*Musca domestica* thyrotropin receptor-like (LOC101887582), mRNA
GMOY003354	2.48	*Ceratitis capitata* elongation of very long chain fatty acids protein AAEL008004-like (LOC101449680), mRNA
GMOY003354	6.3	*Musca domestica* elongation of very long chain fatty acids protein AAEL008004-like (LOC101893043), mRNA
GMOY003443	1.27	*Musca domestica* uncharacterized LOC101889318 (LOC101889318), partial mRNA
GMOY003590	1.77	*Musca domestica* collagen alpha-1(IV) chain-like (LOC101897761), transcript variant X3, mRNA
GMOY003590	1.3	*Musca domestica* collagen alpha-1(IV) chain-like (LOC101897761), transcript variant X3, mRNA and variant X1, X2
GMOY003830	2.75	*Homo sapiens* BAC clone CH17-465I15 from chromosome unknown, complete sequence (=hypothetical)
GMOY003830	3.7	*Volvox carteri f, nagariensis* mRNA for pherophorin-dz1 protein
GMOY003839	0.95	*Musca domestica* putative inorganic phosphate cotransporter-like (LOC101889974), mRNA
GMOY003949	1.01	*M. domestica* glutamine-fructose-6-phosphate aminotransferase [isomerizing] 2-like (LOC101889985), transcript
GMOY004309	2.44	*Musca domestica* fatty acid synthase-like (LOC101893120), mRNA
GMOY004332	2.1	*Drosophila willistoni* GK20732 (Dwil\GK20732), mRNA /Fatty acyl-CoA reductase
GMOY004337	5.8	*D. willistoni* GK20950 (Dwil\GK20950), mRNA Bardet-Biedl syndrome 4 protein homolog (=hypothetical on Gmm genome)
GMOY004337	6.6	*Ceratitis capitata* Bardet-Biedl syndrome 4 protein homolog (LOC101449311), mRNA (=hypothetical on Gmm genome)
GMOY004589	1.09	*Musca domestica* muscle M-line assembly protein unc-89-like (LOC101890868) mRNA
GMOY004712	1.65	*Musca domestica* acyl-protein thioesterase 1-like (LOC101890399), mRNA
GMOY004738	-0.78	*Musca domestica* facilitated trehalose transporter Tret1-like (LOC101891733), transcript variant X1, Mrna
GMOY004873	1.6	*Musca domestica* transmembrane and TPR repeat-containing protein CG4341-like (LOC101893859), mRNA
GMOY005102	6.28	*Musca domestica* N-acetylgalactosaminyltransferase 4-like (LOC101894376), mRNA
GMOY005106	-1.22	*Drosophila willistoni* GK13266 (Dwil\GK13266), mRNA / Major facilitator superfamily transporter
GMOY005278	2.93	*Musca domestica* mucin-5AC-like (LOC101899868), mRNA
GMOY005278	1.9	*Musca domestica* mucin-5AC-like (LOC101899868), mRNA
GMOY005345	-6.5	*Musca domestica* lysosomal aspartic protease-like (LOC101894831), mRNA
GMOY005487	3.48	*Musca domestica* LIM/homeobox protein Lhx4-like (LOC101900654), mRNA
GMOY005488	1.81	*Musca domestica* alpha-methyldopa hypersensitive protein-like (LOC101888467), mRNA
GMOY005527	0.87	*Musca domestica* c-1-tetrahydrofolate synthase, cytoplasmic-like (LOC101891351), transcript variant X2, mRNA
GMOY005606	6.3	*Musca domestica* leucine-rich repeat-containing protein 15-like (LOC101899894), mRNA (=hypothetical on Gmm genome)
GMOY005934	2.72	*Ceratitis capitata* cysteine sulfinic acid decarboxylase-like (LOC101455610), mRNA
GMOY006111	1.1	*Drosophila willistoni* GK14673 (Dwil\GK14673), mRNA (Gonadal trypsine)
GMOY006205	1.2	*Ceratitis capitata* DNA replication licensing factor Mcm5-like (LOC101458261), mRNA
GMOY006406	1.69	*Musca domestica* ecdysteroid-regulated 16 kDa protein-like (LOC101898283), mRNA
GMOY006406	1.7	*Musca domestica* ecdysteroid-regulated 16 kDa protein-like (LOC101898283), mRNA
GMOY006458	-0.78	*Musca domestica* inosine-5′-monophosphate dehydrogenase-like (LOC101895820), mRNA
GMOY006671	4.0	*Musca domestica* uncharacterized LOC101890025 (LOC101890025), mRNA
GMOY006761	1.99	*Musca domestica* cytochrome P450 CYP4G13v2 mRNA, complete cds
GMOY006761	2.4	*Musca domestica* cytochrome P450 CYP4G13v2 mRNA, complete cds
GMOY006761	-2.1	*Musca domestica* cytochrome P450 CYP4G13v2 mRNA, complete cds

(Continued)

TABLE 5 | Continued

Genes	$\log_2$ FC	Homology with other organisms (>60%)
GMOY006875	-2.0	*Musca domestica* membrane-bound alkaline phosphatase-like (LOC101896753), mRNA
GMOY006875	-1.8	*Musca domestica* membrane-bound alkaline phosphatase-like (LOC101896753), mRNA
GMOY006979	1.08	*Musca domestica* phosrestin-2-like (LOC101892743), Mrna
GMOY007046	2.0	*Ceratitis capitata* UDP-glucuronosyltransferase 2B13-like (LOC101462823), transcript variant X2, mRNA
GMOY007131	0.97	*Musca domestica* inositol-3-phosphate synthase-like (LOC101889622), mRNA
GMOY007148	2.10	*Ceratitis capitata* fatty acid synthase-like (LOC101463409), mRNA
GMOY007497	6.3	*Musca domestica* NADH-cytochrome b5 reductase 3-like (LOC101897795), transcript variant X2, mRNA
GMOY007523	1.44	*Musca domestica* collagen alpha-1(IV) chain-like (LOC101895032), transcript variant X3, mRNA
GMOY007523	1.1	*Musca domestica* collagen alpha-1(IV) chain-like (LOC101895032), transcript variant X3, mRNA
GMOY007560	-1.0	*C. capitata* polypeptide N-acetylgalactosaminyltransferase 2-like (LOC101448408), mRNA (=hypothetical on Gmm genome)
GMOY007584	1.1	*Ceratitis capitata* synaptotagmin-1-like (LOC101450559), mRNA (=hypothetical on Gmm genome)
GMOY008017	1.88	*Volvox carteri f. nagariensis* mRNA for pherophorin-dz1 protein (=hypothetical when mapped on Gmm genome)
GMOY008017	1.2	*Volvox carteri f, nagariensis* mRNA for pherophorin-dz1 protein (=hypothetical when mapped on Gmm genome)
GMOY008266	-1.3	*Drosophila willistoni* GK24772 organic anion transporter (Dwil\GK24772), mRNA
GMOY008308	1.9	*Drosophila melanogaster* easter (ea), transcript variant A, mRNA
GMOY008458	5.74	*Musca domestica* actin, indirect flight muscle-like (LOC101895248), mRNA
GMOY008525	0.97	*Drosophila willistoni* GK21885 (Dwil\GK21885), mRNA
GMOY008601	2.58	*Musca domestica* fatty acid synthase-like (LOC101893120), mRNA
GMOY008601	4.1	*Drosophila willistoni* GK12914 (Dwil\GK12914), mRNA
GMOY008602	2.02	*Drosophila pseudoobscura pseudoobscura* GA26263 (Dpse\GA26263), mRNA
GMOY008602	-2.5	*Drosophila willistoni* GK12914 (Dwil\GK12914), mRNA
GMOY008852	0.93	*Musca domestica* myosin heavy chain, non-muscle-like (LOC101892851), transcript variant X1 to X3, Mrna
GMOY008966	4.4	*Loxodonta africana* kallikrein-11-like (LOC100667195), mRNA
GMOY008973	0.80	*Lucilia cuprina* alpha esterase (LcaE7) mRNA, implicated in organophosphate resistance, complete cds
GMOY009018	1.59	*Ceratitis capitata* uncharacterized LOC101448539 (LOC101448539), transcript variant
GMOY009018	1.8	*Musca domestica* uncharacterized LOC101899326 (LOC101899326), mRNA
GMOY009079	1.23	*Musca domestica* fatty acid synthase-like (LOC101893120), mRNA
GMOY009375	7.56	*Musca domestica* uncharacterized LOC101900740 (LOC101900740), mRNA
GMOY009394	-5.56	*Musca domestica* CCAAT/enhancer-binding protein-like (LOC101898926), mRNA
GMOY009447	-1.22	*Ceratitis capitata* calcitonin gene-related peptide type 1 receptor-like (LOC101462563), mRNA
GMOY009600	1.20	*Musca domestica* enkurin-like (LOC101897351), mRNA
GMOY009845	0.6	*Musca domestica* endoplasmic reticulum metallopeptidase 1-like (LOC101898765), transcript variant X3, mRNA
GMOY009903	2.75	*M. domestica* strain rspin nicotinic acetylcholine receptor beta 3 subunit (nAChRbeta3) gene, nAChRbeta3-C allele, complete cds
GMOY009983	1.7	*Drosophila grimshawi* GH17190 (Dgri\GH17190), mRNA
GMOY010224	6.9	*Musca domestica* uncharacterized LOC101889990 (LOC101889990), partial mRNA
GMOY010224	3.6	*Musca domestica* uncharacterized LOC101889990 (LOC101889990), partial mRNA **(=>** Hypothetical**)**
GMOY010241	0.8	*Musca domestica* endoplasmic reticulum metallopeptidase 1-like (LOC101898765), transcript variant X3, mRNA
GMOY010481	-1.53	*Musca domestica* protein Wnt-5-like (LOC101892275), mRNA
GMOY010972	0.73	*Musca domestica* phenoloxidase subunit A3-like (LOC101897997), transcript variant X1 and X2, mRNA
GMOY011232	1.32	*Drosophila melanogaster* PAPS synthetase (Papss), transcript variant A, mRNA variant A to H
GMOY011418	0.87	*Drosophila willistoni* GK13980 (Dwil\GK13980), mRNA / glycogen synthase
GMOY011618	-0.9	*Ceratitis capitata* putative fatty acyl-CoA reductase CG5065-like (LOC101456246), transcript variant X2, mRNA
GMOY012052	3.4	*Drosophila pseudoobscura pseudoobscura* GA30114 Neuropeptide Y (Dpse\GA30114), mRNA
GMOY012069	9.1	*Musca domestica* uncharacterized LOC101891108 (LOC101891108), mRNA
GMOY012069	5.3	*Musca domestica* uncharacterized LOC101891108 (LOC101891108), mRNA
GMOY012075	1.56	*Drosophila melanogaster* CG31663 (CG31663), transcript variant B, mRNA (Major facilitator superfamily transporter)
GMOY012075	-1.7	*Drosophila willistoni* GK15555 (Dwil\GK15555), mRNA (Major facilitator superfamily transporter)
GMOY012352	0.94	*Ceratitis capitata* monocarboxylate transporter 10-like (LOC101448353), transcript variant X1, mRNA

Black fonts, day-3 samples; Blue fonts, day-10 samples; Red fonts, day-20 samples.

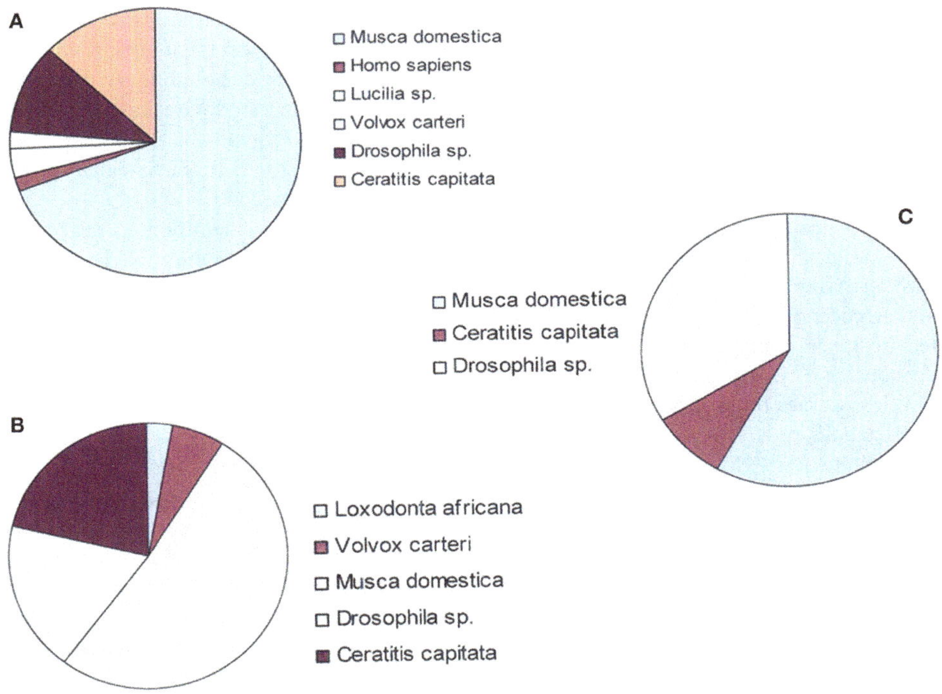

FIGURE 4 | Species on which Gmm genes were mapped in order to characterize genes previously annotated as "hypothetical." (A) Mapping of the 284 Gmm genes heterologous to Gpg DEGs in trypanosome stimulated vs. non-stimulated flies (day-3 sampling). **(B)** Mapping of the 139 Gmm genes heterologous to Gpg DEGs in trypanosome infected vs. non-infected flies (day-10 sampling). **(C)** Mapping of the 59 Gmm genes heterologous to Gpg DEGs in trypanosome infected vs. non-infected flies (day-20 sampling).

vertebrate hosts by the *Glossina* species Gpg and Gmm (Aksoy et al., 2014; Beschin et al., 2014). Nevertheless, the biological cycles, vertebrate transmission processes, and pathogenicity development of the two parasites are similar. Recently, in the context of an anti-vector strategy project to fight the disease, we performed a global transcriptomic analysis of Gpg gene expression associated with fly infection by Tbg. More precisely, we attempted to characterize genes that were differentially expressed according to the status of the fly at several sampling times (i.e., non-infected, infected, or self-cured). This included genes that could be involved in the fly's vector competence, and consequently genes that could possibly be manipulated in order to reduce or even suppress this competence.

The similarities between the Tbg and Tbr life cycles prompted us to determine whether the Gmm genome carried genes that could be heterologous to the Gpg DEGs, which could then allow the development of common molecular approaches. Accordingly, the Gpg sequences resulting from the previous RNA-seq *de novo* assembly (Hamidou Soumana et al., 2015) were mapped on the Gmm genome, the DEGs were characterized, and the corresponding genes were annotated.

When the Gpg sequences were mapped and annotated on a panel of various databases (*C. capitata*, *D. melanogaster*, *D. willistoni*, *D. virilis*, *D. mojavensis*, *Acyrthosiphon pisum*, *Hydra magnipapillata*, *Anopheles* sp., *Bombyx* sp., *Aedes* sp., and *G. morsitans*; Hamidou Soumana et al., 2015) we identified 553 (S vs. NS), 52 (I10 vs. NI10), and 143 (I20 vs. NI20) DEGs. In contrast, we identified 284 (S vs. NS), 139 (I10 vs. NI10) and 59 (I20 vs. NI20) DEGs when sequences were mapped and annotated on the *G. m. morsitans* database (using its whole genome annotated on the *Drosophila melanogaster*, *Aedes aegypti*, *Anopheles gambiae*, *Culex quinquefasciatus*, and *Phlebotomus papatasi* databases; International Glossina Genome Initiative, 2014). The differences in the number of identified DEGs, as well as the high number of "uncharacterized" genes, could be due to differences in the database panels used to annotate Gpg or Gmm. We cannot exclude the possibility that some of the Gpg DEGs do not have heterologous genes in Gmm, or that some of them could be specific to either Gpg or Gmm and consequently cannot be annotated yet. Nevertheless, regarding I10 vs. NI10 sampling (and in contrast to the two other experimental conditions), the number of recorded DEGs was more than 2-fold higher when the Gpg transcripts were mapped on the Gmm genome, prompting questions of how this is possible. However, at this stage of our research we cannot offer a satisfactory explanation.

We examined the potential influence of database panel composition by annotating the Gmm DEGs on a separate set of databases that included *D. melanogaster* as an internal control. The results (**Table 5**) clearly demonstrate the validity of the annotation process, since all Gmm genes (GMOY, etc.) were annotated (best hit description and fold-change) on the novel set of databases as they had been annotated on the former set (**Table 3**), and that several genes could be identified thanks to their annotation primarily on the *Volvox carteri* or *Musca domestica* databases which had never been used before, and despite the fact these organisms (algae and mouse) are genetically distant from the tsetse fly.

The most important observation regarding our objective is that almost all of the Gpg genes previously considered to be potentially involved in tsetse fly vector competence (cf. Hamidou Soumana et al., 2015) had a "countrepart" (i.e., heterologous genes) in the Gmm genome, despite the fact that none of the Gpg DEGs matched with any Gmm genes. This was the case for the large array of genes encoding peptidases, especially serine peptidases (represented by more than 20 genes), identified in the genomes of both fly species. This was similarly observed for ~10 genes present in both genomes that encode chitin binding proteins, since chitin metabolism is involved in the ability of tsetse flies to host trypanosomes (Maudlin and Welburn, 1994; Welburn and Maudlin, 1999), in addition to cecropin (an antimicrobial peptide), among others (Weiss et al., 2014).

Here, we were particularly interested in detecting the presence or not of genes with a reported role in the immunity of tsetse flies or other organisms (Weiss et al., 2014). Genes encoding Pro3 protein (GMOY009756, GMOY000672) and transferrin (GMOY004228) were identified. Pro3 has a potential function as a serine protease (tyrosinase) and is specifically produced by the proventriculus, an organ that plays an important role in the tsetse immune response. This protein could be involved in the immune response via activation of the cascade of prophenol oxidase and melanization (Jiang et al., 1998). Moreover, the gene GMOY0010488 was identified as encoding an "immuno reactive putative protease inhibitor" that is overexpressed in trypanosome stimulated or infected Gpg flies. The transferrin gene was overexpressed in both stimulated and infected Gpg flies; this result is in agreement with Geiser and Winzerling (2012), who reported on the role of transferrin in the immune response of insects, as well as its role in iron transport. By reducing the oxidative stress in tsetse fly guts, transferrin may promote the survival of trypanosomes. Guz et al. (2012) observed transferrin overexpression after challenge with bacteria, even at a higher level than what is typically observed in the case of infection by trypanosomes.

The gene GMOY011809 encodes Pro 1 peritrophin, which is a constituent of the peritrophic membrane (PM). The PM is established after the fly takes its first blood meal, and it is permanently renewed by the proventriculus (Moloo et al., 1970; Tellam et al., 1999). The PM primarily functions to envelop the blood meal and protect the intestinal epithelium against abrasion by ingested matter, although it can also represent an obstacle to the passage of ingested parasites into the ectoperitrophic space (Lehane, 1997; Hegedus et al., 2009). The gene GMOY005278 encodes mucin, which participates with peritrophin in the composition of the PM.

We have also identified genes encoding antimicrobial peptides: in Supplementary Table S1, GMOY01052 through GMOY010524 encode attacin, whereas GMOY0011562 and GMOY0011563 encode cecropin. Furthermore, both attacin and cecropin are overexpressed in Gpg trypanosome stimulated or infected flies.

Our work is the first comparison of its kind between the two *Glossina* species. This is primarily due to the fact that the different scientific teams working on HAT commonly focus on investigating either Gmm (and the acute form of trypanosomiasis) or Gpg (and the chronic form of trypanosomiasis), but not both together. Indeed, one of our most relevant findings is the observation that Gmm has the same genes at its disposal that Gpg may use to control its vector competence. Importantly, this comparison will assist future studies in revealing common molecular targets to increase the refractoriness of either fly species to infection by trypanosomes.

AUTHOR CONTRIBUTIONS

Conceived and designed the experiments: IH, AG. Performed the experiments: IH, BT, SR, HP. Analyzed the data: IH, SR, HP, AG. Wrote the paper: AG.

ACKNOWLEDGMENTS

The authors thank the "Région Languedoc-Roussillon—Appel d'Offre Chercheur d'Avenir 2011" and the "Institut de Recherche pour le Développement" for their support.

REFERENCES

1. Aksoy, S., Weiss, B. L., and Attardo, G. M. (2014). Trypanosome transmission dynamics in tsetse. *Curr. Opin. Insect Sci.* 3, 43–49. doi: 10.1016/j.cois.2014.07.003
2. Anders, S., Pyl, P. T., and Huber, W. (2014). HTSeq - A Python framework to work with high-throughput sequencing data. *Bioinformatics* 31, 166–169. doi: 10.1093/bioinformatics/ btu638
3. Benjamini, Y., and Hochberg, Y. (1995). Controlling the false discovery rate: a practical and powerful approach to multiple testing. *J. R. Stat. Soc. Ser. B* 57, 289–300.
4. Beschin, A., Van Den Abbeele, J., De Baetselier, P., and Pays, E. (2014). African trypanosome control in the insect vector and mammalian host. *Trends Parasitol.* 30, 538–547. doi: 10.1016/j.pt.2014.08.006
5. Bullard, J. H., Purdom, E., Hansen, K. D., and Dudoit, S. (2010). Upper quartile: evaluation of statistical methods for normalization and differential expression in mRNASeq experiments. *BMC Bioinformatics* 11:94. doi: 10.1186/1471-2105-11-94
6. Dennis G. Jr., Sherman, B. T., Hosack, D. A., Yang, J., Gao, W., Lane, H. C., et al. (2003). DAVID: database for annotation, visualization, and integrated discovery. *Genome Biol.* 4:P3. doi: 10.1186/gb-2003-4-5-p3
7. Farikou, O., Njiokou, F., Mbida Mbida, J. A., Njitchouang, G. R., Djeunga, H. N., Asonganyi, T., et al. (2010). Tripartite interactions between tsetse flies, Sodalis glossinidius and trypanosomes-an epidemiological approach in

two historical human African trypanosomiasis foci in Cameroon. *Infect. Genet. Evol.* 10, 115–121. doi: 10.1016/j.meegid.2009.10.008

8. Geiser, D. L., and Winzerling, J. J. (2012). Insect transferrins: multifunctional proteins. *Biochim. Biophys. Acta* 1820, 437–451. doi: 10.1016/j.bbagen.2011.07.011
9. Gentleman, R. C., Carey, V. J., Bates, D. M., Bolstad, B., Dettling, M., Dudoit, S., et al. (2004). Bioconductor: open software development for computational biology and bioinformatics. *Genome Biol.* 5:R80. doi: 10.1186/gb-2004-5-10-r80
10. Guz, N., Kilincer, N., and Aksoy, S. (2012). Molecular characterization of *Ephestia kuehniella* (Lepidoptera: Pyralidae) transferrin and its response to parasitoid Venturia canescens (Hymenoptera: Ichneumonidae Gravenhorst). *Insect Mol. Biol.* 21, 139–147. doi: 10.1111/j.1365-2583.2011.01129.x
11. Hamidou Soumana, I., Klopp, C., Ravel, S., Nabihoudine, I., Tchicaya, B., Parrinello, H., et al. (2015). RNA-seq *de novo* assembly reveals differential gene expression in *Glossina palpalis* gambiensis infected with *Trypanosoma brucei* gambiense vs. non-infected and self-cured flies. *Front. Microbiol.* 6:1259. doi: 10.3389/fmicb.2015.01259
12. Hamidou Soumana, I., Loriod, B., Ravel, S., Tchicaya, B., Simo, G., Rihet, P., et al. (2014a). The transcriptional signatures of *Sodalis glossinidius* in the *Glossina palpalis* gambiensis flies negative for *Trypanosoma brucei* gambiense contrast with those of this symbiont in tsetse flies positive for the parasite: possible involvement of a Sodalis-hosted prophage in fly Trypanosoma refractoriness? *Infect. Genet. Evol.* 24, 41–56. doi: 10.1016/j.meegid.2014.03.005
13. Hamidou Soumana, I., Tchicaya, B., Simo, G., and Geiger, A. (2014b). Comparative gene expression of Wigglesworthia inhabiting non-infected and *Trypanosoma brucei* gambiense-infected *Glossina palpalis* gambiensis flies. *Front. Microbiol.* 5:620. doi: 10.3389/fmicb.2014.00620
14. Hegedus, D., Erlandson, M., Gillott, C., and Toprak, U. (2009). New insights into peritrophic matrix synthesis, architecture, and function. *Annu. Rev. Entomol.* 54, 285–302. doi: 10.1146/annurev.ento.54.110807.090559
15. Hoare, C. A. (1972). *The Trypanosomes of Mammals, A Zoological Monograph*. Oxford: Blackwell Scientific Publications. International Glossina Genome Initiative (2014). Genome sequence of the tsetse fly (*Glossina morsitans*): vector of African trypanosomiasis. *Science* 344, 380–386. doi: 10.1126/science.1249656
16. Jiang, H., Wang, Y., and Kanost, M. R. (1998). Pro-phenol oxidase activating proteinase from an insect, *Manduca sexta*: a bacteria-inducible protein similar to Drosophila easter. *Proc. Natl. Acad. Sci. U.S.A.* 95, 12220–12225. doi: 10.1073/pnas.95.21.12220
17. Kim, D., Pertea, G., Trapnell, C., Pimentel, H., Kelley, R., and Salzberg, S. L. (2013). TopHat2: accurate alignment of transcriptomes in the presence of insertions, deletions and gene fusions. *Genome Biol.* 14:R36. doi: 10.1186/gb-2013-14-4-r36
18. Langmead, B., and Salzberg, S. (2012). Fast gapped-read alignment with Bowtie 2. *Nat. Methods* 9, 357–359. doi: 10.1038/nmeth.1923
19. Lehane, M. J. (1997). Peritrophic matrix structure and function. *Annu. Rev. Entomol.* 42, 525–550. doi: 10.1146/annurev.ento.42.1.525
20. Louis, F. J., Simarro, P. P., and Lucas, P. (2002). Sleeping sickness: one hundred years of control strategy evolution. *Bull. Soc. Pathol. Exot.* 95, 331–336.
21. Maudlin, I., and Welburn, S. C. (1994). Maturation of trypanosome infections in tsetse. *Exp. Parasitol.* 79, 202–205. doi: 10.1006/expr.1994.1081
22. Moloo, S. K., Steiger, R. F., and Hecker, H. (1970). Ultrastructure of the peritrophic membrane formation in Glossina Wiedemann. *Acta Trop.* 274, 378–383.
23. Mount, D. W. (2007). Using the Basic Local Alignment Search Tool (BLAST). *CSH Protoc.* 2007:pdb.top17. doi: 10.1101/pdb.top17
24. Robinson, M. D., McCarthy, D. J., and Smyth, G. K. (2010). EdgeR: a Bioconductor package for differential expression analysis of digital gene expression data. *Bioinformatics* 26, 139–140. doi: 10.1093/bioinformatics/btp616
25. Savage, A. F., Kolev, N. G., Franklin, J. B., Vigneron, A., Aksoy, S., and Tschudi, C. (2016). Transcriptome profiling of *Trypanosoma brucei* development in the tsetse fly vector *Glossina morsitans*. *PLoS ONE* 11:e0168877. doi: 10.1371/journal.pone.0168877
26. Tellam, R. L., Wijffels, G., and Willadsen, P. (1999). Peritrophic matrix proteins. *Insect Biochem. Mol. Biol.* 29, 87–101. doi: 10.1016/S0965-1748(98)00123-4 Van den Abbeele, J., Claes, Y., van Bockstaele, D., Le Ray, D., and Coosemans, M. (1999). *Trypanosoma brucei* spp. development in the tsetse fly: characterization of the post mesocyclic stages in the foregut and proboscis. *Parasitology* 118, 469–478. doi: 10.1017/S0031182099004217
27. Vickerman, K., Tetley, L., Hendry, K. A., and Turner, C. M. (1988). Biology of African trypanosomes in the tsetse fly. *Biol. Cell* 64, 109–119. doi: 10.1016/0248-4900(88)90070-6
28. Weiss, B. L., Savage, A. F., Griffith, B. C., Wu, Y., and Aksoy, S. (2014). The peritrophic matrix mediates differential infection outcomes in the tsetse fly gut following challenge with commensal, pathogenic, and parasitic microbes. *J. Immunol.* 193, 773–782. doi: 10.4049/jimmunol.1400163
29. Welburn, S. C., and Maudlin, I. (1999). Tsetse-trypanosome interactions: rites of passage. *Parasitol. Today* 15, 399–403. doi: 10.1016/S0169-4758 (99)01512-4
Welburn, S. C., Maudlin, I., and Simarro, P. P. (2009). Controlling
30. sleeping sickness-a review. *Parasitology* 136, 1943–1949. doi: 10.1017/S0031182009006416
31. Wixon, J., and Kell, D. (2000). The Kyoto encyclopedia of genes and genomes-KEGG. *Yeast* 17, 48–55. doi: 10.1002/(SICI)1097-0061(200004)17:1<48:: AID-YEA2>3.0.CO;2-H

12

Decoding the Role of Glycans in Malaria

Pollyanna S. Gomes[1], Daniel F. Feijó[2], Alexandre Morrot[1,3] and Celio G. Freire-de-Lima[4]**

[1] Departamento de Imunologia, Instituto de Microbiologia, Universidade Federal do Rio de Janeiro, Rio de Janeiro, Brazil, [2] Instituto Gonçalo Moniz, Fundação Oswaldo Cruz (Fiocruz), Salvador, Brazil, [3] Instituto Oswaldo Cruz, Fiocruz, Rio de Janeiro, Brazil, [4] Instituto de Biofísica Carlos Chagas Filho, Universidade Federal do Rio de Janeiro, Rio de Janeiro, Brazil

***Correspondence:**
Alexandre Morrot
morrot@micro.ufrj.br;
Célio Geraldo Freire-de-Lima
celio@biof.ufrj.br

Complications arising from malaria are a concern for public health authorities worldwide, since the annual caseload in humans usually exceeds millions. Of more than 160 species of *Plasmodium*, only 4 infect humans, with the most severe cases ascribed to *Plasmodium falciparum* and the most prevalent to *Plasmodium vivax*. Over the past 70 years, since World War II, when the first antimalarial drugs were widely used, many efforts have been made to combat this disease, including vectorial control, new drug discoveries and genetic and molecular approaches. Molecular approaches, such as glycobiology, may lead to new therapeutic targets (both in the host and the parasites), since all interactions are mediated by carbohydrates or glycan moieties decorating both cellular surfaces from parasite and host cells. In this review, we address the carbohydrate-mediated glycobiology that directly affects *Plasmodium* survival or host resistance.

Keywords: malaria, glycobiology, carbohydrate-targets, *Plasmodium falciparum*

INTRODUCTION

Malaria is caused by a protozoan of the *Plasmodium* genus, which belongs to the *Apicomplexans* phylum, an obligatory parasite (Kishore et al., 2013). Only in the last two decades has there been a significant reduction in malaria caseloads, and, according to the latest World Health Organization (WHO) records, cases have dropped significantly, i.e., from 262 million in 2000 to 214 million in 2015 (WHO, 2015). It is still a serious condition, however, noteworthy when compared to other pathologies of equal importance worldwide, due to its high prevalence (Binns and Low, 2015). Efforts toward the elimination of malaria involve the extermination of its vectors, and parasites and universal access to prevention (diagnosis and earlier treatment); this includes the discovery of new drugs, to deal with the high number of drug-resistant strains (Tanner and Hommel, 2010; Feng et al., 2016).

The first malaria drug treatments began with the use of quinine as the active ingredient (Parola and Miller, 2002). During World War II, a quinine-derivative, chloroquine, was widely used and treated as a "top secret" (Loff and Cordner, 1999; Skvara, 2004). Chloroquine was associated with many benefits (low cost, efficacy, and safety) (Kofoed et al., 2003; Savarino et al., 2006). Quinine-based drugs were replaced by Artemisinin derivatives and other drugs; and the use of Artemisinin-based Combined Therapies (ACT) is now recommended (Visser et al., 2014; Watsierah and Ouma, 2014; Pousibet-Puerto et al., 2016) to eliminate the blood phases, since in the exoerythrocytic phase (asymptomatic phase), there are no obvious symptoms for early treatment (Imrie et al., 2007).

Most of these drugs are still in use today in different doses, depending on the infective species and host background (Achan et al., 2011). Resistance is usually accompanied by a range of genetic diversity, and a high level of polymorphism, crucial to spreading these infective parasites but also after the widespread use of drugs, the first resistance-cases have appeared, and it seems that drugs have an "expiration date" this has also been observed in different malaria-infected patients in different regions, such as Thailand and Papua New Guinea (Cui et al., 2003; Brito and Ferreira, 2011). For example, *Plasmodium falciparum* shows high antigenic variation, with more than 60 coding variations of the *P. falciparum* erythrocyte membrane protein 1 (*Pf*EMP-1), directly related to the virulence and lethality of the infection of this species (Arnot and Jensen, 2011). On the other hand, may present variations in the merozoite surface protein MSP-3α is a multi-gene family important in *P. falciparum* and *Plasmodium vivax*, acting as "decoys" for antigenic diversity during RBCs invasion (Rice et al., 2014). CSP genes or circumsporozoite protein (CSP) in sporozoite surface, thrombospondin-related anonymous protein/sporozoite surface protein 2 (TRAP) or else in *P. vivax* apical membrane antigen 1 (AMA1) in ectodomain and C-terminal region of MSP-1 as a immunodominant antigen that was studied with recombinant protein (MSP119) as a novel potential vaccine (Rocha et al., 2017) and liver stage antigen (LSA1) also studied in malaria vaccine approaches (Pichyangkul et al., 2008).Thus, these and many more key proteins at each *Plasmodium* stage open up the "branches" for studies of this type of interactions, as seen in glycobiology.

CARBOHYDRATES IN MALARIA: APPROACH FOR POTENTIAL DRUG TARGET DISCOVERY

Glycosaminoglycans (GAGs) are abundant in both host and parasites; they are composed of basic units of carbohydrates that rearrange themselves in various ways, changing function and location (Griffin and Hsieh-Wilson, 2013). Glycobiological approaches investigate the influence of these carbohydrates on host-parasite binding interactions, such as glycolytic enzymes that are adequate in predicting a good understanding of parasite metabolism and glycosylation of malaria proteins. The first evidence about sugars mediatING the parasite-red blood cell invasion was cited by Miller et al. (1977). Experiments determinated that O-linked oligosaccharides, such as NeuNAc and GalNac, were found in high concentration (20 mM) and inhibited the parasite intracellular invasion in RBCs (Pasvol, 1984). Other sugars such as Gal (β1-3) GalNAc disaccharide associated with glycophorin was more inhibitory in the same context (Hermentin et al., 1984).

Thus, these tools give support to studies currently in development in this regard. In addition, some pathogen-associated molecular patterns (PAMPs) consist primarily of carbohydrates structures, although these are not yet well known or understood in malaria parasites (Hoving et al., 2014). However, recently, the most discussed PAMPs are GPI anchores, haemozoin, and immunostimulatory nucleic acid motifs (Gazzinelli et al., 2014).

Other crucial receptor crucial, that requires specific receptor-ligand interactions to RBC invasion and cytoadherence in malaria, is Duffy-binding-like domains (DBLs). In *P. vivax* and *P. knowlesi*, parasites invade RBC exclusively through the DARC receptors (Duffy antigen receptor for chemokines). However, in *P. knowlesi* DBL domain (Pkalpa-DBL) to due a immune pressure they seems development a evasion strategy to run away, mapping to opposite surface of the DBL.

Spitzmuller and Mestres (2013) addressed the design of a generation of new antimalarials drugs. A major challenge is to identify *P. falciparum* proteins, among million possible combinations that can be targeted at the same time by the just one drug. In their studies, they analyzed databases and to identify drugs with multi protein targets, because the drugs until now supported specific protein targets, which in a few time allows the parasite to mutate only at this target reaching. Unlikely, Artemisinin which is regarded as a multi-target drug, maintaining as a new generation drug and which is advocated throughout malaria treatment (Spitzmuller and Mestres, 2013).

Still regarding innate immunity, there are two major families of pattern recognition receptors (PPR) predominantly expressed by cells of innate immune system are TLRs and C-type lectin receptors (CLRs). CLRs are important for the immune response against parasites, and in some studies example has been observed that, for example, CLRs are related with cerebral malaria in mice infected by *Plasmodium berghei*, and CARD9 is upregulated, but CARD9$^{-/-}$ mice were not protected from infection, suggesting that the CARD9 receptor influences infectivity by the plasmodium but in its absence (as demonstrated in knockout animals) does not prevent the disease from occurring (McGuinness et al., 2003). Another study conducted with *P. chabaudi* demonstrated that the mannose receptor C type 2 (MRC2) increased with parasitemia, but toll-like receptors and sialoadhesin decreased in contrast to other MRCs (1 and 2), and that decreased with parasitemia in *P. yoelii*, suggesting the importance of lectin-receptors in the development of mounting of the immune response (Rosanas-Urgell et al., 2012).

Studies regarding parasite sugar supply demand has increased in the last decades, given that *Plasmodium* parasites require a high sugar demand to replicate. These parasites also show the ability to manipulate vector behavior to ensure survival, including increased sugar seeking, although it is unclear how this manipulation affects vector-plant interactions and sugar uptake (Nyasembe et al., 2014). Parasite manipulation in search of sugar supplies has been described as established at the moment of vector infection. *Plasmodium* present in the bloodstream require glucose, which crosses the plasma membranes and enters the parasite cytosol (Coppi et al., 2005; von Itzstein et al., 2008; Bertolino and Bowen, 2015; Swearingen et al., 2016). The parasites are able expose the RBC hexose transporter to facilitate sugar nucleotide uptake, allowing *Plasmodium* to biosynthesize certain glycans for maintenance (Cova et al., 2015). After the release of the sequence in the PlasmoDB, database facilitated the search for tools in interventions in this receptor for therapeutic purposes. The hexoses receptor (PfHT) has been widely studied, because its decrease implies in the lower supply of glucose to parasites and causing the plasmodium elimination (Bahl et al., 2003).

The surface of infected red blood cells (RBCs) are rich in glycophorins and *Plasmodium* possesses some proteins like erythrocytes binding-like (EBL) and reticulocyte binding-like (Rh) protein families that recognize them, playing a critical role in attachment in invasion (Davidson and Gowda, 2001; Salinas et al., 2014), Studies demonstrated that glycophorins as play crucial role in *Plasmodium* invasion, in absence of glycophorins A relatively resistant to the invasion in red blood cells (Pasvol, 1984). Other portion of glycophorin A has sialic acid residues, which is known as EBA-175 (175 kDa), and it mediates binding of *P. falciparum* to RBCs. A part of this, EBA-175 is highly conserved and rich in cysteine, is referred to as F2 (PfF2) and it has receptor binding sites that have been studied as a possible recombinant protein in malaria vaccines trials (Pattnaik et al., 2007).

In Tham et al. (2015) the cytoplasmatic tails of these proteins were phosphorylated *in vitro* and blocked RBC invasion, evidencing the importance of these proteins for invasion (Tham et al., 2015).

In addition to studies on the interactions between the parasite and carbohydrates in RBCs, it has been demonstrated that blood type (ABO, Lewis, Duffy, and others surface antigens) influences erythrocyte parasitism, with certain types more susceptible to *Plasmodium* infection (Cooling, 2015). Studies indicate that individuals of blood group A are highly susceptible to *P. falciparum* induced-malaria, while blood group O has been shown to be protective against complicated cases (Fischer and Boone, 1998; Lell et al., 1999). The CSP and TRAP domains on the sporozoite that mediate the adhesive contact with the sulphated glycoconjugates on the surface of hepatocytes allow plasmodium invasion to the bloodstream. Thus, these proteins are extremely important for the parasite, since it is from the entry in the hepatocytes that the cycle begins. Taking this into account, these same proteins have been studied extensively, including in the manufacturing of anti-malarial vaccines, such as RTS,S (Coppi et al., 2005; Swearingen et al., 2016). Despite having obtained good results in treating mice with anti-CSP, it has been verified that, in the absence of this protein, the cycle of hepatocyte invasion continues normally, since after invasion CSPs are less expressed, while other proteins become highly expressed (Bertolino and Bowen, 2015).

As the *Plasmodium* parasite uses sugar-requirements to ensure survival, approaches with drug-targeting carbohydrates have increasingly been proposed as possible treatments. Regarding *in vitro* studies, Plaimas et al. (2013) investigated a database of genetic information from *Plasmodium* to try to decipher which points of the proteins expressed could be future of therapeutic targets. 22 potential targets, refined the search by removing false positives, leaving only 5 targets, among them, glutamyl-tRNA (gln) aminotransferase and with a known inhibitor of this transferase 6-diazo-5-oxonorleucine (Don). The tests were carried out and the growth of the parasite decreased both *in vitro* and *in vivo* in Swiss mice, despite the side effects related to the dosage (Plaimas et al., 2013). Similar results have recently been observed with DON in experimental cerebral malaria mice models, although this compound has shown inhibitory effects by blocking CD8+ T-cell effector function, which is the highest cause of mice death (Gordon et al., 2015). On the other hand, other studies indicate that mice mortality was attenuated due to GPI anchors, not T cells, since several literature reports indicate the importance of glycophosphatidylinositol (GPI) anchors for the success of *Plasmodium* infection (Naik et al., 2000). CSP have also been associated to GPI, which have a canonical domain in the COOH portion, although this has not yet been demonstrated (Coppi et al., 2005).

Of significance, people living in endemic areas are more resistant to malaria, due to the production of antibodies against GPI anchors (Vijaykumar et al., 2001).

In addition to inhibitors that hinder this type of parasite-host interaction, mice immunized with the glycan moiety of GPIs were able to produce anti-GPI antibodies to prevent progression to cerebral malaria (Schofield et al., 2002). It has been reported that a microbial polyssacharide, Gellan Gum (GG), containing a sugar moiety produced by the *Sphingomonas* (*Pseudomonas*) *elodea* bacterium, strongly inhibited parasite invasion; this also inhibits growth (strains 3D7 and Dd2), demonstrating that "natural" sugars can also contain *Plasmodium* effects (Recuenco et al., 2014). In human malaria, successive pregnancies contribute to resistance against *Plasmodium*, which mediates binding to chondroitin sulfate A (CSA) in the placenta through the VAR2CSA protein (Salanti et al., 2004; Gamain et al., 2005); this leads to accumulation of *Plasmodium* parasites in the placenta, resulting in severe clinical consequences for both mother and child (Resende et al., 2008), such that the investigation of this interaction is a viable target for vaccines (Clausen et al., 2012; Fried and Duffy, 2017). Through all this information about the various receivers composed by sugar and the interactions required these reinforce the importance of deciphering the nature of glycan functions in malaria in order to improve approaches for predicting drug-target interactions for this complex.

AUTHOR CONTRIBUTIONS

PSG, DFF, AM, and CGF-de-L wrote the paper. All authors read and approved the final version of the manuscript.

ACKNOWLEDGMENTS

This work was supported by grants from the Conselho Nacional de Desenvolvimento Científico e Tecnológico do Brasil (CNPq) and the Fundação de Amparo à Pesquisa do Estado do Rio de Janeiro (FAPERJ).

REFERENCES

1. Achan, J., Talisuna, A. O., Erhart, A., Yeka, A., Tibenderana, J. K., Baliraine, F. N., et al. (2011). Quinine, an old anti-malarial drug in a modern world: role in the treatment of malaria. *Malar. J.* 10:144. doi: 10.1186/1475-2875-10-144
2. Arnot, D. E., and Jensen, A. T. (2011). Antigenic variation and the genetics and epigenetics of the PfEMP1 erythrocyte surface antigens in *Plasmodium falciparum* Malaria. *Adv. Appl. Microbiol.* 74, 77–96. doi: 10.1016/B978-0-12-387022-3.00007-0
3. Bahl, A., Brunk, B., Crabtree, J., Fraunholz, M. J., Gajria, B., Grant, G. R., et al. (2003). PlasmoDB: the Plasmodium genome resource. A database integrating experimental and computational data. *Nucleic Acids Res.* 31, 212–215. doi: 10.1093/nar/gkg081
4. Bertolino, P., and Bowen, D. G. (2015). Malaria and the liver: immunological hide-and-seek or subversion of immunity from within? *Front. Microbiol.* 6:41. doi: 10.3389/fmicb.2015.00041
5. Binns, C., and Low, W. Y. (2015). Malaria continues as a major public health problem. *Asia Pac. J. Public Health* 27, 261–262. doi: 10.1177/1010539515583388
6. Brito, C. F., and Ferreira, M. U. (2011). Molecular markers and genetic diversity of *Plasmodium vivax*. *Mem. Inst. Oswaldo Cruz* 106 (Suppl. 1), 12–26. doi: 10.1590/S0074-02762011000900003
7. Clausen, T. M., Christoffersen, S., Dahlback, M., Langkilde, A. E., Jensen, K. E., Resende, M., et al. (2012). Structural and functional insight into how the *Plasmodium falciparum* VAR2CSA protein mediates binding to chondroitin sulfate A in placental malaria. *J. Biol. Chem.* 287, 23332–23345. doi: 10.1074/jbc.M112.348839
8. Cooling, L. (2015). Blood Groups in Infection and Host Susceptibility. *Clin. Microbiol. Rev.* 28, 801–870. doi: 10.1128/CMR.00109-14
9. Coppi, A., Pinzon-Ortiz, C., Hutter, C., and Sinnis, P. (2005). The Plasmodium circumsporozoite protein is proteolytically processed during cell invasion. *J. Exp. Med.* 201, 27–33. doi: 10.1084/jem.20040989
10. Cova, M., Rodrigues, J. A., Smith, T. K., and Izquierdo, L. (2015). Sugar activation and glycosylation in Plasmodium. *Malar. J.* 14, 427. doi: 10.1186/s12936-015-0949-z
11. Cui, L., Mascorro, C. N., Fan, Q., Rzomp, K. A., Khuntirat, B., Zhou, G., et al. (2003). Genetic diversity and multiple infections of *Plasmodium vivax* malaria in Western Thailand. *Am. J. Trop. Med. Hyg.* 68, 613–619. doi: 10.4269/ajtmh.2003.68.613
12. Davidson, E. A., and Gowda, D. C. (2001). Glycobiology of *Plasmodium falciparum*. *Biochimie* 83, 601–604. doi: 10.1016/S0300-9084(01)01316-5
13. Feng, J., Liu, J., Feng, X., Zhang, L., Xiao, H., and Xia, Z. (2016). Towards Malaria Elimination: Monitoring and Evaluation of the "1-3-7" Approach at the China-Myanmar Border. *Am. J. Trop. Med. Hyg.* 95, 806–810. doi: 10.4269/ajtmh.15-0888
14. Fischer, P. R., and Boone, P. (1998). Short report: severe malaria associated with blood group. *Am. J. Trop. Med. Hyg.* 58, 122–123.
15. Fried, M., and Duffy, P. E. (2017). Malaria during pregnancy. *Cold Spring Harb. Perspect. Med.* 7:a025551. doi: 10.1101/cshperspect.a025551
16. Gamain, B., Trimnell, A. R., Scheidig, C., Scherf, A., Miller, L. H., and Smith, J. D. (2005). Identification of multiple chondroitin sulfate A (CSA)-binding domains in the var2CSA gene transcribed in CSA-binding parasites. *J. Infect. Dis.* 191, 1010–1013. doi: 10.1086/428137
17. Gazzinelli, R. T., Kalantari, P., Fitzgerald, K. A., and Golenbock, D. T. (2014). Innate sensing of malaria parasites. *Nat. Rev. Immunol.* 14, 744–757. doi: 10.1038/nri3742
18. Gordon, E. B., Hart, G. T., Tran, T. M., Waisberg, M., Akkaya, M., Kim, A. S., et al. (2015). Targeting glutamine metabolism rescues mice from late-stage cerebral malaria. *Proc. Natl. Acad. Sci. U.S.A.* 112, 13075–13080. doi: 10.1073/pnas.1516544112
19. Griffin, M. E., and Hsieh-Wilson, L. C. (2013). Synthetic probes of glycosaminoglycan function. *Curr. Opin. Chem. Biol.* 17, 1014–1022. doi: 10.1016/j.cbpa.2013.09.015
20. Hermentin, P., Paulsen, H., Kolar, C., and Enders, B. (1984). *Plasmodium falciparum*: carbohydrates as receptor sites of invasion. *Exp. Parasitol.* 58, 290–306.
21. Hoving, J. C., Wilson, G. J., and Brown, G. D. (2014). Signalling C-type lectin receptors, microbial recognition and immunity. *Cell. Microbiol.* 16, 185–194. doi: 10.1111/cmi.12249
22. Imrie, H., Fowkes, F. J., Michon, P., Tavul, L., Reeder, J. C., and Day, K. P. (2007). Low prevalence of an acute phase response in asymptomatic children from a malaria-endemic area of Papua New Guinea. *Am. J. Trop. Med. Hyg.* 76, 280–284. doi: 10.4269/ajtmh.2007.76.280
23. Kishore, S. P., Stiller, J. W., and Deitsch, K. W. (2013). Horizontal gene transfer of epigenetic machinery and evolution of parasitism in the malaria parasite *Plasmodium falciparum* and other apicomplexans. *BMC Evol. Biol.* 13:37. doi: 10.1186/1471-2148-13-37
24. Kofoed, P. E., Poulsen, A., Co, F., Hedegaard, K., Aaby, P., and Rombo, L. (2003). No benefits from combining chloroquine with artesunate for three days for treatment of *Plasmodium falciparum* in Guinea-Bissau. *Trans. R. Soc. Trop. Med. Hyg.* 97, 429–433. doi: 10.1016/S0035-9203(03)90078-2
25. Lell, B., May, J., Schmidt-Ott, R. J., Lehman, L. G., Luckner, D., Greve, B., et al. (1999). The role of red blood cell polymorphisms in resistance and susceptibility to malaria. *Clin. Infect. Dis.* 28, 794–799. doi: 10.1086/515193
26. Loff, B., and Cordner, S. (1999). World War II malaria trials revisited. *Lancet* 353, 1597.
27. McGuinness, D. H., Dehal, P. K., and Pleass, R. J. (2003). Pattern recognition molecules and innate immunity to parasites. *Trends Parasitol.* 19, 312–319. doi: 10.1016/S1471-4922(03)00123-5
28. Miller, L. H., Haynes, J. D., McAuliffe, F. M., Shiroishi, T., Durocher, J. R., and McGinniss, M. H. (1977). Evidence for differences in erythrocyte surface receptors for the malarial parasites, *Plasmodium falciparum* and *Plasmodium knowlesi*. *J. Exp. Med.* 146, 277–281.
29. Naik, R. S., Davidson, E. A., and Gowda, D. C. (2000). Developmental stage-specific biosynthesis of glycosylphosphatidylinositol anchors in intraerythrocytic *Plasmodium falciparum* and its inhibition in a novel manner by mannosamine. *J. Biol. Chem.* 275, 24506–24511. doi: 10.1074/jbc.M002151200
30. Nyasembe, V. O., Teal, P. E., Sawa, P., Tumlinson, J. H., Borgemeister, C., and Torto, B. (2014). *Plasmodium falciparum* infection increases *Anopheles gambiae* attraction to nectar sources and sugar uptake. *Curr. Biol.* 24, 217–221. doi: 10.1016/j.cub.2013.12.022
31. Parola, P., and Miller, R. S. (2002). Quinine in the modern treatment of falciparum malaria. *Lancet Infect. Dis.* 2, 206–207. doi: 10.1016/S1473-3099(02)00237-2 Pasvol, G. (1984). Receptors on red cells for *Plasmodium falciparum* and their interaction with merozoites. *Philos. Trans. R. Soc. Lond. B. Biol. Sci.* 307, 189–200.
32. Pattnaik, P., Shakri, A. R., Singh, S., Goel, S., Mukherjee, P., and Chitnis, C. E. (2007). Immunogenicity of a recombinant malaria vaccine based on receptor binding domain of *Plasmodium falciparum* EBA-175. *Vaccine* 25, 806–813. doi: 10.1016/j.vaccine.2006.09.048
33. Pichyangkul, S., Kum-Arb, U., Yongvanitchit, K., Limsalakpetch, A., Gettayacamin, M., Lanar, D. E., et al. (2008). Preclinical evaluation of the safety and immunogenicity of a vaccine consisting of *Plasmodium falciparum* liver-stage antigen 1 with adjuvant AS01B administered alone or concurrently with the RTS,S/AS01B vaccine in rhesus primates. *Infect. Immun.* 76, 229–238. doi: 10.1128/IAI.00977-07
34. Plaimas, K., Wang, Y., Rotimi, S. O., Olasehinde, G., Fatumo, S., Lanzer, M., et al. (2013). Computational and experimental analysis identified 6-diazo- 5-oxonorleucine as a potential agent for treating infection by *Plasmodium falciparum*. *Infect. Genet. Evol.* 20, 389–395. doi: 10.1016/j.meegid.2013.09.019
35. Pousibet-Puerto, J., Salas-Coronas, J., Sanchez-Crespo, A., Molina-Arrebola, M. A., Soriano-Perez, M. J., Gimenez-Lopez, M. J., et al. (2016). Impact of using artemisinin-based combination therapy (ACT) in the treatment of uncomplicated malaria from *Plasmodium falciparum* in a non-endemic zone. *Malar. J.* 15, 339. doi: 10.1186/s12936-016-1408-1
36. Recuenco, F. C., Kobayashi, K., Ishiwa, A., Enomoto-Rogers, Y., Fundador, N. G., Sugi, T., et al. (2014). Gellan sulfate inhibits *Plasmodium falciparum* growth and invasion of red blood cells *in vitro*. *Sci. Rep.* 4:4723. doi: 10.1038/srep04723
37. Resende, M., Nielsen, M. A., Dahlback, M., Ditlev, S. B., Andersen, P., Sander, A. F., et al. (2008). Identification of glycosaminoglycan binding regions in the *Plasmodium falciparum* encoded placental sequestration ligand, VAR2CSA. *Malar. J.* 7:104. doi: 10.1186/1475-2875-7-104
38. Rice, B. L., Acosta, M. M., Pacheco, M. A., Carlton, J. M., Barnwell, J.

W., and Escalante, A. A. (2014). The origin and diversification of the merozoite surface protein 3 (msp3) multi-gene family in *Plasmodium vivax* and related parasites. *Mol. Phylogenet. Evol.* 78, 172–184. doi: 10.1016/j.ympev.2014.05.013

39. Rocha, M. V., Francoso, K. S., Lima, L. C., Camargo, T. M., Machado, R. L., Costa, F. T., et al. (2017). Generation, characterization and immunogenicity of a novel chimeric recombinant protein based on *Plasmodium vivax* AMA-1 and MSP119. *Vaccine* 35, 2463–2472. doi: 10.1016/j.vaccine.2017. 03.023
40. Rosanas-Urgell, A., Martin-Jaular, L., Ricarte-Filho, J., Ferrer, M., Kalko, S., Kimura, E., et al. (2012). Expression of non-TLR pattern recognition receptors in the spleen of BALB/c mice infected with *Plasmodium yoelii* and *Plasmodium chabaudi* chabaudi AS. *Mem. Inst. Oswaldo Cruz* 107, 410–415. doi: 10.1590/S0074-02762012000300017
41. Salanti, A., Dahlback, M., Turner, L., Nielsen, M. A., Barfod, L., Magistrado, P., et al. (2004). Evidence for the involvement of VAR2CSA in pregnancy-associated malaria. *J. Exp. Med.* 200, 1197–1203. doi: 10.1084/jem.200break41579
42. Salinas, N. D., Paing, M. M., and Tolia, N. H. (2014). Critical glycosylated residues in exon three of erythrocyte glycophorin A engage *Plasmodium falciparum* EBA-175 and define receptor specificity. *MBio* 5, e01606–e01614. doi: 10.1128/mBio.01606-14
43. Savarino, A., Lucia, M. B., Giordano, F., and Cauda, R. (2006). Risks and benefits of chloroquine use in anticancer strategies. *Lancet Oncol.* 7, 792–793. doi: 10.1016/S1470-204570875-0
44. Schofield, L., Hewitt, M. C., Evans, K., Siomos, M. A., and Seeberger, P. H. (2002). Synthetic GPI as a candidate anti-toxic vaccine in a model of malaria. *Nature* 418, 785–789. doi: 10.1038/nature00937
45. Skvara, F. C. (2004). World War II: exhibit pages (The Red Cross society, blood transfusions, discovery of penicillin, malaria). *Scalpel Tongs* 48, 60–64.
46. Spitzmuller, A., and Mestres, J. (2013). Prediction of the *P. falciparum* target space relevant to malaria drug discovery. *PLoS Comput. Biol.* 9:e1003257. doi: 10.1371/journal.pcbi.1003257
47. Swearingen, K. E., Lindner, S. E., Shi, L., Shears, M. J., Harupa, A., Hopp, C. S., et al. (2016). Interrogating the Plasmodium Sporozoite Surface: Identification of Surface-Exposed Proteins and Demonstration of Glycosylation on CSP and TRAP by Mass Spectrometry-Based Proteomics. *PLoS Pathog.* 12:e10 05606. doi: 10.1371/journal.ppat.1005606
48. Tanner, M., and Hommel, M. (2010). Towards malaria elimination–a new thematic series. *Malar. J.* 9:24. doi: 10.1186/1475-2875-9-24
49. Tham, W. H., Lim, N. T., Weiss, G. E., Lopaticki, S., Ansell, B. R., Bird, M., et al. (2015). *Plasmodium falciparum* adhesins play an essential role in signalling and activation of invasion into human erythrocytes. *PLoS Pathog.* 11:e1005343. doi: 10.1371/journal.ppat.1005343
50. Vijaykumar, M., Naik, R. S., and Gowda, D. C. (2001). *Plasmodium falciparum* glycosylphosphatidylinositol-induced TNF-α secretion by macrophages is mediated without membrane insertion or endocytosis. *J. Biol. Chem.* 276, 6909–6912. doi: 10.1074/jbc.C100007200
51. Visser, B. J., Wieten, R. W., Kroon, D., Nagel, I. M., Belard, S., van Vugt, M., et al. (2014). Efficacy and safety of artemisinin combination therapy (ACT) for non-falciparum malaria: a systematic review. *Malar. J.* 13:463. doi: 10.1186/1475-2875-13-463
52. von Itzstein, M., Plebanski, M., Cooke, B. M., and Coppel, R. L. (2008). Hot, sweet and sticky: the glycobiology of *Plasmodium falciparum*. *Trends Parasitol.* 24, 210–218. doi: 10.1016/j.pt.2008.02.007
53. Watsierah, C. A., and Ouma, C. (2014). Access to artemisinin-based combination therapy (ACT) and quinine in malaria holoendemic regions of western Kenya. *Malar. J.* 13:290. doi: 10.1186/1475-2875-13-290
54. WHO (2015). *World Malaria Report 2015.* Geneva: WHO.

13

Canine Macrophage DH82 Cell Line as a Model to Study Susceptibility to *Trypanosoma cruzi* Infection

Pedro Henrique Braz Mendonça[1], Raphael Francisco Dutra Barbosa da Rocha[1], Julliane Brito de Braz Moraes[1], Isabel Ferreira LaRocque-de-Freitas[2], Jorgete Logullo[2], Alexandre Morrot[3], Marise Pinheiro Nunes[4], Celio Geraldo Freire-de-Lima[2] and Debora Decote-Ricardo[1]**

[1] Instituto de Veterinária, Universidade Federal Rural do Rio de Janeiro, Rio de Janeiro, Brazil, [2] Instituto de Biofísica Carlos Chagas Filho, Universidade Federal do Rio de Janeiro, Rio de Janeiro, Brazil, [3] Instituto de Microbiologia Paulo de Góes, Universidade Federal do Rio de Janeiro, Rio de Janeiro, Brazil, [4] Instituto Oswaldo Cruz, FIOCRUZ, Rio de Janeiro, Brazil

***Correspondence:**
Celio Geraldo Freire-de-Lima
celio@biof.ufrj.br;
Debora Decote-Ricardo
decotericardo@ufrrj.br

Trypanosoma cruzi is an obligatory intracellular protozoan parasite, and it is the etiological agent of Chagas' disease that is endemic in the Americas. In addition to humans, a wide spectrum of mammals can be infected by *T. cruzi*, including dogs. Dogs develop acute and chronic disease, similar to human infection. *T. cruzi* can infect almost all cell types and after cell invasion, the metacyclics trypomastigotes localize in the cytoplasm, where they transform into amastigotes, the replicative form of *T. cruzi* in mammals. After amastigote multiplication and differentiation, parasites lyse host cells and spread through the body by blood circulation. In this work, we evaluated the *in vitro* ability of *T. cruzi* to infect a canine macrophage cell line DH82 compared with RAW264.7, a murine tissue culture macrophage. Our results have shown that the *T. cruzi* is able to infect, replicate and differentiate in DH82 cell line. We observed that following treatment with LPS and IFN-γ DH82 cells were more resistant to infection and that resistance was not related reactive oxygen species production in our system. In this study, we also found that DH82 cells became more susceptible to *T. cruzi* infection when cocultured with apoptotic cells. The analysis of cytokine production has showed elevated levels of the TGF-β, IL-10, and TNF-α produced by *T. cruzi*-infected canine macrophages. Additionally, we demonstrated a reduced expression of the MHC class II and CD80 by infected DH82 cell line.

Keywords: *Trypanosoma cruzi*, chagas disease, dogs, macrophages, immunomodulation, infection model, susceptibility

INTRODUCTION

Chagas' disease is caused by the protozoan hemoflagellate *Trypanosoma cruzi*, which is transmitted by a blood-sucking reduviid bugs (1). Although it was described more than 100 years ago, this disease remains a serious public health problem in South and Central America countries, which come to account for 12 million to 14 million of infected people (2).

The *T. cruzi* infection begins when the infective metacyclic trypomastigotes forms are transmitted to humans or other mammals by the infected feces of triatomine bugs. Trypomastigotes are able to invade cells, phagocytic or non-phagocytic, differentiate, and multiply in almost all mammalian nucleated cells, including macrophages, muscle cells, glial cells, neurons, fibroblasts, adipocytes, and endothelial cells. After cell invasion trypomastigotes transform into amastigotes, that multiply intensively, then transform into trypomastigotes and finally break the host-infected cells. After reaching the bloodstream and lymphatic vessels, blood trypomastigotes can invade other tissues, penetrate the cells, and differentiate again into amastigotes, forming new multiplying foci. Due to the cyclical sequence of these events, a rapid increase of circulating trypomastigotes is observed. Thus, during the acute phase of Chagas' disease parasitemia is readily detectable by fresh blood examination. After the acute phase, there is a latent phase of infection, also called indeterminate phase, which can last for long periods of time or can be permanent, then develops into a chronic stage (3).

Trypanosoma cruzi can infect a wide range of wild and domestic mammals that serve as parasite reservoirs. Dogs play an important role in domestic cycle of infection representing a risk factor for humans (4, 5). Naturally infected dogs or seropositive dogs were detected in the United States (6), Mexico, Argentina, Venezuela, and Panama (7, 8). In Brazil, the presence of infected animals was also reported in different areas of the country (5, 9). The canine Chagas' disease is becoming a major veterinarian concern in the Americas (8).

Trypanosoma cruzi-infected dogs reproduce several aspects of the infection observed in humans. In the acute phase of infection, dogs develop lymphadenopathy and hepatosplenomegaly and show circulating blood trypomastigotes (10). In animals that progress to the chronic phase of infection, cardiac involvement with cardiomegaly occurs (11). Recently, it was reported that seropositive dogs exhibit high levels of IgG that correlates with the severity of myocarditis, characterized by mononuclear cell infiltrates (12). In experimentally infected dogs of Beagle breed, it was observed high levels of proinflammatory cytokines such as INF-γ, TNF-α, and low IL-10 levels in the acute phase of infection. These data suggest that the development of chronic heart abnormalities may be related to a strong Th1-type response during the acute phase (10). Using Beagle dogs infected by two distinct genetic groups of parasites, Guedes and coworkers (10) showed that the cardiac type 1/2 chemokines and their receptors expression depend on the genetic diversity of parasites that can determine the migration of Th1 or Th2 cells to the heart during the acute and chronic phases of the disease. In addition, they have showed that infected dogs that develop the cardiac form of disease, have increased expression of CCL5, CCL4, and CXCR3 type 1 chemokines receptors when compared with dogs in the indeterminate phase of the disease (13).

Trypanosoma cruzi invasion strategy demonstrates its ability to subvert the macrophage antimicrobial defense mechanisms. The trypomastigotes interact with host cells by inducing a signal that results in lysosomes recruitment in a Ca^{+}-dependent manner. Initially, parasites enter the cells and are located inside parasitophorous vacuoles, at that time *T. cruzi* releases a hemolysin called TcTox to able escape into the host cell cytoplasm (14).

The intracellular signaling of macrophages can be triggered by the innate immunity receptor is also explored by *T. cruzi*. Parasite-derived molecules, like trypomastigote-derived glycosylphosphatidylinositol anchors of mucin-like glycoproteins, can be recognized by toll-like receptors (TLR2) and initiate a cascade of signals that induces the production of IL-12, TNF-α, and nitric oxide (NO) (15–17). The *T. cruzi* GPI-mucin can induce a state of tolerance phenomena in macrophages *in vitro*, similar to that observed when macrophages were stimulated by LPS (18). These researchers showed that macrophages stimulated with low doses of LPS have a lock response to a second stimulus with LPS. This resulted in suppression of IL-12 and TNF-α production, while the production of NO and IL-10 was not affected.

These mechanisms of tolerance induced by endotoxin interfere with the signaling pathways mediated by TLR4, resulting in decreased activation of MAPK and the p50 subunit NFκB. It has been shown that stimulation of macrophages by LPS then mucin-GPI *T. cruzi* produces a tolerogenic effect associated with defects in phosphorylation of IRAK-1, MAPK activation, and degradation IκB (19). An important aspect of these data is the fact that TLR activation can lead to suppression of another TLR, resulting in blocking the activation of macrophages (20). Thus, the interaction between the parasite and the host cell could modulate the activation process that favors the invasion and persistence of the parasite.

Besides, to directly affect macrophages, infection with *T. cruzi* can produce a modulating effect through the deleterious events affecting other cell populations. An important feature observed during experimental infection with *T. cruzi* is an intense $CD4^{+}$ T cell death by apoptosis (21). The interaction of macrophages with apoptotic bodies leads to TGF-β production that induces the deactivation of macrophages making it more susceptible to infection (22).

Various studies have used cell culture systems derived from mammals to understand the interaction between the host and different *T. cruzi* strains. Spleen and peritoneal macrophages obtained from a variety of mouse strains have been widely used to study *T. cruzi* infectivity *in vitro*. Although the importance of dogs as domestic reservoir, as a model for testing of vaccines and new drugs for the treatment of Chagas' disease is recognized, there is a lack of experimental studies with dog macrophages. Here we have investigated the *in vitro* infectivity rate of trypomastigotes and the replication of amastigotes of *T. cruzi* Dm28c in dog DH82 and mouse RAW264.7 tissue culture macrophages. The DH82 cell is a line isolated from a dog presenting malignant histiocytosis, this lineage shows macrophages morphology and is excellent phagocytic cells. Also, express in the cell surface Fc-gamma receptor and are negative for the C3b receptor (23).

In the present study, we demonstrated that DH82 cells are susceptible to *T. cruzi* infection and the parasites were able to modulate expression of the MHC class II, CD80, and cytokines production.

MATERIALS AND METHODS

Cell Culture

To prepare tissue culture cells for infection, DH82 and RAW264.7 cells (ATCC) were grown in 75 cm^2 tissue culture flasks (T75) (Nunc, Roskilde, Denmark) with Dulbecco's Modified Eagle Medium (DMEM; Sigma-Aldrich) supplemented with 10% fetal calf serum (FCS; Gibco), 100 μg/mL of streptomycin and 100 Units/mL of penicillin, 1% MEM non-essential amino acids (Sigma-Aldrich), and 2 mM of L-glutamine were cultured at

37°C with 5% CO_2. Subcultures of both cell lines were carried out once a week, when they reached a confluence of 95–100%. Cells were released with 0.25% of trypsin (Difco) and 1 mM of EDTA (Sigma-Aldrich), harvested, and washed twice in HBSS by centrifugation at room temperature for 10 min at 250*g*. The supernatant was discarded, cell pellet was resuspended in DMEM containing 10% FCS, cultured into new T75 flasks, and culture medium was changed after 3 days in culture. Prior to use in infectivity assays, cells' viability was assessed by trypan blue exclusion in a hemocytometer.

Parasites and Infection

Infection of DH82 and RAW264.7 cell lines were carried out in 24-well plates at a concentration of 2.0×10^5 macrophages/well. Cells were infected overnight with chemically induced metacyclic trypomastigotes forms of *T. cruzi* clone Dm28c, obtained as previously described (24), at a 1:1, 3:1, and 5:1 parasite-to-cell ratios in 1 mL of DMEM 10% FCS and incubated at 37°C in 5% CO_2. In the following day (day 1), monolayers were extensively washed to remove extracellular parasites and cultured with complete culture medium containing 1% Nutridoma (Sigma-Aldrich) instead of FCS. Some cultures were stimulated with 400 ng/mL of lipopolysaccharides from *Salmonella enterica* serotype typhimurium (LPS, Sigma-Aldrich) and 1.5 ng/mL of recombinant canine or murine IFN-γ (Serotech) 24 h after infection. DH82 and RAW264.7 were also seeded in 24-well plate containing glass coverslips for parasite burden evaluation. Three days after infection, coverslips were washed with HBSS, fixed with methanol, and stained with Diff-Quick (Thermo Fisher, Waltham, MA, USA). Amastigotes were counted at 100× oil immersion on a (Olympus) microscope. The number of amastigotes was estimated in 100 infected cells per coverslip, and the frequency of infection was compared among six coverslips per time point. The number of viable trypomastigotes released in the supernatants was evaluated each 2 days of culture for 9 days, using a Neubauer chamber. We also conducted experiments using *T. cruzi* of CL strain transfected with green fluorescent protein (GFP) (25) obtained from Vero cells. The DH82 cells were infected overnight (ON). After that, the monolayers were washed, and DH82 cells were stained with DAPI 1.5 μg/mL (VECTASHIELD®) at room temperature for 30 min before examination by confocal microscopy Zeiss Axioplan.

Detection of Reactive Oxygen Species (ROS)

Intracellular levels of ROS were quantified by oxydation of non-fluorescent 2′,7′-dichlorofluorescein probe, delivered as diacetate form (DCFH-DA), to the fluorescent product 2′,7′-dichlorofluorescein (26). DH82 cells were seeded in 96-well plate (5.0×10^4 cells/well), infected with metacyclic trypomastigotes at a ratio of 5:1 (parasite/cell), stimulated or not with LPS (400 ng/mL, Sigma-Aldrich) and recombinant IFN-γ (1.5 ng/mL, Serotech) and after 1, 2, 3, and 4 h later cells were washed and loaded with 10 μM DCFH-DA (Invitrogen) for 20 min at 37°C. Uninfected cells were used as negative control. In different checkpoints, the cells were washed, and fluorescence was measured (excitation = 485 nm excitation; λ emission = 535 nm) in an FLx800 Fluorescence Microplate Reader (BioTek).

Detection of Nitric Oxide (NO)

Quantification of NO DH82 and RAW264.7 (2.5×10^5/mL) was cultivated in the presence of LPS (200 or 400 ng/mL) and INF-γ (1.5 ng/mL). After 12 and 24 h of incubation, NO production was evaluated by the presence of the nitrite accumulated in the supernatant of cultures using Griess colorimetric method.

Apoptotic Lymphocytes and Coculture with DH82

In order to evaluate the effect of apoptotic lymphocytes in *T. cruzi* growth *in vitro*, we have used two approaches. In both approaches, DH82 macrophages were seeded into 24-well plate at a concentration of 2.0×10^5 cells/well, incubated for 1 h at 37°C in a humidified atmosphere with 5% CO_2 and the adherent monolayer was washed to remove non-adherent cells. Apoptotic cells were prepared as previously described (27). Briefly, single cell suspension of the Jurkat human lymphoblastoid cells was prepared and irradiated with 30 Gy (Apo-2) as previous described (27). We first performed experiments with *T. cruzi*-infected DH82 monolayers at a 5:1 parasite/cell ratio. Extracellular parasites were removed by washing the wells with HBSS and then apoptotic lymphocytes were added to the cultures at a 5:1 apoptotic lymphocyte:macrophage ratio, and kept at 37°C with 5% CO_2 for 9 days. In other experiments, prior to *T. cruzi* infection, the DH82 monolayer were incubated with apoptotic lymphocytes at a 5:1 apoptotic lymphocyte:macrophage ratio for 2 h at 37°C with 5% CO_2. After that period non-internalized apoptotic cells were removed and adherent macrophages were infected with *T. cruzi* at 5:1 parasite:macrophage ratio for ON at 37°C. After removing free parasites, the medium was replaced and infected DH82 cells were further incubated at 37°C with 5% CO_2. In both experiments, the extracellular motile trypomastigotes were determined in cell supernatants after 9 days in culture by counting parasites in Neubauer chambers (28).

Cytokine Determination

Cell supernatants were collected at 24 h postinfection for cytokine determination. TNF-α, TGF-β, and IL-10 concentration was estimated by the method of sandwich immunoassay (ELISA) according to methodology recommended by the manufacturer (R&D). The optical density was evaluated by reading in a microplate spectrophotometer (Versamax Microplates Reader Molecular Devices, USA), with filter of 405 nm.

Flow Cytometric Analysis

To assess the expression of MHC class II and CD80 on DH82 macrophage cell line by flow cytometric analysis, cells were infected or not with *T. cruzi* Dm28c and were activated or not in the presence of recombinant IFN-γ and LPS. Cells were detached at 24 h postinfection, washed, adjusted to a concentration of 5.0×10^5 cells/tube and blocked with anti-CD16/CD32 (Calbiochem) at concentration of the 1 μg/10^6 cells to prevent non-specific antibody binding to Fc-receptors. Cells were stained with MHC class II-FITC, and CD80-PE antibodies (Serotech). All washing steps were performed with phosphate-buffered saline containing 3% bovine serum albumin and 0.02% of sodium azide. Data were acquired (10,000 events), evaluated on FACSCalibur™ cytometer, and analyzed using Cell-Quest® software (BD Biosciences, Heidelberg, Germany). Analyzed gates of scattered dot plots were adjusted not to exceed 2% of positive staining cells related to the particular negative controls (29).

Statistical Analysis

Statistical analysis was performed in the program GraphPad InStat version 3.01 (San Diego, USA). Data were analyzed by the method of Student's *t*-test. Differences at *p*-value 0.05 or lower were reported as significant for a given comparison.

RESULTS

DH82 Canine Macrophages Are Infected by *T. cruzi*

Previously published studies report *T. cruzi* infection of various mouse macrophage cell lines to study the infectivity of *T. cruzi* strains *in vitro* (30), but infection of dog macrophages has not been showed. In order to evaluate the susceptibility of DH82, a canine macrophage cell line, to *T. cruzi* Dm 28c infection, cells were plated and infected at different parasite:cell ratios. We found that canine macrophages were infected and after 5 days in culture parasite intracellular multiplication was observed (**Figures 1A–C**). Analyzing the rate of infected cells, we found that 33% of DH82 cells were infected at a parasite-to-cell ratio of 5:1. (**Figure 1D**). After 7 days in culture a large number of trypomastigotes were counted in the supernatants (**Figures 1E,F**). To further confirm DH82 macrophage cell line infection, we have also used *T. cruzi* of CL strain transfected with GFP and observed the adhesion, internalization (data not shown) and differentiation into intracellular amastigotes 5 days after infection (**Figure 1C**). Our results showed, for the first time, that the DH82, a canine macrophage cell line is susceptible to infection with *T. cruzi*, being able to provide an enabling environment for replication and differentiation of the parasite and the release of viable infective forms.

Canine Macrophages DH82 Are More Susceptible to Infection by *T. cruzi* than Murine Macrophage RAW264.7

Since we have found that dog DH82 tissue culture macrophages could be infected with *T. cruzi* Dm28c, we decided to compare the rate of infection, the replication of amastigotes, and the number of trypomastigotes released in cultures of dog DH82 and mouse RAW264.7 macrophages. For this purpose, DH82 cells and RAW264.7 cells were infected at a parasite/cell ratio of 10:1 and cultivated for 9 days. At the first 3 days of infection, motile trypomastigotes forms were observed in supernatants of DH82 macrophages cell line, but not in RAW264.7 cells. After 8 to 10 days postinfection, it was observed a higher number of trypomastigotes in DH82 culture supernatants than in RAW264.7. It is important to point out that canine DH82 cells infected with *T. cruzi* were able to support the infection for the entire infection period. In contrast, *T. cruzi* replication inside murine macrophage RAW264.7 cells died 7 days after infection whereas the DH82 cells showed loss of viable morphology after 9 days of infection. These findings indicate that DH82 cells are more susceptible to infection by *T. cruzi* than RAW264.7 cell line (**Figure 2**).

Activation of the DH82 Macrophage Decrease the Infectivity of *T. cruzi*

The outcome of infection is determined by the activation status of macrophages. In the present study, we have used classical macrophage activators such as LPS and INF-γ. Therefore, DH82 cells were plated, pretreated or not with LPS or LPS + IFN-γ, and were infected with *T. cruzi*. Following incubation for 9 days, the trypomastigotes forms released in the supernatants were counted. We demonstrated that LPS stimulated macrophages showed a reduced parasite burden in 50%. Furthermore, we demonstrated that pretreatment of mouse macrophages with LPS and IFN-γ resulted in low levels of macrophage infection by *T. cruzi*, suggesting that previous macrophage stimulation was able to effectively control parasite replication (**Figure 3**).

Reactive Species of Oxygen Produced by DH82 Macrophages Is Not Responsible for the Decrease to Infection

Since ROS production is a crucial event associated with *in vitro* microbicidal activity in macrophages (17), we measured the production of ROS to evaluate if it could interfere in intracellular parasite replication of DH82 cells infected by *T. cruzi*. The amount of ROS produced was measured in cultures that were infected or not, in the presence or absence of LPS and IFN-γ. Increased ROS production was similar in activated and non-activated infected cells as well as in uninfected and activated cells (**Figure 4**). Taking into consideration that stimulation of DH82 canine macrophages with LPS and IFN-γ restricted intracellular replication and ROS production was elevated, associated with the fact that ROS release was also observed in *T. cruzi*-infected and unactivated DH82 cells at similar level suggests that, in our system, ROS is not involved in limiting parasite replication inside DH82 cells infected by *T. cruzi*.

Profile of Cytokines of DH82 Cells after Infection with *T. cruzi*

Cytokines play a fundamental role in mediating interaction between macrophages, T lymphocytes, and other cells from the immune system in order to establish an immune response to control disease progression or in maintaining a persistent infection. Depending on the type of cytokines produced, intracellular parasites can be eliminated or can favor its permanence in the infected host (31). Here, we analyzed the TNF-α, TGF-β, and IL-10 cytokines production in the supernatants of *T. cruzi*-infected DH82 cells after overnight stimulation or not with LPS and IFN-γ. Our results showed that secretion of TNF-α production was detected in *T. cruzi*-infected DH82 macrophages at similar levels observed in stimulated

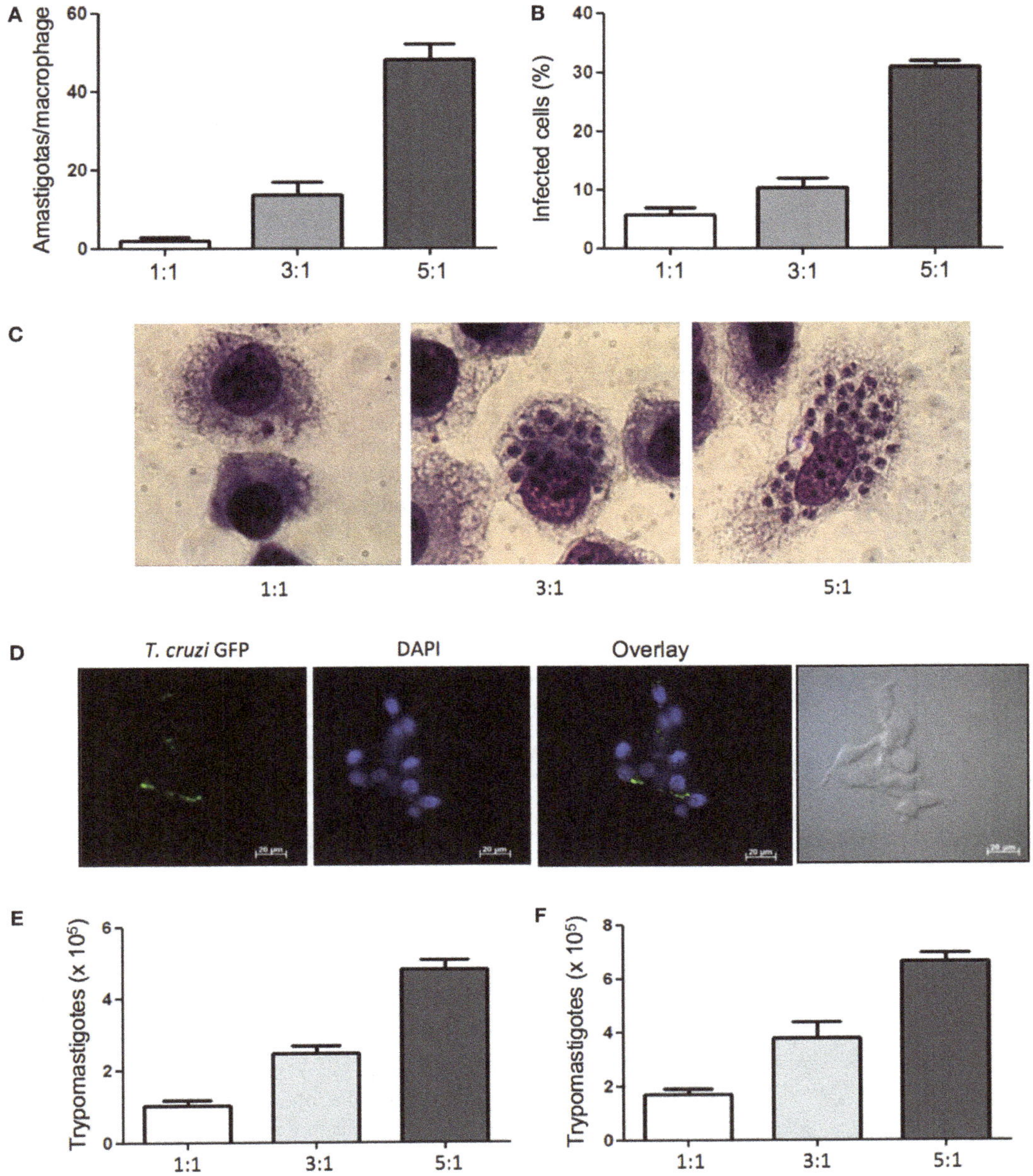

FIGURE 1 | Infectivity of *Trypanosoma cruzi* in canine macrophage DH82 cell line. DH82 cells were cultured (2.5 × 10^5/mL) with trypomastigotes forms of *T. cruzi* Dm28c clone. After overnight incubation, the cell culture was washed, and phagocyte was cultured for another 3 days with Dulbecco's Modified Eagle Medium (DMEM) at 37°C. After this period, cells were stained and amastigotes inside the macrophages were counted under the light microscope **(A)** and set the percentage of infected cells **(B)**. Infected macrophage displaying amastigotes after 3 days of infection with *T. cruzi* staining with Diff-Quick **(C)** and infection with CL strain green fluorescent protein (GFP) **(D)** observed by confocal microscope. To quantify trypomastigotes forms in the supernatants, the cells were infected with trypomastigotes forms of *T. cruzi* Dm28c clone. After overnight incubation the cell culture was washed and phagocyte were cultured for another 9 days with DMEM at 37°C. The trypomastigotes forms were quantified in the supernatant of the cultures of infected DH82 macrophages after 7 days **(E)** and 9 days **(F)**. All cultures were performed in triplicate and bars show the mean + SD.

macrophages (**Figure 5A**). However, with stimulation by LPS and IFN-γ, infected cells exhibited TNF-α production and reached higher levels as seen in **Figure 5A**. With regard to IL-10, maximal production was also detected in stimulated and infected DH82 macrophages (**Figure 5C**). LPS and IFN-γ treatment of DH82 resulted in TGF-β secretion but *T. cruzi*-infected and stimulated macrophages triggered a substantially higher level of release TGF-β in DH82 cell than was observed with in *T. cruzi*-infected macrophages only (**Figure 5B**). The increased TGF-β production observed in infected DH82 cells indicate that TGF-β might be involved in the success of DH82 cell infection by *T. cruzi*.

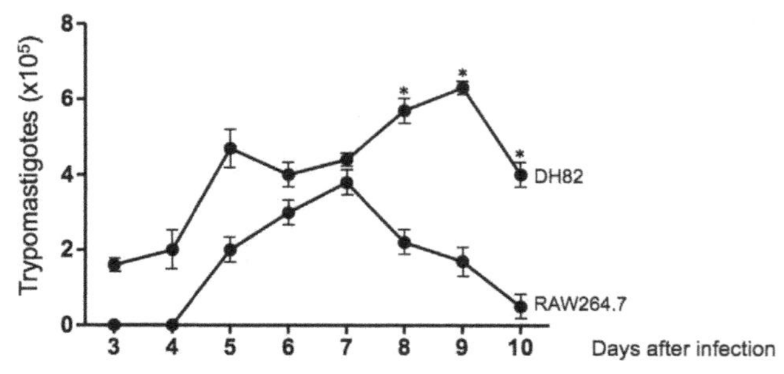

FIGURE 2 | Curve of growth of *Trypanosoma cruzi* in DH82 and RAW264.7 cell line. DH82 and RAW 264.7 macrophages were cultured (2.5×10^5/mL) with trypomastigotes forms of *T. cruzi* Dm28c clone. After overnight incubation, the cell culture was washed, and phagocyte was cultured for another 3 days with Dulbecco's Modified Eagle Medium (DMEM) at 37°C. After 3 days, we start the quantification of the trypomastigotes forms in the supernatants of the cultures. All cultures were performed in triplicate and bars show the mean + SD. Statistical analysis was performed by *t*-test from representative results of three similar experiments ($^*p \leq 0.05$).

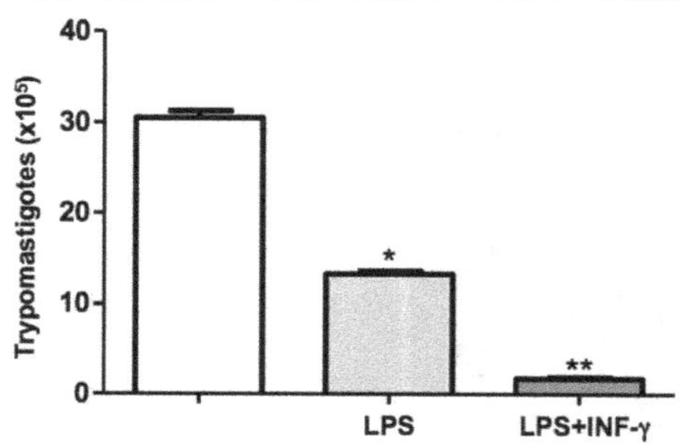

FIGURE 3 | Activated DH82 macrophages decreased trypomastigotes release. DH82 macrophages were cultured (2.5×10^5/mL). The macrophages were infected with *Trypanosoma cruzi* Dm28c clone. Some cultures were stimulated with LPS (400 ng/mL) and INF-γ (1.5 ng/mL) for 24 h. After 9 days of infection was quantified the number of the trypomastigotes forms in the supernatants of the cultures. All cultures were performed in triplicate and bars show the mean + SD. Statistical analysis was performed by *t*-test from representative results of three similar experiments ($^*p \leq 0.05$).

MHC Class II and CD80 Are Modulated after Infection

The ability to express MHC class II and CD80 on surface confer to macrophage the status of antigen-presenting cell (APC). To be efficient APC during infection is very important to maintain unchanged the expression levels of these molecules (32). In order to study possible alterations resulting from *T. cruzi* infection that could lead to any modification in these molecules expression, DH82 canine macrophage cell line was infected or not and cultured in the presence or not of some activating factors, such as LPS and IFN-γ. After 24 h in culture, cells were harvested and labeled with monoclonal antibodies directed against MHC-II and CD80 and the expression was evaluated by flow cytometry analysis. The results showed that upon stimulation, the levels of surface MHC-II molecules increased but when DH82 macrophages were infected with *T. cruzi* the cells expressed lower levels of MHC II (**Figures 6A,B**). Upregulated surface expression of CD80 was also observed in DH82 stimulated and uninfected cells. On the other hand, low level of CD80 expression could be detected in *T. cruzi*-infected cells (**Figures 6C,D**). These data suggest that parasite infection inhibit the ability of DH82 canine macrophage cells to up regulate the expression of both molecules crucial to act as effective APCs.

Taken together, our results indicate that the DH82 canine macrophage cell line is susceptible to infection by *T. cruzi*, able to sustain the infection for long time when compare with RAW264.7, a murine macrophage cell line, support replication and differentiation to the parasite, culminating with the release of the infective forms that can be used as *in vitro* study to explore parasite-host interaction. Furthermore, the infection of activated cells induced production of cytokines known as deactivating factors for macrophage like TGF-β and IL-10, that when associated with decreased expression of MHC II and CD80 represent a powerful mechanism to modulate parasite growth in this cell line.

Interaction between DH2 and Apoptotic Cells Increases Susceptibility to *T. cruzi* Infection

Phagocytosis of apoptotic cells by *T. cruzi*-infected macrophages has the potential to down modulate macrophages leading to an

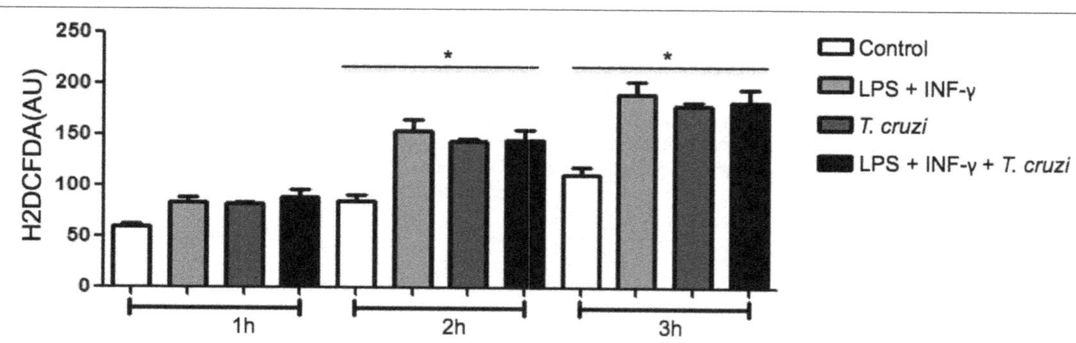

FIGURE 4 | The production of reactive species of oxygen (ROS) does not affect the infectivity of *Trypanosoma cruzi* in DH82 cells. DH82 macrophages were cultured (5.0×10^4/mL) and incubated with H2DCFDA, followed by washing and some cultures were stimulated with LPS (400 ng/mL) or LPS and INF-γ (1.5 ng/mL) in indicated time. All cultures were performed in triplicate are shown as the mean arbitrary fluorescence units (AU) + SD. Statistical analysis was performed by *t*-test from representative results of three similar experiments ($^*p \leq 0.05$).

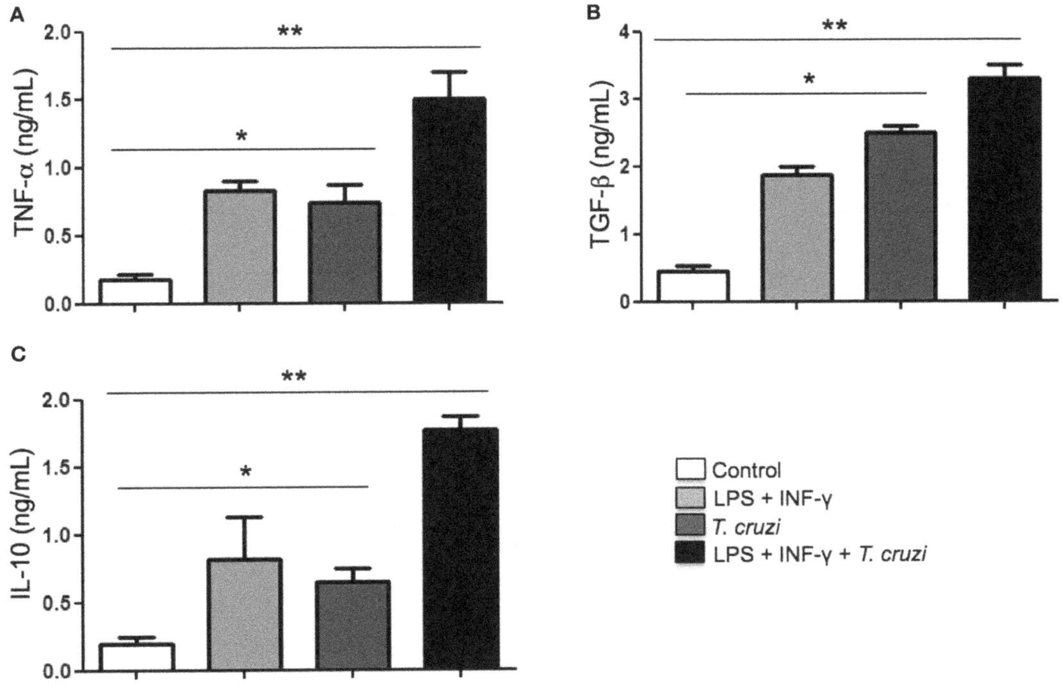

FIGURE 5 | Modulation of cytokines production in DH82 cells by *Trypanosoma cruzi* infection. DH82 macrophages (2.5 × 10^5/mL) were infected with trypomastigotes forms of *T. cruzi* Dm28c clone. After infection the cells were washed and some cultures were stimulated with LPS (400 ng/mL) and INF-γ (1.5 ng/mL). After 24 h, the supernatant was collected and TNF-α **(A)**, TGF-β **(B)**, and IL-10 **(C)** were measured by ELISA. All cultures were performed in triplicate and bars show the mean + SD. Statistical analysis was performed by *t*-test from representative results of three similar experiments ($^*p \leq 0.05$, $^{**}p \leq 0.01$).

anti-inflammatory response that results in increased parasite replication (22). In this context, we tested the modulatory effect of apoptotic cells on *T. cruzi*-infected DH82 canine macrophages. DH82 cell monolayers were cocultivated with apoptotic Jurkat T cells before or after infection with *T. cruzi*. As seen in **Figure 4**, the quantification of viable parasites released in the supernatants was made 9 days after infection. Cultures that received apoptotic cells before or after *T. cruzi* infection showed a significant increase in the number of released parasites (**Figure 7**), indicating similar modulation as previously described for mouse peritoneal macrophages.

DISCUSSION

Different cultured cells from mammal origin have been extensively used *in vitro* to study host-parasite interaction (33). Various studies have described the use of murine macrophage cell lines to analyze the infection of *T. cruzi* strains *in vitro* (34, 35) but infections of canine macrophages have not been evaluated. In the present work, we investigated whether the canine macrophage cell line DH82 is susceptible to *T. cruzi* infection *in vitro*. To determine the DH82 cells susceptibility to *T. cruzi* Dm 28c infection, macrophages monolayers were infected with metacyclic trypomastigotes differentiated *in vitro*. Our results showed that DH82 cells experienced infection rate of 30%. We found that trypomastigotes differentiated in amastigotes forms, replicated, and transform in trypomastigote before being released in cultures supernatants. To compare intracellular parasitism of *T. cruzi* in macrophages from a different host we also used mouse RAW264.7 tissue cultured macrophages. Microscopically, trypomastigotes free in the supernatants were detected earlier in DH82 than in RAW264.7 cells, as well as the number of parasites was higher in canine than in mouse macrophages. We also noted that DH82 macrophages were able to support infection for a prolonged period of time. This finding favors the use of DH82 cells as a model to study the *in vitro* interaction between *T. cruzi* and canine macrophages. The current study is the first to describe that DH82 cells are infected by *T. cruzi*, reproduce intracellular parasite replication, transformation into trypomastigotes and can be used as model to investigate host-pathogen interaction *in vitro* or can contribute in experiments to identify new drugs for the treatment of Chagas' disease.

In the presence of the cytokines or bacterial products such as LPS or CPG DNA, macrophages exhibited an increase in NO and ROS production that represent a key defensive element in various infectious disease (36). In *in vitro* models of macrophages infection by *T. cruzi*, the resistance to infection is closely associated with activation and consequent increase in the microbicidal activity of macrophages (37, 38). Our results showed that resistance of the DH82 cells to *T. cruzi* infection was increased after stimulation, indicating that pretreatment with classical activators can modulate these macrophages. An opposite effect was seen when *T. cruzi*-infected DH82 cells were cocultured with apoptotic lymphocytes. After interact with apoptotic cells

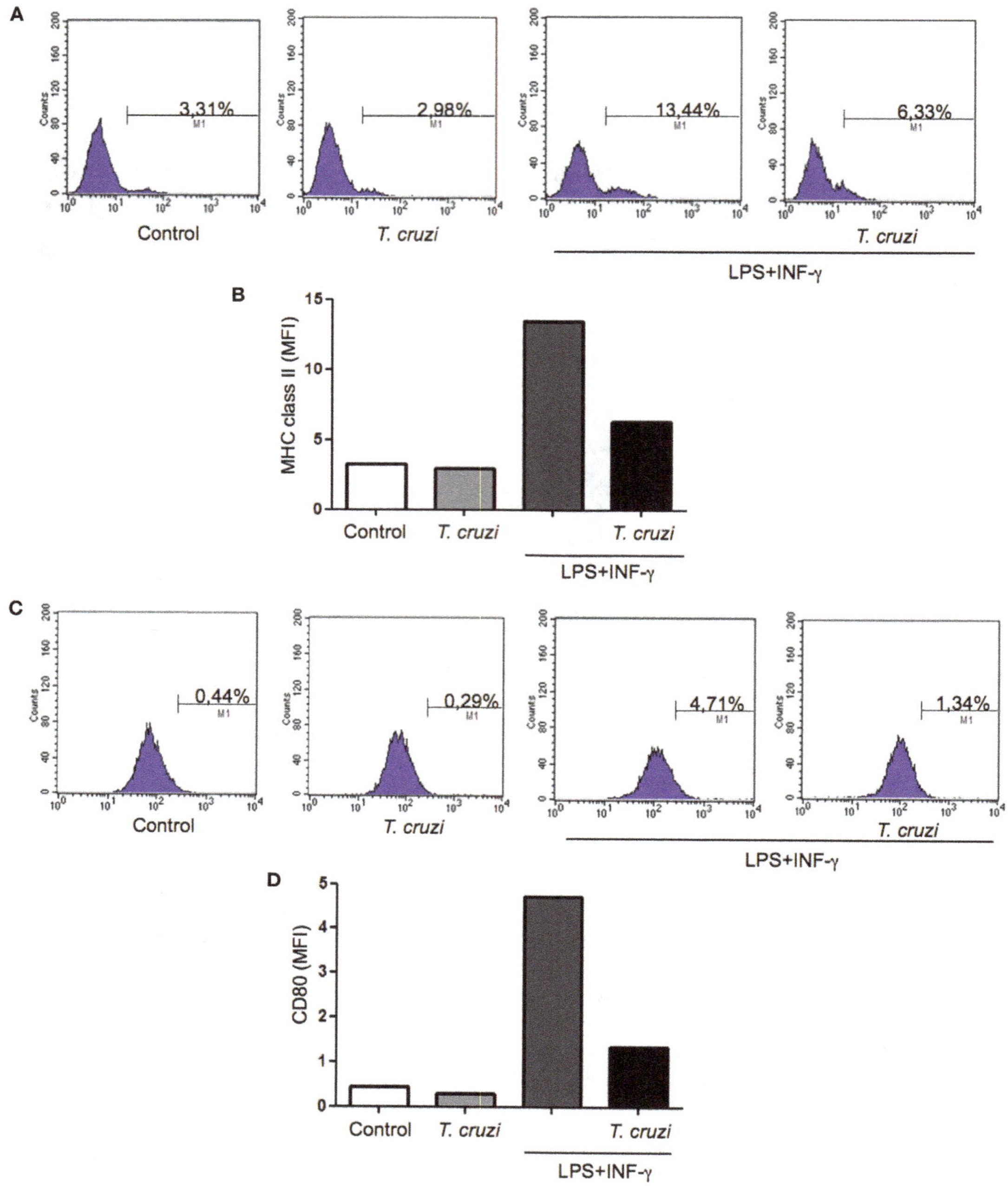

FIGURE 6 | Measurement of MHC class II and CD80 expression in infected DH82 by *Trypanosoma cruzi*. DH82 macrophages (5.0×10^5/mL) were infected with trypomastigotes forms of *T. cruzi* Dm28c clone. After infection the cells were washed and some cultures were stimulated with LPS (400 ng/mL) and INF-γ (1.5 ng/mL). After 24 h, the cells were prepared for analysis by flow cytometry. The M1 marker shows the percentage of cells identified by MHC calss II **(A,B)** or CD80 **(C,D)**. The data are representative of three independent experiments.

canine macrophages became more susceptible to infection, independently if apoptotic lymphocytes were added to the culture before or after infection. Interaction with apoptotic cells lead macrophages to secrete TGF-β, which in turn suppresses their proinflammatory cytokine response. In addition, TGF-β renders both phagocytic and non-phagocytic cells permissive to *T. cruzi* infection (39) and antagonizes INF-γ-induced NO production and macrophage trypanocidal activity (22). Based on these, ours results suggest that canine macrophage DH82 can be driven to the resistance or susceptibility depending on stimulus received that might increase their microbicidal activity or become permissive to cell invasion.

Since our results showed that DH82 cells become more resistant to infection after being stimulated with LPS and

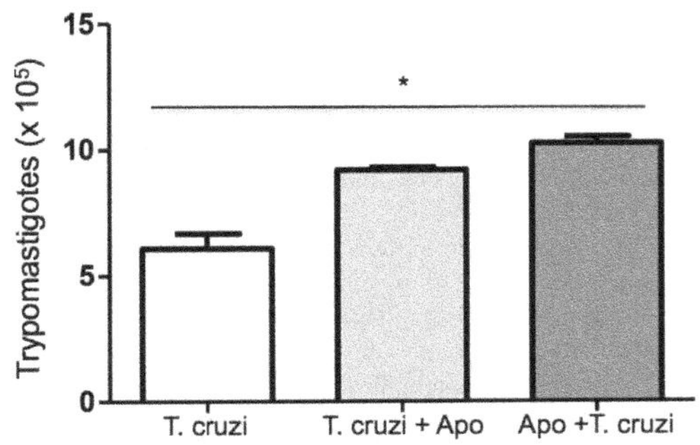

FIGURE 7 | Coculture of apoptotic cells with DH82 cells exacerbates infection by *Trypanosoma cruzi*. DH82 macrophages (2.5×10^5/mL) were exposed to apoptotic T cells (five apoptotic cells for each DH82) 1 h before infection (Apo + *T. cruzi*) or infected and exposed to apoptotic T cells (*T. cruzi* + Apo). After 9 days, the trypomastigotes forms in the supernatants were counted. All cultures were performed in triplicate and bars show the mean + SD. Statistical analysis was performed by *t*-test from representative results of three similar experiments ($^*p \leq 0.05$).

IFN-γ, we investigated which molecules could be involved. We attempted to quantify NO production; however, the cells were not able to increase NO even after stimulation with LPS and INF-γ (Figure S1 in Supplementary Material). Similar results were described in a previous study (40) that shown unchanged levels in NO production by DH82 cells. On the other hand, ROS production by canine macrophages was evident after stimulation. In our model, *T. cruzi*-infected cells were capable of producing ROS at similar levels detected in stimulated cells only and the production was markedly enhanced in the presence of LPS + IFN-γ. Despite the production of high levels of ROS by *T. cruzi*-infected DH82 macrophages, intracellular parasite replication was not effectively affected. It is noteworthy to mention that a recent report showed that to withstand such variable sources of oxidative stress, *T. cruzi* has developed complex defense mechanisms. This includes ROS detoxification pathways that are distinct from the ones in the mammalian host, DNA repair pathways and specialized polymerases, which not only protect its genome from the resulting oxidative damage but also contribute to the generation of genetic diversity within the parasite population (41).

When stimulated DH82 macrophages were infected, we detected a strong increase in TNF-α production accompanied by TGF-β and IL-10. This profile suggests that DH82 canine macrophages infected by *T. cruzi* are modulated to produce anti-inflammatory cytokines and this phenomenon can be increased in stimulated cells. In fact, high levels of TGF-β were detected in stimulated and infected cells, as well as in uninfected cells. TGF-β is an important anti-inflammatory mediator and participates in the metabolism of L-arginine, which favors the production of arginase and is involved in the activity of ornithine decarboxylase. The intracellular stage of *T. cruzi* requires this host cell enzyme and the synthesis of polyamines to multiply inside the cell (42). We suggest that this mechanism is involved in the successful infection of DH82 canine macrophage by *T. cruzi*.

Protozoan parasites such as *T. cruzi* can modulate the function of dendritic cells by interfering with recognition, migration, and antigen presentation (43). It is known that *T. cruzi* inhibits the expression of MHC II, CD40, CD80, and CD86, hampers the production and secretion of IL-12, TNF-α, and IL-6, increases the production of the cytokine IL-10, and inhibits antigen presentation in murine and human dendritic cells *in vitro* (44). Corroborating the *in vitro* findings, *in vivo* experiments have also demonstrated that *T. cruzi* is able to impair many aspects of dendritic cells biology. Additionally during acute infection, splenic dendritic cells migration and expression of the CD86 are inhibited in infected mice with *T. cruzi* (45). Interestingly, the same correlation was observed in our study with DH82 canine macrophages. These cells showed a reduction in MHC II and CD80 expression following infection with *T. cruzi*. The MHC II and CD80 expression was increased in LPS and IFN-γ stimulated cells, while infection by *T. cruzi* affected the ability of previously activated cells to increase MHC II and CD80 expression in DH82 cells. Taken together, our results reinforce the relevance of *T. cruzi* infection in modulating canine macrophages and the role in the infection establishment and disease progression. In addition, our results suggest that canine macrophages DH82 are more susceptible to infection by *T. cruzi* when compared with RAW264.7 murine macrophages.

AUTHOR CONTRIBUTIONS

DD-R, CGF-de-L, and PHBM conceived and designed the experiments. PHBM, RFDBR, JBBM, IFLRF, and JL performed the experiments. DD-R, CGF-de-L, MPN, and AM analyzed the data. DD-R and CGF-de-L wrote the article.

ACKNOWLEDGMENTS

This work was supported by grants from Conselho Nacional de Desenvolvimento Científico e Tecnológico do Brasil (CNPq), Fundação de Amparo à Pesquisa do Estado do Rio de Janeiro (FAPERJ).

SUPPLEMENTARY MATERIAL

FIGURE S1 | DH82 canine macrophage do not upregulate nitric oxide. RAW264.7 and DH82 macrophages were cultured (2.5×10^5/mL) in the absence or presence of LPS (200 or 400 ng/mL) and INF-γ (1.5 ng/mL). After 12 and 24 h of incubation, NO production was evaluated by Griess colorimetric method. All cultures were performed in triplicate and bars show the mean + SD. Statistical analysis was performed by *t*-test from representative results of three similar experiments ($^{***}p \leq 0.0001$).

REFERENCES

1. Rodrigues Coura J, De Castro SL. A critical review on Chagas disease chemotherapy. *Mem Inst Oswaldo Cruz* (2002) 97(1):3–24. doi:10.1590/S0074-02762002000100001
2. Rocha MO, Teixeira MM, Ribeiro AL. An update on the management of Chagas cardiomyopathy. *Expert Rev Anti Ifect Ther* (2007) 5(4):727–43. doi:10.1586/14787210.5.4.727
3. Rassi A Jr, Rassi A, Marin-Neto JA. Chagas disease. *Lancet* (2010) 375(9723):1388–402. doi:10.1016/S0140-6736(10)60061-X
4. Cohen JE, Gurtler RE. Modeling household transmission of American trypanosomiasis. *Science* (2001) 293(5530):694–8. doi:10.1126/science.1060638
5. Xavier SC, Roque AL, Lima VS, Monteiro KJ, Otaviano JC, Ferreira, et al. Lower richness of small wild mammal species and Chagas disease risk. *PLoS Negl Trop Dis* (2012) 6(5):e1647. doi:10.1371/journal.pntd.0001647
6. Bradley KK, Bergman DK, Woods JP, Crutcher JM, Kirchhoff LV. Prevalence of American trypanosomiasis (Chagas disease) among dogs in Oklahoma. *J Am Vet Med Assoc* (2000) 217(12):1853–7. doi:10.2460/javma.2000.217.1853
7. Estrada-Franco JG, Bhatia V, Diaz-Albiter H, Ochoa-Garcia L, Barbosa A, Vazquez-Chagoyan JC, et al. Human *Tryapanosoma cruzi* infection and seropositivity in dogs, México. *Emerg Infect Dis* (2006) 12(4):624–30. doi:10.3201/eid1204.050450
8. Esch KJ, Petersen CA. Transmission and epidemiology of zoonotic protozoal diseases of companion animals. *Clin Microbiol Rev* (2013) 26(1):58–85. doi:10.1128/CMR.00067-12
9. Pinto AGS, Schubach TMP, Figueiredo FB, Baptista C, Fagundes A, Barros JHS, et al. Isolation of *Trypanosoma caninum* in domestic dogs in Rio de Janeiro, Brazil. *Parasitology* (2010) 137(11):1653–60. doi:10.1017/S0031182010000417
10. Guedes PMM, Veloso VM, Afonso LCC, Caliari MV, Carneiro CM, Diniz LF, et al. Development of chronic cardiomyopathy in canine Chagas disease correlates with high INF-γ, TNF-α, and low IL-10 production during the acute infection phase. *Vet Immunol Immunopathol* (2009) 130(1–2):43–52. doi:10.1016/j.vetimm.2009.01.004
11. Montenegro VM, Jimenez M, Pinto-Dias JC, Zeledon R. Chagas disease in dogs from endemic areas of Costa Rica. *Mem Inst Oswaldo Cruz* (2002) 97(4):491–4. doi:10.1590/S0074-02762002000400006
12. Cruz-Chan JV, Bolio-González M, Colín-Flores R, Ramirez-Sierra MJ, Quijano-Hernandez I, Dumonteli E. Immunopathology of natural infection with *Trypanosoma cruzi* in dogs. *Vet Parasitol* (2009) 162(1–2):151–5. doi:10.1016/j.vetpar.2009.02.024
13. Guedes PMM, Veloso, Talvini A, Diniz LF, Caldas IS, Do Vale Mata MA, et al. Increased type 1 chemokine expression in experimental Chagas disease correlates with cardiac pathology in Beagles dogs. *Vet Immunol Immunopathol* (2010) 138(1–2):106–13. doi:10.1016/j.vetimm.2010.06.010
14. Idone V, Tam C, Goss JW, Toomore D, Pypaert M, Andrews NW. Repair of injured plasma membrane by rapid $Ca2^{+}$-dependent endocytosis. *J Cell Biol* (2008) 180(5):905–14. doi:10.1083/jcb.200708010
15. Gazzinelli RT, Denkers EY. Protozoan encounters with toll-like receptor signaling pathways: implications for host parasitism. *Nat Rev Immunol* (2006) 6(12):895–906. doi:10.1038/nri1978
16. Kayama H, Takeda K. The innate immune response to *Trypanosoma cruzi* infection. *Microbes Infect* (2010) 12(7):511–7. doi:10.1016/j.micinf.2010.03.005
17. Gomes JA, Campi-Azevedo AC, Teixeira-Carvalho A, Silveira-Lemos D, Vitelli-Avelar D, Sathler-Oliveira R, et al. Impaired phagocytic capacity driven by downregulation of major phagocytosis-related cell surface molecules elicits and overall modulatory cytokine profile in neutrophils and monocytes from the indeterminate clinical form of Chagas disease. *Immunobiology* (2012) 217(10):1006–16. doi:10.1016/j.imbio.2012.01.014
18. Medvedev AE, Kopydlowski KM, Vogel SN. Inhibition of lipopolysaccharide-induced signal transduction in endotoxina-tolerized mouse macrophages: dysregulation of cytokine, chemokine and toll-like receptor 2 and 4 gene expression. *J Immunol* (2000) 164(11):5564–74. doi:10.4049/jimmunol.164.11.5564
19. Ropert C, Closel M, Chaves AC, Gazzinelli RT. Inhibition of a p38/stress-activation protein kinase-2-dependent phosphatase restores function of IL-1 receptor-associate kinase-1 and reverses toll-like receptor 2-and 4-dependent tolerance of macrophages. *J Immunol* (2003) 171(3):1456–65. doi:10.4049/jimmunol.171.3.1456
20. Fukao T, Koyasu S. PI3K and negative regulation of TLR signaling. *Trends Immunol* (2003) 24(7):358–63. doi:10.1016/S1471-4906(03)00139-X
21. Lopes MF, da Veiga VF, Santos AR, Fonseca ME, DosReis GA. Activation-induced CD4+ T cell death by apoptosis in experimental Chagas disease. *J Immunol* (1995) 154(2):744–52.
22. Freire de Lima CG, Nascimento DO, Soares MB, Bozza P, Castro-Faria-Neto HC, DosReis AG, et al. Uptake of apoptotic cells drives the growth of a pathogenic trypanosome in macrophages. *Nature* (2000) 403(6766):199–203. doi:10.1038/35003208
23. Heinrich F, Contioso VB, Stein VM, Carlson R, Tipold A, Reiner U, et al. Passage-dependent morphological and phenotypical changes of a canine histiocytic sarcoma cell line (DH82). *Vet Immunol Immunopathol* (2015) 163(2015):86–92. doi:10.1016/j.vetimm.2014.11.006
24. Contreras VT, Salles JM, Thomas N, Morel CM, Goldenberg S. *In vitro* differentiation of *Trypanosoma cruzi* under chemically defined conditions. *Mol Biochem Parasitol* (1985) 16(3):315–27. doi:10.1016/0166-6851(85)90073-8
25. Gluenz E, Taylor MC, Kelly JM. The *Trypanosoma cruzi* metacyclic-specific protein Met-III associates with the nucleolus and contains independent amino and carboxyl terminal targeting elements. *Int J Parasitol* (2007) 37(6):617–25. doi:10.1016/j.ijpara.2006.11.016
26. Sandaresan M, Yu ZX, Ferrans VJ, Irani K, Finkel T. Requirement for generation of H_2O_2 for platelet-derived growth factor signal transduction. *Science* (1995) 270(5234):296–9. doi:10.1126/science.270.5234.296
27. Griffith TS, Yu X, Herndon JM, Green DR, Ferguson TA. CD95-induced apoptosis of lymphocytes in an immune privileged site induces immunological tolerance. *Immunity* (1996) 5(1):7–16. doi:10.1016/S1074-7613(00)80305-2
28. Nunes MP, Andrade RM, Lopes MF, DosReis GA. Activation-induced T cell death exacerbates *Trypanosoma cruzi* replication in macrophages cocultured with $CD4^{+}$ T lymphocytes from infected hosts. *J Immunol* (1998) 160(3):1313–9.
29. Stein VM, Czub M, Hansen R, Leibold W, Moore PF, Zurbriggen A, et al. Characterization of canine microglial cells isolated *ex vivo*. *Vet Immunol Immunopathol* (2004) 99(1–2):73–85. doi:10.1016/j.vetimm.2004.01.002
30. Buscaglia CA, Di Noia JM. *Trypanosoma cruzi* clonal diversity and the epidemiology of Chagas disease. *Microbes Infect* (2003) 5(5):419–27. doi:10.1016/S1286-4579(03)00050-9
31. Mege JL, Capo C. Is macrophage polarization the Gordian knot of bacterial infection? *Med Sci (Paris)* (2010) 26(1):83–8. doi:10.1051/medsci/201026183
32. Knowlton ER, Lepone LM, Li J, Rappocciolo G, Jenkins FJ, Rinaldo CR. Professional antigen presenting cells in human herpevirus 8 infection. *Front Immunol* (2013) 3(427):1–17. doi:10.3389/fimmu.2012.00427
33. Martínez-Díaz RA, Escario JA, Nogal-Ruiz JJ, Gómez-Barrio A. Biological characterization of *Trypanosoma cruzi* strains. *Mem Inst Oswaldo Cruz* (2001) 96(1):53–9. doi:10.1590/S0074-02762001000100006
34. De Souza W, De Carvalho TM, Barrias ES. Review on *Trypanosoma cruzi*: host cell interaction. *Int J Cell Biol* (2010) 2010:295394. doi:10.1155/2010/295394
35. Junqueira C, Caetano B, Bartholomeu DC, Melo MB, Ropert C, Rodrigues MM, et al. The endless race between *Trypanosoma cruzi* and host immunity:lessons for beyond Chagas disease. *Expert Rev Mol Med* (2010) 12:e29. doi:10.1017/S1462399410001560
36. Gordon S. Alternative activation of macrophages. *Nat Rev Immunol* (2003) 3(1):23–35. doi:10.1038/nri978
37. Garrido VV, Dulgerian LR, Stempin CC, Cerbán FM. The increase in mannose receptor recycling favors arginase induction and *Trypanosoma cruzi* survival in macrophages. *Int J Biol Sci* (2011) 7(9):1257–72. doi:10.7150/ijbs.7.1257
38. Vázquez A, Ruiz-Rosado JD, Terrazas LI, Juárez I, Gomez-Garcia L, Calleja E, et al. Mouse macrophage galactose-type lectin (mMGL) is critical for host resistance against *Trypanosoma cruzi* infection. *Int J Biol Sci* (2014) 10(8):909–20. doi:10.7150/ijbs.9214
39. Silva JS, Twardzik DR, Reed SG. Regulation of *Trypanosoma cruzi* infection *in vitro* and *in vivo* by transforming growth factor beta (TGF-beta). *J Exp Med* (1991) 174(3):539–45. doi:10.1084/jem.174.3.539

40. Wasserman J, Diese L, VanGundy Z, London C, Carson WE, Papenfuss TL. Suppression of canine myeloid cells by soluble factors from cultured canine tumor cells. *Vet Immunol Immunopathol* (2012) 145(1–2):420–30. doi:10.1016/j.vetimm.2011.12.018
41. Machado-Silva A, Cerqueira PG, Grazielle-Silva V, Gadelha FR, Peloso EF, Teixeira SM, et al. How *Trypanosoma cruzi* deals with oxidative stress: antioxidant defence and DNA repair pathways. *Mutat Res Rev Mutat Res* (2016) 767:8–22. doi:10.1016/j.mrrev.2015.12.003
42. Gazzinelli RT, Oswald IP, Hieny S, James SL, Sher A. The microbicidal activity of interferon-gamma-treated macrophages against *Trypanosoma cruzi* involves an L-arginine-dependent, nitrogen-mediated mechanism inhibitable by interleukin-10 and transforming growth factor-beta. *Eur J Immunol* (1992) 22(10):2501–6. doi:10.1002/eji.1830221006
43. Poncini CV, Soto CDA, Batalla E, Solana ME, Cappa SMG. Trypanosoma cruzi induces regulatory dendritic cells *in vitro*. *Infect Immun* (2008) 76(6):2633–41. doi:10.1128/IAI.01298-07
44. Van Overtvelt L, Vanderheyde N, Verhasselt V, Ismaili J, De Vos L, Goldman M, et al. *Trypanosoma cruzi* infects human dendritic cells and prevents their maturation: inhibition of cytokines, HLA-DR, and costimulatory molecules. *Infect Immun* (1999) 67(8):4033–40.
45. Chaussabel D, Pajak B, Vercruysse V, Bisseyé C, Garzé V, Habib M, et al. Alteration of migration and maturation of dendritic cells and T-cell depletion in the course of experimental *Trypanosoma cruzi* infection. *Lab Invest* (2003) 83(9):1373–82. doi:10.1097/01.LAB.0000087587.93781.6F

14

African Trypanosomes Undermine Humoral Responses and Vaccine Development: Link with Inflammatory Responses?

Benoit Stijlemans[1,2*†], *Magdalena Radwanska*[3†], *Carl De Trez*[1,4‡] *and Stefan Magez*[1,3‡]

[1] Laboratory of Cellular and Molecular Immunology, Vrije Universiteit Brussel (VUB), Brussels, Belgium, [2] Myeloid Cell Immunology Lab, VIB-UGent Center for Inflammation Research, Ghent, Belgium, [3] Laboratory for Biomedical Research, Ghent University Global Campus, Yeonsu-Gu, Incheon, South Korea, [4] Structural Biology Research Centre (SBRC), VIB, Brussels, Belgium

***Correspondence:**
Benoit Stijlemans
benoit.stijlemans@vub.be

†These authors share co-first authorship.
‡These authors share co-last authorship.

African trypanosomosis is a debilitating disease of great medical and socioeconomical importance. It is caused by strictly extracellular protozoan parasites capable of infecting all vertebrate classes including human, livestock, and game animals. To survive within their mammalian host, trypanosomes have evolved efficient immune escape mechanisms and manipulate the entire host immune response, including the humoral response. This report provides an overview of how trypanosomes initially trigger and subsequently undermine the development of an effective host antibody response. Indeed, results available to date obtained in both natural and experimental infection models show that trypanosomes impair homeostatic B-cell lymphopoiesis, B-cell maturation and survival and B-cell memory development. Data on B-cell dysfunctioning in correlation with parasite virulence and trypanosome-mediated inflammation will be discussed, as well as the impact of trypanosomosis on heterologous vaccine efficacy and diagnosis. Therefore, new strategies aiming at enhancing vaccination efficacy could benefit from a combination of (i) early parasite diagnosis, (ii) anti-trypanosome (drugs) treatment, and (iii) anti-inflammatory treatment that collectively might allow B-cell recovery and improve vaccination.

Keywords: B-cell lymphopoiesis, African trypanosomosis, vaccination strategies, inflammation, T-cells, macrophage migration inhibitory factor (MIF)

INTRODUCTION

African trypanosomes are strictly extracellular single-celled protozoan parasites belonging to the genus *Trypanosoma*, which cause debilitating diseases in humans and livestock and consequently significantly affect the socioeconomic development of sub-Saharan Africa (1). About 70 million people distributed over a surface of one and a half million square kilometers are estimated to be at risk for contracting sleeping sickness in Africa (2). The distribution of African trypanosomes coincides mostly with the distribution of the habitat of the hematophagic insect vector, i.e., the tsetse "fly" (*Glossina* sp.), with tsetse meaning "fly" in the Tswana language of Southern Africa (3). Human African trypanosomosis (HAT) or sleeping sickness is caused by *Trypanosoma brucei gambiense* (west and central Africa) and *Trypanosoma brucei rhodesiense* (eastern and southern Africa) (4, 5).

Both parasites cause infections that exhibit clinically diverse patterns and hence require different patient management, with the less prevalent *T. b. rhodesiense* HAT considered to be the more acute and virulent/lethal form of the disease (6, 7). HAT mainly affects remote rural communities where the health infrastructure is often minimal. In general, the disease is characterized by two stages: the early hemolymphatic stage whereby parasites proliferate in the blood and lymphatic system and the late meningoencephalitic stage whereby parasites penetrate the blood–brain barrier and proliferate in the cerebral spinal fluid (8). When patients in the meningoencephalitic stage remain untreated, an encephalitic reaction can occur resulting in coma and subsequent death (9–11). However, it is important to mention that in recent years a number of reports have indicated that HAT is not always lethal and that both *T. b. gambiense* and *T. b. rhodesiense* can result in chronic human infections with little or no symptoms (12, 13). Limited surveillance in particular of non-symptomatic cases, however, make it hard to assess how widespread these non-lethal cases are, or what the molecular and genetic underlying factors are that account for HAT resistance in certain individuals (14).

According to WHO, recent successes in the fight against HAT have brought the annual new cases to less than 10,000 (5, 7, 8). To design and maintain future control strategies, it is important to indicate that *T. b. gambiense* is an anthroponotic disease with a minor role for animal reservoirs that accounts for 98% of the reported HAT cases and causes a chronic, gradually progressing disease, whereby the late meningoencephalitic stage is not reached before months or even years of infection (10, 15). *T. b. rhodesiense* on the other hand is a zoonotic disease affecting mainly animals (livestock and wildlife), with humans being only accidentally infected, and represents only 2% of the reported HAT cases, whereby the infections are acute and progress rapidly (within weeks) to the late meningoencephalitic stage (10, 16). The zoonotic nature of *T. b. rhodesiense* infections make them more difficult to control compared to *T. b. gambiense* infections (15, 17, 18). Animal African trypanosomosis (AAT) also known as Nagana is a second form of trypanosomosis that affects sub-Saharan Africa. It is mainly caused by *Trypanosoma congolense*, *Trypanosoma vivax*, and to a lesser extent *Trypanosoma brucei brucei*, while surra and dourine are also forms of AAT caused by *Trypanosoma evansi* and *Trypanosoma equiperdum*, respectively (19–21). Of note, some parasites acquired a mechanical transmission mode (hence, they can reside outside the tsetse/vector belt) and are also found in South/Latin America (*T. vivax* and *T. evansi*) and Asia (*T. evansi* and *T. equiperdum*) (19, 21–23). Yet, *T. congolense* forms a major constraint on livestock production and remains the leading cause of livestock morbidity and mortality in sub-Saharan Africa. Hereby, cattle succumb to infection primarily due to parasite-induced anemia or complications resulting from secondary, opportunistic infections (24). Progressive disease for a prolonged time will weaken these animals, thereby preventing them to be used as draft animals or for food/milk production. As a result, farming in the tsetse belt remains challenging and hampers the development of poor societies, leading to great economic losses in terms of productivity (25, 26). Indeed, AAT accounts for an estimated annual loss of about US$5 billion, whereby Africa invests every year at least US$30 million to control cattle trypanosomosis in term of curative and prophylactic treatments (27, 28). The total losses for the total tsetse-infested lands in terms of agricultural gross domestic product are US$4.75 billion per year (1). In fact, the impact of AAT on the affected areas is the combined result of environmental, political, sociocultural, entomological, and livestock management factors (29), whereby (i) the political instability of the areas hampers controlled intervention strategies and subsequently discourages commercial investment in control strategies, (ii) pharmaceutical companies are less prone to engage/invest in drug discovery/development against diseases that affect the poorest people, (iii) wild animals function as reservoir of the parasite and therefore hamper the control of the disease, and (iv) the inappropriate use of the available drugs resulting in the emergence of drug resistance (30, 31). Up till now, not a single-field applicable vaccine exists, and chemotherapy is the only strategy available to treat the disease, which is associated with high drug toxicity. Nevertheless, so far chemotherapy remains the only therapeutic choice for these diseases, whereby they target unique organelles of trypanosomes such as glycosomes and the kinetoplast that are absent in the mammalian host or trypanosome metabolic pathways that differ from the host counterparts [carbohydrate metabolism, protein and lipid modifications, and programmed cell death (PCD)] (32–34). Unlike the situation with HAT, where the nifurtimox–eflornithine combination therapy is the preferred first-line treatment for second-stage disease (35, 36), no drug combinations are currently used for AAT (27). Instead, alternating use of compounds, particularly diminazene and isometamidium (called a "sanative pair"), with low risk of cross-resistance, is recommended where possible. Hence, there is an urgent need to optimize trypanocide usage/delivery such as extending the half-life of current trypanocides to use lower quantities of trypanocide in a more effective way and, consequently, pose a decreased risk of toxicity and possibly decreased resistance development (37, 38). However, there is some optimism since progress in HAT/AAT control measures were made over the past decade due to the establishment of the Pan-African tsetse and trypanosome eradication campaign, funded by the African Development Bank, which was established in the year 2000. This organization has set tsetse elimination as its goal and has strengthened renewed interest in the research and development of control/intervention options (29, 39). Overall, "elimination" of *T. b. gambiense* HAT has been targeted for 2020 under leadership of the WHO (40).

One crucial factor that stands in the way of total eradication of trypanosomosis in general is inefficient diagnosis of the infection. To date, microscopy detection of the parasite remains the only available tool to diagnose AAT and *T. b. rhodesiense* HAT in a reliable way. Only for *T. b. gambiense*, monitoring tools are available for both detection of exposure and staging of the disease (41). The latter is important to reduce the risk of treatment-associated complications occurring during treatment of the second stage of the disease (42). In this context, improvement in staging diagnosis and early screening methods are current challenges, which would avoid delayed patient treatment. Diagnosis is often hampered due to lack of positive predictive value of existing field applicable techniques and the fact that antibody (Ab)-based detection cannot differentiate between active or passed—but cured—infections (41). Immunodiagnostics based on antigen detection in this case would be preferable but are currently non-existent for trypanosomosis in the field (41, 43). An additional complication resides in the recent finding that tsetse-transmissible *T. b. gambiense* parasites can be found in human skin biopsies from undiagnosed individuals (44). Hence, this suggests that the current diagnostic methods and control policies need to be reevaluated.

In the next sections, we will give an overview of (i) the different escape mechanisms used by African trypanosomes to survive within their mammalian host and (ii) their strategies to undermine the entire host immune response, including the humoral response, which in turn hampers vaccine development. This review will focus on two most relevant AAT species *T. brucei* and *T. congolense*, given that for both parasites, established murine models and field studies in the economically and clinically relevant host (cattle) are available (45). While for *T. vivax*, field study information is scanty, hardly any representative experimental data are available as these parasites do not grow in mice unless they are carefully adapted (23, 46, 47). However, there is prospect since Minoprio and coworkers were able to establish a murine model for *T. vivax* (48). Although rodents are not natural hosts for these pathogens, murine models can be considered valuable tools to unravel the interactions and the immune evasion mechanisms of these parasites with their mammalian host.

HOST–PARASITE INTERACTIONS

Life Cycle of African Trypanosomes

African trypanosomes have a digenetic/heteroxenous complex life cycle alternating between the intestine of the tsetse fly vector and the blood/tissues of the mammalian host, whereby they progress through different developmental stages, i.e., procyclic or trypomastigote forms, respectively (49, 50). Yet, to survive in each of these hosts, they undergo essential changes at the level of morphology, energy metabolism, and surface coat protein expression (51, 52). Hereby, trypanosomes feed by absorbing nutrients (proteins, carbohydrates, and fats) as well as iron and oxygen from the body fluids of the host to generate the energy necessary for the vital processes (53). Within the bloodstream of the mammalian host, they subsist as bloodstream forms (BSFs) that are ingested by tsetse flies during a blood meal, wherein they differentiate into procyclic forms in the insect midgut. Next, they migrate to the proboscis (mouth parts) where they differentiate into epimastigote forms and finally into infective metacyclic forms (MCFs) that can be transmitted to a new mammalian host during the next blood meal. Although within the tsetse fly both *T. brucei* and *T. congolense* parasites have a similar migratory life cycle (i.e., initial establishment of midgut infection and invasion of the proventriculus), they exhibit differences in transitional developmental stages with production of infective MCFs in the proboscis for *T. congolense* and in the salivary glands for *T. brucei* (54–56). Within the mammalian host, *T. congolense* is a strictly intravascular parasite, whereby they bind to circulating erythrocytes and endothelial cells through their flagellum, causing damage at the adhesion site (57, 58). In contrast, *T. brucei* can also extravasate blood vessels and invade tissues and cause severe tissue injury (44, 59, 60). Hence, this implies differences in virulence mechanisms, host–pathogen relationships, and pathogenic effects between the two species (61). In addition, *T.* congolense exists strictly as a long slender (LS) dividing form, whereas *T. brucei* parasites are pleomorphic (i.e., can exhibit two forms); a LS dividing form and a short stumpy (SS) non-dividing form that is preadapted for transmission to the fly (62, 63). This transition, which involves a quorum sensing factor (i.e., an enigmatic stumpy inducing factor), is suggested to help control parasitemia and to increase the host survival time, thereby increasing the probability for successful transmission of the trypanosomes to a new host (50, 64). It is suggested that this removal of the majority of the population is an altruistic form of PCD and the counterpart of apoptosis in metazoan (65, 66). Hereby, increased intracellular reactive oxygen species and prostaglandin D2, which is produced principally by stumpy forms, are promoting this PCD that can be considered as a second control point in terminal differentiation to the SS form (67, 68). Moreover, it is suggested that the SS form is heterogeneous, whereby one part is altruistic and undergoes apoptosis-like events, thereby stimulating the host's immune response and eliminating the major LS and SS antigen population, while the other is tsetse infective (69). Both the LS and SS forms are covered by a dense variant surface glycoprotein (VSG) coat, which protects them from both the innate and the adaptive host immune systems. Of note, within the tsetse fly, the parasites are covered by a procyclin coat, and only when they differentiate into the MCF (infective form), they express a metacyclic VSG coat (70).

Parasite Escape Mechanisms in the Mammalian Host

To survive as extracellular parasites within the mammalian host environment (i.e., blood or extravascular tissues), African trypanosomes have developed efficient immune evasion mechanisms, at both the parasite level and the level of modulating host responses. Indeed, during millions of years of coevolution with their mammalian host, these parasites have "learned" to divert and sculpture the host immune system to prevent the generation of an effective response. The most predominant changes at the level of the host occurring during African trypanosomosis are massive splenomegaly coinciding with destruction of the lymphoid architecture and hepatomegaly. These modulations are followed by lymphadenopathy and hypergammaglobulinemia, leading to systemic multiple organ failure and death in experimental mouse models (71). In this section, we will give an overview of the most prominent escape mechanisms trypanosomes developed to allow successful infection within their mammalian host.

Parasite-Associated Escape Mechanisms

Already at the onset of infection, i.e., inoculation of trypanosome-containing saliva upon the bite of a tsetse fly, components present in the saliva are able to (i) dampen local host inflammatory immune responses characterized by the release of trypanolytic molecules, i.e., tumor necrosis factor (TNF) and nitric oxide (NO), thereby favoring parasite development and (ii) trigger mast cell degranulation resulting in release of histamine and increased vasodilatation, thereby allowing parasite dissemination/extravasation into the blood circulation [reviewed in Stijlemans et al. (72)]. Within the mammalian host, trypanosomes are very proficient in avoiding and subsequently reorchestrating host immune responses. Being extracellular parasites, they are confronted with the host's humoral immune response; hence, to allow infection to occur, they have to overcome this major obstacle. In first instance, these parasites are covered with a very dense coat composed of approximately 5×10^6 identical VSG homodimers of 50–60 kDa subunits that are anchored in the plasma membrane by a glycosylphosphatidylinositol (GPI) anchor, which functions as a ~15-nm thick barrier and protects the cell from Abs that might bind to buried conserved proteins (73, 74). Second, to prevent Ab-mediated elimination by Abs raised against the immunodominant/immunogenic VSGs, these parasites acquired a system of antigenic variation, whereby they are equipped with a battery of more than 1,000 different VSG genes and pseudogenes in their genome that in turn can undergo segmental gene recombination to encode an estimated 10,000 different VSG surface coats during infection (75). Hence, at regular time points [i.e., upon recognition by the host's humoral response or when a maximal density is reached (Quorum sensing)], they switch their coat into a different variable antigen type, thereby allowing escaping Ab-mediated elimination (76). This antigenic variation is accomplished by (i) *in situ* switching of transcriptional control (i.e., changing the VSG expression site) or (ii) gene replacement resulting in a switch of the terminal telomeric VSG gene itself (77, 78). Besides antigenic variation, these parasites were shown to express a mosaic VSG during the process of VSG switching (i.e., changing from metacyclic to BSFs, or during the course of infection), which in turn might be an efficient way to prevent effective Ab recognition (79, 80). Also the infective MCFs use this differential VSG expression to generate diversity and counter existing partial immunity/enhance transmission, while BSF use this to prolong infection (see **Figure 1**). Interestingly, the MCFs initiate VSG expression by each cell, activating at random one from a small subset of metacyclic VSG (M-VSG) genes, resulting in a heterogenous population, whereby each trypanosome expresses a single VSG (81, 82). Hereby, the M-VSG expression is regulated exclusively at the transcriptional level, while the bloodstream VSG expression is regulated mainly at the posttranscriptional levels and transcribed polycistronically (83). Third, trypanosomes also exhibit a very high endocytosis rate as an efficient way to acquire nutrients and at the same time to remove Ab-bound VSG molecules and thereby prevent Ab-mediated or even complement-mediated opsonization/elimination (84, 85). This might allow parasites to transiently escape T-cell-independent B-cell-mediated

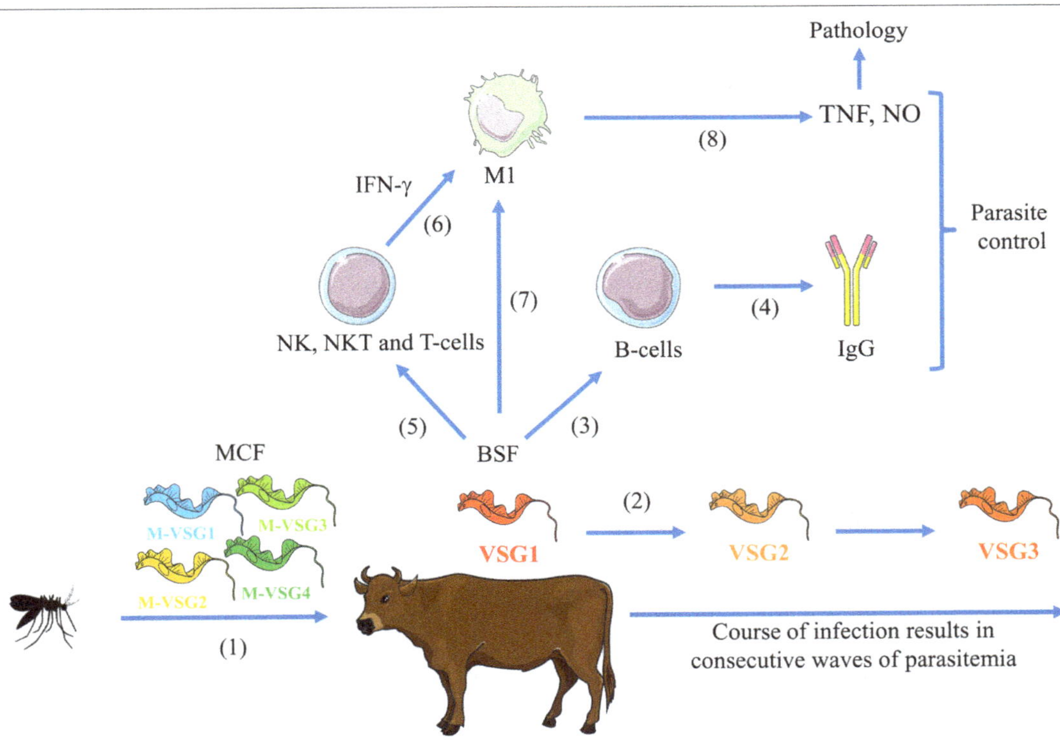

FIGURE 1 | Model for African trypanosomosis within the mammalian host. (1) Upon the bite of a trypanosome-infected tsetse fly, metacyclic form (MCF) parasites are inoculated within the mammalian host. (2) These parasites differentiate into bloodstream forms (BSFs) and switch their metacyclic VSG (M-VSG) into a bloodstream uniform VSG (VSG1) giving rise to the first parasitemia peak. During the course of infection, there is antigenic variation (VSG2, VSG3, etc.) giving rise to different peaks of parasitemia. (3,4) Parasites-derived components trigger B-cell activation and production of antiparasite IgG needed for parasitemia control. (5,6) Parasite-derived components trigger NK, NKT, and T-cell activation resulting in the production of interferon-gamma (IFN-γ). (7) Parasite-derived components in concert with IFN-γ trigger the induction of classically activated macrophages (M1 cells). (8) These M1 cells release pro-inflammatory cytokines [like tumor necrosis factor (TNF)] that are needed for parasite control, but at the same time contribute to pathology development if maintained during the course of infection.

elimination, which is the first line of defense. This immunological escape also gives time to transform into trypomastigote forms, which are adapted to survive in the mammalian host during the initiation of infection and gives the parasites an immunological advantage during the process of antigenic variation.

Although mainly IgMs play a key role during *T. brucei* infection, while in *T. congolense* infections, IgGs are mostly important (86, 87), it could be assumed that complement-mediated lysis is also an important innate defense mechanism. However, trypanosomes have developed efficient mechanisms to avoid complement-mediated elimination. First, trypanosomes are able to avoid elimination *via* the complement pathway, which is typically activated *via* immune complexes with Abs. Indeed, by releasing vast amounts of soluble VSG (mainly at the peak of parasitemia), Abs and complement factors will be scavenged and thereby induce a state of hypocomplementemia that can favor the survival of the parasites (88). Second, besides undermining the classical activation of the complement pathway that could contribute to trypanosome clearance through Ab-mediated trypanolysis and/or phagocytosis, the alternative pathway of complement activation occurring in the absence of specific Abs (i.e., during early stages of infection) is also impaired. Indeed, by masking sites on the VSG plasma membrane, which are capable of promoting alternative pathway activation, the cascade is blocked at the C3 convertase stage, thereby impairing the generation of the terminal complex (C5–C9) that normally induces trypanolysis (89, 90). However, it seems that the later stages of the complement activation cascade do not play a detrimental role in parasite control. Indeed, in AKR mice, which are natural C5 KO mice (91), the absence of the complement lysis pathway does not prevent periodic trypanosome clearance and does not hamper long-term survival in case of *T. congolense* infections (92, 93). However, soluble complement molecules, such as C3a and C5a, secreted during early stages of trypanosome infection, can contribute to the initiation of the early inflammatory immune response and also act as (i) chemotactic agents attracting phagocytes to the site of infection and (ii) release histamine from mast cells, thereby increasing microvascular permeability (94), which would allow/enable parasite extravasation into the blood circulation.

Parasite-Induced Escape Mechanisms

Besides being equipped with tools to avoid elimination by the host's "innate" humoral response, trypanosomes also undermine the host cellular immune responses to allow chronic infection. Moreover, the data in literature suggest that the efficiency to modulate the innate immune response is crucial for the progression of trypanosomosis (95). Hereby, the suppression of cellular immune responses is an efficient mechanism to evade host defense mechanisms and a general feature of trypanosomosis in bovine, human, and murine hosts. To this end, these parasites are equipped with a battery of molecules able to modulate early antiparasite responses to allow establishment. It is important to mention that the course of an African trypanosome infection can be characterized by an early release of interferon-gamma (IFN-γ) by activated NK-, NKT- and T-cells required to induce classically activated macrophages (M1) (see **Figure 1**). In turn, these activated M1 develop upon exposure to parasite-derived molecules such as VSG and CpG a type-1 inflammatory immune response leading to the production of the potential trypanocidal molecules such as TNF and NO that in conjunction with Abs will contribute to parasite control (96, 97). Yet, persistence of this type-1 immune response and hyperactivated M1 cells will culminate in trypanosusceptible animals into immunopathological features such as the systemic immune response syndrome and anemia (98). Trypanotolerant animals on the other hand are able to switch to a more type-2 immune response and the induction of alternatively activate macrophages (M2), whereby the anti-inflammatory cytokine interleukin (IL)-10 was shown to play a pivotal "dampening" role (99, 100).

Undermining Macrophage Functionality

To sustain the development of the first (most prominent) peak of parasitemia in the blood and its control by the host, some parasite-derived molecules are able to dampen pro-inflammatory responses (TNF, NO) by these M1. Most research so far has been performed using *T. brucei* infections and indicate that these parasites release components such as adenylate cyclase (AdC) and kinesin heavy chain (TbKHC-1) to dampen initial host responses, thereby allowing early parasite establishment (101, 102). Indeed, AdC released by altruistic parasites upon parasite phagocytosis by liver-associated myeloid cells prevents production of the trypanolytic cytokine TNF (*via* a protein kinase A pathway), which promotes early establishment of trypanosomes within the mammalian host (101). On the other hand, the release of TbKHC-1 by parasites induces IL-10 and arginase release by myeloid cells in a SIGN-R1-dependent manner and favors initial parasite seeding by inducing the production of polyamines, which constitute trypanosome essential nutrients (102, 103). Recently, it was also shown that metabolites produced by trypanosomes such as indolepyruvate (i.e., a transamination product of tryptophan) can dampen macrophage pro-inflammatory responses that prevent elimination (104). Finally, the order of exposure to parasite-derived versus host-derived macrophage-activating components as well as the relative concentration of these mediators may influence the ability of the host to respond to trypanosome infections. Indeed, early during infection, exposure of macrophages to soluble VSG (encompassing the glycosylinositolphosphate substituent) before IFN-γ priming downregulated the level of signal transducer and activator of transcription 1 phosphorylation, which in turn reduced transcription of pro-inflammatory cytokines such as TNF (105). So far, nothing is known about such mechanisms for *T. congolense*. In summary, it seems that trypanosomes have developed a system whereby altruistic parasites are phagocytosed, thereby disabling the M1-mediated innate immune response required for parasite control and paving the way for initiation and establishment of the first wave of parasitemia.

Modulation of T-Cell Functionality

Besides undermining the antitrypanosomal potential of the myeloid system, the parasite is also impairing T-cell help required to mount a more efficient response during the course of infection. Early during *T. brucei* and *T. congolense* infection, T-cell suppression is occurring *via* suppressive myeloid cells by inhibiting

IL-2 secretion and downregulation of IL-2 receptor expression (106–108), whereby prostaglandins were found to play an important role in the murine model, but not in the bovine model (109). In addition, early data on T cell regulation and trypanosomosis showed that both IFN-γ and TNF play a key role in the suppressive effects on CD4 and CD8 T-cells (107). Furthermore, this suppressive phenotype of the host cells during the early stages of *T. brucei* infection is due to a combination of (i) trypanosome-released macrophage-activating factors leading to secretion of immunosuppressive factors such as NO, prostaglandins, and TNF and (ii) host-derived IFN-γ needed for optimal macrophage activation (110, 111). Moreover, this work also showed that within the *T. brucei* model, there is a compartmentalization of the suppressive effect in murine models during the later stages of infection, whereby NO plays a key role in macrophage-mediated splenic suppression, whereas the macrophage-mediated lymph node suppression occurred in an IFN-γ-dependent manner (110). Hence, at this stage of infection, an IFN-γ-independent suppressive mechanism is elicited in the spleen, whereas in the lymph nodes, IFN-γ is required yet not sufficient to inhibit T cell proliferation. In this context, it was shown that the trypanosome suppression-inducing factor (TSIF) released by *T. brucei* during the course of infection induces TNF and NO secretion by classically activated macrophages (i.e., M1), which is a prerequisite for parasite control. However, at the same time, it blocks T-cell proliferation in a NO, IFN-γ, and cell contact-dependent manner as well as downregulates type-2 immune responses required to dampen M1-mediated pathogenicity (112). Moreover, TSIF was shown to be essential for parasite biology given that TSIF knockdown parasites die within 2 days. In the *T. congolense* model, it was shown that besides IFN-γ, the anti-inflammatory cytokine IL-10 also contributed to T-cell suppression (113). Finally, although both murine and bovine African trypanosomosis induce suppression, it seems that NO does not play a role in the loss of T-cell proliferative function in the bovine trypanosomosis model and that, in contrast to the mouse model, the capacity of monocytes and macrophages to produce NO is actually downregulated in infected cattle (114). In summary, these results suggest that the T-cell suppression is multifactorial, tissue and infection stage dependent, and host/parasite dependent. However, T-cells are dispensable for parasite control, which was evidenced by the fact that mice lacking a functional T-cell compartment are as efficient as immune-competent animals in controlling trypanosome infection (86). These data indicate that T-cell-independent B-cell-mediated elimination is the driving factor implicated in controlling parasitemia. Nevertheless, T-cells play a key role in the development of African trypanosomosis-associated pathogenicity, such as anemia (115).

Undermining B-Cell Functionality

Given that trypanosomes are extracellular parasites, it is not surprising that the host–parasite coevolution resulted in a subtle equilibrium between suppression of B-cell and Ab functionality and parasite persistence. Indeed, besides suppression of myeloid cells and T-cells, B-cells were also found to be negatively affected during the early stages of trypanosome infection. Accordingly, trypanosomes exert full control of the different types of host immune responses to establish chronic infection. In this context, in cattle, it was found that there are also differences in humoral responses between *T. congolense*-infected trypano-resistant (N'Dama) and trypanosusceptible Boran cattle, further highlighting the importance of the humoral immune response in parasitemia control (116). In the following section, the effect of African trypanosome infections at the level of the B-cell compartment will be scrutinized.

In homeostatic conditions, B-cells develop from bone marrow (BM)-derived hematopoietic stem cells (HSCs) that initially differentiate into multipotent progenitor cells and subsequently into common lymphoid progenitor cells (117). Next, B-cell lymphopoiesis occurs through several developmental stages, such as pre-pro-B, pro-B, pre-B, and, finally immature B-cells, which is a highly regulated process with alternating phases of cell proliferation and differentiation (118, 119). During this process, these different B-cell subsets rearrange their immunoglobulin heavy-chain and light-chain gene loci and express different surface markers that can be identified *via* flow cytometry (see **Table 1**; **Figure 2**, left panel). Within the BM, these B-cells also undergo a positive and negative selection procedure, whereby the B-cell receptor (BCR) plays a checkpoint role (120). If the BCRs do not bind their antigen, they stop their development, i.e., during positive selection, while during negative selection, binding of self-antigens to the BCR triggers either clonal deletion, receptor editing, anergy, or ignorance, resulting in central tolerance (121). At the last stage of differentiation within the BM, these immature B-cells exhibit a high IgM expression and low or no expression of the IgD maturation marker. To complete their

TABLE 1 | B-cell surface marker expression used to track cellular alterations during infection.

	Marker expression
Hematopoietic stem cell (Lin$^-$)	(Terll9, CD3, CDllb, GR1, NK1.1)$^-$, B220$^+$, CD93$^+$, IL7r, ckit$^+$, CD34$^+$
Common lymphoid progenitor (Lin$^-$)	(Ter119, CD3, CD11b, GR1, NK1.1)$^-$, B220$^+$, CD93$^+$, IL7r$^+$, ckit$^+$, CD34$^-$
Pre-proB (Lin$^-$)	(Ter119, CD3, CD11b, GR1, NK1.1)$^-$, B220$^+$, CD93$^+$, CD19$^-$, IgM$^-$, CD43^{high}
ProB (Lin$^-$)	(Ter119, CD3, CD11b, GR1, NK1.1)$^-$, B220$^+$, CD93$^+$, CD19$^+$, IgM$^-$, CD43^{high}
PreB (Lin$^-$)	(Ter119, CD3, CD11b, GR1, NK1.1)$^-$, B220$^+$, CD93$^+$, CD19$^+$, IgM$^-$, CD43$^{low/-}$
Immature B (BM) (Lin$^-$)	(Ter119, CD3, CD11b, GR1, NK1.1)$^-$, B220$^+$, CD93$^+$, CD19$^+$, IgM$^+$, CD43$^{low/-}$
Transitional B (Lin$^-$) (blood/spleen)	(Ter119, CD3, CD11b, GR1, NK1.1)$^-$, B220$^+$, CD93$^+$, CD19$^+$, IgM$^+$, IgD$^+$, CD21$^+$
Immature B (spleen) (Lin$^-$)	(Ter119, CD3, CD11b, GR1, NK1.1)$^-$, B220$^+$, CD93$^+$, CD19$^+$, IgM$^+$, IgD$^+$, CD21$^+$
Mature B	(Ter119, CD3, CD11b, GR1, NK1.1)$^-$, B220$^+$, CD93$^-$, CD19$^+$, IgM$^+$, IgD$^+$, CD21$^+$
Marginal zone B	(Ter119, CD3, CD11b, GR1, NK1.1)$^-$, B220$^+$, CD93$^-$, CD19$^+$, IgM$^+$, IgD$^+$, CD21$^+$, CD1d^{high}
Follicular B	(Ter119, CD3, CD11b, GR1, NK1.1)$^-$, B220$^+$, CD93$^-$, CD19$^+$, IgM$^+$, IgD$^+$, CD21$^+$, CD1d$^-$

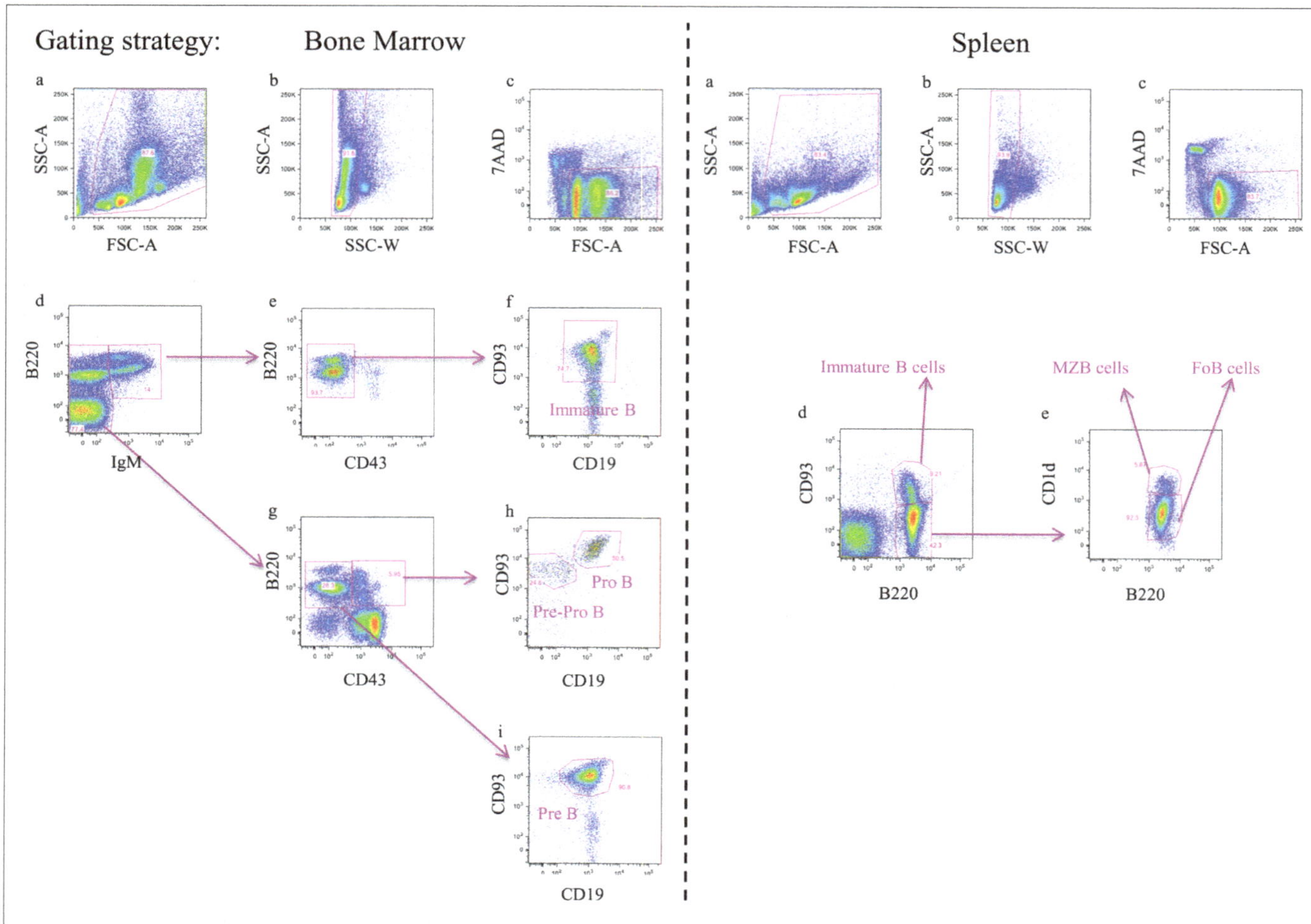

FIGURE 2 | FACS gating strategy to track B-cell alterations during infection within the bone marrow (BM) and spleen. BM (left panel): **(A,B)** In an FSC-A versus SSC-A plot, a life gate was selected followed by gating on singlets in an SSC-A versus SSC-W plot, respectively. **(C,D)** Following gating on 7AAD$^-$ cells and plotting in a B220 versus IgM allow identification of IgM$^+$ and IgM$^-$ cells. **(E,F)** The IgM$^+$ cells are plotted in a B220 versus CD43 plot to identify B220$^+$CD43$^-$ cells and subsequently plotted in a CD93 versus CD19 to identify immature B-cells (CD93$^+$CD19$^+$). **(G)** The IgM$^-$ cells are plotted in a B220 versus CD43 plot to identify B220$^+$CD43$^-$ cells and B220$^+$CD43$^+$ cells. **(H)** The B220$^+$CD43$^-$ cells are plotted in a CD93 versus CD19 to identify pre B-cells (CD93$^+$CD19$^+$). **(I)** The B220$^+$CD43$^+$ cells are plotted in a CD93 versus CD19 to identify pro B-cells (CD93$^+$CD19$^+$) and pre-pro B-cells (CD93$^+$CD19$^-$). Spleen (right panel): **(A,B)** In an FSC-A versus SSC-A plot, a life gate was selected followed by gating on singlets in an SSC-A versus SSC-W plot, respectively. **(C,D)** Following gating on 7AAD$^-$ cells and plotting in a CD93 versus B220 allow identification of immature B-cells (CD93$^+$B220$^+$). **(E)** The CD93$^+$B220$^-$ cells are subsequently plotted in a CD1d versus B220 plot to identify marginal zone B (MZB) cells (CD1d$^+$B220$^+$) and follicular B (FoB) cells (CD1d$^-$B220$^+$). It is important to mention that during infection, the expression levels of typical splenic B-cell subset markers can be modulated, which substantially complicates the identification of the different B-lymphocyte subsets.

development, immature B cells migrate to the spleen *via* the blood as transitional B cells (T1 type). In the spleen, these transitional B (T1) cells differentiate into T2 cells before they develop into two types of mature naïve B-cells (122), namely follicular B (FoB) or marginal zone B (MZB) cells (see **Figure 2**, right panel). In homeostatic conditions, B (FoB) cells are mainly located in the white pulp area of the spleen where they form primary B-cell follicles, preferentially undergo T-cell-dependent activation (upon activation *via* proteins and glycoproteins), and can give rise to both short-lived plasma cells (i.e. plasmablasts) for immediate protection and high-affinity class-switched IgG long-lived plasma cells and memory B cells for persistent protection. In contrast, MZB cells are concentrated outside the splenic marginal sinus surrounding the white pulp. Most of the time, they initiate a fast and preferentially T-cell-independent activation (upon activation *via* polysaccharides or unmethylated CpG DNA) giving rise to not only short-lived plasma cells that rapidly produce low-affinity Abs of IgM isotype but also some populations of long-lived plasma cells (123). Overall, B-cell activation is considered a very efficient defense system against invading "extracellular/blood-borne" pathogens. However, African trypanosomes have developed efficient ways to undermine the host's humoral response to establish chronic infection and allow completion of its life cycle/transmission. Indeed, using murine models, it was shown that African trypanosomes (both *T. brucei* and *T. congolense*) already during the early stages of infection trigger polyclonal B-cell activation in an attempt to dilute-out VSG-specific Abs during the course of infection. For example, it was shown that the CpG motifs of the *T. brucei* trypanosomal genomic DNA triggers TLR-9 signaling events and contributes to polyclonal B-cell activation (96). This phenomenon might contribute to parasite immune evasion by driving unselective differentiation of B cells into short-lived plasma cells. In addition, Fcγ-receptors on phagocytes become saturated by poly-specific Abs, thereby reducing the efficiency of opsonization-mediated parasite clearance. Besides polyclonal B-cell activation, trypanosomes also undermine the "protective" humoral response by ablating B cell lymphopoiesis in primary and secondary lymphoid organs during both *T. brucei* and *T. congolense* infections. This was reflected by a depletion of all developmental B-cell stages in the BM and the spleen as well as previous effector B cells, such as memory B cells (124–126), thereby preventing the development of a B-cell memory required for permanent elimination (**Figure 3**). Similar results were obtained in the experimental *T. vivax* model (127). In addition, experimental results obtained in mice and livestock animals have shown that trypanosome infections exert detrimental effects on non-pathogen-related vaccines, by preventing the occurrence of memory recall responses (126, 128–130), or on the maintenance of the antigen-specific plasma B cell pool driving the development of collagen-induced arthritis (CIA) in DBA/1 prone mice (131). This destruction of the B-cell compartment at the level of both the BM and the spleen could be attributed to either parasite-derived components and/or host-derived (infection-induced) components. Interestingly, a recent work by Cnops et al. (132), revealed that during murine infection with a chronic low-virulent *T. b. gambiense* field isolate, FoB cells are retained, which coincided with reduced production of TNF and IFN-γ pro-inflammatory cytokines during the acute stage of infection compared to *T. brucei* and *T. congolense* infections. This finding was paralleled by the finding of Lejon et al. (133), which showed that in *T. b. gambiense*, HAT patients' low parasite levels seem to be associated with limited B cell dysfunction, whereby B-cell memory responses are only slightly reduced; however, the functionality of these memory B cells was not verified in rechallenge studies. These findings indicate that in both experimental trypanosomosis and natural infection, the inflammation stage linked to the acuteness of infection could be a major determinant in the

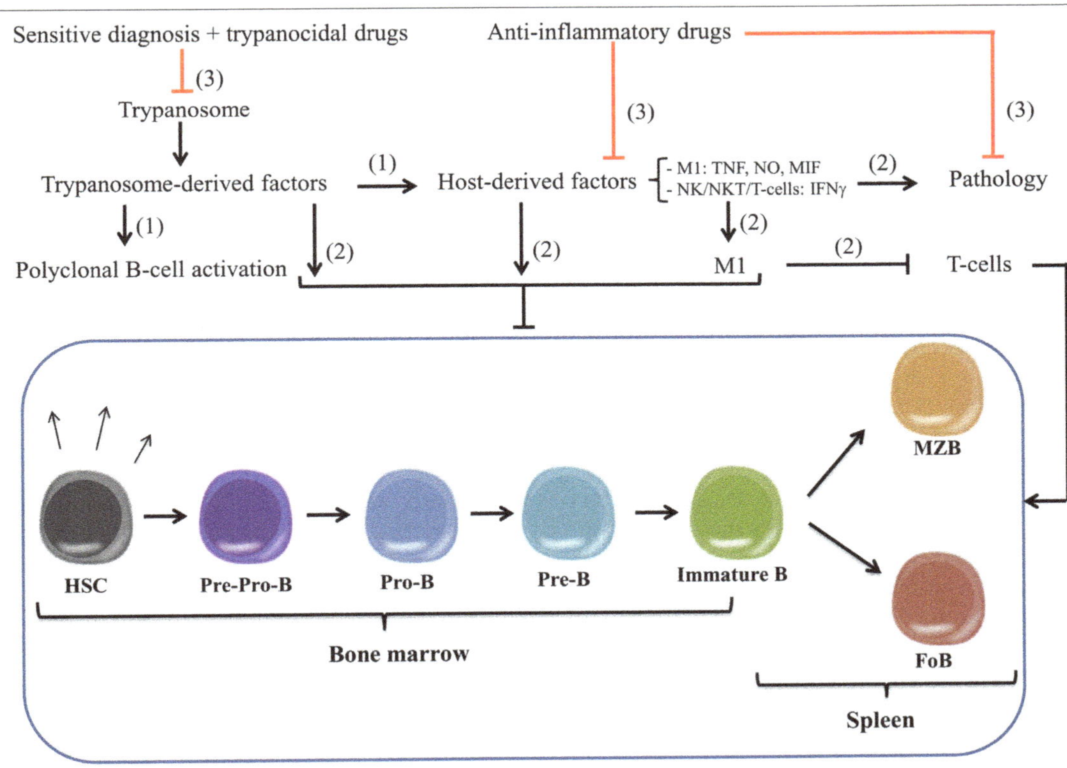

FIGURE 3 | Model for African trypanosomosis-associated impaired B-cell lymphopoiesis and improved vaccine development. (1) During the course of African trypanosomosis (AT), parasite-derived components are released that trigger besides polyclonal B-cell activation also the production of host-derived pro-inflammatory factors (i.e., NK-, NKT-, and T-cell-derived IFN-γ, M1-cell-derived TNF, NO, MIF) needed directly/indirectly for early parasite control. Yet, following control of the first parasitemia peak, polyclonal B-cell activation leads to dilution of parasite-specific antibodies, whereas the persistent pro-inflammatory response contributes to suppression of host responses and pathology. (2) Both parasite- and host-derived components can lead to a general state of impaired B-cell lymphopoiesis in (i) the bone marrow (BM), ranging from pre-pro-B-cell, pro-B-cell, pre-B-cell, and immature B-cell and (ii) the spleen, ranging from immature B-cell till MZB cell and FoB cell. In addition, also host-derived factors (involving M1) can contribute to T-cell suppression that in turn can affect B-cell homeostasis. (3) Hence, a more efficient therapeutic intervention strategy for AT should consist of a combination of (i) more reliable/sensitive diagnosis systems allowing early-stage parasite detection, (ii) more efficient trypanocidal/toxic drugs allowing improved parasite treatment, and (iii) pro-inflammatory-blocking molecules that could lead to a reduced pathology and a restoration of normal B-cell responses, thereby allowing more efficient/optimal vaccination. M1, classically activated myeloid cells; MIF, macrophage migration inhibitory factor; IFN, interferon; TNF, tumor necrosis factor; NO, nitric oxide; MZB, marginal zone B; FoB, follicular B.

processes that drive B-cell compartment destruction. This hypothesis is reinforced by the fact that both IFN-$\gamma^{(-/-)}$ and IFN-$\gamma R^{(-/-)}$ mice are protected from early trypanosomosis-associated FoB cell depletion (134). This phenotype coincided with a drastic inhibition of B-cell apoptosis and a reduced activation of FoB cells and inflammatory responses during the first week postinfection. These data demonstrated that IFN-γ is an important cytokine involved in undermining trypanosomosis-associated B-cell responses. So far, the cellular source of early IFN-γ production involved in triggering impaired B-cell lymphopoiesis remains to be fully elucidated. However, it was recently suggested that NK-cells, an important early source of IFN-γ, are involved in B-cell killing and suppressing humoral immunity within the *T. brucei* model (115, 135). Yet, it cannot be excluded that other sources of IFN-γ, such as NKT, $CD8^+$, and $CD4^+$ T-cells, are also involved in IFN-γ-mediated B-cell apoptosis given that there is a transition of IFN-γ production by these cells during the course of *T. brucei* infection (115). Interestingly, upon drug treatment [suramin and diminazene aceturate (Berenil)] of *T. brucei*- and *T. congolense*-infected mice, the BM B-cell lymphopoiesis is reinitiated, and the splenic B-cell subsets are repopulated, suggesting that an active chronic infection (i.e., parasite–host interaction) is involved in undermining the humoral responses *via* either parasite-released components and/or inflammatory-based mechanism(s) (136, 137). However, Uzonna and coworkers (137) showed that Berenil besides exerting trypanolytic effects could also modulate the host immune response to the parasite by dampening excessive immune activation and production of pathology-promoting pro-inflammatory cytokines. Hence, it cannot be excluded that the beneficial effects of Berenil for treatment of AT are multifactorial: (i) eliminate parasites thereby resulting in reduced triggering of host inflammatory immune responses and (i) reduce the host's pro-inflammatory potential to respond to pro-inflammatory/parasite-derived components. In both cases, this will result in a more efficient host-mediated parasite control due to a recovery from the impaired B-cell lymphopoiesis and protection from infection-associated pathogenicity due to lower inflammatory responses (138). In this context, it was recently shown within the *T. congolense* experimental model that also host molecules such as macrophage migration inhibitory factor (MIF) can play a key role in regulating trypanosomosis-associated pro-inflammatory responses and B-cell homeostasis (139). In this work, it was shown that *T. congolense*-infected MIF-deficient mice exhibited increased Ab titers that correlated with reduced B-cell apoptosis. Hence, MIF could be considered as a target to alleviate the impaired B-cell lymphopoiesis.

CONCLUSIONS AND PERSPECTIVES

The extracellular African trypanosomes have acquired efficient immune evasion mechanisms to undermine protective host immune responses and allow survival in the host's extracellular environment. Hereby, they are proficient in avoiding elimination *via* the host's humoral immune response by destroying the B-cell compartment/memory and shielding-off conserved epitope, thereby paving the way for chronic infection. This destruction of B-cell memory already very early during infection might explain the failure of developing an effective vaccine. Indeed, immunization with the immunodominant VSG did not yield any universal protection. So far, attempts to immunize with trypanosome molecules (VSG, beta tubulin, etc.), such as conserved membrane proteins or receptors for uptake of nutrients, have resulted in limited protective effects because such molecules are either concealed beneath the surface coat or are expressed at a to low level to induce protective host immunity (140, 141). However, some protection against AT-associated pathological features (i.e., anemia, tissue injury) has been achieved upon vaccination with pathology-inducing factors such as the VSG-derived GPI moiety (*T. brucei*, *T. congolense*) or the cysteine proteinase congopain (*T. congolense*), yet the animals were never fully cured (142, 143). Moreover, as far as the GPI-based strategy in the murine model was concerned, there was no effect on parasitemia but rather the protective effect correlated with reduced pro-inflammatory immune responses and was independent of the Ab response. This is in line with the observation that pathogenicity did not correlate with Ab levels at least for the experimental murine *T. brucei* model (86). In contrast, for the congopain vaccination strategy in experimental bovine *T. congolense* models, there was a correlation between reduced pathogenicity and increased Ab titers (143, 144). This is in line with the observation that *T. congolense*-infected N'Dama cattle (a trypanotolerant breed showing natural resistance to trypanosomosis) exhibited higher antiparasite Ab titers than the susceptible Boran breeds (145, 146), suggesting that there are differences in the frequency of trypanosome-specific Ab-secreting cells in the spleen and in the activation state of B-cells in the blood between both cattle breeds during infection. Interestingly, the sera from *T. congolense*-infected N'Dama cattle specifically recognized dimer-associated epitopes on the congopain antigen (147).

The current research on vaccine development has switched toward identification of invariant surface glycoproteins or conserved *c*-terminal VSG epitopes/peptides that are predicted to contain several MHC II recognition sites (148–150). Whether these latter approaches will lead to the development of an effective protective and antipathology vaccine will be challenging and possibly not achievable given that African trypanosomes undermine B-cell memory responses. In addition, also the whole genome transcriptome analysis (i.e., SAGE technique) that enables to (i) explore the full transcriptome of trypanosusceptible and trypanotolerant cattle might lead to the identification of interesting gene variations linked to the trypanotolerance status of the animal (151–153) and (ii) understand the molecular aspects of the trypanosome dialog with its tsetse and mammalian hosts (i.e., interaction with the salivary glands and LS versus SS differentiation, respectively) might pave the way to develop novel diagnostic/therapeutic intervention strategies (154, 155). Furthermore, although the loss of B-cell responses/memory during AT might rely on either a parasite-induced or a host-induced effect or a combination of both, understanding the molecular mechanisms used by the trypanosomes to dampen B cell responses might lead to the development of new therapeutics not only for AT but also for other diseases such as autoimmune diseases (i.e., CIA) or malaria, where B-cell dysfunction is contributing to the disease outcome (131, 156–158). In this context, it was shown that the B-cell adaptor molecule Bam32 plays a pivotal role in optimal Ab responses and resistance during *T. congolense* infections in mice (159). Besides parasite-derived molecules, also host-derived molecule could be considered as a potential target for intervention strategies. In this context, MIF can be proposed as potential candidate given that it can play a role both in innate as adaptive immunity *via* interaction with its main receptor CD74 to regulate the host inflammatory response (160, 161). Indeed, MIF was shown to play a pivotal role in stimulating/inflammatory responses and regulating T- and B-cell recruitment as well as B-cell proliferation/survival and thereby contribute to pathology development (162–164). Hence, blocking MIF-signaling could reduce inflammatory responses, thereby alleviating suppression of B-cell lymphopoiesis, which in turn might favor vaccine efficacy.

In the future, most likely, a combination of (i) more sensitive/reliable diagnosis techniques needed for early-stage parasite detection and (ii) anti-parasite intervention strategies (trypanocidal/trypanotoxic drugs) and (iii) antidisease/pathology (anti-inflammatory) intervention strategies will be required to combat AT (see **Figure 3**).

AUTHOR CONTRIBUTIONS

All authors contributed to writing the manuscript. However, BS and MR are co-first and CT and SM share co-last authorship.

ACKNOWLEDGMENTS

We acknowledge the financial support of the Interuniversity Attraction Pole Program (PAI-IAP N. P7/41, http://www.belspo.be/belspo/iap/index_en.stm) and grants from the FWO (FWO G015016N and G.0.028.10.N.10) and the Bill and Melinda Gates Foundation grant 641K760. BS is a research fellow supported by the Strategic Research Program (SRP3, VUB): Targeting inflammation linked to infectious diseases and cancer (Nanobodies for Health). We would like to thank Prof. Dr. Patrick De Baetselier for the constructive discussions and help in writing the manuscript. The funders had no role in study design, data collection and analysis, decision to publish, or preparation of the manuscript.

REFERENCES

1. Yaro M, Munyard KA, Stear MJ, Groth DM. Combatting African Animal Trypanosomiasis (AAT) in livestock: the potential role of trypanotolerance. *Vet Parasitol* (2016) 225:43–52. doi:10.1016/j.vetpar.2016.05.003
2. Simarro PP, Cecchi G, Franco JR, Paone M, Diarra A, Ruiz-Postigo JA, et al. Estimating and mapping the population at risk of sleeping sickness. *PLoS Negl Trop Dis* (2012) 6:e1859. doi:10.1371/journal.pntd.0001859
3. Welburn SC, Molyneux DH, Maudlin I. Beyond tsetse – implications for research and control of Human African trypanosomiasis epidemics. *Trends Parasitol* (2016) 32:230–41. doi:10.1016/j.pt.2015.11.008
4. World Health Organization. *Trypanosomiasis, Human African (Sleeping Sickness)*. World Health Organization (2013). 259 p. Available from: http://www.who.int/mediacentre/factsheets/fs259/en/
5. Brun R, Blum J, Chappuis F, Burri C. Human African trypanosomiasis. *Lancet* (2010) 375:148–59. doi:10.1016/S0140-6736(09)60829-1
6. Simarro PP, Diarra A, Ruiz Postigo JA, Franco JR, Jannin JG. The Human African trypanosomiasis control and surveillance programme of the world health organization 2000–2009: the way forward. *PLoS Negl Trop Dis* (2011) 5(2):e1007. doi:10.1371/journal.pntd.0001007
7. Franco JR, Simarro PP, Diarra A, Jannin JG. Epidemiology of Human African trypanosomiasis. *Clin Epidemiol* (2014) 6:257–75. doi:10.2147/CLEP.S39728
8. Kennedy PG. Clinical features, diagnosis, and treatment of Human African trypanosomiasis (sleeping sickness). *Lancet Neurol* (2013) 12:186–94. doi:10.1016/S1474-4422(12)70296-X
9. Rodgers J. Trypanosomiasis and the brain. *Parasitology* (2010) 137:1995–2006. doi:10.1017/S0031182009991806
10. MacLean L, Reiber H, Kennedy PG, Sternberg JM. Stage progression and neurological symptoms in *Trypanosoma brucei* rhodesiense sleeping sickness: role of the CNS inflammatory response. *PLoS Negl Trop Dis* (2012) 6:e1857. doi:10.1371/journal.pntd.0001857
11. Tiberti N, Matovu E, Hainard A, Enyaru JC, Lejon V, Robin X, et al. New biomarkers for stage determination in *Trypanosoma brucei* rhodesiense sleeping sickness patients. *Clin Transl Med* (2013) 2:1. doi:10.1186/2001-1326-2-1
12. Jamonneau V, Ilboudo H, Kabore J, Kaba D, Koffi M, Solano P, et al. Untreated human infections by *Trypanosoma brucei* gambiense are not 100% fatal. *PLoS Negl Trop Dis* (2012) 6:e1691. doi:10.1371/journal.pntd.0001691
13. MacLean LM, Odiit M, Chisi JE, Kennedy PG, Sternberg JM. Focus-specific clinical profiles in Human African trypanosomiasis caused by *Trypanosoma brucei* rhodesiense. *PLoS Negl Trop Dis* (2010) 4:e906. doi:10.1371/journal.pntd.0000906
14. Bucheton B, Macleod A, Jamonneau V. Human host determinants influencing the outcome of *Trypanosoma brucei* gambiense infections. *Parasite Immunol* (2011) 33:438–47. doi:10.1111/j.1365-3024.2011.01287.x
15. WHO. Control and surveillance of Human African trypanosomiasis. *World Health Organ Tech Rep Ser* (2013) (984):1–237.
16. Lejon V, Bentivoglio M, Franco JR. Human African trypanosomiasis. *Handb Clin Neurol* (2013) 114:169–81. doi:10.1016/B978-0-444-53490-3.00011-X
17. Ruiz-Postigo JA, Franco JR, Lado M, Simarro PP. Human African trypanosomiasis in South Sudan: how can we prevent a new epidemic? *PLoS Negl Trop Dis* (2012) 6:e1541. doi:10.1371/journal.pntd.0001541
18. Hasker E, Mpanya A, Makabuza J, Mbo F, Lumbala C, Kumpel J, et al. Treatment outcomes for Human African trypanosomiasis in the Democratic Republic of the Congo: analysis of routine program data from the world's largest sleeping sickness control program. *Trop Med Int Health* (2012) 17:1127–32. doi:10.1111/j.1365-3156.2012.03042.x
19. Desquesnes M, Dargantes A, Lai DH, Lun ZR, Holzmuller P, Jittapalapong S. *Trypanosoma evansi* and surra: a review and perspectives on transmission, epidemiology and control, impact, and zoonotic aspects. *Biomed Res Int* (2013) 2013:321237. doi:10.1155/2013/321237
20. Brun R, Hecker H, Lun ZR. *Trypanosoma evansi* and *T. equiperdum*: distribution, biology, treatment and phylogenetic relationship (a review). *Vet Parasitol* (1998) 79:95–107. doi:10.1016/S0304-4017(98)00146-0
21. Claes F, Büscher P, Touratier L, Goddeeris BM. *Trypanosoma equiperdum*: master of disguise or historical mistake? *Trends Parasitol* (2005) 21:316–21. doi:10.1016/j.pt.2005.05.010
22. Jones TW, Dávila AMR. *Trypanosoma vivax* – out of Africa. *Trends Parasitol* (2001) 17:99–101. doi:10.1016/S1471-4922(00)01777-3
23. Osório AL, Madruga CR, Desquesnes M, Soares CO, Ribeiro LR, Costa SC. *Trypanosoma (Duttonella) vivax*: its biology, epidemiology, pathogenesis, and introduction in the New World – a review. *Mem Inst Oswaldo Cruz* (2008) 103:1–13. doi:10.1590/S0074-02762008000100001
24. Naessens J. Bovine trypanotolerance: a natural ability to prevent severe anaemia and haemophagocytic syndrome? *Int J Parasitol* (2006) 36:521–8. doi:10.1016/j.ijpara.2006.02.012
25. Disease T. African Animal trypanosomiasis African Animal trypanosomiasis. *In Vitro* (2009):1–5. Available from: http://www.cfsph.iastate.edu/Factsheets/pdfs/trypanosomiasis_african.pdf

26. Swallow B. *Impacts of Trypanosomiasis on African Agriculture*. Nairobi, Kenya: Int Livest Res Institute (1999). p. 1–46. Available from: http://www.cabdirect.org/abstracts/20003010139.html
27. Giordani F, Morrison LJ, Rowan TG, de Koning HP, Barrett MP. The animal trypanosomiases and their chemotherapy: a review. *Parasitology* (2016) 143(14):1862–89. doi:10.1017/S0031182016001268
28. Gilbert M, Jenner C, Pender J, Rogers D, Slingenbergh J, Wint W. The programme against African trypanosomiasis information system (PAATIS). *The African Trypanosomes*, Vol. 1 (2002). p. 11–24.
29. Bouyer J, Bouyer F, Donadeu M, Rowan T, Napier G. Community- and farmer-based management of animal African trypanosomosis in cattle. *Trends Parasitol* (2013) 29:519–22. doi:10.1016/j.pt.2013.08.003
30. Baker N, de Koning HP, Maser P, Horn D. Drug resistance in African trypanosomiasis: the melarsoprol and pentamidine story. *Trends Parasitol* (2013) 29:110–8. doi:10.1016/j.pt.2012.12.005
31. Delespaux V, de Koning HP. Drugs and drug resistance in African trypanosomiasis. *Drug Resist Updat* (2007) 10:30–50. doi:10.1016/j.drup.2007.02.004
32. Naula C, Burchmore R. A plethora of targets, a paucity of drugs: progress towards the development of novel chemotherapies for human African trypanosomiasis. *Expert Rev Anti Infect Ther* (2003) 1:157–65. doi:10.1586/14787210.1.1.157
33. Wenzler T, Schumann Burkard G, Schmidt RS, Mäser P, Bergner A, Roditi I, et al. A new approach to chemotherapy: drug-induced differentiation kills African trypanosomes. *Sci Rep* (2016) 6:22451. doi:10.1038/srep22451
34. Haanstra JR, Gerding A, Dolga AM, Sorgdrager FJH, Buist-homan M, Toit F, et al. Targeting pathogen metabolism without collateral damage to the host. *Sci Rep* (2017) 7:40406. doi:10.1038/srep40406
35. Priotto G, Kasparian S, Mutombo W, Ngouama D, Ghorashian S, Arnold U, et al. Nifurtimox-eflornithine combination therapy for second-stage African *Trypanosoma brucei* gambiense trypanosomiasis: a multicentre, randomised, phase III, non-inferiority trial. *Lancet* (2009) 374:56–64. doi:10.1016/S0140-6736(09)61117-X
36. Alirol E, Schrumpf D, Amici Heradi J, Riedel A, de Patoul C, Quere M, et al. Nifurtimox-eflornithine combination therapy for second-stage gambiense Human African trypanosomiasis: medecins Sans Frontieres experience in the Democratic Republic of the Congo. *Clin Infect Dis* (2013) 56:195–203. doi:10.1093/cid/cis886
37. Unciti-Broceta JD, Arias JL, Maceira J, Soriano M, Ortiz-Gonzalez M, Hernandez-Quero J, et al. Specific cell targeting therapy bypasses drug resistance mechanisms in African trypanosomiasis. *PLoS Pathog* (2015) 11:e1004942. doi:10.1371/journal.ppat.1004942
38. Kroubi M, Karembe H, Betbeder D. Drug delivery systems in the treatment of African trypanosomiasis infections. *Expert Opin Drug Deliv* (2011) 8:735–47. doi:10.1517/17425247.2011.574122
39. Holt HR, Selby R, Mumba C, Napier GB, Guitian J. Assessment of animal African trypanosomiasis (AAT) vulnerability in cattle-owning communities of sub-Saharan Africa. *Parasit Vectors* (2016) 9:53. doi:10.1186/s13071-016-1336-5
40. Simarro PP, Cecchi G, Franco JR, Paone M, Diarra A, Priotto G, et al. Monitoring the progress towards the elimination of gambiense Human African trypanosomiasis. *PLoS Negl Trop Dis* (2015) 9:e0003785. doi:10.1371/journal.pntd.0003785
41. Bonnet J, Boudot C, Courtioux B. Overview of the diagnostic methods used in the field for Human African trypanosomiasis: what could change in the next years? *Biomed Res Int* (2015) 2015:583262. doi:10.1155/2015/583262
42. Kennedy PG. Human African trypanosomiasis-neurological aspects. *J Neurol* (2006) 253:411–6. doi:10.1007/s00415-006-0093-3
43. Odongo S, Sterckx YG, Stijlemans B, Pillay D, Baltz T, Muyldermans S, et al. An anti-proteome nanobody library approach yields a specific immunoassay for *Trypanosoma congolense* diagnosis targeting glycosomal aldolase. *PLoS Negl Trop Dis* (2016) 10:e0004420. doi:10.1371/journal.pntd.0004420
44. Capewell P, Cren-Travaillé C, Marchesi F, Johnston P, Clucas C, Benson RA, et al. The skin is a significant but overlooked anatomical reservoir for vector-borne African trypanosomes. *Elife* (2016) 5:e17716. doi:10.7554/eLife.17716
45. Morrison LJ, Vezza L, Rowan T, Hope JC. Animal African trypanosomiasis: time to increase focus on clinically relevant parasite and host species. *Trends Parasitol* (2016) 32:599–607. doi:10.1016/j.pt.2016.04.012
46. Delafosse A, Thébaud E, Desquesnes M, Michaux Y. Epidemiology of *Trypanosoma vivax* infection in cattle in the tsetse free area of Lake Chad. *Prev Vet Med* (2006) 74:108–19. doi:10.1016/j.prevetmed.2005.10.006
47. La Greca F, Haynes C, Stijlemans B, De Trez C, Magez S. Antibody-mediated control of *Trypanosoma vivax* infection fails in the absence of tumour necrosis factor. *Parasite Immunol* (2014) 36:271–6. doi:10.1111/pim.12106
48. Blom-Potar MC, Chamond N, Cosson A, Jouvion G, Droin-Bergere S, Huerre M, et al. *Trypanosoma vivax* infections: pushing ahead with mouse models for the study of Nagana. II. Immunobiological dysfunctions. *PLoS Negl Trop Dis* (2010) 4:e793. doi:10.1371/journal.pntd.0000793
49. Rotureau B, Van Den Abbeele J. Through the dark continent: African trypanosome development in the tsetse fly. *Front Cell Infect Microbiol* (2013) 3:53. doi:10.3389/fcimb.2013.00053
50. Achcar F, Kerkhoven EJ, Barrett MP. *Trypanosoma brucei*: meet the system. *Curr Opin Microbiol* (2014) 20:162–9. doi:10.1016/j.mib.2014.06.007
51. MacGregor P, Szoor B, Savill NJ, Matthews KR. Trypanosomal immune evasion, chronicity and transmission: an elegant balancing act. *Nat Rev Microbiol* (2012) 10:431–8. doi:10.1038/nrmicro2779
52. Fenn K, Matthews KR. The cell biology of *Trypanosoma brucei* differentiation. *Curr Opin Microbiol* (2007) 10:539–46. doi:10.1016/j.mib.2007.09.014
53. Stijlemans B, Beschin A, Magez S, Van Ginderachter JA, De Baetselier P. Iron homeostasis and *Trypanosoma brucei* associated immunopathogenicity development: a battle/quest for iron. *Biomed Res Int* (2015) 2015:819389. doi:10.1155/2015/819389
54. Peacock L, Cook S, Ferris V, Bailey M, Gibson W. The life cycle of *Trypanosoma (Nannomonas) congolense* in the tsetse fly. *Parasit Vectors* (2012) 5:109. doi:10.1186/1756-3305-5-109
55. Ooi C-P, Bastin P. More than meets the eye: understanding *Trypanosoma brucei* morphology in the tsetse. *Front Cell Infect Microbiol* (2013) 3:71. doi:10.3389/fcimb.2013.00071
56. Van Den Abbeele J, Rotureau B. New insights in the interactions between African trypanosomes and tsetse flies. *Front Cell Infect Microbiol* (2013) 3:63. doi:10.3389/fcimb.2013.00063
57. Banks KL. Injury induced by *Trypanosoma congolense* adhesion to cell membranes. *J Parasitol* (1980) 66:34–7. doi:10.2307/3280584
58. Hemphill A, Frame I, Ross CA. The interaction of *Trypanosoma congolense* with endothelial cells. *Parasitology* (1994) 109(Pt 5):631–41. doi:10.1017/S0031182000076514
59. Trindade S, Rijo-Ferreira F, Carvalho T, Pinto-Neves D, Guegan F, Aresta-Branco F, et al. *Trypanosoma brucei* parasites occupy and functionally adapt to the adipose tissue in mice. *Cell Host Microbe* (2016) 19:837–48. doi:10.1016/j.chom.2016.05.002
60. Mogk S, Meiwes A, Shtopel S, Schraermeyer U, Lazarus M, Kubata B, et al. Cyclical appearance of African trypanosomes in the cerebrospinal fluid: new insights in how trypanosomes enter the CNS. *PLoS One* (2014) 9:e91372. doi:10.1371/journal.pone.0091372
61. Beschin A, Van Den Abbeele J, De Baetselier P, Pays E. African trypanosome control in the insect vector and mammalian host. *Trends Parasitol* (2014) 30:538–47. doi:10.1016/j.pt.2014.08.006
62. MacGregor P, Szöőr B, Savill NJ, Matthews KR. Trypanosomal immune evasion, chronicity and transmission: an elegant balancing act. *Nat Rev Microbiol* (2012) 10:431–8. doi:10.1038/nrmicro2779
63. Rico E, Rojas F, Mony BM, Szoor B, Macgregor P, Matthews KR. Bloodstream form pre-adaptation to the tsetse fly in *Trypanosoma brucei*. *Front Cell Infect Microbiol* (2013) 3:78. doi:10.3389/fcimb.2013.00078
64. Mony BM, Matthews KR. Assembling the components of the quorum sensing pathway in African trypanosomes. *Mol Microbiol* (2015) 96:220–32. doi:10.1111/mmi.12949
65. Welburn SC, Macleod E, Figarella K, Duzensko M. Programmed cell death in African trypanosomes. *Parasitology* (2006) 132(Suppl):S7–18. doi:10.1017/S0031182006000825
66. Duszenko M, Figarella K, Macleod ET, Welburn SC. Death of a trypanosome: a selfish altruism. *Trends Parasitol* (2006) 22:536–42. doi:10.1016/j.pt.2006.08.010
67. Vassella E, Reuner B, Yutzy B, Boshart M. Differentiation of African trypanosomes is controlled by a density sensing mechanism which signals cell cycle arrest via the cAMP pathway. *J Cell Sci* (1997) 110(Pt 2):2661–71.

68. Figarella K, Rawer M, Uzcategui NL, Kubata BK, Lauber K, Madeo F, et al. Prostaglandin D2 induces programmed cell death in *Trypanosoma brucei* bloodstream form. *Cell Death Differ* (2005) 12:335–46. doi:10.1038/sj.cdd.4401564
69. Seed JR, Wenck MA. Role of the long slender to short stumpy transition in the life cycle of the African trypanosomes. *Kinetoplastid Biol Dis* (2003) 2:3. doi:10.1186/1475-9292-2-3
70. Barry JD, Graham SV, Fotheringham M, Graham VS, Kobryn K, Wymer B. VSG gene control and infectivity strategy of metacyclic stage *Trypanosoma brucei*. *Mol Biochem Parasitol* (1998) 91:93–105. doi:10.1016/S0166-6851(97)00193-X
71. Takeya M, Reinwald E, Risse HJ. Pathobiochemical alterations in experimental chronic and acute trypanosomal infection in mice. *Clin Chem Lab Med* (1987) 25:665–74. doi:10.1515/cclm.1987.25.10.665
72. Stijlemans B, Caljon G, Van Den Abbeele J, Van Ginderachter JA, Magez S, De Trez C. Immune evasion strategies of *Trypanosoma brucei* within the mammalian host: progression to pathogenicity. *Front Immunol* (2016) 7:233. doi:10.3389/fimmu.2016.00233
73. Schwede A, Macleod OJ, MacGregor P, Carrington M. How does the VSG coat of bloodstream form African trypanosomes interact with external proteins? *PLoS Pathog* (2015) 11:e1005259. doi:10.1371/journal.ppat.1005259
74. Schwede A, Jones N, Engstler M, Carrington M. The VSG C-terminal domain is inaccessible to antibodies on live trypanosomes. *Mol Biochem Parasitol* (2011) 175:201–4. doi:10.1016/j.molbiopara.2010.11.004
75. Morrison LJ, Marcello L, McCulloch R. Antigenic variation in the African trypanosome: molecular mechanisms and phenotypic complexity. *Cell Microbiol* (2009) 11:1724–34. doi:10.1111/j.1462-5822.2009.01383.x
76. *Collection S. HHS Public Access.* (2016) 8:583–92.
77. Pays E, Vanhamme L, Pérez-Morga D. Antigenic variation in *Trypanosoma brucei*: facts, challenges and mysteries. *Curr Opin Microbiol* (2004) 7:369–74. doi:10.1016/j.mib.2004.05.001
78. Borst P. Antigenic variation and allelic exclusion. *Cell* (2002) 109:5–8. doi:10.1016/S0092-8674(02)00711-0
79. Hall JPJ, Wang H, David Barry J. Mosaic VSGs and the scale of *Trypanosoma brucei* antigenic variation. *PLoS Pathog* (2013) 9:e1003502. doi:10.1371/journal.ppat.1003502
80. Dubois ME, Demick KP, Mansfield JM. Trypanosomes expressing a mosaic variant surface glycoprotein coat escape early detection by the immune system. *Infect Immun* (2005) 73:2690–7. doi:10.1128/IAI.73.5.2690-2697.2005
81. Graham SV, Barry JD. Transcriptional regulation of metacyclic variant surface glycoprotein gene expression during the life cycle of *Trypanosoma brucei*. *Mol Cell Biol* (1995) 15:5945–56. doi:10.1128/MCB.15.11.5945
82. Graham SV, Terry S, Barry JD. A structural and transcription pattern for variant surface glycoprotein gene expression sites used in metacyclic stage *Trypanosoma brucei*. *Mol Biochem Parasitol* (1999) 103:141–54. doi:10.1016/S0166-6851(99)00128-0
83. Barry JD, McCulloch R. Antigenic variation in trypanosomes: enhanced phenotypic variation in a eukaryotic parasite. *Adv Parasitol* (2001) 49:1–70. doi:10.1016/S0065-308X(01)49037-3
84. Engstler M, Pfohl T, Herminghaus S, Boshart M, Wiegertjes G, Heddergott N, et al. Hydrodynamic flow-mediated protein sorting on the cell surface of trypanosomes. *Cell* (2007) 131:505–15. doi:10.1016/j.cell.2007.08.046
85. Field MC, Carrington M. The trypanosome flagellar pocket. *Nat Rev Microbiol* (2009) 7:775–86. doi:10.1038/nrmicro2221
86. Magez S, Schwegmann A, Atkinson R, Claes F, Drennan M, De Baetselier P, et al. The role of B-cells and IgM antibodies in parasitemia, anemia, and VSG switching in *Trypanosoma brucei*-infected mice. *PLoS Pathog* (2008) 4:e1000122. doi:10.1371/journal.ppat.1000122
87. Magez S, Radwanska M, Drennan M, Fick L, Baral TN, Brombacher F, et al. Interferon-gamma and nitric oxide in combination with antibodies are key protective host immune factors during *Trypanosoma congolense* Tc13 Infections. *J Infect Dis* (2006) 193:1575–83. doi:10.1086/503808
88. Balber AE, Bangs JD, Jones SM, Proia RL. Inactivation or elimination of potentially trypanolytic, complement-activating immune complexes by pathogenic trypanosomes. *Infect Immun* (1979) 24:617–27.
89. Ferrante A, Allison AC. Alternative pathway activation of complement by African trypanosomes lacking a glycoprotein coat. *Parasite Immunol* (1983) 5:491–8. doi:10.1111/j.1365-3024.1983.tb00763.x
90. Devine DV, Falk RJ, Balber AE. Restriction of the alternative pathway of human complement by intact *Trypanosoma brucei* subsp. gambiense. *Infect Immun* (1986) 52:223–9.
91. Ooi YM, Colten HR. Genetic defect in secretion of complement C5 in mice. *Nature* (1979) 282:207–8. doi:10.1038/282207a0
92. Jarvinen JA, Dalmasso A. *Trypanosoma musculi* infections in normocomplementemic, C5-deficient, and C3-depleted mice. *Infect Immun* (1977) 16:557–63.
93. Morrison WI, Roelants GE, Mayor-Withey KS, Murray M. Susceptibility of inbred strains of mice to *Trypanosoma congolense*: correlation with changes in spleen lymphocyte populations. *Clin Exp Immunol* (1978) 32:25–40.
94. Mekori YA, Metcalfe DD. Mast cells in innate immunity. *Immunol Rev* (2000) 173:131–40. doi:10.1016/j.jaci.2004.04.045
95. Paulnock DM, Freeman BE, Mansfield JM. Modulation of innate immunity by African trypanosomes. *Parasitology* (2010) 137:2051–63. doi:10.1017/S0031182010001460
96. Drennan MB, Stijlemans B, Van den Abbeele J, Quesniaux VJ, Barkhuizen M, Brombacher F, et al. The induction of a type 1 immune response following a *Trypanosoma brucei* infection is MyD88 dependent. *J Immunol* (2005) 175:2501–9. doi:10.4049/jimmunol.175.4.2501
97. Mansfield JM, Paulnock DM. Regulation of innate and acquired immunity in African trypanosomiasis. *Parasite Immunol* (2005) 27:361–71. doi:10.1111/j.1365-3024.2005.00791.x
98. Stijlemans B, Guilliams M, Raes G, Beschin A, Magez S, De Baetselier P. African trypanosomosis: from immune escape and immunopathology to immune intervention. *Vet Parasitol* (2007) 148:3–13. doi:10.1016/j.vetpar.2007.05.005
99. Stijlemans B, Vankrunkelsven A, Caljon G, Bockstal V, Guilliams M, Bosschaerts T, et al. The central role of macrophages in trypanosomiasis-associated anemia: rationale for therapeutical approaches. *Endocr Metab Immune Disord Drug Targets* (2010) 10:71–82. doi:10.2174/187153010790827966
100. Bosschaerts T, Morias Y, Stijlemans B, Hérin M, Porta C, Sica A, et al. IL-10 limits production of pathogenic TNF by M1 myeloid cells through induction of nuclear NF-κB p50 member in *Trypanosoma congolense* infection-resistant C57BL/6 mice. *Eur J Immunol* (2011) 41:3270–80. doi:10.1002/eji.201041307
101. Salmon D, Vanwalleghem G, Morias Y, Denoeud J, Krumbholz C, Lhomme F, et al. Adenylate cyclases of *Trypanosoma brucei* inhibit the innate immune response of the host. *Science* (2012) 337:463–6. doi:10.1126/science.1222753
102. De Muylder G, Daulouède S, Lecordier L, Uzureau P, Morias Y, Van Den Abbeele J, et al. A *Trypanosoma brucei* kinesin heavy chain promotes parasite growth by triggering host arginase activity. *PLoS Pathog* (2013) 9:e1003731. doi:10.1371/journal.ppat.1003731
103. Willert E, Phillips MA. Regulation and function of polyamines in African trypanosomes. *Trends Parasitol* (2012) 28:66–72. doi:10.1016/j.pt.2011.11.001
104. McGettrick AF, Corcoran SE, Barry PJ, McFarland J, Crès C, Curtis AM, et al. *Trypanosoma brucei* metabolite indolepyruvate decreases HIF-1α and glycolysis in macrophages as a mechanism of innate immune evasion. *Proc Natl Acad Sci U S A* (2016) 113(48):E7778–87. doi:10.1073/pnas.1608221113
105. Coller SP, Mansfield JM, Paulnock DM. Glycosylinositolphosphate soluble variant surface glycoprotein inhibits IFN-gamma-induced nitric oxide production via reduction in STAT1 phosphorylation in African trypanosomiasis. *J Immunol* (2003) 171:1466–72. doi:10.4049/jimmunol.171.3.1466
106. Sileghem M, Darji A, Hamers R, Van De Winkel M, De Baetselier P. Dual role of macrophages in the suppression of interleukin 2 production and interleukin 2 receptor expression in trypanosome-infected mice. *Eur J Immunol* (1989) 19:829–35. doi:10.1002/eji.1830190508
107. Darji A, Beschin A, Sileghem M, Heremans H, Brys L, De Baetselier P. In vitro simulation of immunosuppression caused by *Trypanosoma brucei*: active involvement of gamma interferon and tumor necrosis factor in the pathway of suppression. *Infect Immun* (1996) 64:1937–43.
108. Uzonna JE, Kaushik RS, Gordon JR, Tabel H. Immunoregulation in experimental murine *Trypanosoma congolense* infection: anti-IL-10 antibodies reverse trypanosome-mediated suppression of lymphocyte proliferation in vitro and moderately prolong the lifespan of genetically susceptible BALB/c mice. *Parasite Immunol* (1998) 20:293–302. doi:10.1046/j.1365-3024.1998.00156.x
109. Sileghem M, Norman Flynn J. Suppression of interleukin 2 secretion and interleukin 2 receptor expression during tsetse-transmitted trypanosomiasis in cattle. *Eur J Immunol* (1992) 22:767–73. doi:10.1002/eji.1830220321

110. Beschin A, Brys L, Magez S, Radwanska M, De Baetselier P. *Trypanosoma brucei* infection elicits nitric oxide-dependent and nitric oxide-independent suppressive mechanisms. *J Leukoc Biol* (1998) 63:429–39.
111. Millar AE, Sternberg J, McSharry C, Wei XQ, Liew FY, Turner CM. T-Cell responses during *Trypanosoma brucei* infections in mice deficient in inducible nitric oxide synthase. *Infect Immun* (1999) 67:3334–8.
112. Gomez-Rodriguez J, Stijlemans B, De Muylder G, Korf H, Brys L, Berberof M, et al. Identification of a parasitic immunomodulatory protein triggering the development of suppressive M1 macrophages during African trypanosomiasis. *J Infect Dis* (2009) 200:1849–60. doi:10.1086/648374
113. Uzonna JE, Kaushik RS, Zhang Y, Gordon JR, Tabel H. Experimental murine *Trypanosoma congolense* infections. II. Role of splenic adherent CD3+Thy1.2+ TCR-alpha beta gamma delta- CD4+8- and CD3+Thy1.2+ TCR-alpha beta gamma delta- CD4-8-cells in the production of IL-4, IL-10, and IFN-gamma and in trypanosom. *J Immunol* (1998) 161:6189–97.
114. Taylor K, Lutje V, Mertens B. Nitric oxide synthesis is depressed in *Bos indicus* cattle infected with *Trypanosoma congolense* and *Trypanosoma vivax* and does not mediate T-cell suppression. *Infect Immun* (1996) 64:4115–22.
115. Cnops J, De Trez C, Stijlemans B, Keirsse J, Kauffmann F, Barkhuizen M, et al. NK-, NKT- and CD8-derived IFNγ drives myeloid cell activation and erythrophagocytosis, resulting in trypanosomosis-associated acute anemia. *PLoS Pathog* (2015) 11:e1004964. doi:10.1371/journal.ppat.1004964
116. Taylor KA, Lutje V, Kennedy D, Authié E, Boulangé A, Logan-Henfrey L, et al. *Trypanosoma congolense*: B-lymphocyte responses differ between trypanotolerant and trypanosusceptible cattle. *Exp Parasitol* (1996) 83:106–16. doi:10.1006/expr.1996.0054
117. Kondo M. Lymphoid and myeloid lineage commitment in multipotent hematopoietic progenitors. *Immunol Rev* (2010) 238:37–46. doi:10.1111/j.1600-065X.2010.00963.x
118. Boller S, Grosschedl R. The regulatory network of B-cell differentiation: a focused view of early B-cell factor 1 function. *Immunol Rev* (2014) 261:102–15. doi:10.1111/imr.12206
119. Reth M, Nielsen P. Signaling circuits in early B-cell development. *Adv Immunol* (2014) 122:129–75. doi:10.1016/B978-0-12-800267-4.00004-3
120. Mårtensson I-L, Almqvist N, Grimsholm O, Bernardi AI. The pre-B cell receptor checkpoint. *FEBS Lett* (2010) 584:2572–9. doi:10.1016/j.febslet.2010.04.057
121. Lebien TW, Tedder TF. B lymphocytes: how they develop and function. *Blood* (2008) 112:1570–80. doi:10.1182/blood-2008-02-078071
122. Allman D, Pillai S. Peripheral B cell subsets. *Curr Opin Immunol* (2008) 20:149–57. doi:10.1016/j.coi.2008.03.014
123. Nutt SL, Hodgkin PD, Tarlinton DM, Corcoran LM. The generation of antibody-secreting plasma cells. *Nat Rev Immunol* (2015) 15:160–71. doi:10.1038/nri3795
124. Bockstal V, Guirnalda P, Caljon G, Goenka R, Telfer JC, Frenkel D, et al. *T. brucei* infection reduces B lymphopoiesis in bone marrow and truncates compensatory splenic lymphopoiesis through transitional B-cell apoptosis. *PLoS Pathog* (2011) 7:e1002089. doi:10.1371/journal.ppat.1002089
125. Obishakin E, de Trez C, Magez S. Chronic *Trypanosoma congolense* infections in mice cause a sustained disruption of the B-cell homeostasis in the bone marrow and spleen. *Parasite Immunol* (2014) 36:187–98. doi:10.1111/pim.12099
126. Radwanska M, Guirnalda P, De Trez C, Ryffel B, Black S, Magez S. Trypanosomiasis-induced B cell apoptosis results in loss of protective anti-parasite antibody responses and abolishment of vaccine-induced memory responses. *PLoS Pathog* (2008) 4:e1000078. doi:10.1371/journal.ppat.1000078
127. Chamond N, Cosson A, Blom-Potar MC, Jouvion G, D'Archivio S, Medina M, et al. *Trypanosoma vivax* infections: pushing ahead with mouse models for the study of Nagana. I. Parasitological, hematological and pathological parameters. *PLoS Negl Trop Dis* (2010) 4:e792. doi:10.1371/journal.pntd.0000792
128. Holland WG, Do TT, Huong NT, Dung NT, Thanh NG, Vercruysse J, et al. The effect of *Trypanosoma evansi* infection on pig performance and vaccination against classical swine fever. *Vet Parasitol* (2003) 111:115–23. doi:10.1016/S0304-4017(02)00363-1
129. Holland WG, My LN, Dung TV, Thanh NG, Tam PT, Vercruysse J, et al. The influence of *T. evansi* infection on the immuno-responsiveness of experimentally infected water buffaloes. *Vet Parasitol* (2001) 102:225–34. doi:10.1016/S0304-4017(01)00534-9
130. Sharpe RT, Langley AM, Mowat GN, Macaskill JA, Holmes PH. Immunosuppression in bovine trypanosomiasis: response of cattle infected with *Trypanosoma congolense* to foot-and-mouth disease vaccination and subsequent live virus challenge. *Res Vet Sci* (1982) 32:289–93.
131. De Trez C, Katsandegwaza B, Caljon G, Magez S. Experimental African trypanosome infection by needle passage or natural tsetse fly challenge thwarts the development of collagen-induced arthritis in DBA/1 prone mice via an impairment of antigen specific B cell autoantibody titers. *PLoS One* (2015) 10:e0130431. doi:10.1371/journal.pone.0130431
132. Cnops J, Kauffmann F, De Trez C, Baltz T, Keirsse J, Radwanska M, et al. Maintenance of B cells during chronic murine *Trypanosoma brucei gambiense* infection. *Parasite Immunol* (2016) 38:642–7. doi:10.1111/pim.12344
133. Lejon V, Mumba Ngoyi D, Kestens L, Boel L, Barbé B, Kande Betu V, et al. Gambiense human African trypanosomiasis and immunological memory: effect on phenotypic lymphocyte profiles and humoral immunity. *PLoS Pathog* (2014) 10:e1003947. doi:10.1371/journal.ppat.1003947
134. Cnops J, De Trez C, Bulte D, Radwanska M, Ryffel B, Magez S. IFN-gamma mediates early B-cell loss in experimental African trypanosomosis. *Parasite Immunol* (2015) 37:479–84. doi:10.1111/pim.12208
135. Frenkel D, Zhang F, Guirnalda P, Haynes C, Bockstal V, Radwanska M, et al. *Trypanosoma brucei* co-opts NK cells to kill splenic B2 B cells. *PLoS Pathog* (2016) 12:e1005733. doi:10.1371/journal.ppat.1005733
136. Cnops J, Bockstal V, De Trez C, Miquel MC, Radwanska M, Magez S. Curative drug treatment of trypanosomosis leads to the restoration of B-cell lymphopoiesis and splenic B-cell compartments. *Parasite Immunol* (2015) 37:485–91. doi:10.1111/pim.12209
137. Kuriakose S, Muleme HM, Onyilagha C, Singh R, Jia P, Uzonna JE. Diminazene aceturate (Berenil) modulates the host cellular and inflammatory responses to *Trypanosoma congolense* infection. *PLoS One* (2012) 7:e48696. doi:10.1371/journal.pone.0048696
138. Wellde BT, Preston JM, Kovatch RM, Higgs J, Chumo DA. *Trypanosoma congolense*: erythrocyte indices, plasma iron turnover and effects of treatment in infected cattle. *Ann Trop Med Parasitol* (1989) 83(Suppl 1):201–6. doi:10.1080/00034983.1989.11812425
139. Stijlemans B, Brys L, Korf H, Bieniasz-Krzywiec P, Sparkes A, Vansintjan L, et al. MIF-mediated hemodilution promotes pathogenic anemia in experimental African trypanosomosis. *PLoS Pathog* (2016) 12:e1005862. doi:10.1371/journal.ppat.1005862
140. Magez S, Radwanska M. African trypanosomiasis and antibodies: implications for vaccination, therapy and diagnosis. *Future Microbiol* (2009) 4:1075–87. doi:10.2217/fmb.09.65
141. La Greca F, Magez S. Vaccination against trypanosomiasis: can it be done or is the trypanosome truly the ultimate immune destroyer and escape artist? *Hum Vaccin* (2011) 7:1225–33. doi:10.4161/hv.7.11.18203
142. Stijlemans B, Baral TN, Guilliams M, Brys L, Korf J, Drennan M, et al. A glycosylphosphatidylinositol-based treatment alleviates trypanosomiasis-associated immunopathology. *J Immunol* (2007) 179:4003–14. doi:10.4049/jimmunol.179.6.4003
143. Authié E, Boulangé A, Muteti D, Lalmanach G, Gauthier F, Musoke AJ. Immunisation of cattle with cysteine proteinases of *Trypanosoma congolense*: targetting the disease rather than the parasite. *Int J Parasitol* (2001) 31:1429–33. doi:10.1016/S0020-7519(01)00266-1
144. Lalmanach G, Boulange A, Serveau C, Lecaille F, Scharfstein J, Gauthier F, et al. Congopain from *Trypanosoma congolense*: drug target and vaccine candidate. *Biol Chem* (2002) 383:739–49. doi:10.1515/BC.2002.077
145. Authie E, Duvallet G, Robertson C, Williams DJ. Antibody responses to a 33 kDa cysteine protease of *Trypanosoma congolense*: relationship to "trypanotolerance" in cattle. *Parasite Immunol* (1993) 15:465–74. doi:10.1111/j.1365-3024.1993.tb00632.x
146. Taylor KA, Lutje V, Kennedy D, Authie E, Boulange A, Logan-Henfrey L, et al. *Trypanosoma congolense*: B-lymphocyte responses differ between trypanotolerant and trypanosusceptible cattle. *Exp Parasitol* (1996) 83:106–16. doi:10.1006/expr.1996.0054
147. Boulange AF, Khamadi SA, Pillay D, Coetzer TH, Authie E. Production of congopain, the major cysteine protease of *Trypanosoma (Nannomonas) congolense*, in *Pichia pastoris* reveals unexpected dimerisation at physiological pH. *Protein Expr Purif* (2011) 75:95–103. doi:10.1016/j.pep.2010.09.002

148. Lanca AS, de Sousa KP, Atouguia J, Prazeres DM, Monteiro GA, Silva MS. *Trypanosoma brucei*: immunisation with plasmid DNA encoding invariant surface glycoprotein gene is able to induce partial protection in experimental African trypanosomiasis. *Exp Parasitol* (2011) 127:18–24. doi:10.1016/j.exppara.2010.06.017
149. Dagenais TR, Demick KP, Bangs JD, Forest KT, Paulnock DM, Mansfield JM. T-cell responses to the trypanosome variant surface glycoprotein are not limited to hypervariable subregions. *Infect Immun* (2009) 77:141–51. doi:10.1128/IAI.00729-08
150. Radwanska M, Magez S, Dumont N, Pays A, Nolan D, Pays E. Antibodies raised against the flagellar pocket fraction of *Trypanosoma brucei* preferentially recognize HSP60 in cDNA expression library. *Parasite Immunol* (2000) 22:639–50. doi:10.1046/j.1365-3024.2000.00348.x
151. Berthier D, Chantal I, Thevenon S, Sakande H, Maillard J-C, Bengaly Z, et al. Study of bovine trypanotolerance by whole transcriptome analysis. *Ann N Y Acad Sci* (2008) 1149:71–6. doi:10.1196/annals.1428.062
152. O'Gorman GM, Park SD, Hill EW, Meade KG, Coussens PM, Agaba M, et al. Transcriptional profiling of cattle infected with *Trypanosoma congolense* highlights gene expression signatures underlying trypanotolerance and trypanosusceptibility. *BMC Genomics* (2009) 10:207. doi:10.1186/1471-2164-10-207
153. Auty H, Torr SJ, Michoel T, Jayaraman S, Morrison LJ. Cattle trypanosomosis: the diversity of trypanosomes and implications for disease epidemiology and control. *Rev Sci Tech* (2015) 34:587–98. doi:10.20506/rst.34.2.2382
154. Mulindwa J, Mercé C, Matovu E, Enyaru J, Clayton C. Transcriptomes of newly-isolated *Trypanosoma brucei* rhodesiense reveal hundreds of mRNAs that are co-regulated with stumpy-form markers. *BMC Genomics* (2015) 16:1118. doi:10.1186/s12864-015-2338-y
155. Telleria EL, Benoit JB, Zhao X, Savage AF, Regmi S, e Silva TLA, et al. Insights into the trypanosome-host interactions revealed through transcriptomic analysis of parasitized tsetse fly salivary glands. *PLoS Negl Trop Dis* (2014) 8:e2649. doi:10.1371/journal.pntd.0002649
156. Ng DH, Skehel JJ, Kassiotis G, Langhorne J. Recovery of an antiviral antibody response following attrition caused by unrelated infection. *PLoS Pathog* (2014) 10:e1003843. doi:10.1371/journal.ppat.1003843
157. Bockstal V, Geurts N, Magez S. Acute disruption of bone marrow B lymphopoiesis and apoptosis of transitional and marginal zone B cells in the spleen following a blood-stage plasmodium chabaudi infection in mice. *J Parasitol Res* (2011) 2011:11. doi:10.1155/2011/534697
158. Keitany GJ, Kim KS, Krishnamurty AT, Hondowicz BD, Hahn WO, Dambrauskas N, et al. Blood stage malaria disrupts humoral immunity to the pre-erythrocytic stage circumsporozoite protein. *Cell Rep* (2016) 17:3193–205. doi:10.1016/j.celrep.2016.11.060
159. Onyilagha C, Jia P, Jayachandran N, Hou S, Okwor I, Kuriakose S, et al. The B cell adaptor molecule Bam32 is critically important for optimal antibody response and resistance to *Trypanosoma congolense* infection in mice. *PLoS Negl Trop Dis* (2015) 9:e0003716. doi:10.1371/journal.pntd.0003716
160. Leng L, Metz CN, Fang Y, Xu J, Donnelly S, Baugh J, et al. MIF signal transduction initiated by binding to CD74. *J Exp Med* (2003) 197:1467–76. doi:10.1084/jem.20030286
161. Calandra T, Roger T. Macrophage migration inhibitory factor: a regulator of innate immunity. *Nat Rev Immunol* (2003) 3:791–800. doi:10.1038/nri1200
162. Stijlemans B, Leng L, Brys L, Sparkes A, Vansintjan L, Caljon G, et al. MIF contributes to *Trypanosoma brucei* associated immunopathogenicity development. *PLoS Pathog* (2014) 10:e1004414. doi:10.1371/journal.ppat.1004414
163. Klasen C, Ohl K, Sternkopf M, Shachar I, Schmitz C, Heussen N, et al. MIF promotes B cell chemotaxis through the receptors CXCR4 and CD74 and ZAP-70 signaling. *J Immunol* (2014) 192:5273–84. doi:10.4049/jimmunol.1302209
164. Alampour-Rajabi S, El Bounkari O, Rot A, Müller-Newen G, Bachelerie F, Gawaz M, et al. MIF interacts with CXCR7 to promote receptor internalization, ERK1/2 and ZAP-70 signaling, and lymphocyte chemotaxis. *FASEB J* (2015) 29:4497–511. doi:10.1096/fj.15-273904

15

Implication of Apoptosis for the Pathogenesis of *Trypanosoma cruzi* Infection

Débora Decote-Ricardo[1], Marise P. Nunes[2], Alexandre Morrot[3]* and Celio G. Freire-de-Lima[4]*

[1] Instituto de Veterinária, Universidade Federal Rural do Rio de Janeiro, Seropédica, Brazil, [2] Instituto Oswaldo Cruz, Fundação Oswaldo Cruz, Rio de Janeiro, Brazil, [3] Instituto de Microbiologia Paulo de Góes, Universidade Federal do Rio de Janeiro, Rio de Janeiro, Brazil, [4] Instituto de Biofísica Carlos Chagas Filho, Universidade Federal do Rio de Janeiro, Rio de Janeiro, Brazil

***Correspondence:**
Alexandre Morrot
morrot@micro.ufrj.br;
Celio G. Freire-de-Lima
celio@biof.ufrj.br

Apoptosis is induced during the course of immune response to different infectious agents, and the ultimate fate is the recognition and uptake of apoptotic bodies by neighboring cells or by professional phagocytes. Apoptotic cells expose specific ligands to a set of conserved receptors expressed on macrophage cellular surface, which are the main cells involved in the clearance of the dying cells. These scavenger receptors, besides triggering the production of anti-inflammatory factors, also block the production of inflammatory mediators by phagocytes. Experimental infection of mice with the parasite *Trypanosoma cruzi* shows many pathological changes that parallels the evolution of human infection. Leukocytes undergoing intense apoptotic death are observed during the immune response to *T. cruzi* in the mouse model of the disease. *T. cruzi* replicate intensely and secrete molecules with immunomodulatory activities that interfere with T cell-mediated immune responses and secretion of pro-inflammatory cytokine secretion. This mechanism of immune evasion allows the infection to be established in the vertebrate host. Under inflammatory conditions, efferocytosis of apoptotic bodies generates an immune-regulatory phenotype in phagocytes, which is conducive to intracellular pathogen replication. However, the relevance of cellular apoptosis in the pathology of Chagas' disease requires further studies. Here, we review the evidence of leukocyte apoptosis in *T. cruzi* infection and its immunomodulatory mechanism for disease progression.

Keywords: *Trypanosoma cruzi*, apoptosis, immunomodulation, infection, macrophages

INTRODUCTION

Chagas disease or American trypanosomiasis was discovered by Carlos Chagas in the early twentieth century. The disease is caused by the protozoan parasite *Trypanosoma cruzi*. It is estimated that 18–20 million people in Latin America are infected with *T. cruzi*, and approximately 100 million people are living in areas at risk of infection (1). *T. cruzi* is an obligate intracellular parasite that infects a variety of the mammalian host cells but shows preference for cells of the macrophage and muscle lineage.

The biological cycle in man has two evolutionary forms (1) trypomastigotes, the flagellate form of the parasite that invades cells, where they differentiate into (2) amastigotes that have no free flagellum and replicate inside almost all nucleated cells of the vertebrate host (2). Soon after infection, trypomastigotes have the ability to escape the parasitophorous vacuole and differentiate into amastigotes in the host cell cytoplasm. After several rounds of binary divisions inside the infected cells, amastigotes differentiate to trypomastigotes forms, lyse the infected cells, and reinvade adjacent cells (3, 4).

An important successful factor that allows *T. cruzi* to survive in the vertebrate host is the evasion of the cellular immune response (5–7). Many studies in this area describe the existence of different strategies developed by the parasite to modulate the immune response of the vertebrate host in its favor (4, 8–12).

One of the most efficient mechanisms that *T. cruzi* parasites use to establish a persistent infection is the induction of T and B cell apoptosis, and such process has immunomodulatory effects on the host immune response (8, 13).

APOPTOSIS AS A HALLMARK OF *T. cruzi* INFECTION

Apoptosis is crucial for normal tissue homeostasis and for modulation of immune response. During parasitic infections, apoptosis or programmed cell death can be triggered by antigens, factors secreted and/or released by pathogens, by chronic infection, and by intense cellular activation (14–16). Recent evidences have shown that in order to survive in their hosts, intracellular protozoan parasites have to limit the defense mechanisms and are taking advantage of cell death to facilitate parasite spreading. It was described that *T. cruzi* infection triggers activation-induced cell death (AICD) of $CD4^+$ T lymphocytes during the acute phase of infection (8, 17). The AICD occurs after stimulation with anti-TCR and anti-CD3 agonist antibodies *in vitro*. When cultured in the presence of anti-Fas agonist antibody, $CD4^+$ T cells from infected mice, but not from normal mice, undergo apoptosis (17, 18).

The interaction between the Fas molecule (CD95) and its ligand, the Fas ligand (FasL) molecule (CD95L) induces death by apoptosis (19). The involvement of Fas/FasL molecules was confirmed during the acute phase of *T. cruzi* experimentally infected mice. It was found that there is an increased expression and function of the Fas/FasL in $CD4^+$ T cells, and cells from FasL-deficient mice (*gld* mice) do not undergo AICD during *T. cruzi* infection (20). It has been suggested that AICD could have a deleterious role in *T. cruzi* infection, causing early elimination of effector T cells and supporting parasite escape (13). In agreement with these results, Rodrigues et al. (21) observed high levels of FasL in the serum of *T. cruzi* chronically infected patients (21). In addition, studies by Guillermo et al. (22) and Vasconcelos et al. (23) have revealed more information about the kinetics of Fas/FasL expression and T lymphocytes apoptosis during *T. cruzi* experimental infection (22). Splenic $CD4^+$ and $CD8^+$ T cells showed an upregulation in CD95/CD95L expression in a time-dependent manner during *T. cruzi* acute infection, which was associated with activation-induced cell death (AICD). *In vivo* injection of anti-FasL, but not anti-TNF-alpha or anti-TRAIL antibodies, blocked activation-induced cell death of $CD8^+$ T cells, improved type 1 immune responses, and reduced the infection severity as estimated by parasitemia (22, 23). Recently, Chaves et al. (24) demonstrated that T cell apoptosis was related to decreased cell proliferative and modulation of genes associated with apoptosis and caspase family receptors in chagasic patients with heart problems. Thus, the authors concluded that the T cell death was interfering with the clinical manifestations of the disease (24).

Infection caused by *T. cruzi* results in polyclonal lymphocyte activation (24–27), which, by itself, triggers T cell apoptosis (28, 29). *T. cruzi* released molecules such as *trans*-sialidase, an enzyme that catalyzes the transfer of exogenous sialic acid residues from the host acceptor molecules on the *T. cruzi* surface, induces a strong cell death by apoptosis and resulted in increasing parasite infectivity (30–32).

The *T. cruzi* surface expresses an unusual family of glycoinositolphospholipid (GIPL) molecules that are present in all *T. cruzi* evolutionary forms (33). Studies from our group have shown that in the presence of the cytokine IFN-γ, the ceramide portion of the GIPL induced intense macrophage apoptosis, independent of nitric oxide production. This effect was not observed when macrophages were treated with intact *T. cruzi* GIPL or with the GIPL-derived glycan chain. In *T. cruzi*-infected macrophages, apoptosis also increased the release of infective trypomastigotes and spheromastigotes (34). The pro-apoptotic action of ceramide had been described in previous studies, in which permeable ceramides were shown to promote a strong cytotoxic effect of this molecule (35, 36). Recently, the α-galactosylceramide molecule derived from *T. cruzi* induced NK T cell anergy and IL-33-mediated myeloid-derived suppressor cell accumulation (37).

Clearance of apoptotic cells involves the recognition of the dying cell by the phagocytes, internalization, the immunological consequences to host–parasite interaction, and pathogenesis of disease (38). In recent years, the term "efferocytosis" has been introduced to specifically refer to the engulfment or phagocytosis of apoptotic cells (39–42). Macrophages undergo specific molecular and functional changes upon encounter, interaction with, and uptake of apoptotic cells (efferocytosis) that control both phagocytosis and immune signaling (42).

In vitro studies showed that engulfment of apoptotic $CD4^+$ T lymphocytes from infected mice by *T. cruzi* experimentally infected macrophages exacerbate parasite replication. When apoptosis of $CD4^+$ T cells from infected mice was blocked with anti-FasL mAb, parasite growth was also blocked. Prevention of parasite growth was observed in a transwell coculture system, where $CD4^+$ T cells were cultured and separated from infected macrophages, showing that the contact and phagocytosis of apoptotic cells ensures parasite replication. This finding was also associated with decreased IFN-γ production, suggesting that AICD was occurring on Th1 $CD4^+$ cell population (18). Apoptotic cells trigger production of anti-inflammatory cytokines such as IL-10 and TGF-β by the phagocytes (41, 43–47). The process of apoptotic cells uptake by *T. cruzi*-infected macrophages is associated with the release of TGF-β IL-10 and prostaglandin PGE_2 (8, 9, 12). Together, these mediators would deactivate macrophages and favor the growth of *T. cruzi* amastigotes and other intracellular parasites (8, 18, 48).

Phagocytic cells express on the cell surface a group of receptors that actively participate in the recognition and capture of apoptotic bodies, the vast majority of these receptors have affinity to phosphatidylserine (PtdSer) expressed by apoptotic cells (49). The integrin αVβ3 is one of these receptors, which recognizes PtdSer through molecules that act as bridges, such as lactadherin, glycoprotein produced by phagocytes, and the fat globule of opsonin-factor-8 EGF (MFG-E8) (50). In addition, the αvβ3 integrin express on phagocytes can bind to thrombospondin, helping the recognition of PS on the surface of apoptotic cells (51). Other apoptotic cell recognition receptors, such as the family of receptor tyrosine kinases Tyro3, Axl, and MerTK (TAM), also need to bind to bridge molecule to interact with PtdSer on the surface of apoptotic cells (52–54).

Because *T. cruzi* is an intracellular pathogen that can not produce putrescine, and is an auxotrophic parasite for polyamines, because of its incapacity to produce putrescine due to the lack of both, ornithine decarboxylase (ODC) and arginine. *T. cruzi* needs to capture exogenous putrescine for the proliferation of amastigote forms within the cells (55, 56). Besides the fact that binding of apoptotic lymphocytes to $\alpha_V\beta_3$ expressed by macrophages results in secretion of PGE_2 and TGF-β, the engulfment of apoptotic cells is also followed by induction of ODC and synthesis of putrescine: this functions as a growth factor for intracellular forms of *T. cruzi* (8, 9). In addition, this deleterious effect of apoptotic cells is eradicated by inhibitors of prostaglandin synthesis (NSAIDs drugs) and neutralizing antibodies for TGF-β (11, 12). Injection of apoptotic cells increases parasitemia *in vivo*, and treatment with the cyclooxygenase inhibitors aspirin or indomethacin reduces parasitemia (8).

The use of NSAIDs in *T. cruzi* experimental infection has been used by different groups. However, it is important to emphasize that the use of cyclooxygenase blockers in experimental infection may lead to conflicting results, depending on the experimental model (8, 11, 57, 58). Recently, it was described that aspirin in low doses decreased mortality, parasitemia, and heart damage in *T. cruzi*-infected mice, and they suggested that the protective effect was established to the generation of anti-inflammatory mediator 15-epi-LXA4 (59). However, when aspirin was given in high doses, this protective effect disappeared (59). Also, it has been characterized that the use of COX inhibitors inhibits *T. cruzi* infection of murine cardiac cells (60). The results presented by Michelin and collaborators suggest that the prostaglandins produced mainly by the activation of the COX-2 enzyme favor the immunosuppression of the acute phase of infection (61). These data reinforce our hypothesis that NSAIDs may somehow favor the immune response of the vertebrate host (8, 11).

The contribution of apoptotic T cell pathways in the outcome of *T. cruzi* infection *in vivo* was addressed by injection of caspase 8 inhibitor or by the use of caspase 8-deficient mice. However, blockade of the initiator caspase 8 *in vivo* was unable to inhibit apoptosis, and mice that have received treatment demonstrated a profound $CD8^+$ T cell depletion. Furthermore, caspase 8-deficient mice upregulated Th2 cytokine responses and increased susceptibility to *T. cruzi* infection (62). Therapy with zIETG (caspase 8 inhibitor), initiated 4 days after infection, resulted in inhibition of T cell expansion and increased parasitemia (62). In contrast, administration of zVAD, a pan caspase inhibitor (or anti-FasL antibody) initiated at day 7 after *T. cruzi* infection was shown to reduce T cell death, promotes type 1 immune response and reduced parasitemia. Spleen cells produced more IFN-γ when stimulated with parasite antigens, while peritoneal macrophages showed a reduced parasite load (63). The number of inflammatory cells in the hearts of acutely infected mice injected with zVAD was not affected (63). Treatment with anti-FasL mAb starting at 11 days after infection, but not anti-TNF or anti-TRAIL antibodies, protect CD8 T cells from AICD, improved cytokine production by CD4 T cells, activate CD8 T cells, upregulate Fas expression by CD8 T cells earlier than CD4 T cells, and decreased parasitemia (22). Mice vaccinated with an adenoviral vector expressing two *T. cruzi*-dominant epitopes improved CD8 T cell functionality and decreased parasitemia after parasite challenge, a phenotype attributed to the lack of CD95 expression in parasite-specific CD8 T cells (23). Recently, Cabral-Piccin and collaborators demonstrated that treatment of *T. cruzi*-infected mice with anti-FasL prevents $CD8^+$ T lymphocytes apoptosis, upregulates type 1 responses to parasite antigens, and reduces macrophages infection when cocultured with CD8 T cells (64). Further analysis showed that injection of anti-FasL mAb resulted in a polarized M1 macrophage phenotype, both *in vitro* and *in vivo*. The authors suggested that rescuing CD8 T cells from death with anti-FasL treatment prevents the negative effects of efferocytosis on macrophage activation.

CONCLUDING REMARKS

The role of T cells-mediated immune response in controlling intracellular protozoan parasite infection is well established. In the acute phase of infection, *T. cruzi* proliferates within the cells of the vertebrate host, besides producing and secreting molecules with immunomodulatory activities that obstruct the immune response mediated by T lymphocytes. The final result of this important modulatory mechanism is the propagation of *T. cruzi* to different organs of the vertebrate host (13). It is also clear that T cell apoptosis occurs during human and experimental infection with *T. cruzi* (8, 24). Some studies showed evidences that parasites have adapted to their hosts modulating or even taking advantage of cell death in order to facilitate their own survival in a hostile environment and promoting disease. In this context, elucidation of apoptotic cell-mediated signaling mechanisms would help to discover new effective therapies and vaccines.

The modulation of host immune response is an important approach in the efficacy of treatment against *T. cruzi* in the experimental acute models of Chagas disease. The quality of response could be an important factor, not only in T cell disease progression but also in chemotherapy responsiveness. Apoptosis modulation has a beneficial therapeutic effect in various cardiovascular diseases, as well as infectious diseases (65). There appears to be an association between apoptosis and heart failure, as well as in disease severity in Chagas patients, such that pharmacological use of apoptosis inhibitors could be an attractive choice for adjuvant therapy in the chronic treatment phase; this restores an efficient T cell immune response to parasite infection, thus diminishing the pathological signals of disease.

AUTHOR CONTRIBUTIONS

DD-R, MN, AM, and CGF-de-L wrote the paper. All authors read and approved the final version of the manuscript.

ACKNOWLEDGMENTS

This work was supported by grants from Fundação de Amparo à Pesquisa do Estado do Rio de Janeiro (FAPERJ) and Conselho Nacional de Desenvolvimento Científico e Tecnológico do Brasil (CNPq).

REFERENCES

1. Costa J, Peterson AT. Ecological niche modeling as a tool for understanding distributions and interactions of vectors, hosts, and etiologic agents of Chagas disease. *Adv Exp Med Biol* (2012) 710:59–70. doi:10.1007/978-1-4419-5638-5_7
2. Goldenberg S, Avila AR. Aspects of *Trypanosoma cruzi* stage differentiation. *Adv Parasitol* (2011) 75:285–305. doi:10.1016/B978-0-12-385863-4.00013-7
3. Rubin-de-Celis SS, Uemura H, Yoshida N, Schenkman S. Expression of trypomastigote trans-sialidase in metacyclic forms of *Trypanosoma cruzi* increases parasite escape from its parasitophorous vacuole. *Cell Microbiol* (2006) 8:1888–98. doi:10.1111/j.1462-5822.2006.00755.x
4. Cardoso MS, Reis-Cunha JL, Bartholomeu DC. Evasion of the immune response by *Trypanosoma cruzi* during acute infection. *Front Immunol* (2016) 6:659. doi:10.3389/fimmu.2015.00659
5. Akbar AN, Henson SM. Are senescence and exhaustion intertwined or unrelated processes that compromise immunity? *Nat Rev Immunol* (2011) 11:289–95. doi:10.1038/nri2959
6. Gigley JP, Bhadra R, Moretto MM, Khan IA. T cell exhaustion in protozoan disease. *Trends Parasitol* (2012) 28:377–84. doi:10.1016/j.pt.2012.07.001
7. Albareda MC, De Rissio AM, Tomas G, Serjan A, Alvarez MG, Viotti R, et al. Polyfunctional T cell responses in children in early stages of chronic *Trypanosoma cruzi* infection contrast with monofunctional responses of long-term infected adults. *PLoS Negl Trop Dis* (2013) 7:e2575. doi:10.1371/journal.pntd.0002575
8. Freire-de-Lima CG, Nascimento DO, Soares MB, Bozza PT, Castro-Faria-Neto HC, de Mello FG, et al. Uptake of apoptotic cells drives the growth of a pathogenic trypanosome in macrophages. *Nature* (2000) 403:199–203. doi:10.1038/35003208
9. Lopes MF, Freire-de-Lima CG, DosReis GA. The macrophage haunted by cell ghosts: a pathogen grows. *Immunol Today* (2000) 21:489–94. doi:10.1016/S0167-5699(00)01713-8
10. DosReis GA, Freire-de-Lima CG, Nunes MP, Lopes MF. The importance of aberrant T-cell responses in Chagas disease. *Trends Parasitol* (2005) 21:237–43. doi:10.1016/j.pt.2005.03.008
11. D'Avila H, Freire-de-Lima CG, Roque NR, Teixeira L, Barja-Fidalgo C, Silva AR, et al. Host cell lipid bodies triggered by *Trypanosoma cruzi* infection and enhanced by the uptake of apoptotic cells are associated with prostaglandin E(2) generation and increased parasite growth. *J Infect Dis* (2011) 204:951–61. doi:10.1093/infdis/jir432
12. Luna-Gomes T, Filardy AA, Rocha JD, Decote-Ricardo D, LaRocque-de-Freitas IF, Morrot A, et al. Neutrophils increase or reduce parasite burden in *Trypanosoma cruzi*-infected macrophages, depending on host strain: role of neutrophil elastase. *PLoS One* (2014) 9:e90582. doi:10.1371/journal.pone.0090582
13. DosReis GA. Evasion of immune responses by *Trypanosoma cruzi*, the etiological agent of Chagas disease. *Braz J Med Biol Res* (2011) 44:84–90. doi:10.1590/S0100-879X2011007500005
14. Cohen TS, Jones-Nelson O, Hotz M, Cheng L, Miller LS, Suzich J, et al. *S. aureus* blocks efferocytosis of neutrophils by macrophages through the activity of its virulence factor alpha toxin. *Sci Rep* (2016) 6:35466. doi:10.1038/srep35466
15. Green DR, Oguin TH, Martinez J. The clearance of dying cells: table for two. *Cell Death Differ* (2016) 23:915–26. doi:10.1038/cdd.2015.172
16. Greenlee-Wacker MC. Clearance of apoptotic neutrophils and resolution of inflammation. *Immunol Rev* (2016) 273:357–70. doi:10.1111/imr.12453
17. Lopes MF, da Veiga VF, Santos AR, Fonseca ME, DosReis GA. Activation-induced CD4+ T cell death by apoptosis in experimental Chagas' disease. *J Immunol* (1995) 154:744–52.
18. Nunes MP, Andrade RM, Lopes MF, DosReis GA. Activation-induced T cell death exacerbates *Trypanosoma cruzi* replication in macrophages cocultured with CD4+ T lymphocytes from infected hosts. *J Immunol* (1998) 160:1313–9.
19. Alderson MR, Tough TW, Davis-Smith T, Braddy S, Falk B, Schooley KA, et al. Fas ligand mediates activation-induced cell death in human T lymphocytes. *J Exp Med* (1995) 181:71–7. doi:10.1084/jem.181.1.71
20. Lopes MF, Nunes MP, Henriques-Pons A, Giese N, Morse HC III, Davidson WF, et al. Increased susceptibility of Fas ligand-deficient gld mice to *Trypanosoma cruzi* infection due to a Th2-biased host immune response. *Eur J Immunol* (1999) 29:81–9. doi:10.1002/(SICI)1521-4141(199901)29:01<81::AID-IMMU81>3.3.CO;2-P
21. Rodrigues V Jr, Agrelli GS, Leon SC, Silva Teixeira DN, Tostes S Jr, Rocha-Rodrigues DB. Fas/Fas-L expression, apoptosis and low proliferative response are associated with heart failure in patients with chronic Chagas' disease. *Microbes Infect* (2008) 10:29–37. doi:10.1016/j.micinf.2007.09.015
22. Guillermo LV, Silva EM, Ribeiro-Gomes FL, De Meis J, Pereira WF, Yagita H, et al. The Fas death pathway controls coordinated expansions of type 1 CD8 and type 2 CD4 T cells in *Trypanosoma cruzi* infection. *J Leukoc Biol* (2007) 81:942–51. doi:10.1189/jlb.1006643
23. Vasconcelos JR, Bruna-Romero O, Araujo AF, Dominguez MR, Ersching J, de Alencar BC, et al. Pathogen-induced proapoptotic phenotype and high CD95 (Fas) expression accompany a suboptimal CD8+ T-cell response: reversal by adenoviral vaccine. *PLoS Pathog* (2012) 8:e1002699. doi:10.1371/journal.ppat.1002699
24. Chaves AT, de Assis Silva Gomes Estanislau J, Fiuza JA, Carvalho AT, Ferreira KS, Fares RC, et al. Immunoregulatory mechanisms in Chagas disease: modulation of apoptosis in T-cell mediated immune responses. *BMC Infect Dis* (2016) 16:191. doi:10.1186/s12879-016-1523-1
25. Minoprio PM, Coutinho A, Joskowicz M, D'Imperio Lima MR, Eisen H. Polyclonal lymphocyte responses to murine *Trypanosoma cruzi* infection. II. Cytotoxic T lymphocytes. *Scand J Immunol* (1986) 24:669–79. doi:10.1111/j.1365-3083.1986.tb02186.x
26. Flavia Nardy A, Santos L, Freire-de-Lima CG, Morrot A. Modulation of intrathymic sphingosine-1-phosphate levels promotes escape of immature thymocytes to the periphery with a potential proinflammatory role in Chagas disease. *Biomed Res Int* (2015) 2015:709846. doi:10.1155/2015/709846
27. Tarleton RL. CD8+ T cells in *Trypanosoma cruzi* infection. *Semin Immunopathol* (2015) 37:233–8. doi:10.1007/s00281-015-0481-9
28. Green DR, Droin N, Pinkoski M. Activation-induced cell death in T cells. *Immunol Rev* (2003) 193:70–81. doi:10.1034/j.1600-065X.2003.00051.x
29. Sikora E. Activation-induced and damage-induced cell death in aging human T cells. *Mech Ageing Dev* (2015) 151:85–92. doi:10.1016/j.mad.2015.03.011
30. Leguizamon MS, Mocetti E, Garcia Rivello H, Argibay P, Campetella O. Trans-sialidase from *Trypanosoma cruzi* induces apoptosis in cells from the immune system in vivo. *J Infect Dis* (1999) 180:1398–402. doi:10.1086/315001
31. Mendonca-Previato L, Penha L, Garcez TC, Jones C, Previato JO. Addition of alpha-O-GlcNAc to threonine residues define the post-translational modification of mucin-like molecules in *Trypanosoma cruzi*. *Glycoconj J* (2013) 30:659–66. doi:10.1007/s10719-013-9469-7
32. Freire-de-Lima L, da Fonseca LM, da Silva VA, da Costa KM, Morrot A, Freire-de-Lima CG, et al. Modulation of cell sialoglycophenotype: a stylish

mechanism adopted by *Trypanosoma cruzi* to ensure its persistence in the infected host. *Front Microbiol* (2016) 7:698. doi:10.3389/fmicb.2016.00698
33. Previato JO, Jones C, Xavier MT, Wait R, Travassos LR, Parodi AJ, et al. Structural characterization of the major glycosylphosphatidylinositol membrane-anchored glycoprotein from epimastigote forms of *Trypanosoma cruzi* Y-strain. *J Biol Chem* (1995) 270:7241–50. doi:10.1074/jbc.270.13.7241
34. Freire-de-Lima CG, Nunes MP, Corte-Real S, Soares MP, Previato JO, Mendonca-Previato L, et al. Proapoptotic activity of a *Trypanosoma cruzi* ceramide-containing glycolipid turned on in host macrophages by IFN-gamma. *J Immunol* (1998) 161:4909–16.
35. Wyllie AH. Apoptosis and carcinogenesis. *Eur J Cell Biol* (1997) 73:189–97.
36. Kuzmenko DI, Klimentyeva TK. Role of ceramide in apoptosis and development of insulin resistance. *Biochemistry (Mosc)* (2016) 81:913–27. doi:10.1134/S0006297916090017
37. Huang JR, Tsai YC, Chang YJ, Wu JC, Hung JT, Lin KH, et al. alpha-Galactosylceramide but not phenyl-glycolipids induced NKT cell anergy and IL-33-mediated myeloid-derived suppressor cell accumulation via upregulation of egr2/3. *J Immunol* (2014) 192:1972–81. doi:10.4049/jimmunol.1302623
38. Schaumburg F, Hippe D, Vutova P, Luder CG. Pro- and anti-apoptotic activities of protozoan parasites. *Parasitology* (2006) 132 Suppl:S69–85. doi:10.1017/S0031182006000874
39. Erwig LP, Henson PM. Clearance of apoptotic cells by phagocytes. *Cell Death Differ* (2008) 15:243–50. doi:10.1038/sj.cdd.4402184
40. Hermetet F, Jacquin E, Launay S, Gaiffe E, Couturier M, Hirchaud F, et al. Efferocytosis of apoptotic human papillomavirus-positive cervical cancer cells by human primary fibroblasts. *Biol Cell* (2016) 108:189–204. doi:10.1111/boc.201500090
41. Janssen WJ, Bratton DL, Jakubzick CV, Henson PM. Myeloid cell turnover and clearance. *Microbiol Spectr* (2016) 4. doi:10.1128/microbiolspec.MCHD-0005-2015
42. Elliott MR, Koster KM, Murphy PS. Efferocytosis signaling in the regulation of macrophage inflammatory responses. *J Immunol* (2017) 198:1387–94. doi:10.4049/jimmunol.1601520
43. Voll RE, Herrmann M, Roth EA, Stach C, Kalden JR, Girkontaite I. Immunosuppressive effects of apoptotic cells. *Nature* (1997) 390:350–1. doi:10.1038/37022
44. Fadok VA, Bratton DL, Konowal A, Freed PW, Westcott JY, Henson PM. Macrophages that have ingested apoptotic cells in vitro inhibit proinflammatory cytokine production through autocrine/paracrine mechanisms involving TGF-beta, PGE2, and PAF. *J Clin Invest* (1998) 101:890–8. doi:10.1172/JCI1112
45. Freire-de-Lima CG, Xiao YQ, Gardai SJ, Bratton DL, Schiemann WP, Henson PM. Apoptotic cells, through transforming growth factor-beta, coordinately induce anti-inflammatory and suppress pro-inflammatory eicosanoid and NO synthesis in murine macrophages. *J Biol Chem* (2006) 281:38376–84. doi:10.1074/jbc.M605146200
46. Xiao YQ, Freire-de-Lima CG, Janssen WJ, Morimoto K, Lyu D, Bratton DL, et al. Oxidants selectively reverse TGF-beta suppression of proinflammatory mediator production. *J Immunol* (2006) 176:1209–17. doi:10.4049/jimmunol.176.2.1209
47. Xiao YQ, Freire-de-Lima CG, Schiemann WP, Bratton DL, Vandivier RW, Henson PM. Transcriptional and translational regulation of TGF-beta production in response to apoptotic cells. *J Immunol* (2008) 181:3575–85. doi:10.4049/jimmunol.181.5.3575
48. Arcanjo AF, LaRocque-de-Freitas IF, Rocha JD, Zamith D, Costa-da-Silva AC, Nunes MP, et al. The PGE2/IL-10 axis determines susceptibility of B-1 cell-derived phagocytes (B-1CDP) to *Leishmania major* infection. *PLoS One* (2015) 10:e0124888. doi:10.1371/journal.pone.0124888
49. Ravichandran KS, Lorenz U. Engulfment of apoptotic cells: signals for a good meal. *Nat Rev Immunol* (2007) 7:964–74. doi:10.1038/nri2214
50. Hanayama R, Tanaka M, Miwa K, Shinohara A, Iwamatsu A, Nagata S. Identification of a factor that links apoptotic cells to phagocytes. *Nature* (2002) 417:182–7. doi:10.1038/417182a
51. Savill J, Hogg N, Ren Y, Haslett C. Thrombospondin cooperates with CD36 and the vitronectin receptor in macrophage recognition of neutrophils undergoing apoptosis. *J Clin Invest* (1992) 90:1513–22. doi:10.1172/JCI116019
52. Grabiec AM, Hussell T. The role of airway macrophages in apoptotic cell clearance following acute and chronic lung inflammation. *Semin Immunopathol* (2016) 38:409–23. doi:10.1007/s00281-016-0555-3
53. Penberthy KK, Ravichandran KS. Apoptotic cell recognition receptors and scavenger receptors. *Immunol Rev* (2016) 269:44–59. doi:10.1111/imr.12376
54. Roszer T. Transcriptional control of apoptotic cell clearance by macrophage nuclear receptors. *Apoptosis* (2017) 22:284–94. doi:10.1007/s10495-016-1310-x
55. Ariyanayagam MR, Oza SL, Mehlert A, Fairlamb AH. Bis(glutathionyl)spermine and other novel trypanothione analogues in *Trypanosoma cruzi*. *J Biol Chem* (2003) 278:27612–9. doi:10.1074/jbc.M302750200
56. Reigada C, Saye M, Vera EV, Balcazar D, Fraccaroli L, Carrillo C, et al. *Trypanosoma cruzi* polyamine transporter: its role on parasite growth and survival under stress conditions. *J Membr Biol* (2016) 249:475–81. doi:10.1007/s00232-016-9888-z
57. Moraes KC, Diniz LF, Bahia MT. Role of cyclooxygenase-2 in *Trypanosoma cruzi* survival in the early stages of parasite host-cell interaction. *Mem Inst Oswaldo Cruz* (2015) 110:181–91. doi:10.1590/0074-02760140311
58. Cossentini LA, Da Silva RV, Yamada-Ogatta SF, Yamauchi LM, De Almeida Araujo EJ, Pinge-Filho P. Aspirin treatment exacerbates oral infections by *Trypanosoma cruzi*. *Exp Parasitol* (2016) 164:64–70. doi:10.1016/j.exppara.2016.01.008
59. Molina-Berrios A, Campos-Estrada C, Henriquez N, Faundez M, Torres G, Castillo C, et al. Protective role of acetylsalicylic acid in experimental *Trypanosoma cruzi* infection: evidence of a 15-epi-lipoxin A(4)-mediated effect. *PLoS Negl Trop Dis* (2013) 7:e2173. doi:10.1371/journal.pntd.0002173
60. Malvezi AD, Panis C, da Silva RV, de Freitas RC, Lovo-Martins MI, Tatakihara VL, et al. Inhibition of cyclooxygenase-1 and cyclooxygenase-2 impairs *Trypanosoma cruzi* entry into cardiac cells and promotes differential modulation of the inflammatory response. *Antimicrob Agents Chemother* (2014) 58:6157–64. doi:10.1128/AAC.02752-14
61. Michelin MA, Silva JS, Cunha FQ. Inducible cyclooxygenase released prostaglandin mediates immunosuppression in acute phase of experimental *Trypanosoma cruzi* infection. *Exp Parasitol* (2005) 111:71–9. doi:10.1016/j.exppara.2005.05.001
62. Silva EM, Guillermo LV, Ribeiro-Gomes FL, De Meis J, Pereira RM, Wu Z, et al. Caspase-8 activity prevents type 2 cytokine responses and is required for protective T cell-mediated immunity against *Trypanosoma cruzi* infection. *J Immunol* (2005) 174:6314–21. doi:10.4049/jimmunol.174.10.6314
63. Silva EM, Guillermo LV, Ribeiro-Gomes FL, De Meis J, Nunes MP, Senra JF, et al. Caspase inhibition reduces lymphocyte apoptosis and improves host immune responses to *Trypanosoma cruzi* infection. *Eur J Immunol* (2007) 37:738–46. doi:10.1002/eji.200636790
64. Cabral-Piccin MP, Guillermo LV, Vellozo NS, Filardy AA, Pereira-Marques ST, Rigoni TS, et al. Apoptotic CD8 T-lymphocytes disable macrophage-mediated immunity to *Trypanosoma cruzi* infection. *Cell Death Dis* (2016) 7:e2232. doi:10.1038/cddis.2016.135
65. Favaloro B, Allocati N, Graziano V, Di Ilio C, De Laurenzi V. Role of apoptosis in disease. *Aging (Albany NY)* (2012) 4:330–49. doi:10.18632/aging.100459

16

Dependency of B-1 Cells in the Maintenance of Splenic Interleukin-10 Producing Cells and Impairment of Macrophage Resistance in Visceral Leishmaniasis

Angélica Fernandes Arcanjo[1], Dirlei Nico[2], Gabriellen Menezes Migliani de Castro[2], Yasmin da Silva Fontes[2], Paula Saltarelli[2], Debora Decote-Ricardo[3], Marise P. Nunes[4], Antônio Ferreira-Pereira[2], Clarisa B. Palatnik-de-Sousa[2], Célio G. Freire-de-Lima[1] and Alexandre Morrot[4,5]**

[1] Instituto de Biofísica Carlos Chagas Filho, Universidade Federal do Rio de Janeiro, Rio de Janeiro, Brazil, [2] Departamento de Microbiologia Geral, Universidade Federal do Rio de Janeiro, Rio de Janeiro, Brazil, [3] Instituto de Veterinária, Universidade Federal Rural do Rio de Janeiro, Rio de Janeiro, Brazil, [4] Instituto Oswaldo Cruz, Fiocruz, Rio de Janeiro, Brazil, [5] Departamento de Imunologia, Instituto de Microbiologia, Universidade Federal do Rio de Janeiro, Rio de Janeiro, Brazil

***Correspondence:**
Alexandre Morrot
morrot@micro.ufrj.br
Célio G. Freire-de-Lima
celio@biof.ufrj.br

Visceral leishmaniasis is a neglected disease caused by *Leishmania* protozoa parasites transmitted by infected sand fly vectors. This disease represents the second in mortality among tropical infections and is associated to a profound immunosuppression state of the host. The hallmark of this infection-induced host immunodeviation is the characteristic high levels of the regulatory interleukin-10 (IL-10) cytokine. In the present study, we investigated the role of B-1 cells in the maintenance of splenic IL-10 levels that could interfere with resistance to parasite infection. Using an experimental murine infection model with *Leishmania (L.) infantum chagasi* we demonstrated an improved resistance of B-1 deficient BALB/XID mice to infection. BALB/XID mice developed a reduced splenomegaly with diminished splenic parasite burden and lower levels of IL-10 secretion of purified splenocytes at 30 days post-infection, as compared to BALB/c wild-type control mice. Interestingly, we found that resident peritoneal macrophages isolated from BALB/XID mice were more effective to control the parasite load in comparison to cells isolated from BALB/c wild-type mice. Our findings point to a role of B-1 cells in the host susceptibility to visceral leishmaniasis.

Keywords: visceral leishmaniasis, *Leishmania (L.) infantum chagasi*, B-1 cells, host protective responses

INTRODUCTION

Visceral leishmaniasis (VL), also known as Kala Azar is a neglected tropical disease caused by the intracellular protozoan *Leishmania donovani* and *Leishmania (L.) infantum chagasi* parasites (Kaye and Scott, 2011). Over 90% of the annual incidence of new cases occurs in Bangladesh, India, Nepal, Sudan, South Sudan, Ethiopia, and Brazil. In these countries, the outbreaks and prevalence of infection, from which are reported clinical cases, differ in their eco-epidemiology and sand fly vectors involved. This disease is fatal if not treated, and can kill between 20,000 and 40,000 people a year worldwide.

The treatment is often performed on the basis of pentavalent antimony compounds and amphotericin B lipid formulations, and its symptoms include: hepatosplenomegaly, fever, anemia, weight loss, and hyperglobulinemia (Kaye and Scott, 2011; Matlashewski et al., 2011; McCall et al., 2013; Ready, 2014).

The immune system works as a crucial barrier in the hosts to the establishment of natural infections. The initial steps of a immune response against *Leishmania* infection is triggered from the activation of innate receptors pattern recognition receptors (PRRs) by molecules associated with pathogens (MMAPs) such as lipophosphoglycans, glycoinositolphospholipid, and metalloproteinase GP63, all expressed on parasite cell surface (Liu and Uzonna, 2012). Activation of PRRs is crucial for induction of interleukin-12 (IL-12) by antigen presenting cells necessary to promote the secretion of interferon-gamma (IFN-γ) by $CD4^+$ T lymphocytes and natural killer cells. IFN-γ is a type-1 pro-inflammatory cytokine extremely important to activate the microbicidal activity of macrophages, the major reservoir of *Leishmania* parasites. Once activated, macrophages are able to secrete reactive oxygen species (ROS) and nitric oxide (NO), both involved in the destruction of parasites (Kaye and Scott, 2011; Liu and Uzonna, 2012).

In natural and experimental VL infection, cell-mediated immune responses are suppressed causing a decrease in IFN-γ levels. This subversion of the immune response is associated with production of regulatory cytokines such as interleukin-10 (IL-10) and transforming growth factor-beta (TGF-β), associated with the progression of disease (Kumar and Nylén, 2012). In human infection, significantly higher levels of IL-10 produced by regulatory T cells are present in patients that do not respond to chemotherapeutic treatment, suggesting an important role of this cytokine in the suppression of host immunity during disease (Guha et al., 2014). Increased levels of IL-10 negatively modulate innate immunity via macrophage inhibition of ROS and NO expression (Kumar and Nylén, 2012).

The expression of IL-10 is not specific to cells of the innate immune system but also lymphocytes, including B cells that mediate suppressive responses in VL (Murphy et al., 2001; Deak et al., 2010; Gautam et al., 2011; Bankoti et al., 2012). It has been shown that IL-10-derived from B cells is capable to promote the development of suppressive responses associated with susceptibility to infection (Bankoti et al., 2012; Arcanjo et al., 2015). However, the identification of the B cell population involved in the susceptibility to VL is still vague and needs further studies. Recently it has been demonstrated that B-1 cells contribute to susceptibility to infection with *L. (L.) infantum chagasi* (Gonzaga et al., 2015). B-1 cells represent the major population of B lymphocytes in the pleural and peritoneal cavity. These cells are able to secrete high levels of IL-10 that could modulate the phagocytic activity of macrophages (Aziz et al., 2015). The impairment of the mononuclear phagocyte system is a key factor in the disease progression thus contributing to splenic dysfunction and symptoms of splenomegaly (Kaye et al., 2004). In the present study, we aimed to investigate the role of B-1 cells in the resistance of macrophages to *Leishmania* infection.

MATERIALS AND METHODS

Ethics Statement

All mouse studies followed the guidelines set by the National Institutes of Health, United States. The study was approved by the Research Ethics Committee of Federal University of Rio de Janeiro (protocol IMPPG040-07/16). Protocols for animal were approved by the Institutional Ethical Committees in accordance with international guidelines. All animal experimentation was performed in accordance with the terms of the Brazilian guidelines for the animal welfare regulations.

Animals, Infection, and Evaluation of Host Responses

BALB/c wild-type control mice and BALB/XID mice (X-linked BALB/c immunodeficient mice genetically deficient in B-1 cells) originated from breeding colonies kindly donated by Professor Mário Mariano (UNIFESP, Brazil) were maintained in our animal facilities (UFRJ). Experimental infection was performed by inoculating 4- to 8-week-old female BALB/c and B-1 cell-deficient BALB/XID mice intravenously with 5×10^7 *L. (L.) infantum chagasi* amastigotes (IOC-L 3324) obtained from infected hamster spleens. Thirty days after infection, mice were euthanized and the liver and splenic parasite load were evaluated in Giemsa-stained smears and expressed in LDU values (*Leishman–Donovan* units of Stauber = number of amastigotes per 1000 liver cell nuclei/mg of liver weight).

Anti-*Leishmania (L.) infantum chagasi* ELISA

Immunoglobulin isotypes and IgG subtype profiles were monitored by an enzyme-linked immunosorbent assay (ELISA) using the freeze and thawed lysate of stationary phase promastigotes of *L. (L.) infantum chagasi* (MHOM/BR/74/PP/75) as antigen. Whole parasite antigens (2 μg/ml) were plated at 100 μl/well to 96-well plates and, after overnight incubation at 4°C, the plates were washed three times using PBS containing 0.05% (vol/vol) Tween 20 (Sigma, Gillingham, United Kingdom). Serial twofold 1:100 to 1:800 dilutions of serum samples from mice diluted in PBS containing 0.05% Tween were added to the plates and incubated at 37°C for 1 h. Afterward the plates were washed three times with PBS containing 0.05% Tween, and the 1:5,000 dilution of peroxidase-labeled each goat anti-mouse Ig isotypes (Jackson ImmunoResearch, West Grove, United States) were added at 100 μl/well and incubated at 37°C for 1 h. The reaction was developed with 50 mM phosphate/citrate buffer (pH 5.0) containing 2 mM *o*-phenylenediamine HCl and 0.007% (vol/vol) H_2O_2 (Sigma, United Kingdom), and interrupted with the addition of 2 M H_2SO_4 (50 μl/well). The ELISA plates were read at 490 nm (Spectra Max 190, Molecular Devices, Sunnyvale, United States).

Cytokine Assays

Splenocytes (1×10^6/0.5 mL) obtained from control or infected mice at 30 days post-infection (DPI) were cultured in 48 well at

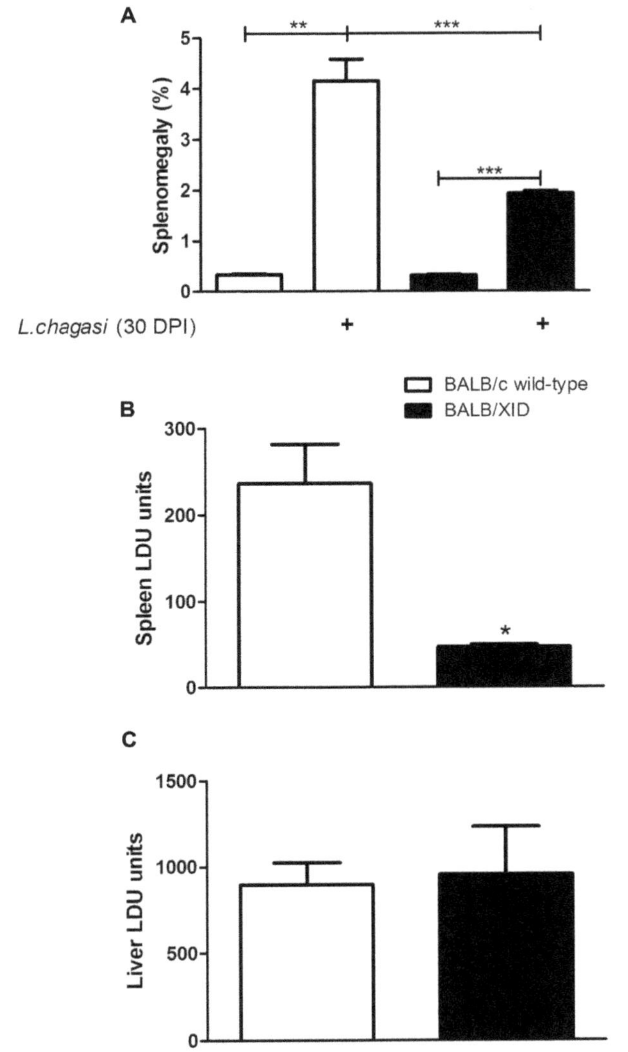

FIGURE 1 | B-1 cell-deficient BALB/XID mice show resistance to visceral leishmaniasis. BALB/c and BALB/XID mice were intravenously injected with 5×10^7 amastigotes of *Leishmania (L.) infantum chagasi*, and 30 days after infection the clinical signs of disease were examined. **(A)** Spleen/body relative weights are attenuated in B-1 cell-deficient BALB/XID mice. The body weight was measured in grams and the spleen/body relative weights (grams of organ weight × 100/grams of body weight) were determined in BALB/c and BALB/XID mice. **(B)** Decreased parasite burden in the spleen of BALB/XID mice. The vertical axis in the histogram represents the average parasite load from spleen or **(C)** liver tissues in Leishman–Donovan units of Stauber (LDU = number of amastigotes/1000 cell nuclei × organ weight in mg) obtained at 30 days post-infection (DPI). Data are means ± SE and represent the results of two independent experiments performed with five to six mice per group. Differences between groups are significant $^{*}p < 0.05$, $^{**}p < 0.01$, $^{***}p < 0.001$.

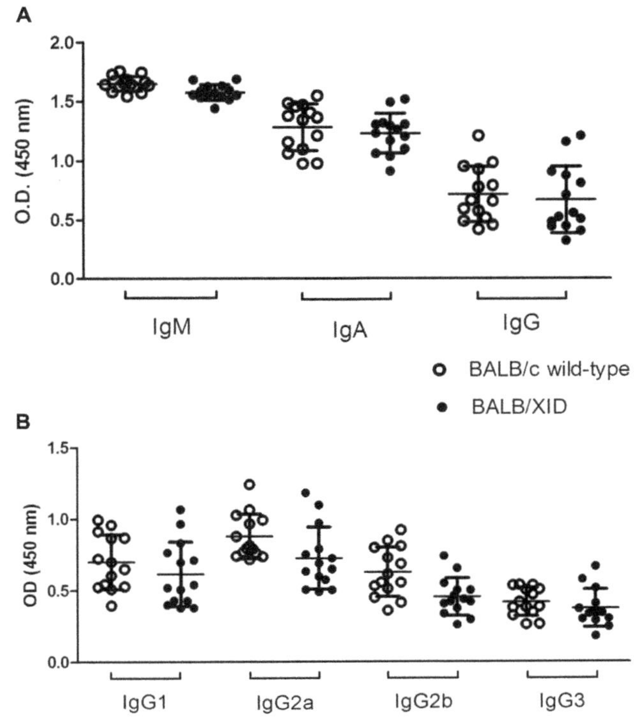

FIGURE 2 | Isotype and IgG subclass profiles of serum antibodies to *Leishmania (L.) infantum chagasi* of B-1 cell-deficient mice. Sera from wild type BALB/c and B-1 cell-deficient BALB/XID mice infected with 5×10^7 amastigote forms of *Leishmania (L.)* infantum chagasi were collected at 30 DPI and the absorbance values of **(A)** antibody Isotypes (IgM, IgA and IgG); and **(B)** IgG antibody subclasses (IgG1, IgG2a, IgG2b and IgG3) were determined by ELISA using *Leishmania (L.) infantum chagasi* promastigote lysates as parasite antigens. Bars show levels of immunoglobulin isotypes and IgG subclasses as the individual absorbancy values of 1/100 diluted sera. Data represent the individual results for each group of mice obtained from two independent experiments.

37°C/5% CO_2 in complete RPMI medium, stimulated or not with 10^6 freeze–thawed stationary phase *L. (L) infantum chagasi* (L579 Fiocruz) promastigotes. After 3 days, supernatants were collected and cytokine levels (IFN-γ, TNF-α, IL-10, and TGF-β) were assayed by ELISA (R&D Systems). Plates were read at 405 nm and values are presented as pg cytokine/mL [mean ± standard error (SE)]. Statistical differences between mean values were evaluated by ANOVA, and pair-wise comparisons were done by the Tukey test.

In Vitro Infection of Macrophages and Detection of ROS

Resident peritoneal macrophages isolated from BALB/c or BALB/XID mice cultured at 1.0×10^5 cells/well in 48-well plates received 10^6 *L. (L.) infantum chagasi* promastigote forms (MHOM/BR/74/PP/75) in the stationary phase at 37°C in complete Dulbecco's Modified Eagle's Medium (DMEM) containing 10% fetal bovine serum (FBS). After 4 h, the cell monolayers were extensively washed for the removal of extracellular parasites, and the cultures were then maintained for 3 days at 37°C. Afterward, infected macrophages were cultured in Schneider medium (Life Technologies) supplemented with 20% FBS at 26°C for an additional 3 days in order to estimate the *L. chagasi* load by counting the promastigotes

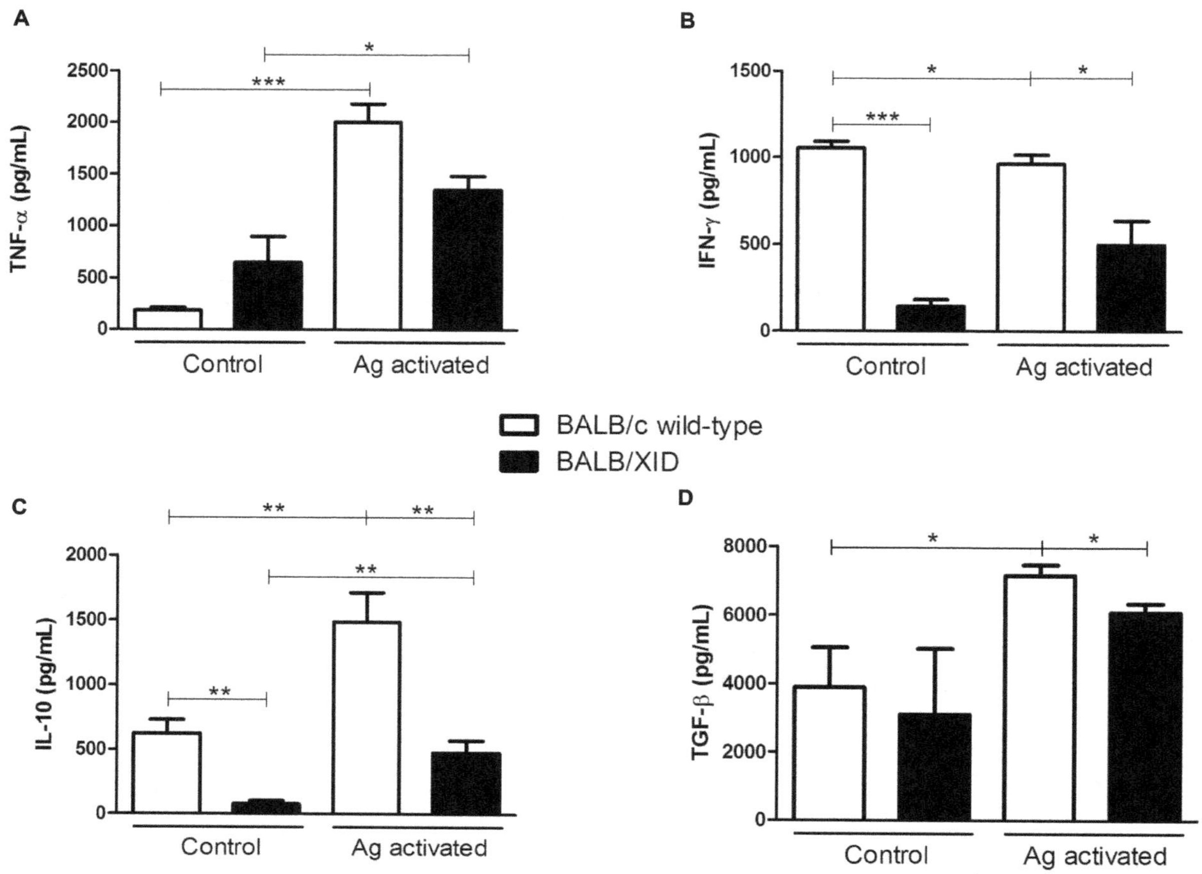

FIGURE 3 | Splenocytes from B-1 cell-deficient BALB/XID mice produce low levels of IL-10. BALB/c and BALB/XID mice were intravenously infected with 5×10^7 amastigotes of *Leishmania (L.) infantum chagasi*, and 30 days after infection splenocytes were isolated and assayed for cytokine production upon parasite antigen (Ag) stimulation. After 3 days of *in vitro* culture with freeze and thawed lysates of *Leishmania (L.) infantum chagasi* promastigotes, as described elsewhere (Popi et al., 2012), splenocyte supernatants were harvested for determination of **(A)** TNF-α, **(B)** IFN-γ, **(C)** IL-10, and **(D)** TGF-β by ELISA. The *y*-axis represents the levels of cytokines, detected by specific ELISA assays, expressed in ng/ml. Data are means ± SE and represent the results of two independent experiments performed with five to six mice per group. Asterisks represent statistical significance between groups $*p < 0.05$, $**p < 0.01$, $***p < 0.001$.

forms, as described elsewhere (Ribeiro-Gomes et al., 2004). For detection of ROS, cells were incubated with 10 μM H_2DCFDA probe (Invitrogen) prior to parasite infection and/or activation stimuli (200 ng/ml LPS, 2 ng/ml IFN-γ). A change in fluorescence was assessed with a fluorimeter (Spectramax M3).

Statistical Analysis

Statistical analyses were performed with GraphPad Prism 4 software, using one-way ANOVA test. Results were expressed as mean ± SE, differences between control and treated group were considered statistically significant when $p \leq 0.05$.

RESULTS AND DISCUSSION

In our study, we used a murine model of VL in which infection of BALB/c mice with *L. (L.) infantum chagasi* amastigotes gives rise to a higher parasite load in the first weeks of infection, after which it is controlled by the host immune response. The infection of BALB/c and B-1 cell-deficient BALB/XID mice was performed by inoculating 4- to 8-week-old females intravenously with 5×10^7 *L. (L.) infantum chagasi* amastigotes (IOC-L 3324) obtained from infected hamster spleens. Thirty days after infection, mice were euthanized and the splenic and intrahepatic parasite burdens were evaluated in Giemsa-stained smears and expressed in LDU values. Our results demonstrated an increased resistance of BALB/XID mice correlating with lower increases in the spleen/body weight ratio as compared to BALB/c wild-type control mice (**Figure 1A**). These results were in line with the demonstration of a reduced splenic parasite burden at 30 DPI in B-1 cell-deficient mice (**Figure 1B**). In contrast, infection in both mice groups yielded similar intrahepatic parasite burden indexes 1 month after intravenously inoculation with *L. (L.) infantum chagasi* amastigotes (**Figure 1C**), corroborating previous findings using an infection experimental model with lower parasite dose (Gonzaga et al., 2015). The higher susceptibility of infected BALB/XID mice was not due to any alteration of antibody-mediated responses as we did not observe any significant change in the immunoglobulin isotypes nor in the IgG subtype profiles from both groups at 30 DPI (**Figure 2**).

A major factor contributing to susceptibility in leishmaniasis is the development of a strong IL-10 response (Murphy et al., 2001; Gautam et al., 2011; Bankoti et al., 2012). We therefore compared the cytokine responses to infection with *L. (L.) infantum chagasi* parasites by analyzing the supernatants of splenocytes isolated from both infected BALB/XID mice and BALB/c wild-type control groups that were stimulated with whole parasite antigens for 3 days. Splenocytes obtained from both infected mice groups at 30 DPI showed increased levels of protective pro-inflammatory response characterized by high levels of TNF-α, when antigen-stimulated (**Figure 3A**). However when compared the ratio of antigen-stimulated/control indexes for the TNF-α values, we observed a higher increase for BALB/c wild-type control groups as compared to BALB/XID mice. Analysis of IFN-γ expression also indicated an increased levels of this pro-inflammatory cytokine upon stimulation of splenocytes with parasite antigens in BALB/XID mice, although basal levels of this cytokine were secreted in the controls of BALB/c wild-type mice (**Figure 3B**). Increased basal levels of IFN-γ may indicate a progressive disease with high parasite load and infection-induced pathology (Goto and Prianti, 2009). In contrast, the splenocytes from infected BALB/XID mice produced lower levels of IL-10 upon stimulation with parasite antigens (**Figure 3C**). The same pattern was obtained for the regulatory TGF-β cytokine, as the splenocytes from infected BALB/XID mice produced slightly lower amounts of TGF-β upon stimulation with parasite antigens in comparison to controls of BALB/c wild-type mice (**Figure 3D**). However, although statistically significant, the differences observed for TGF-β between both mice groups have not yielded striking results.

We next tested the capacity of resident peritoneal macrophages isolated from BALB/XID mice to control de parasite load in comparison to their counterparts isolated from infected BALB/c wild-type mice. In these assays, macrophages were *in vitro* infected with *L. (L.) infantum chagasi* promastigote forms and the parasite load was measured to determine the macrophage resistance to *Leishmania* infection. According to our results, resident peritoneal macrophages obtained from BALB/XID mice were more effective in eliminating *Leishmania* parasites as compared to macrophages isolated from BALB/c wild-type mice (**Figure 4**). The differences in the innate resistance from resident peritoneal macrophages isolated from both mice groups were not due to any chance in the production of ROS, which are important effector agents against intracellular pathogens. Our results showed that *in vitro*-infected IFN-γ/LPS-activated macrophages from both mice groups produced ROS within first hours of infection with *L. (L.) infantum chagasi* promastigotes (**Supplementary Figure S1**). The data point to the interference of inhibitory effect of homeostatic IL-10 produced by B1-cells on the resident peritoneal macrophages derived from BALB/XID mice.

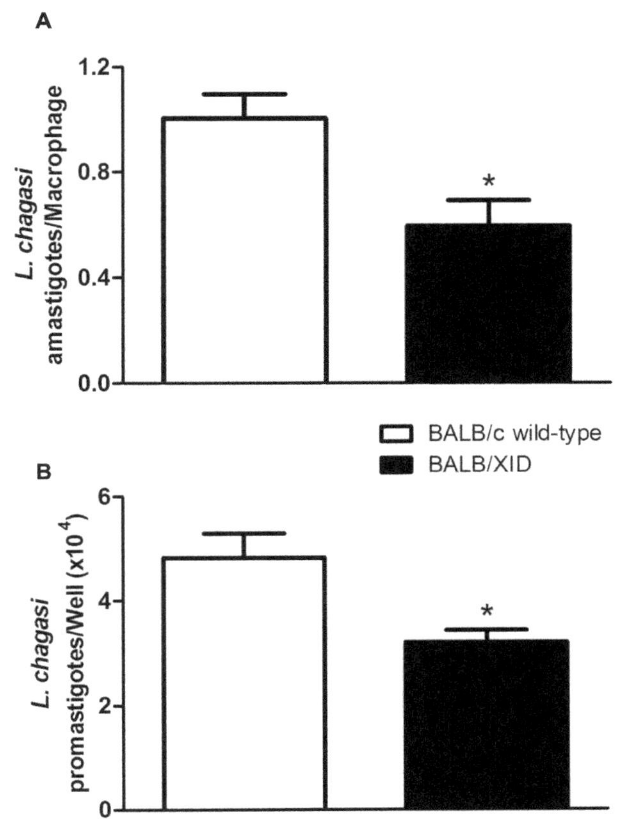

FIGURE 4 | *Leishmania (L.) infantum chagasi* infection of tissue-resident macrophages obtained from BALB/c and BALB/XID mice. Intraperitoneal macrophage cells purified from BALB/c and BALB/XID mice were cultured at 1.0×10^5 cells/well in 48-well plates and infected with 10^6 *Leishmania (L.) infantum chagasi* promastigotes at a 10:1 ratio of parasites:host cells in DMEM containing 10% FBS at 37°C. The infected cells were washed 4 h to remove extracellular parasites and then maintained for 3 days at 37°C to determine the intracellular amastigote load **(A)**. Following intracellular parasitism, infected macrophages were cultured in Schneider medium supplemented with 20% FBS at 26°C for an additional 3 days to estimate the *L. chagasi* load by counting the promastigotes forms derived from released parasites **(B)**. Histograms represent the means ± SE of total number of *Leishmania (L.) infantum chagasi* forms of triplicate assays and are representative from two independent experiments. Differences between groups are significant $^*p < 0.05$.

Taken together, our results clearly indicate that BALB/c mice have an impaired immune response upon infection with *L. (L.) infantum chagasi* as compared to BALB/XID mice. The maintenance of low levels of IL-10 in BALB/XID mice due to the loss of B-1 cells is associated with an improved control of the parasite in spleen tissues and enhanced innate resistance of macrophages to *Leishmania* infection. These results indicate a potentiation of the anti-parasitic activity in B-1 cell-deficient BALB/XID mice. The role of B-1 cells in protective mediated-immunity of the host depends on the nature of the pathogen as well as the infection experimental models (Minoprio et al., 1993; Hoerauf et al., 1994; Babai et al., 1999; Gaubert et al., 1999; Herbert et al., 2002; Popi et al., 2008; Crane et al., 2013;

Szymczak et al., 2013; Gonzaga et al., 2015). Intracelular parasites such as *Trypanosoma cruzi* and *Francisella tularensis* that target macrophage cells are susceptible to negative modulation of the mononuclear phagocyte system by B-1 cells (Minoprio et al., 1993; Crane et al., 2013). In fact these cells can be programmed to differentiate into phagocytes (Popi et al., 2012) that could promote immunosurveillance in the different tissues affected by the parasitism thus contributing to the outcome of infection.

Alternatively, B-1 cells can differentiate into IgM-secreting cells working as an innate-like B cell populations with distinct repertoire and tissue location from the conventional B lymphocytes or B-2 cells (Aziz et al., 2015). Interestingly, it has been proposed that the production and activation of a polyclonal B-lymphocyte responses expressing IgM are the major cause of disease susceptibility in animals infected with *L. infantum* (Deak et al., 2010). In addition, it has been shown that B cells in the marginal zone are able to suppress antigen-specific responses from both $CD8^+$ and $CD4^+$ lymphocytes during the early stages of VL, thereby preventing the generation of protective effector and memory T cells in *L. donovani* infection (Bankoti et al., 2012). The properties of B-1 cells to act as rapid immune responders that promptly migrate and redistribute to secondary lymphoid tissues where they can be resident as cytokine and antibody-secreting differentiated cells (Aziz et al., 2015) could be determinant to the development of infection. Understanding the role of B-1 cells and the control of infection-induced signals that activate these cells in VL could lead to better strategies to control this devastating disease.

AUTHOR CONTRIBUTIONS

AM, CF conceived and designed the experiments. AA, DN, GC, YS, PS performed the experiments. AA, DN, PS, DD, MN, CF and AM analyzed the data. DD, AF, CP and CF contributed reagents/materials/analysis tools. CF and AM wrote the paper.

SUPPLEMENTARY MATERIAL

FIGURE S1 | ROS production during *Leishmania (L.) infantum chagasi* promastigote infection. Resident peritoneal macrophages isolated from BALB/c or BALB/XID mice were infected with *Leishmania (L.) infantum chagasi* promastigote forms (at 1:10 host–parasite ratio. The infection was done in the presence or absence of activation stimuli (200 ng/ml LPS, 2 ng/ml IFN-γ) and the ROS production was measured with fluorometric assay using H_2DCFDA probe. The values represent the mean ± SEM of three independents experiments. Indicated differences between groups are significant $*p < 0.05$, $**p < 0.01$, $***p < 0.001$.

REFERENCES

1. Arcanjo, A. F., La Rocque-de-Freitas, I. F., Rocha, J. D., Zamith, D., Costa-da-Silva, A. C., Nunes, M. P., et al. (2015). The PGE2 /IL-10 axis determines susceptibility of B-1 cell-derived phagocytes (B-1CDP) to *Leishmania major* infection. *PLoS ONE* 10:e0124888. doi: 10.1371/journal.pone.0124888
2. Aziz, M., Holodick, N. E., Rothstein, T. L., and Wang, P. (2015). The role of B- 1 cells in inflammation. *Immunol. Res.* 63, 153–166. doi: 10.1007/s12026-015- 8708-3
3. Babai, B., Louzir, H., Cazenave, P. A., and Dellagi, K. (1999). Depletion of peritoneal CD5+ B cells has no effect on the course of *Leishmania major* infection in susceptible and resistant mice. *Clin. Exp. Immunol.* 117, 123–129. doi: 10.1046/j.1365-2249.1999.00953.x
4. Bankoti, R., Gupta, K., Levchenko, A., and Stäger, S. (2012). Marginal zone B cells regulate antigen-specific T cell responses during infection. *J. Immunol.* 188, 3961–3971. doi: 10.4049/jimmunol.1102880
5. Crane, D. D., Griffin, A. J., Wehrly, T. D., and Bosio, C. M. (2013). B1a cells enhance susceptibility to infection with virulent *Francisella tularensis* via modulation of NK/NKT cell responses. *J. Immunol.* 190, 2756–2766. doi: 10.4049/jimmunol. 1202697
6. Deak, E., Jayakumar, A., Cho, K. W., Goldsmith-Pestana, K., Dondji, B., and Lambris, J. D. (2010). Murine visceral leishmaniasis: IgM and polyclonal B-cell activation lead to disease exacerbation. *Eur. J. Immunol.* 40, 1355–1368. doi: 10.1002/eji.200939455
7. Gaubert, S., Viana da Costa, A., Maurage, C. A., Lima, E. C., Fontaine, J., Lafitte, S., et al. (1999). X-linked immunodeficiency affects the outcome of *Schistosoma mansoni* infection in the murine model. *Parasite Immunol.* 21, 89–101. doi: 10.1046/j.1365-3024.1999.00205.x
8. Gautam, S., Kumar, R., Maurya, R., Nylén, S., Ansari, N., Rai, M., et al. (2011). IL-10 neutralization promotes parasite clearance in splenic aspirate cells from patients with visceral leishmaniasis. *J. Infect. Dis.* 204, 1134–1137. doi: 10.1093/ infdis/jir461
9. Gonzaga, W. F., Xavier, V., Vivanco, B. C., Lopes, J. D., and Xander, P. (2015). B-1 cells contribute to susceptibility in experimental infection with *Leishmania (Leishmania) chagasi*. *Parasitology* 142, 1506–1515. doi: 10.1017/ S0031182015000943
10. Goto, H., and Prianti, M. D. (2009). Immunoactivation and immunopathogeny during active visceral leishmaniasis. *Rev. Inst. Med. Trop. Sao Paulo* 51, 241–246. doi: 10.1590/S0036-46652009000500002
11. Guha, R., Das, S., Ghosh, J., Sundar, S., Dujardin, J. C., and Roy, S. (2014). Antimony resistant *Leishmania donovani* but not sensitive ones drives greater frequency of potent T-regulatory cells upon interaction with human PBMCs: role of IL-10 and TGF-β in early immune response. *PLoS Negl. Trop. Dis.* 8:e2995. doi: 10.1371/journal.pntd.0002995
12. Herbert, D. R., Nolan, T. J., Schad, G. A., and Abraham, D. (2002). The role of B cells in immunity against larval *Strongyloides stercoralis* in mice. *Parasite Immunol.* 24, 95–101. doi: 10.1046/j.0141-9838.2001.00441.x
13. Hoerauf, A., Solbach, W., Lohoff, M., and Röllinghoff, M. (1994). The Xid defect determines an improved clinical course of murine leishmaniasis in susceptible mice. *Int. Immunol.* 6, 1117–1124. doi: 10.1093/intimm/6.8.1117
14. Kaye, P., and Scott, P. (2011). Leishmaniasis: complexity at the host-pathogen interface. *Nat. Rev. Microbiol.* 9, 604-615. doi: 10.1038/nrmicro2608
15. Kaye, P. M., Svensson, M., Ato, M., Maroof, A., Polley, R., Stager, S., et al. (2004). The immunopathology of experimental visceral leishmaniasis. *Immunol. Rev.* 201, 239–253. doi: 10.1111/j.0105-2896.2004.00188.x
16. Kumar, R., and Nylén, S. (2012). Immunobiology of visceral leishmaniasis. *Front. Immunol.* 3:251. doi: 10.3389/fimmu.2012.00251
17. Liu, D., and Uzonna, J. E. (2012). The early interaction of Leishmania with macrophages and dendritic cells and its influence on the host immune response. *Front. Cell. Infect. Microbiol.* 2:83. doi: 10.3389/fcimb.2012.00083
18. Matlashewski, G., Arana, B., Kroeger, A., Battacharya, S., Sundar, S., Das, P., et al. (2011). Visceral leishmaniasis: elimination with existing interventions. *Lancet Infect. Dis.* 11, 322-325. doi: 10.1016/S1473-3099(10) 70320-0
19. McCall, L. I., Zhang, W. W., and Matlashewski, G. (2013). Determinants for

the development of visceral leishmaniasis disease. *PLoS Pathog.* 9:e1003053. doi: 10.1371/journal.ppat.1003053

20. Minoprio, P., el Cheikh, M. C., Murphy, E., Hontebeyrie-Joskowicz, M., Coffman, R., Coutinho, A., et al. (1993). Xid-associated resistance to experimental Chagas' disease is IFN-gamma dependent. *J. Immunol.* 151, 4200–4208.
21. Murphy, M. L., Wille, U., Villegas, E. N., Hunter, C. A., and Farrell, J. P. (2001). IL-10 mediates susceptibility to Leishmania donovani infection. *Eur. J. Immunol.* 31, 2848–2856. doi: 10.1002/1521-4141(2001010)31:10<2848::AID-IMMU2848>3.0.CO;2-T
22. Popi, A. F., Godoy, L. C., Xander, P., Lopes, J. D., and Mariano, M. (2008). B-1 cells facilitate *Paracoccidioides brasiliensis* infection in mice via IL-10 secretion. *Microbes Infect.* 10, 817–824. doi: 10.1016/j.micinf.2008. 04.012
23. Popi, A. F., Osugui, L., Perez, K. R., Longo-Maugéri, I. M., and Mariano, M. (2012). Could a B-1 cell derived phagocyte "be one" of the peritoneal macrophages during LPS-driven inflammation? *PLoS ONE* 7:e34570. doi: 10.1371/journal. pone.0034570
24. Ready, P. D. (2014). Epidemiology of visceral leishmaniasis. *Clin. Epidemiol.* 6, 147-154. doi: 10.2147/clep.s44267
25. Ribeiro-Gomes, F. L., Otero, A. C., Gomes, N. A., Moniz-De-Souza, M. C., Cysne- Finkelstein, L., Arnholdt, A. C., et al. (2004). Macrophage interactions with neutrophils regulate *Leishmania major* infection. *J. Immunol.* 172, 4454–4462. doi: 10.4049/jimmunol.172.7.4454
26. Szymczak, W. A., Davis, M. J., Lundy, S. K., Dufaud, C., Olszewski, M., and Pirofski, L. A. (2013). X-linked immunodeficient mice exhibit enhanced susceptibility to *Cryptococcus neoformans* Infection. *MBio* 4:e00265-13. doi: 10.1128/mBio. 00265-13

17

Intestinal Bacterial Communities of Trypanosome-Infected and Uninfected *Glossina palpalis palpalis* from Three Human African Trypanomiasis Foci in Cameroon

*Franck Jacob[1], Trésor T. Melachio[2], Guy R. Njitchouang[2], Geoffrey Gimonneau[1], Flobert Njiokou[2], Luc Abate[3], Richard Christen[4], Julie Reveillaud[5,6] and Anne Geiger[1]**

[1] UMR INTERTRYP, Institut de Recherche pour le Développement-CIRAD, CIRAD TA A-17/G, Montpellier, France, [2] Parasitology and Ecology Laboratory, Department of Animal Biology and Physiology, Faculty of Science, University of Yaounde 1, Yaounde, Cameroon, [3] UMR MIVEGEC, Institut de Recherche pour le Développement 224-Centre National de la Recherche Scientifique 5290, Montpellier, France, [4] UMR 7138, Systématique Adaptation Evolution, Université de Nice-Sophia Antipolis, Nice, France, [5] Institut National de la Recherche Agronomique, UMR 1309 ASTRE, Montpellier, France, [6] CIRAD, UMR ASTRE, Montpellier, France

***Correspondence:**
Anne Geiger
anne.geiger@ird.fr

Glossina sp. the tsetse fly that transmits trypanosomes causing the Human or the Animal African Trypanosomiasis (HAT or AAT) can harbor symbiotic bacteria that are known to play a crucial role in the fly's vector competence. We hypothesized that other bacteria could be present, and that some of them could also influence the fly's vector competence. In this context the objectives of our work were: (a) to characterize the bacteria that compose the *G. palpalis palpalis* midgut bacteriome, (b) to evidence possible bacterial community differences between trypanosome-infected and non-infected fly individuals from a given AAT and HAT focus or from different foci using barcoded Illumina sequencing of the hypervariable V3-V4 region of the *16S rRNA gene*. Forty *G. p. palpalis* flies, either infected by *Trypanosoma congolense* or uninfected were sampled from three trypanosomiasis foci in Cameroon. A total of 143 OTUs were detected in the midgut samples. Most taxa were identified at the genus level, nearly 50% at the species level; they belonged to 83 genera principally within the phyla Actinobacteria, Bacteroidetes, Firmicutes, and Proteobacteria. Prominent representatives included *Wigglesworthia* (the fly's obligate symbiont), *Serratia,* and *Enterobacter hormaechei*. *Wolbachia* was identified for the first time in *G. p. palpalis*. The average number of bacterial species per tsetse sample was not significantly different regarding the fly infection status, and the hierarchical analysis based on the differences in bacterial community structure did not provide a clear clustering between infected and non-infected flies. Finally, the most important result was the evidence of the overall very large diversity of intestinal bacteria which, except for *Wigglesworthia*, were unevenly distributed over the sampled flies regardless of their geographic origin and their trypanosome infection status.

Keywords: ***Glossina*****, trypanosome, microbiome, meta-taxonomics, sleeping sickness, nagana**

INTRODUCTION

Animal African Trypanosomiasis (AAT), or Nagana, is primarily caused by *Trypanosoma brucei brucei* (Tbb), *Trypanosoma vivax,* and *Trypanosoma congolense*, which are transmitted to their mammalian hosts by tsetse flies belonging to the species *Glossina palpalis* and *Glossina morsitans*. This disease is responsible for significant economic losses in areas where cattle are exposed to parasites (Shaw et al., 2013). Human African Trypanosomiasis (HAT), or sleeping sickness, is endemic to Sub-Saharan Africa, where it causes significant health and economic impacts (Welburn and Maudlin, 2012). The chronic form of HAT is caused by *Trypanosoma brucei gambiense* (Tbg), whereas *Trypanosoma brucei rhodesiense* (Tbr) causes the acute form; the two forms are transmitted to humans by *G. palpalis* and *G. morsitans*, respectively.

Currently, about 60 million people continue to be at risk for HAT in 36 Sub-Saharan African countries. Several factors complicate the treatment of HAT. The medications that are currently used to treat human patients can generate many side effects (reviewed in Geiger et al., 2011a). In addition, the emergence of drug-resistant trypanosomes was recently reported (Baker et al., 2013). These factors are pertinent, since epidemiological modeling of the impact of global change on HAT expansion predicts that 46–70 million more people will be at risk by 2090 (Moore et al., 2012). Thus, the search for new control strategies is a priority to impede the spread of the disease. In this context, identifying the factors involved in fly vector competence (as well as understanding how they work) may open new perspectives.

Trypanosomes ingested by the tsetse fly during a blood meal on an infected host passively reach the tsetse intestine, where they differentiate into their procyclic form, mature, and multiply. Then, depending on the species, the trypanosomes migrate toward either the fly's salivary glands (in the case of *T. brucei* sp.) or the mouth parts, where they undergo the maturation step into their infective metacyclic form. The trypanosomes may then be transmitted to a mammalian host during a subsequent blood meal ingested by the fly (Vickerman et al., 1988). This ability of tsetse flies to acquire trypanosomes and to subsequently favor their maturation and transmit them to a vertebrate host, known as the fly's vector competence, depends on several factors including the production of antimicrobial peptides (e.g., cecropin and attacin; Hu and Aksoy, 2006), reactive oxygen species (MacLeod et al., 2007), EP-protein [Glutamic acid (E)—Proline (P) rich protein, an immune responsive protein], (Haines et al., 2010), intestinal lectin (Welburn et al., 1994), as well as the peritrophic matrix (Weiss et al., 2013, 2014; Rose et al., 2014; Aksoy et al., 2016).

As previously reported, tsetse flies can harbor three different symbionts that play a crucial role in the physiology of their host. First, the obligate Enterobacteria *Wigglesworthia glossinidia* is present intracellularly in the bacteriocytes, specialized cells of the intestine that form the bacteriome (Aksoy, 1995). This ancient host association (Chen et al., 1999) is involved in the tsetse fly's fertility, nutrition, and the development of its immune system (Akman et al., 2002; Weiss et al., 2011; Rio et al., 2012). Second, the facultative symbiont *Sodalis glossinidius* is present in the cells of the intestine, but it can also be found extracellularly and in other tissues of the fly (Cheng and Aksoy, 1999; Balmand et al., 2013). There is substantial evidence that certain *S. glossinidius* genotypes favor the establishment of trypanosomes in the fly's gut (Geiger et al., 2007; Farikou et al., 2010a; Hamidou Soumana et al., 2014). *W. glossinidia* and *S. glossinidius* are both transmitted maternally to the progeny *via* milk secretions during the intra-uterine development of the larvae (Aksoy, 1995). Third, the facultative symbiont *Wolbachia* can be detected very early in oocytes, embryos and larvae (Cheng et al., 2000). This symbiont acts on the reproductive process of tsetse flies by inducing cytoplasmic incompatibility (Alam et al., 2011). *Wolbachia* infection has been negatively correlated with the prevalence of trypanosome and of salivary gland hypertrophy virus (Alam et al., 2012). This indicates that *Wolbachia* may have a role in preventing infection of tsetse flies from trypanosomes (Aksoy et al., 2013), which interestingly has not been revealed for plasmodium infection in mosquitoes that harbor *Wolbachia* (Zélé et al., 2014). This symbiont is trans-ovary transmitted to the progeny (Cheng and Aksoy, 1999).

The presence of bacteria (other than symbionts) in the gut of field-collected tsetse flies has been assessed by bacterial isolation and culture approaches (Geiger et al., 2009, 2011b; Lindh and Lehane, 2011), as well as by direct molecular identification methods. Using deep sequencing of the V4 hypervariable region of the *16S rRNA* gene, Aksoy et al. (2014) revealed the limited diversity of gut-specific microbiota in wild tsetse flies from Uganda. Surprisingly, bacteria belonging to the genera *Enterobacter*, *Acinetobacter*, and *Enterococcus* were found in the gut of the blood-sucking fly, despite the fly feeds on animals which blood is normally devoid of any bacteria. The source of these bacteria is unknown, but their presence could be due to the fact that tsetse flies can occasionally feed on nutrients other than blood that may be contaminated by diverse bacteria (Colman et al., 2012). Flies may also ingest bacteria present on the skin surface of the hosts when taking their bloodmeal (Poinar et al., 1979). Finally, differences in their diet that may depend on the environmental conditions could lead to differences in the fly's gut bacteriome as it was shown for other insects (Colman et al., 2012). Finding such bacteria in an organ where trypanosomes are localized raised the question whether these bacteria could be involved, besides the known symbionts, in fly infection by trypanosomes, inasmuch as certain bacteria species have been shown to produce antiparasitic molecules (Lazaro et al., 2002; Moss, 2002). In this context, a novel bacterial species, *Serratia glossinae*, has been identified in the gut of insects reared in insectarium (Geiger et al., 2010). This bacterium is related to *Serratia marcescens* (Enterobacteriaceae) a bacterium involved in the production of pigments that are toxic for *Trypanosoma cruzi* (Azambuja et al., 2004). In *Anopheles*, the abundance of intestinal Enterobacteriaceae has been associated to the presence of the parasite *Plasmodium falciparum* (Boissière et al., 2012). This illustrates the need for a better understanding of the composition of the tsetse fly bacteriome and its potential variations, since differences in the environment could induce differences in the bacteriome composition which, in turn, could induce differences in the fly vector competence.

Using bar-coded Illumina sequencing of the hypervariable V3-V4 region of the *16S rRNA* gene, we aimed to characterize bacterial communities in the midgut of *G. p. palpalis* sampled from three different sleeping sickness foci in Cameroon, and to verify the hypotheses that the composition of the midgut bacterial communities of trypanosome-infected *G. p. palpalis* might be different from that of non-infected flies across these three HAT foci. Finally we aimed to identify bacteria that could be associated with the infection status of the fly. Those, if any, associated with fly refractoriness would be of particular interest inasmuch if they would be maternally transmitted to offspring. In the case they would not be maternally transferred, their trypanocidal compound(s) should be identified and possibly delivered via the paratransgenic approach described by Rio et al. (2004). Both approaches may offer the possibility to block the fly vector competence, hence the spread of the sleeping disease.

MATERIALS AND METHODS

Sampling Areas

The study was performed in three sleeping sickness foci (Bipindi, Campo, and Fontem) located in the forest region of southern-Cameroon (**Figure 1**).

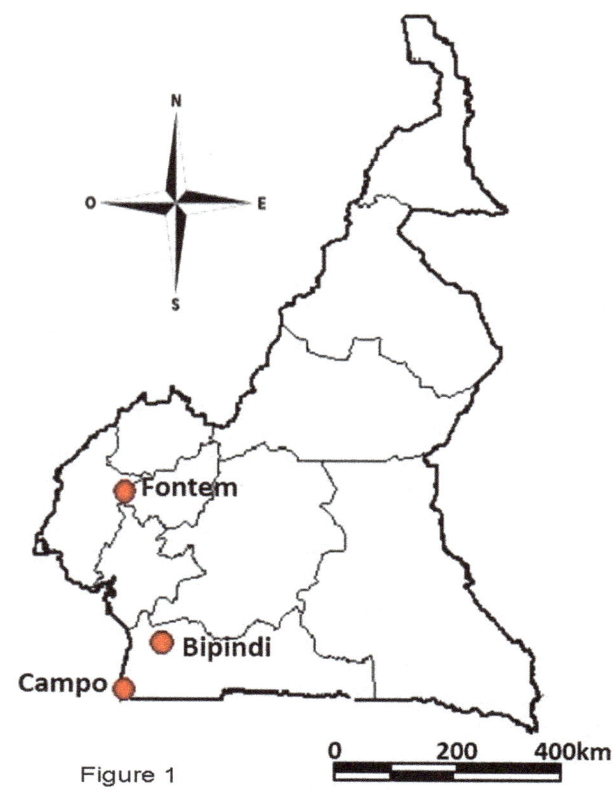

FIGURE 1 | Geographical map showing the three described Cameroonian HAT foci.

Bipindi (3°2′N, 10°22′E) is a historical sleeping sickness focus originally described in 1920 (Grébaut et al., 2001). It is situated between Lolodorf and Kribi, 75 km from the Atlantic Ocean. Although, a 2004 survey identified four tsetse fly species (Grébaut et al., 2004), *G. p. palpalis* was the only species found in this focus since 2007 (Farikou et al., 2010a,b; Melachio et al., 2011; Tchouomene-Labou et al., 2014). Bipindi is surrounded by hills and covers several villages, mainly located along the roads. The focus has a typical forest bioecological environment, including equatorial forest and farmland along the roads and surrounding the villages. Bipindi is home to highly diverse wild fauna (Njiokou et al., 2004, 2006) and it has a dense network of rivers crossing cocoa farms, all of which offer suitable habitats for tsetse flies.

Campo (2°20′N, 9°52′E) is a hypo-endemic focus where several cases of sleeping sickness are diagnosed every year. It is located along the Ntem River, which separates Cameroon from Equatorial Guinea. Several tsetse fly species (including *G. p. palpalis*, and to a lesser extent *G. pallicera*, *G. caliginea*, and *G. nigrofusca*) can be encountered in this focus (Simo et al., 2008). Several biotopes are found in the Campo focus, including farmland, marshes, swampy areas, and rainy forest.

Fontem (5°40′N, 9°55′E), in the Southwest Region of Cameroon, has been recognized as a sleeping sickness focus since 1949. Since that time, the prevalence of HAT has decreased considerably. The landscape is characterized by the presence of hills and valleys that are crossed by rivers with fast currents. *G. p. palpalis* is the only tsetse fly species found in this area (Simo et al., 2008). The focus is divided into the North, Center and South sub-foci. The Center sub-focus (comprising the villages of Menji, Fotabong, Nsoko, and Azi), where flies were sampled, has only had a few sleeping sickness cases in the past decade. In the Northern sub-focus (comprising the villages of Bechati, Folepi, and Besali) no new HAT patients have been diagnosed in the last 20 years (Ebo'o Eyenga, personal communication), although 15% of all pigs were infected with *T. b. gambiense* group 1 in 1999 (Nkinin et al., 2002).

Fly Sampling and Experimental Design

Entomological surveys were conducted in the Campo focus in March 2008, and in the Bipindi and Fontem foci in November 2013. Pyramidal traps (Gouteux and Lancien, 1986) were placed for 4 consecutive days in suitable tsetse fly biotopes of each village located within each focus. The geographical position of the sampling sites was determined by GPS. Trapped tsetse flies were harvested twice a day (before 12 a.m. and before 3 p.m.).

The *Glossina* species were first identified according to morphological criteria (Grébaut et al., 2004), and then sorted into two groups of teneral (young flies that had never taken a blood meal) and non-teneral flies, respectively. Among the 599 non-teneral flies that were caught in the Campo focus, 200 were randomly sampled, their midguts dissected (see below) and observed under a light microscope (magnification x100) to detect the presence of motile trypanosomes (infected flies) or the absence of trypanosomes (non-infected flies). The trypanosomes from infected flies were subsequently identified (species or sub-species) by PCR using specific primers (**Table 1**). The absence

TABLE 1 | Primers used for PCR amplification of trypanosome DNA (Farikou et al., 2010a).

Specificity	Primer sequence	Amplified product (bp)	References
T. congolense (forest type)	5′-GGACACGCCAGAAGGTACTT-3′ 5′-GTTCTCGCACCAAATCCAAC-3′	350	Masiga et al., 1992
T. congolense (savannah type)	5′-TCGAGCGAGAACGGGCACTTTGCGA-3′ 5′-ATTAGGGACAAACAAATCCCGCACA-3′	341	Moser et al., 1989
T. brucei s.l.	5′-CGAATGAATATTAAACAATGCGCAG-3′ 5′-AGAACCATTTATTAGCTTTGTTGC-3′	164	Masiga et al., 1992
T. vivax	5′-CGACTCCGGGCGACCGT-3′ 5′-CATGCGGCGGACCGTGG-3′	600	Majiwa et al., 1994

of any trypanosomes (negative PCR assay) was confirmed in all non-infected flies using the same specific primers. Among the 300 flies caught in Bipindi, 200 were sampled and processed as for the Campo flies. Only 27 non-teneral flies could be caught in Fontem; as shown after dissection, microscopy, and PCR analyses, they all were non-infected by trypanosomes.

The microbiota analysis was performed on *G. p. palpalis* flies that had undergone further selection. The midguts from the 200 sampled flies from Campo were separated into two groups composed, respectively, of trypanosome infected and non-infected midguts. Among the infected midguts, only those harboring *T. congolense* (either the forest or savannah type; mixed infections were discarded) were taken into account. Finally, from the non-infected group and from the *T. congolense* infected group, respectively, eight midguts were randomly selected and identified by numbering. The 200 samples from Bipindi were processed similarly. Among the midguts from the 27 flies from Fontem, eight were randomly selected, which formed a unique group of non-infected samples. In total, five groups were formed that differed from each other regarding the infection status of the flies and/or their geographic origin. The "sex ratio" (12.5, 37.5, 37.5, 75, and 25% male flies in, respectively group 1–5) was recorded but not taken into account in the subsequent analyses. The characteristics of each group, including sample numbering, are the followings: "Group 1/Campo infected flies: number 1–8; Group 2/Campo non-infected flies: number 9–16; Group 3/Bipindi infected flies: number 17–24; Group 4/Bipindi non-infected flies: number 25–32; Group5/Fontem non-infected flies: number 33–40 (**Figure 2**).

Dissection of Tsetse Flies, DNA Extraction, and Trypanosome PCR Amplification

The non-teneral flies were surface-sterilized (once with 5% sodium hypochlorite for 10 min and twice with 70% ethanol, each for 10 min) and the midgut of each fly was dissected under sterile conditions using a Bunsen burner, and in sterile NaCl 0.9%. The instruments used were carefully cleaned after the dissection of each fly to prevent cross-contamination. Midguts were recovered and then separately transferred into tubes containing 95° ethanol for further DNA extraction. During the field surveys (10 days for each mission), tubes containing the samples were maintained at −20°C; thereafter, in the laboratory, the midgut samples were immediately processed and subjected to DNA extraction using the DNeasy kit (Qiagen, Paris, France) according to Geiger et al. (2007). Genomic DNA was quantified using NanoDrop (Thermo Scientific, Paris).

PCR amplification was performed as previously described (Farikou et al., 2010a) using trypanosome-specific primers (**Table 1**; Moser et al., 1989; Masiga et al., 1992; Majiwa et al., 1994; Herder et al., 2002). This procedure allowed detection of *T. brucei s.l.*, *T. congolense* (both forest and savannah types), and *T. vivax*.

Meta-Barcoding Analysis

Amplification of the highly variable V3-V4 region of the *16S rRNA* gene, using the forward primer 5′-CCTACGGGNGGC WGCAG-3′ and the reverse primer 5′-GACTACHVGGGTHTC TAATCC-3′ (N representing A, C, G, or T; V representing A, C, or G; H representing A, C, or T; W representing A or T; IUPAC codes), was performed to evaluate the bacterial communities of tsetse midguts on the Illumina MiSeq (MR DNA Laboratory-http://www.mrdnalab.com/shallowater, USA). The primers were specifically designed by one of the co-authors of the current study. As previously described in the method of Porter et al. (2016), each PCR amplifying medium contained 2 μL DNA template, 17.5 μL molecular biology-grade water, 2.5 μL 10× reaction buffer, 1 μL 50× MgCl2 (50 mM), 0.5 μL dNTPs mix (10 mM), 0.5 μL forward primer (10 mM), 0.5 μL reverse primer (10 mM), and 0.5 μL Invitrogen Platinum *Taq* polymerase (5 U/μL) in a total volume of 25 μL. The amplification program was: 95°C for 5 min, followed by 25 cycles of 94°C for 40 s, 55°C for 1 min, and 72°C for 30 s, and lasted at 72°C for 5 min. Amplicons were purified using MiniElute PCR purification columns (Qiagen, Paris, France) and were eluted in 50 μL molecular biology-grade water. The purified amplicons from the first PCR round served as templates for the second PCR round, using Illumina adaptor-tailed primers in a 10-cycle amplification regime. All PCR reactions were performed in an Eppendorf Mastercycler ep gradient S thermal cycler. Negative controls (containing all reagents except the midgut DNA that was replaced by water) were included in all experiments. Amplicons were quantified using a Bioanalyzer (Agilent Technologies, Paris) and then the KAPA Quantification Kit (Roche, Paris). Equimolar amounts of the generated libraries were dual-indexed, combined, and sequenced on an Illumina MiSeq platform (MRDNA Laboratory, Shallowater, USA) using

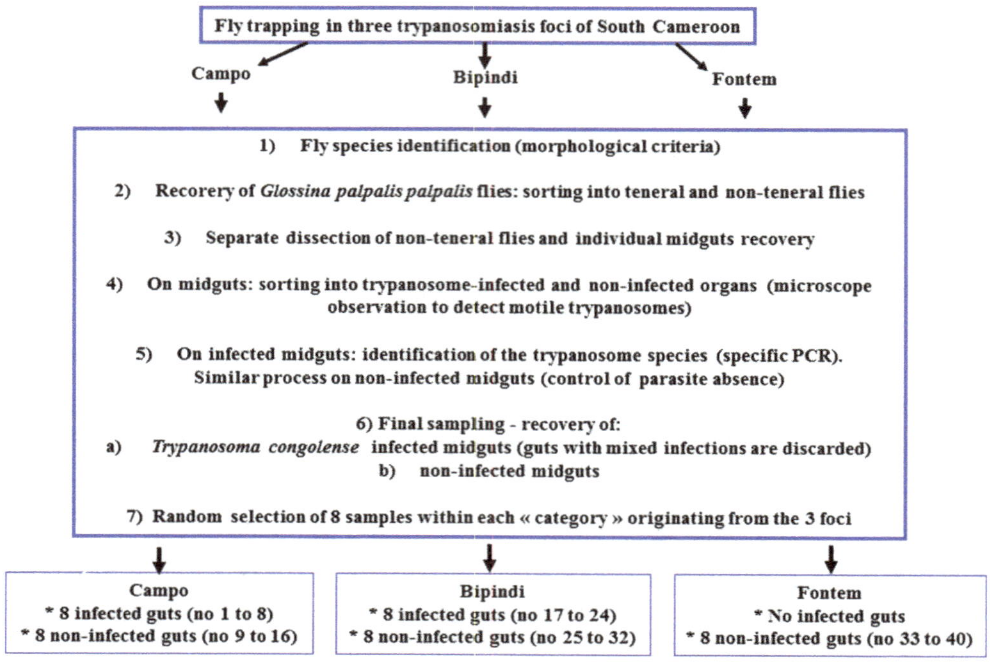

FIGURE 2 | *Glossina* sampling and selection process.

MiSeq Reagent kits (300 cycles), following the 2 × 300-bp paired-end sequencing protocol. The generated sequences have been deposited in the EMBL-EBI (Study accession number PRJEB14010; Secondary study accession number ERP015605 and Locus tag prefix BN6929).

Quality Filtering and Taxonomic Classification of Sequencing Data

Illumina MiSeq reads were analyzed using in-house pipelines (Richard Christen; described in Boissière et al., 2012; Hartmann et al., 2012; Gimonneau et al., 2014; Massana et al., 2015). Briefly, Silva 119 NR (analyses performed in 2014) was used as the reference database for taxonomic identification (Quast et al., 2012). An *in silico* extraction of Silva amplicons using forward: 5′-CCTACGGGNGGCWGCAG-3′ and reverse: 5′-GACTACHVG GGTHTCTAATCC-3′ primers, followed by an analysis by length/number of amplicons, yielded the following results: 1–50/0; 51–100/0; 101–150/2; 151–200/1; 201–250/1; 251–300/11; 301–350/40; 351–400/21,669; 401–450/448,575; 451–500/450; 501–550/192; 551–600/1,198; 601–650/0. This demonstrates that most amplicons were between 350 and 450 nucleotides in length. The extracted database is referenced below as the refseq. Each sequence identifier was reformatted to eight taxonomic fields as in PR2 (Guillou et al., 2012) making it easier to use a pipeline for analyses.

In order to assemble paired-end reads, the software programs PEAR (Zhang et al., 2014) and FLASH (Magoc and Salzberg, 2011) were both tested. PEAR using default parameters merged more pairs, and paired-end reads were therefore assembled and quality filtered (using Illumina quality scores) with PEAR. 94.26% (3,622,233 reads) of the total reads (3,842,672 reads) were assembled; 0.003% were discarded and 5.734% were not assembled.

Reads were then sorted by length using a dedicated python script, yielding the following results: 0–0/0; 1–50/3; 51–100/1,556; 101–150/1,435; 151–200/1,535; 201–250/1,578; 251–300/2,251; 301–350/9,401; 351–400/38,323; 401–450/132,487; 451–500/3,433,239; 501–550/381; 551–600/44; 601–650/0. Reads shorter than 300 nucleotides (0.23% out of the overall number of reads) were discarded, resulting in the extraction of 3,613,875 reads. The fasta file was then demultiplexed using a dedicated C++ program. Primer trimming was performed using CutAdapt v1.8.1 (Martin, 2011).

Each file was dereplicated, sorted by decreasing abundance, chimera checked with UCHIME (Edgar et al., 2011) and then clustered using Crunchclust (Mondani et al., 2011; Gimonneau et al., 2014; Massana et al., 2015; Tchioffo et al., 2016; available from https://github.com/dumaatravaie/crunchclust/blob/master/Documentation; at a Levenstein distance of 5). After this clustering step, clusters that contained <2 reads were discarded as artifacts (see Boissière et al., 2012). All these steps resulted in 2,562,144 high-quality sequences contained in clusters with at least two reads (70.73% of the total assembled reads) that were subsequently used for taxonomic assignment. In each cluster, the most abundant sequence was kept as the representative one, since it was assumed to have the least errors in a cluster. Taxonomic assignment was done as in Pawlowski et al. (2011). Briefly, a Needleman–Wunsch algorithm to search for the 30 most similar sequences to each representative sequence from the refseq was employed. The reference sequences with the highest percentage were then used, and taxonomy to a given level was obtained. When more than one result emerged, the two highest hits were reported. When similarity was <80%, sequences were not assigned. Abundance matrices were generated for statistical analyses at each taxonomic level. Several abundant Operational Taxonomic Units (OTUs) could not be identified satisfactorily down to the genus or species level. In these cases (rough estimation: 1%), reads sequences and similar refseq sequences were selected and then aligned using ClustalO (Sievers et al., 2011) and SeaView (Gouy et al., 2010). Trees were plotted using TreeDyn (Chevenet et al., 2006) or MetaPhlAn (Segata et al., 2012), and distinct robust subtrees were annotated as distinct species whenever possible.

Data and Statistical Analysis

Statistical analyses were performed using the R package vegan. Rarefaction curves (**Figure S1**) were performed prior to comparative analyses between infected and uninfected flies, and between the sampling sites. Significant differences in bacterial richness between the infected and uninfected flies, and between the three sampling sites were tested using non-parametric Kruskal–Wallis test. We used vegdist and hclust using single, average, and complete linkage methods for hierarchical clustering and then compared them for the presence of sub-trees. Nonmetric multidimensional scaling (nMDS) were generated using the R packages ggplot2 and phyloseq (McMurdie and Holmes, 2013).

RESULTS

Distribution of Tsetse Flies by Infected vs. Non-infected Status

The distribution of trypanosome species and/or subspecies in the midgut of tsetse flies from Campo (200 flies) and Bipindi (200 flies) is displayed in **Figure 3**. Nearly half of all flies, whether from Campo (51.4%) or from Bipindi (48.6%), were infected with at least one of the four studied trypanosome species and/or subspecies. The prevalence of the four trypanosome species was highly dependent on the sampling site. In flies sampled from Campo, *T. congolense* (both forest and savannah types) displayed the highest prevalence, accounting for 83% of all infected flies (including mixed infections), while *T. brucei sensu lato* displayed the lowest prevalence (12%, including mixed infections). In contrast, *T. brucei s.l.* displayed the highest prevalence (43%) in infected flies from Bipindi, with *T. congolense* accounting for 42%. As for the Fontem focus, the low number of collected flies (27 flies) prevented any reliable statistical analysis regarding the prevalence of the infected flies in this focus, inasmuch as all of the 27 flies were uninfected (which does not imply that the overall population of flies is uninfected).

Bacterial Communities in the *G. p. palpalis* Midgut

Illumina sequencing of *16S rDNA* gene generated a total of 2,562,144 high-quality sequence reads across the V3–V4 region in 40 tsetse flies, for the 40 samples randomly selected. The average number of tags/sample for the V3–V4 region was 12,988 (ranging from 6,525 to 19,694 per gut), with read length varying from 300 to 600 nucleotides. After taxonomic assignation, a total of 13 phyla were identified from the 40 gut samples (**Table S1**); 12 phyla belonged to the Bacterial kingdom and one phylum belonged to the Archaea. Proteobacteria were present in all 40 samples and had a relative abundance higher than 68% in each sample (even higher than 97% in 37 out of 40 samples), while the other phyla (as well as their respective relative abundances) were unevenly distributed among the different samples. The Bacteroidetes phylum was detected in 26 samples, Firmicutes was observed in 19 samples, Proteobacteria/Actinobacteria was detected in 14 samples, and Actinobacteria was found in 7 samples. The 7 other phyla could only be detected in 4 samples or less. Samples from groups 1 and 2 (infected and non-infected midguts from Campo; sample numbers 1–16) harbored 1 to 4 different phyla; samples from group 3 (infected midguts from Bipindi; sample numbers 17–24) contained 2–5 different phyla; samples from group 4 (non-infected midguts from Bipindi; sample numbers 25–32) contained 3–7 different phyla; and samples from group 5 (non-infected midguts from Fontem;

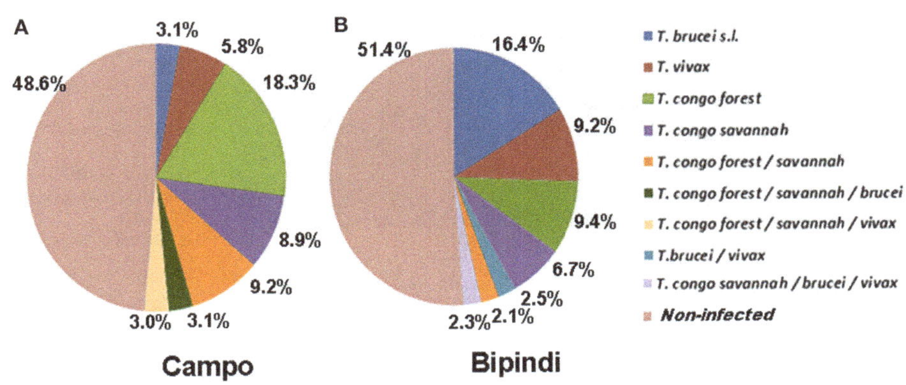

FIGURE 3 | Prevalence of the different trypanosome species or subspecies infecting tsetse flies collected in the Campo **(A)** and Bipindi **(B)** foci. Single as well as mixed infections have been considered.

sample numbers 33–40) harbored 1–4 different phyla (**Table S1**). A heat map analysis of the distribution and abundance of the bacterial phyla showed the sampled midgut did not cluster together, confirming that bacterial communities at the phylum level were unevenly distributed among the samples (**Figure 4**).

The distribution of bacterial taxa among the 40 samples at the class and genus levels and their relative abundance in each sample are reported in **Table S1**. Twenty-four classes and 83 genera could be distinguished. The gut microbiota presented a large inter-individual variability, although only a few taxa were prominent.

Bacteria Classes

As reported above, all 40 samples contained Proteobacteria, accounting for more than 97% of all microbiota in 37 samples. The Gammaproteobacteria, present in all 40 samples and accounting for more than 95% of the total microbiota in 38 samples, was the most prominent class in this phylum. Alpha-proteobacteria (maximal abundance per sample: 11.08%) were found in 32 samples. In contrast, Beta-proteobacteria were present in only 7 samples (maximal abundance per sample: 2.38%). Flavobacteria were present in 26 samples (maximum abundance per sample: 31.09%). Bacteroidia, Mollicutes, Actinobacteria/Gammaproteobacteria, and Bacilli were present in 1, 4, 14, and 19 samples, respectively [maximum abundance (%) of the total microbiota per sample: 0.6, 4.96, 1.88, and 4.11, respectively]. Finally, Actinobacteria were present in 7 samples (maximum abundance per sample: 0.19%). The heat map analysis in **Figure 5** shows the distribution of the most abundant classes (those that were present in at least 7 samples) among the different samples. The other identified classes, such as Negativicutes, Rubrobacteria, Sphingobacteriia, and Clostridia, were present in <7 samples at a frequency of <0.25% per sample. In general, bacterial classes were very unevenly distributed among the samples. For example, whereas the abundance of Gammaproteobacteria was 100% in sample 15 and sample 32, sample 20 harbored representatives of Gammaproteobacteria, Flavobacteria, and Alphaproteobacteria (respective abundance: 57.74, 31.11, and 11.10%).

Bacterial Genera

Out of the 40 samples, 83 different bacteria genera (**Table S1**) were detected. The heat map analysis (**Figure S2**) performed on genera present in at least four samples, displays the distribution of genera, and their respective abundance, among the 40 samples. Midgut bacteria were unevenly distributed among individual tsetse flies and between the different sampled localities. Several genera were found in all (or most of) tsetse flies, possibly representing the midgut core microbiota. This was the case for the genus *Wigglesworthia*, as well as for several genera belonging to the Enterobacteriaceae family. The relative abundance of *Wigglesworthia* ranged from 34.5 to 99.8% across the 40 samples. Other genera widely distributed included two *Enterobacter* that were present, respectively, in 40 (relative abundance: 0.02–61.1%) and in 21 samples (relative abundance: 0.02–1.11%); *Candidatus Sulcia muelleri*, present in 26 samples (relative abundance: 0.01–31.09%); two *Serratia* present in 29 samples (relative abundance: 0.01–14%) and in 20 samples (relative abundance: 0.01–4.95%).

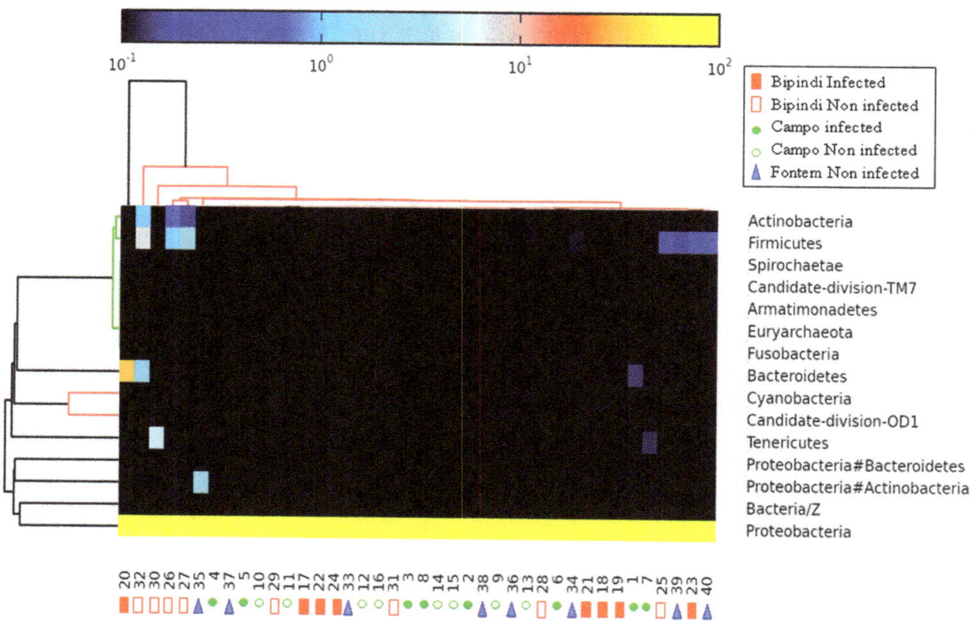

FIGURE 4 | Heat map analysis of the distribution and abundance of the bacterial phyla in midgut samples. The samples did not cluster together, indicating highly variable bacterial communities. Numbers 1–8: infected samples from the Campo focus; Numbers 9–16: non-infected samples from the Campo focus; Numbers 17–24: infected samples from the Bipindi focus; Numbers 25–32: non-infected samples from the Bipindi focus; Numbers 33–40: non infected samples from the Fontem focus.

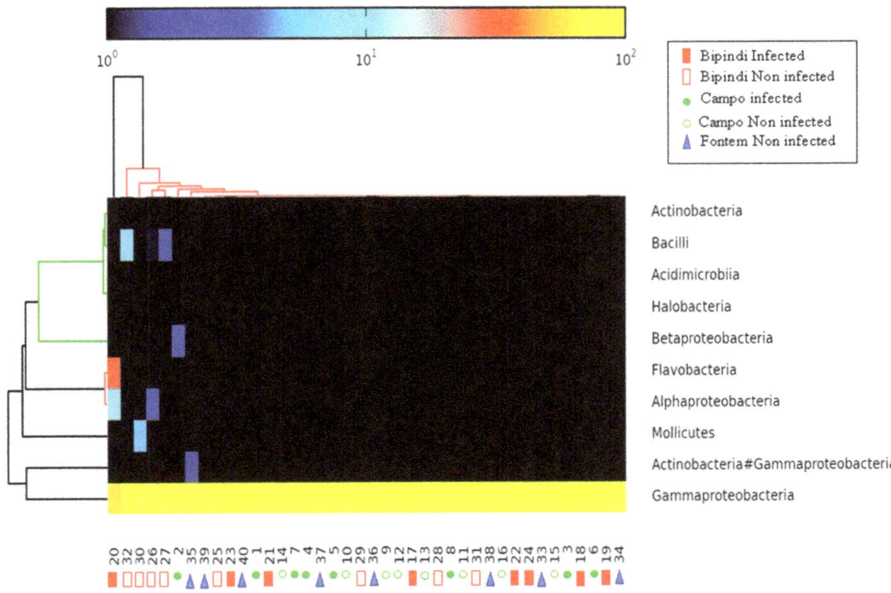

FIGURE 5 | Heat map analysis of the distribution and abundance of the bacterial classes in midgut samples. The samples did not cluster together, indicating highly variable bacterial communities. Sample numbering as in **Figure 4**.

Furthermore, *Wolbachia* was present in 25 samples (relative abundance: 0.01–11.08%), while *Sodalis* was only present in 4 samples, with a maximum relative abundance of 0.06%.

These results indicate that the midgut bacterial flora was mainly composed of gram-negative communities. Gram-positive bacteria belonged to the Bacilli, Mollicutes, Actinobacteria, Rubrobacteria, Clostridia, Fusobacteriia, Acidimicrobiia, and Thermoleophilia classes, and represented 10% of the total bacteria.

Finally, a total of 103 bacterial species (**Table S1**) and one Miscellaneous Euryarchaeotic Group (MEG, archeae) were detected. Only a few genera were shown to include more than one species, including *Bacillus*, *Burkholderia*, *Enterobacter*, *Neisseria*, *Prevoltella*, *Providencia*, and *Serratia*.

Of note, sequences assigned to *W. glossinidia* showed a relative abundance higher than 80% in all except two samples (samples 20 and 35, relative abundance 51.27 and 34.55%, respectively; **Figure S3**). A high number of sequences assigned to the *Pseudomonas*, *Sphingomonas*, and Hyphomicrobiaceae were detected in sample 26, and 74 species were found in sample 32.

Bacterial Communities between Infected and Uninfected Flies from the Different Geographic Located HAT

The average number of bacterial species per tsetse sample was not significantly different regarding their group (Kruskal-Wallis *p-value* = 0.342), their geographical origin (Kruskal-Wallis *p-value* = 0.167), or their status (infected vs. non-infected; Kruskal–Wallis *p-value* = 0.836).

We investigated potential relationships between the structure of the gut microbial communities of tsetse flies from Campo, Bipindi, and Fontem foci and the fly's trypanosome infection status. A hierarchical clustering using the Bray–Curtis indice did not discriminate unambiguously the different groups (**Figure 6**). It however showed a trend of infected flies from a given focus to be separated from non-infected flies of the same focus. One can also notice that infected flies from Bipindi are closely related to non-infected flies from Campo and vice versa. In contrast, the non-infected samples from Fontem were distributed over the different clusters. These results were reinforced by the nonmetric multidimensional scaling plots shown in **Figures S4A,B**.

Novel Bacteria Taxa

A phylogenetic tree was inferred to further investigate the potential dissimilarities between the bacteria sequences identified in this study and the sequences currently available in public databases, thereby illustrating the taxonomic relationships between the representative OTU sequences (**Figures S5A–D**). The most abundant OTU present in each of the 40 samples showed sequence similarities with *Wigglesworthia* sp. We identified 60 different genotypes of *Wigglesworthia*, similar to those from *G. morsitans* or *G. brevipalpis*. Depending on the sample, there were one to four genotypes per sample. However, most samples harbored one genotype, except those from Fontem that harbored two to four different genotypes in the same sample.

Some OTU-representative sequences did not match known targets in the NCBI database (analyses performed in 2014) and had to be annotated manually. Sample 20 (**Figure 7**) was shown to harbor four different genotypes of several bacteria species, including *Candidatus Nasuia* sp., *Wigglesworthia* sp., and *Wolbachia* sp. Similarly, four different genotypes of

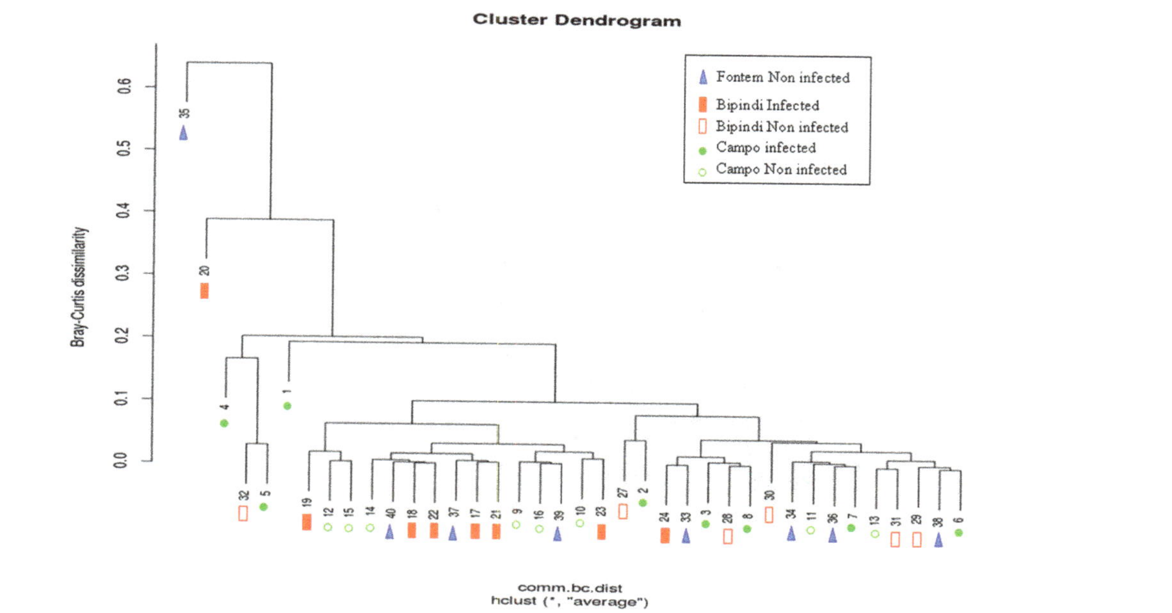

FIGURE 6 | Hierarchical cluster dendrogram based on Bray-Curtis Index values, showing the relationship between different samples (represented by numbers) and foci. Sample numbering as in **Figure 4**.

Enterobacteriaceae sp., *Wigglesworthia* sp., *Wolbachia* sp., and *Spiroplasma* sp. were detected in sample 30 (**Figure 8**).

Presence of Symbionts

Special attention was paid to symbionts, due to their role in tsetse physiology and their interaction with trypanosomes. *Wigglesworthia glossinidia* was once again characterized by its high density in most samples and groups; this was assessed by the high percentages (more than 80% in each sample), except in two samples from groups 4 and 5 (Bipindi and Fontem, non-infected flies). *Wolbachia* sp. sequences were also present in all groups, but in smaller amounts. Nevertheless, a very high number of *Wolbachia* sequences were observed in sample 20 (11.08%). In addition, we detected, at low relative abundance, the presence of the symbiont *S. glossinidius* in four samples distributed over all groups, except Bipindi-uninfected (group 4).

DISCUSSION

The main objective of this study was to characterize the bacterial communities inhabiting the midgut of field-collected tsetse flies from sleeping sickness foci in Cameroon using deep sequencing. Trypanosome-infected and non-infected flies were sampled in three sleeping sickness foci in Cameroon (Bipindi, Campo, and Fontem) that differ in their natural environment, thus offering the possibility to investigate the potential association between specific bacterial communities composition and the environment and/or the ability of the flies to be infected by trypanosomes. In this study the targeted trypanosome species was *T. congolense* (causing AAT) since, as shown in **Figure 3**, its prevalence was large enough in both Campo and Bipindi sampled flies. In contrast, *T. brucei* (*sensu lato*, Tb *sl* hereafter) had a much lower prevalence. Indeed, only 6 Tb *sl* infected flies were recorded in the sampled sites which, furthermore, included the two sub-species, *T. brucei brucei* and *T. brucei gambiense*—the former causing AAT and the second being responsible for the chronic form of HAT.

The Campo sampling campaign was performed in 2008, while the ones regarding Bipindi and Fontem were performed in 2013. A reduced but significant gene flow, due to fly migration, was previously reported between Campo and Bipindi (Farikou et al., 2011b), raising the question whether the 5 years delay between the sampling periods could affect the fly infection status and the microbiota profiles. One may consider that in the case of an important and/or continuous migration flow for years, differences in fly population diversity between the two foci would have been reduced or even suppressed. This was clearly not the case, and was never recorded (Farikou et al., 2010a,b). Although, the possibility that the 5 years delay could marginally affect the comparison between the 3 foci cannot be totally excluded, it could not affect the intra-foci comparison between trypanosome infected and non-infected flies.

Diversity of the Bacterial Communities and Its Origin

We detected a very large, unexpected number of different bacterial taxa (103 species), among which 26 were found in more than one sample. The number of different species identified in the present study was clearly much higher than in previous reports. For instance, three species were identified in *G. p. palpalis* in Angola (Geiger et al., 2009); one, three and eight species were, respectively, found in *G. nigrofusca*, *G. pallicera*, and *G. p. palpalis*

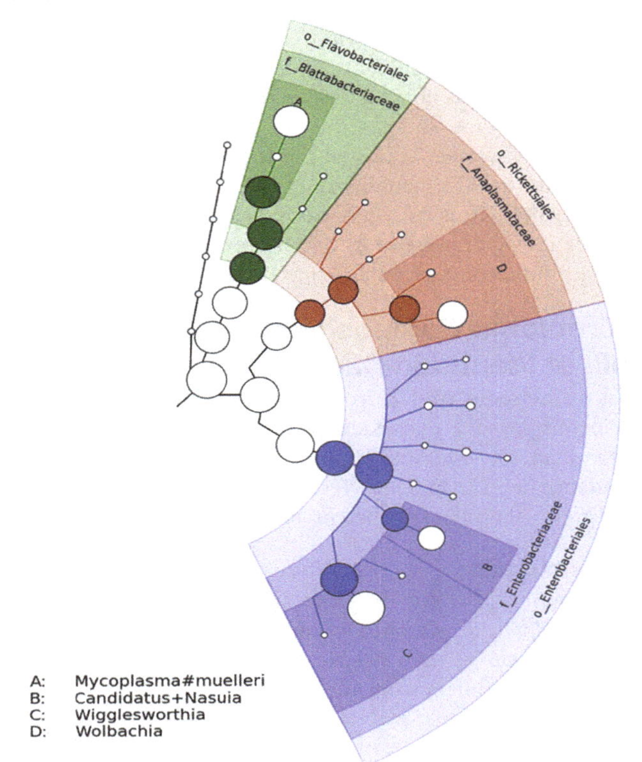

FIGURE 7 | Phylogenetic diversity of bacterial *16S rRNA* sequences found in sample 20 (infected tsetse fly midguts from Bipindi).

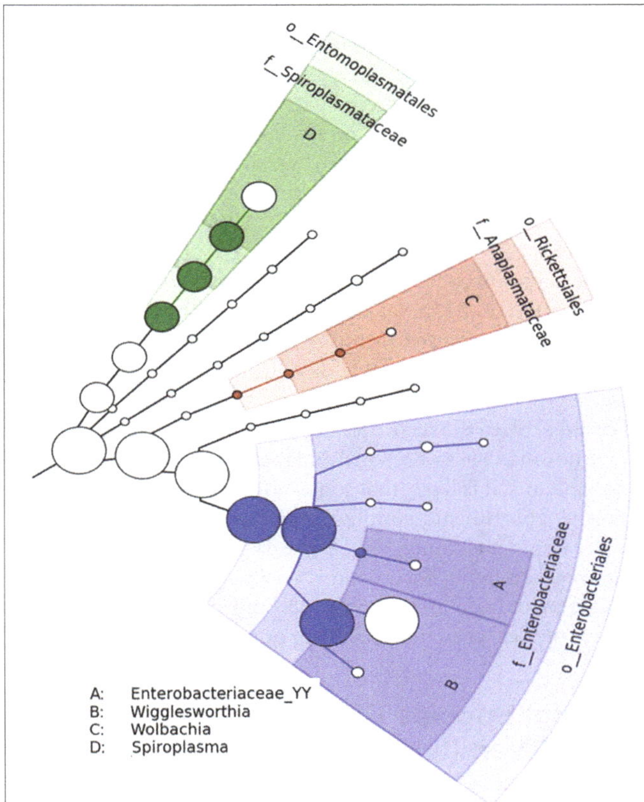

FIGURE 8 | Phylogenetic diversity of bacterial *16S rRNA* sequences found in sample 30 (uninfected tsetse fly midguts from Bipindi).

in Cameroon (Geiger et al., 2011b); one species was identified in *G. p. gambiensis*; and 24 species were found in *G. f. fuscipes* in Kenya (Lindh and Lehane, 2011). With the exception of two bacterial species, all species detected in these previous studies were identified using culture-dependent methods. Many bacteria species are difficult to culture and the density of some species may be too low for proper isolation. This could explain the low number of bacteria identified in other studies as compared to the high number of species we characterized in the gut of tsetse flies using molecular approach.

A more recent study (Aksoy et al., 2014) identified a high number of bacteria species in the gut microbiota of several tsetse fly species collected in Uganda using molecular approaches, although the bacteriome of Uganda flies was less diverse than the one of flies from Cameroon.

Compared to the bacterial communities of flies from Uganda, flies from Cameroon revealed both similarities (namely Enterobacteriaceae and an unexpected high abundance of *Wigglesworthia*) and differences (bacteria belonging to the genus *Delftia*, *Stenotrophomonas*, *Thermoanaerobacterium*, *Proteus*, and *Ochrobactrum*, among others, were not found in flies from Cameroon). These differences may be due to differences in the respective investigated fly species, *G. f. fuscipes*, *G. m. morsitans*, *G pallidipes* vs. *G. p. palpalis*, and/or the respective environmental factors and the geographic locations of the HAT/AAT foci in Uganda vs. Cameroon.

Aside from the question of what effect these gut bacteria may have on tsetse fly physiology and/or on their ability to become trypanosomes infected (i.e., their vector competence), there is also the question of how tsetse flies can acquire such a large diversity of bacterial species. In their report, Aksoy et al. (2014) mentioned the possibility that some of the low abundant bacteria "may have arisen from contamination from environmental sources, such as during field-based dissection processes,...." Although, the occurrence of contamination can never be totally excluded, our data do not support this comment since it would be expected, in such case, that several bacteria species from the environment would be detected, at low abundance, in all or most of the samples, inasmuch the 40 fly were processed at the same time. As shown in **Table S1**, this is not the case; most of the low abundant bacteria (74 out of 103) are present in only one sample and, in contrast, one of the samples (number 32) was shown to harbor 59 species. Nevertheless, further independent studies should be undertaken to confirm the finding. An alternative explanation could account for the complexity of the microbiota as it was recently reported, that is, tsetse flies are not strictly hematophagous; they can occasionally feed on nectar from a broad range of plants growing within their different ecological environments, and, thus, may ingest bacteria colonizing this nutriment (Colman et al., 2012; Solano et al., 2015). Such effect of diet differences and their links to environmental conditions, on bacteriome community structure of insects has been documented by Colman et al. (2012). Finally, as reported by Poinar et al. (1979), adult flies may be contaminated with bacteria present on the epidermis of humans or animals they bite during blood meal. This could lead to a large diversity of the fly bacteriome since tsetse flies are known to ingest their blood meals from a variety of vertebrates (Moloo et al., 1988; Simo et al., 2008; Farikou et al., 2010b). Thus, despite the viviparous reproduction of tsetse flies (in contrast to other dipterans) that prevent fly contamination at the larval stage (except for the symbionts that are vertically transmitted from the mother to the larva *via* milk gland secretions), the modes of acquiring "exogenous" bacteria by tsetse flies seems to be more diverse than previously believed and could explain the recorded large microbiota diversity herein.

One however has to keep in mind that in addition to true tsetse gut inhabitants, it is likely that some—or many—of the 143 OTUs are solely opportunistic, simply in transit or possibly present only as DNA fragments. Since dead bacteria provide the same DNA signature as do living bacteria, further investigations should aim to isolate bacteria of interest; only such approach will provide best evidence of their presence as a living organism in the tsetse gut.

Bacterial Species Richness of the Samples (Alpha Diversity)

Although, the analyzed midgut bacteriome of adult tsetse flies included 103 species belonging to 13 phyla, only 4 of them were dominant (Proteobacteria, Bacteroidetes, Actinobacteria, and Firmicutes), showing some similarities with gut microbial communities from other invertebrates such as cattle tick (Andreotti et al., 2011), several species of *Anopheles* (Rani et al., 2009; Boissière et al., 2012) and of *Aedes* (Zouache et al., 2011; Terenius et al., 2012); Acridid (Dillon et al., 2008); Asian longhorned beetle (Geib et al., 2009); *Lutzomyia longipalpis* (Gouveia et al., 2008); honey and bumble bees (Martinson et al., 2011). However, there is a major difference between the bacteriome of all these invertebrates and those of tsetse flies, namely the presence, in the latter, of *W. glossinidia* in all samples. *W. glossinidia*'s presence is not surprising as it is the tsetse fly's obligate symbiont; its abundance in the different samples was however remarkable as the mean relative abundance over the 40 samples was as high as 95.3% (even higher than 99% in all but five samples—see below), while that of *Enterobacter homaechei*, also present in all samples, was only 1.8%. Such an "overabundance" of *Wigglesworthia* was previously reported by Aksoy et al. (2014) who estimate that it may disrupt proper identification of low abundant bacteria thus leading to an underestimation of the alpha diversity (species richness). In order to decrease the abundance of this bacterium—and thus overcoming the difficulty related to its overabundance—the group of Aksoy et al. (2014) excised part of the bacteriome organ harboring *Wigglesworthia* and was able to discover some bacteria previously non-identified when analyzing the whole bacteriome. In our study, five samples showed smaller *Wigglesworthia* relative abundance than the 35 others; these are [sample number and (relative *Wigglesworthia* abundance)] sample 2 (88.83%), 4 (80.52%), 20 (51.27%), 32 (86.96%), and 35 (34.55%) while the numbers of hosted bacteria were, respectively, 16, 9, 8, 73, 10 (*Wigglesworthia* excluded). Thus, concerning our study, it seems that there was no relationship between the *Wigglesworthia* relative abundance and the species richness of the samples [for example, sample 32 hosted the largest number of bacteria although the relative abundance of *Wigglesworthia* was rather high (86.96%)]. Thus, as suggested by Aksoy et al. (2014), further investigations on the tsetse fly bacteriome should be performed using genomic/complementary functional approaches.

Microbiome Composition and the Possible Role of Identified Bacteria

Most of the sequence tags corresponded to few taxa. Only 16 species displayed a maximum relative abundance per sample higher than 1%, whereas 78 species had a maximum relative abundance lower than 0.2%. Nevertheless, some members of the latter group of bacteria are potentially of great interest.

The Symbionts

This group of bacteria includes in particular three species *W. glossinidia*, *S. glossinidius,* and *Wolbacchia*. Besides its prominent role as an obligate symbiont of the tsetse fly, *Wigglesworthia* differs from the other bacteria by the fact that 60 genotypes of this species have been identified, whereas most other bacteria were represented by only one genotype, or at least by a limited number of genotypes. In samples from Uganda, differences were also detected in the sequences of the *Wigglesworthia* V4 region (Aksoy et al., 2014) that confirmed the existence of several genotypes, although the authors reported small amounts of *Wigglesworthia* carryover between the different tsetse species sampled; thus they do not exclude completely the occurrence of a cross contamination. Nevertheless, the occurrence of multiple genotypes of a given species is not a surprise and may not be considered as an artifact generated along the technical process. For example, we have previously identified number of *S. glossinidius* genotypes when using other approaches than amplicon sequencing (Illumina MiSeq) such as AFLP (Geiger et al., 2005, 2007) or microsatellite (Farikou et al., 2011a,b) genotyping on either insectary-reared or field sampled tsetse flies. This finding could be of great interest, as until now only the density of *Wigglesworthia*, not its potential genetic diversity, was considered to be involved in the modulation of tsetse fly infection by trypanosomes (Wang et al., 2009). In fact, the genetic diversity within populations of *W. glossinidia* that infect tsetse flies could play a prominent role, as previously demonstrated for the facultative symbiont *S. glossinidius* (Geiger et al., 2007). However, investigating a possible association between trypanosome infection and specific *W. glossinidia* genotypes (60 have been identified) will require a much larger sampling size.

Attention was paid to *Sodalis* that was previously shown to be involved in modulating the tsetse fly's ability to acquire trypanosomes (Farikou et al., 2010a; Hamidou Soumana et al., 2014). In the present study this symbiont was identified in 10% of the samples, a finding markedly different from the 30% average prevalence we found previously in nearly the same sampling sites (Farikou et al., 2010a), and from that recorded for example by Aksoy et al. (2014) who suggest the variations could be a matter of sensitivity of the analytical approach. However, this could be only part of an explanation since we used in our study similar analytical approaches and instruments (including the Illumina MiSeq platform). Overall, these data confirm the existence of a very high symbiont variability in natural populations of flies, as previously reported by Farikou et al. (2010a). These variations could be linked to a multitude of factors including differences in tsetse individual flying times, field environment modifications or, as suggested by Aksoy et al. (2014) the competition between *Sodalis* and other intestinal bacteria which diversity and respective abundance may vary.

Wolbachia sp. was previously characterized in field populations of *G. morsitans morsitans*, *G. morsitans centralis*, *G. austeni* flies, *G. brevipalpis*, *G. pallidipes*, and *G. p. gambiensis* (Doudoumis et al., 2012). Interestingly, *Wolbachia* has not been characterized in *G. fuscipes fuscipes* or *G. tachinoides* and, until now in *G. p. palpalis*. The bacterium was detected in 25 out of 40 flies (62.5%) and was distributed over the 5 groups (thus across the three sampling sites, and the fly trypanosome infection status): 5, 4, 7, 5, and 4 *Wolbachia* positive flies in groups 1–5, respectively. At this stage of the investigation we cannot suggest any explanation for its presence; we can only report its relatively high prevalence. The fact that until now *Wolbacchia* was never characterized in *G. palpalis palpalis* does not mean such infection does not occur in other fly individuals; further studies should focus on surveys of larger *G. p. palpalis* populations from the studied HAT foci, or on populations from HAT foci located elsewhere than in Cameroon (for example flies from HAT foci located in RDC—République Démocratique du Congo—or in Angola). In a recent report, Ji et al. (2015) highlight the extreme variability (from 1.54 to 66.67%) of the prevalence of *Wolbacchia* across 25 *Bemisia tabaci* populations from China. The frequency of *Bemisia* infection was shown to be affected by a large panel of factors (putative *B. tabaci* species, geographic location, sex of the host ...). Finally, a cystoplasmic incompatibility occurs when a *Wolbacchia* negative (W−) female fly mates with a *Wolbacchia* positive (W+) male, and the embryos degenerate (Alam et al., 2011). In contrast, when a (W+) female mates with a (W+) or a (W−) male, the offspring is not only fertile but also more numerous than in the case of a (W−) female with (W−) male mating. As *Wolbacchia* is transmitted by the female fly to its offspring, the presence of *Wolbacchia* in a female gives them a reproductive advantage. Could this explain the high prevalence of *Wolbacchia* in the studied Gpp populations?

In contrast to *Anopheles gambiae* whose susceptibility to *Plasmodium* infection increased with the presence of *Wolbachia* under natural conditions (Zélé et al., 2014); the presence of this symbiont was not found to be associated with the infection status of the tsetse flies.

We also identified in tsetse fly midguts the presence of bacteria that are known to be symbionts when infecting other organisms. This is the case of *Candidatus Sulcia muelleri* (Flavobacteriaceae), which displayed an ancient symbiotic relationship with the hemipteran *Auchenorrhyncha* (Moran et al., 2005). The identified bacterium *Candidatus Zinderia* is also a symbiont of the tick *Haemaphysalis longicornis* (McCutcheon and Moran, 2010). Finally, we observed the cohabitation of four symbionts in some of our analyzed samples, although it is unknown if they develop a synergistic effect on the fly's physiology. Given the current state of our investigation, large-scale analyses (including attempts to isolate the two *Candidatus* species) deserve to be undertaken, as until now only three symbionts have been described in tsetse flies.

Other Bacteria of Interest

S. marcescens and *Serratia odorifera* (Enterobacteriaceae) were present in more than 50% of the samples. Both species are considered to be opportunistic pathogens for humans (Chmel, 1988; Hejazi and Falkiner, 1997; Grimont and Grimont, 2015). *Serratia marcescens* is also responsible for the increased mortality in tsetse flies (Poinar et al., 1979) such as *Glossina pallidipes* (Gonzalez-Ceron et al., 2003); it secretes trypanolytic compounds and reduces the establishment of *T. cruzi* in the midgut of its vector, *Rhodnius prolixus* (Triatominae), vector of *T. cruzi* causing the Chagas disease; Azambuja et al., 2004). One previous work reported the presence of the novel species *S. glossinae* in the gut of insectary-reared *G. palpalis gambiensis* flies (Geiger et al., 2010), although this species has never been identified in field-collected *Glossina* flies. Surprisingly, the same situation was observed for mosquitoes where the bacterium *Elizabethkingia* was found only in insectary-reared *Anopheles* sp. (Boissière et al., 2012; Gimonneau et al., 2014). However, this phenomenon cannot be currently explained. The presence of *Serratia* in the guts of *G. f. fuscipes* flies from western Kenya has also been reported (Lindh and Lehane, 2011). In *Anopheles gambiae* mosquito midguts, multiple strains of *Serratia* have been identified, some of which are able to reduce mosquito infections by *Plasmodium* (Bando et al., 2013). *Serratia* has also been identified as a newly acquired symbiotic partner in aphids (Burke and Moran, 2011). Currently, we did not evidence a clear association between the presence of some bacterial and trypanosome infection. However, as suggested previously by Aksoy et al. (2014), understanding the association of *Serratia* with tsetse flies and its functional role in tsetse physiology could provide critical knowledge about trypanosome transmission dynamics in tsetse flies. Similar investigations could be performed with other bacteria.

In addition to *Serratia*, other identified bacteria have the ability to produce antiparasitic compounds, including members of *Acinetobacter*. This genus was previously characterized in the gut of tsetse flies from Cameroon (Geiger et al., 2009). The presence of *Acinetobacter* (*guillouiae* and spp.) was observed in 6 samples in the present study.

Association between the Composition of the Intestinal Communities and the Fly Infection Status and/or the Environmental Differences

The characterization of the composition of the intestinal bacterial communities was an important objective of the work. However, the statistical analyses of the identified bacteria in this study did not reveal any significant differences in the sample bacterial species richness between the different groups (Campo and Bipindi infected and uninfected flies as well as Fontem uninfected flies), or the status of the flies (infected vs. uninfected). A hierarchical clustering neither discriminate properly the different groups, nor the infected flies from the non-infected flies of the same focus. At the level of individual bacteria, some of them seem to display an association with a given group or a sampling site. However, most often they concern species that are poorly represented. The possibly that environmental differences between the three sampling sites (especially the climate, wildlife, and flora) were too weak to induce significant differences in the flies' microbiome composition may be considered. These data suggest future fly microbiome research should aim for greater numbers of flies and target more ecologically contrasted sites, in order to identify bacteria involved in (or at least associated with) the fly vector competence.

In conclusion the meta-barcoding analysis that we performed on DNA extracted from *G. p. palpalis* collected from three different HAT foci in Cameroon resulted in the detection of 143 OTUs belonging to 83 genera and 13 phyla. Part of these bacteria could be identified at the species level (103 annotated OTUs). However, some species were not identifiable since the corresponding sequences did not match any available sequence libraries; they may correspond to novel species, and need to undergo further identification process. The presence of such a variety of bacteria was unexpected and raises many questions regarding how they are acquired by tsetse flies, and the role they may play regarding the fly's physiology and vector competence. In addition, it would be of interest, in a following investigation campaign, to enlarge the sampling scheme and include teneral flies as a supplementary control besides non-infected non-teneral flies. The former are expected to host a more limited microbiota and to have a less developed immunity compared to the latter. On the other hand, it should be noted that, when teneral flies undergo artificial infection process, about 70% do not develop trypanosome infection (Geiger et al., 2007). This suggests that within a collection of teneral flies most of them, even considered as "naïve," are physiologically and genetically "programmed" to be/become refractory to trypanosome infection.

AUTHOR CONTRIBUTIONS

Conceived and designed the experiments: FJ, AG. Performed the experiments: FJ, TM, GN, FN, AG. Analyzed the data: FJ, RC, AG. Contributed reagents/materials/analysis tools: AG. Wrote the paper: GG, FN, LA, JR, AG.

ACKNOWLEDGMENTS

The authors thank the "Région Languedoc-Roussillon—Appel d'Offre Chercheur d'Avenir 2011," the "Institut de Recherche pour le Développement" and the International Atomic Energy Agency (IAEA) for their support.

SUPPLEMENTARY MATERIAL

Table S1 | Classification of the total bacteria detected in the 40 tsetse samples from the Campo, Bipindi, and Fontem foci in Cameroon. The table provides, for each sample, the relative abundance (in %) of each bacterium present in this sample. Several of the detected bacteria could not be identified at the species level. The suffix "X or Y" refers to "unclassified" at that rank.

Figure S1 | Rarefaction analysis on the studied samples (Renyi diversity plots); **(A)** Samples 1–24 and 27–40; **(B)** Samples 25 and 26 that were processed apart.

Figure S2 | Heat map analysis of the distribution and abundance of the bacterial genera in midgut samples. The samples did not cluster together, indicating that the bacterial community among them is highly variable. Sample numbering as in **Figure 4**.

Figure S3 | Heat map analysis of the repartition and abundance of bacterial species in midgut samples. The samples did not cluster together, indicating that the bacterial community among them is highly variable. Sample numbering as in **Figure 4**.

Figure S4 | (A) NMDS plot comparing bacterial OTUs in tsetse fly midguts of different foci (Bipindi, Campo, Fontem) using Bray-Curtis dissimilarity indice. **(B)** NMDS plot comparing bacterial OTUs of infected vs. non infected tsetse fly midguts using Bray-Curtis dissimilarity indice.

Figure S5 | Phylogenetic diversity of bacterial *16S rRNA* sequences in tsetse fly midguts. NJ tree clustering of OTU representatives based on homology with known sequences is shown. The width of the branch is proportional to the number of samples exhibiting a given OTU. Colors correspond to different phyla. **(A–D)** Expended scale of four regions from this figure in order to make it easier to read (the corresponding regions are indicated in this figure).

REFERENCES

1. Akman, L., Yamashita, A., Watanabe, H., Oshima, K., Shiba, T., Hattori, M., et al. (2002). Genome sequence of the endocellular obligate symbiont of tsetse flies, *Wigglesworthia glossinidia*. *Nat. Genet.* 32, 402–407. doi: 10.1038/ng986
2. Aksoy, E., Telleria, E. L., Echodu, R., Wu, Y., Okedi, L. M., Weiss, B. L., et al. (2014). Analysis of multiple tsetse fly populations in Uganda reveals limited diversity and species-specific gut microbiota. *Appl. Environ. Microbiol.* 80, 4301–4312. doi: 10.1128/AEM.00079-14
3. Aksoy, E., Vigneron, A., Bing, X., Zhao, X., O'Neill, M., Wu, Y. N., et al. (2016). Mammalian African trypanosome VSG coat enhances tsetse's vector competence. *Proc. Natl. Acad. Sci. U.S.A.* 113, 6961–6966. doi: 10.1073/pnas.1600304113
4. Aksoy, S. (1995). *Wigglesworthia* gen. nov. and *Wigglesworthia glossinidia* sp. nov., taxa consisting of the mycetocyte-associated, primary endosymbionts of tsetse flies. *Int. J. Syst. Bacteriol.* 45, 848–851. doi: 10.1099/00207713-45-4-848
5. Aksoy, S., Caccone, A., Galvani, A. P., and Okedi, L. M. (2013). Glossina fuscipes populations provide insights for human African trypanosomiasis transmission in Uganda. *Trends Parasitol.* 29, 394–406. doi: 10.1016/j.pt.2013.06.005
6. Alam, U., Hyseni, C., Symula, R. E., Brelsfoard, C., Wu, Y., Kruglov, O., et al. (2012). Implications of microfauna-host interactions for trypanosome transmission dynamics in Glossina fuscipes fuscipes in Uganda. *Appl. Environ. Microbiol.* 78, 4627–4637. doi: 10.1128/AEM.00806-12
7. Alam, U., Medlock, J., Brelsfoard, C., Pais, R., Lohs, C., Balmand, S., et al. (2011). Wolbachia symbiont infections induce strong cytoplasmic incompatibility in the tsetse fly *Glossina morsitans*. *PLoS Pathog.* 7:e1002415. doi: 10.1371/journal.ppat.1002415
8. Andreotti, R., Pérez de León, A. A., Dowd, S. E., Guerrero, F. D., Bendele, K.

G., and Scoles, G. A. (2011). Assessment of bacterial diversity in the cattle tick Rhipicephalus (Boophilus) microplus through tag-encoded pyrosequencing. *BMC Microbiol.* 11:6. doi: 10.1186/1471-2180-11-6

9. Azambuja, P., Feder, D., and Garcia, E. S. (2004). Isolation of *Serratia marcescens* in the midgut of *Rhodnius prolixus*: impact on the establishment of the parasite *Trypanosoma cruzi* in the vector. *Exp. Parasitol.* 107, 89–96. doi: 10.1016/j.exppara.2004.04.007
10. Baker, N., de Koning, H. P., Mäser, P., and Horn, D. (2013). Drug resistance in African trypanosomiasis: the melarsoprol and pentamidine story. *Trends Parasitol.* 29, 110–118. doi: 10.1016/j.pt.2012.12.005
11. Balmand, S., Lohs, C., Aksoy, S., and Heddi, A. (2013). Tissue distribution and transmission routes for the tsetse fly endosymbionts. *J. Invertebr. Pathol.* 112, S116–S122. doi: 10.1016/j.jip.2012.04.002
12. Bando, H., Okado, K., Guelbeogo, W. M., Badolo, A., Aonuma, H., Nelson, B., et al. (2013). Intra-specific diversity of *Serratia marcescens* in Anopheles mosquito midgut defines Plasmodium transmission capacity. *Sci. Rep.* 3:1641. doi: 10.1038/srep01641
13. Boissière, A., Tchioffo, M. T., Bachar, D., Abate, L., Marie, A., Nsango, S. E., et al. (2012). Midgut microbiota of the malaria mosquito vector Anopheles gambiae and interactions with *Plasmodium falciparum* infection. *PLoS Pathog.* 8:e1002742. doi: 10.1371/journal.ppat.1002742
14. Burke, G. R., and Moran, N. A. (2011). Massive genomic decay in Serratia symbiotica, a recently evolved symbiont of aphids. *Genome Biol. Evol.* 3, 195–208. doi: 10.1093/gbe/evr002
15. Chen, X., Song, L., and Aksoy, S. (1999). Concordant evolution of a symbiont with its host insect species: molecular phylogeny of genus Glossina and its bacteriome associated endosymbiont, *Wigglesworthia glossinidia*. *J. Mol. Evol.* 48, 49–58. doi: 10.1007/PL00006444
16. Cheng, Q., and Aksoy, S. (1999). Tissue tropism, transmission and expression of foreign genes *in vivo* in midgut symbionts of tsetse flies. *Insect Mol. Biol.* 8, 125–132. doi: 10.1046/j.1365-2583.1999.810125.x
17. Cheng, Q., Ruel, T. D., Zhou, W., Moloo, S. K., Majiwa, P., O'Neill, S. L., et al. (2000). Tissue distribution and prevalence of Wolbachia infections in tsetse flies, *Glossina* spp. *Med. Vet. Entomol.* 14, 44–50. doi: 10.1046/j.1365-2915.2000.00202.x
18. Chevenet, F., Brun, C., Ba-uls, A. L., Jacq, B., and Christen, R. (2006). TreeDyn: towards dynamic graphics and annotations for analyses of trees. *BMC Bioinformatics* 7:439. doi: 10.1186/1471-2105-7-439
19. Chmel, H. (1988). Serratia odorifera biogroup 1 causing an invasive human infection. *J. Clin. Microbiol.* 26, 1244–1245.
20. Colman, D. R., Toolson, E. C., and Takacs-Vesbach, C. D. (2012). Do diet and taxonomy influence insect gut bacterial communities? *Mol. Ecol.* 21, 5124–5137. doi: 10.1111/j.1365-294X.2012.05752.x
21. Dillon, R. J., Webster, G., Weightman, A. J., Dillon, V. M., Blanford, S., and Charnley, A. K. (2008). Composition of Acridid gut bacterial communities as revealed by 16S rRNA gene analysis. *J. Invertebr. Pathol.* 97, 265–272. doi: 10.1016/j.jip.2007.09.010
22. Doudoumis, V., Tsiamis, G., Wamwiri, F., Brelsfoard, C., Alam, U., Aksoy, E., et al. (2012). Detection and characterization of Wolbachia infections in laboratory and natural populations of different species of tsetse flies (genus Glossina). *BMC Microbiol.* 12(Suppl. 1):S3. doi: 10.1186/1471-2180-12-S1-S3
23. Edgar, R. C., Haas, B. J., Clemente, J. C., Quince, C., and Knight, R. (2011). UCHIME improves sensitivity and speed of chimera detection. *Bioinformatics* 27, 2194–2200. doi: 10.1093/bioinformatics/btr381
24. Farikou, O., Njiokou, F., Cuny, G., and Geiger, A. (2011a). Microsatellite genotyping reveals diversity within populations of *Sodalis glossinidius*, the secondary symbiont of tsetse flies. *Vet. Microbiol.* 150, 207–210. doi: 10.1016/j.vetmic.2011.01.021
25. Farikou, O., Njiokou, F., Mbida Mbida, J. A., Njitchouang, G. R., Djeunga, H. N., Asonganyi, T., et al. (2010a). Tripartite interactions between tsetse flies, *Sodalis glossinidius* and trypanosomes–an epidemiological approach in two historical human African trypanosomiasis foci in Cameroon. *Infect. Genet. Evol.* 10, 115–121. doi: 10.1016/j.meegid.2009.10.008
26. Farikou, O., Njiokou, F., Simo, G., Asonganyi, T., Cuny, G., and Geiger, A. (2010b). Tsetse fly blood meal modification and trypanosome identification in two sleeping sickness foci in the forest of southern Cameroon. *Acta Trop.* 116, 81–88. doi: 10.1016/j.actatropica.2010.06.002
27. Farikou, O., Thevenon, S., Njiokou, F., Allal, F., Cuny, G., and Geiger, A. (2011b). Genetic diversity and population structure of the secondary symbiont of tsetse flies, *Sodalis glossinidius*, in sleeping sickness foci in Cameroon. *PLoS Negl. Trop. Dis.* 5:e1281. doi: 10.1371/journal.pntd.0001281
28. Geib, S. M., Jimenez-Gasco Mdel, M., Carlson, J. E., Tien, M., and Hoover, K. (2009). Effect of host tree species on cellulase activity and bacterial community composition in the gut of larval Asian longhorned beetle. *Environ. Entomol.* 38, 686–699. doi: 10.1603/022.038.0320
29. Geiger, A., Cuny, G., and Frutos, R. (2005). Two Tsetse fly species, *Glossina palpalis* gambiensis and *Glossina morsitans* morsitans, carry genetically distinct populations of the secondary symbiont *Sodalis glossinidius*. *Appl. Environ. Microbiol.* 71, 8941–8943. doi: 10.1128/AEM.71.12.8941-8943.2005
30. Geiger, A., Fardeau, M. L., Falsen, E., Ollivier, B., and Cuny, G. (2010). *Serratia glossinae* sp. nov., isolated from the midgut of the tsetse fly *Glossina palpalis* gambiensis. *Int. J. Syst. Evol. Microbiol.* 60, 1261–1265. doi: 10.1099/ijs.0.013441-0
31. Geiger, A., Fardeau, M. L., Grebaut, P., Vatunga, G., Josénando, T., Herder, S., et al. (2009). First isolation of *Enterobacter*, *Enterococcus*, and *Acinetobacter* spp. as inhabitants of the tsetse fly (*Glossina palpalis* palpalis) midgut. *Infect. Genet. Evol.* 9, 1364–1370. doi: 10.1016/j.meegid.2009.09.013
32. Geiger, A., Fardeau, M. L., Njiokou, F., Joseph, M., Asonganyi, T., Ollivier, B., et al. (2011b). Bacterial diversity associated with populations of *Glossina* spp. from Cameroon and distribution within the Campo sleeping sickness focus. *Microb. Ecol.* 62, 632–643. doi: 10.1007/s00248-011-9830-y
33. Geiger, A., Ravel, S., Mateille, T., Janelle, J., Patrel, D., Cuny, G., et al. (2007). Vector competence of *Glossina palpalis* gambiensis for *Trypanosoma brucei* s.l. and genetic diversity of the symbiont *Sodalis glossinidius*. *Mol. Biol. Evol.* 24, 102–109. doi: 10.1093/molbev/msl135
34. Geiger, A., Simo, G., Grébaut, P., Peltier, J. B., Cuny, G., and Holzmuller, P. (2011a). Transcriptomics and proteomics in human African trypanosomiasis: current status and perspectives. *J. Proteomics* 74, 1625–1643. doi: 10.1016/j.jprot.2011.01.016
35. Gimonneau, G., Tchioffo, M. T., Abate, L., Boissière, A., Awono-Ambéné, P. H., Nsango, S. E., et al. (2014). Composition of Anopheles coluzzii and Anopheles gambiae microbiota from larval to adult stages. *Infect. Genet. Evol.* 28, 715–724. doi: 10.1016/j.meegid.2014.09.029
36. Gonzalez-Ceron, L., Santillan, F., Rodriguez, M. H., Mendez, D., and Hernandez- Avila, J. E. (2003). Bacteria in midguts of field-collected Anopheles albimanus block Plasmodium vivax sporogonic development. *J. Med. Entomol.* 40, 371–374. doi: 10.1603/0022-2585-40.3.371
37. Gouteux, J. P., and Lancien, J. (1986). Le piège pyramidal à tsé-tsé (Diptera: Glossinidae) pour la capture et la lutte. Essais comparatifs et description de nouveaux systèmes de capture. *Trop. Med. Parasitol.* 37, 61–66.
38. Gouveia, C., Asensi, M. D., Zahner, V., Rangel, E. F., and Oliveira, S. M. (2008). Study on the bacterial midgut microbiota associated to different Brazilian populations of *Lutzomyia longipalpis* (Lutz & Neiva) (Diptera: Psychodidae). *Neotrop. Entomol.* 37, 597–601. doi: 10.1590/S1519-566X200800 0500016
39. Gouy, M., Guindon, S., and Gascuel, O. (2010). SeaView version 4: a multiplatform graphical user interface for sequence alignment and phylogenetic tree building. *Mol. Biol. Evol.* 27, 221–224. doi: 10.1093/molbev/msp259
40. Grébaut, P., Mbida, J. A., Kondjio, C. A., Njiokou, F., Penchenier, L., and Laveissiere, C. (2004). Spatial and temporal patterns of human African trypanosomiasis (HAT) transmission risk in the Bipindi focus, in the forest zone of southern Cameroon. *Vector Borne Zoonotic Dis.* 4, 230–238. doi: 10.1089/vbz.2004.4.230
41. Grébaut, P., Wang, S., Bodo, J. M., Ebo'o Eyenga, V., Binzouli, J. J., Ndong Ngoe, C., et al. (2001). Aspects épidémiologiques d'un foyer de la maladie du sommeil mal connu: le foyer de Bipindi au Cameroun. *Bull. Liaison Document. de l'OCEAC.* 33, 16.
42. Grimont, F., and Grimont, P. A. (2015). *Serratia. Bergey's Manual of Systematics of Archaea and Bacteria.* (Oxford: John Wiley & Sons, Inc., in association with Bergey's Manual Trust).
43. Guillou, L., Bachar, D., Audic, S., Bass, D., Berney, C., Bittner, L., et al. (2012). The Protist Ribosomal Reference database (PR2): a catalog of unicellular eukaryote small sub-unit rRNA sequences with curated taxonomy. *Nucleic Acids Res.* 41, D597–D604. doi: 10.1093/nar/gks1160
44. Haines, L. R., Lehane, S. M., Pearson, T. W., and Lehane, M. J. (2010). Tsetse EP protein protects the fly midgut from trypanosome establishment. *PLoS Pathog.* 6:e1000793. doi: 10.1371/journal.ppat.1000793
45. Hamidou Soumana, I., Loriod, B., Ravel, S., Tchicaya, B., Simo, G., Rihet, P., et al. (2014). The transcriptional signatures of *Sodalis glossinidius* in the *Glossina*

palpalis gambiensis flies negative for *Trypanosoma brucei* gambiense contrast with those of this symbiont in tsetse flies positive for the parasite: possible involvement of a Sodalis-hosted prophage in fly Trypanosoma refractoriness? *Infect. Genet. Evol.* 24, 41–56. doi: 10.1016/j.meegid.2014.03.005

46. Hartmann, M., Howes, C. G., VanInsberghe, D., Yu, H., Bachar, D., Christen, R., et al. (2012). Significant and persistent impact of timber harvesting on soil microbial communities in Northern coniferous forests. *ISME J.* 6, 2199–2218. doi: 10.1038/ismej.2012.84
47. Hejazi, A., and Falkiner, F. R. (1997). *Serratia marcescens*. *J. Med. Microbiol.* 46, 903–912. doi: 10.1099/00222615-46-11-903
48. Herder, S., Simo, G., Nkinin, S., and Njiokou, F. (2002). Identification of trypanosomes in wild animals from southern Cameroon using the polymerase chain reaction (PCR). *Parasite* 9, 345–349. doi: 10.1051/parasite/2002094345
49. Hu, C., and Aksoy, S. (2006). Innate immune responses regulate trypanosome parasite infection of the tsetse fly *Glossina morsitans* morsitans. *Mol. Microbiol.* 60, 1194–1204. doi: 10.1111/j.1365-2958.2006.05180.x
50. Ji, H. L., Qi, L. D., Hong, X. Y., Xie, H. F., and Li, Y. X. (2015). Effects of host sex, plant species, and putative host species on the prevalence of wolbachia in natural populations of *Bemisia tabaci* (Hemiptera: Aleyrodidae): a modified nested PCR study. *J. Econ. Entomol.* 108, 210–218. doi: 10.1093/jee/tou004
51. Lazaro, J. E., Nitcheu, J., Predicala, R. Z., Mangalindan, G. C., Nesslany, F., Marzin, D., et al. (2002). Heptyl prodigiosin, a bacterial metabolite, is antimalarial *in vivo* and non-mutagenic *in vitro*. *J. Nat. Toxins* 11, 367–377.
52. Lindh, J. M., and Lehane, M. J. (2011). The tsetse fly Glossina fuscipes fuscipes (Diptera: Glossina) harbours a surprising diversity of bacteria other than symbionts. *Antonie Van Leeuwenhoek* 99, 711–720. doi: 10.1007/s10482-010-9546-x
53. MacLeod, E. T., Maudlin, I., Darby, A. C., and Welburn, S. C. (2007). Antioxidants promote establishment of trypanosome infections in tsetse. *Parasitology* 134, 827–831. doi: 10.1017/S0031182007002247
54. Magocˇ T., and Salzberg, S. L. (2011). FLASH: fast length adjustment of short reads to improve genome assemblies. *Bioinformatics* 27, 2957–2963. doi: 10.1093/bioinformatics/btr507
55. Majiwa, P. A. O., Thatthi, R., Moloo, S. K., Nyeko, J. H. P., Otieno, L. H., and Maloo, S. (1994). Detection of trypanosome infections in the saliva of tsetse flies and buffy-coat samples from antigenaemic but aparasitaemic cattle. *Parasitology* 108, 313–322. doi: 10.1017/S0031182000076150
56. Martin, M. (2011). Cutadapt removes adapter sequences from high-throughput sequencing reads. *EMBnet J.* 17.1, 1–3. doi: 10.14806/ej.17.1.200
57. Martinson, V. G., Danforth, B. N., Minckley, R. L., Rueppell, O., Tingek, S., and Moran, N. A. (2011). A simple and distinctive microbiota associated with honey bees and bumble bees. *Mol. Ecol.* 20, 619–628. doi: 10.1111/j.1365-294X.2010.04959.x
58. Masiga, D. K., Smyth, A. J., Ayes, P., Bromidge, T. J., and Gibson, W. C. (1992). Sensitive detection of trypanosomes in tsetse flies by DNA amplification. *Int. J. Parasitol.* 22, 909–918. doi: 10.1016/0020-7519(92)90047-O
59. Massana, R., Gobet, A., Audic, S., Bass, D., Bittner, L., Boutte, C., et al. (2015). Marine protist diversity in European coastal waters and sediments as revealed by high-throughput sequencing. *Environ. Microbiol.* 17, 4035–4049. doi: 10.1111/1462-2920.12955
60. McCutcheon, J. P., and Moran, N. A. (2010). Functional convergence in reduced genomes of bacterial symbionts spanning 200 My of evolution. *Genome Biol. Evol.* 2, 708–718. doi: 10.1093/gbe/evq055
61. McMurdie, P. J., and Holmes, S. (2013). phyloseq: an R package for reproducible interactive analysis and graphics of microbiome census data. *PLoS ONE* 8:e61217. doi: 10.1371/journal.pone.0061217
62. Melachio, T. T., Simo, G., Ravel, S., De Meeûs, T., Causse, S., Solano, P., et al. (2011). Population genetics of *Glossina palpalis* palpalis from central African sleeping sickness foci. *Parasit. Vectors* 4:140. doi: 10.1186/1756-3305-4-140
63. Moloo, S. K., Grootenhuis, J. G., Kar, S. K., and Karstad, L. (1988). Survival and reproductive performance of female *Glossina morsitans* morsitans when maintained on the blood of different species of wild mammals. *Med. Vet. Entomol.* 2, 347–350. doi: 10.1111/j.1365-2915.1988.tb00207.x
64. Mondani, L., Benzerara, K., Carrière, M., Christen, R., Mamindy-Pajany, Y., Février, L., et al. (2011). Influence of uranium on bacterial communities: a comparison of natural uranium-rich soils with controls. *PLoS ONE* 6:e25771. doi: 10.1371/journal.pone.0025771
65. Moore, S., Shrestha, S., Tomlinson, K. W., and Vuong, H. (2012). Predicting the effect of climate change on African trypanosomiasis: integrating epidemiology with parasite and vector biology. *J. R. Soc. Interface* 9, 817–830. doi: 10.1098/rsif.2011.0654
66. Moran, N. A., Tran, P., and Gerardo, N. M. (2005). Symbiosis and insect diversification: an ancient symbiont of sap-feeding insects from the bacterial phylum Bacteroidetes. *Appl. Environ. Microbiol.* 71, 8802–8810. doi: 10.1128/AEM.71.12.8802-8810.2005
67. Moser, D. R., Cook, G. A., Ochs, D. E., Bailey, C. P., McKane, M. R., and Donelson, J. E. (1989). Detection of *Trypanosoma congolense* and *Trypanosoma brucei* subspecies by DNA amplification using the polymerase chain reaction. *Parasitology* 99, 57–66. doi: 10.1017/S0031182000061023
68. Moss, M. (2002). Bacterial pigments. *Microbiologist* 3, 10–12.
69. Njiokou, F., Laveissière, C., Simo, G., Nkinin, S., Grébaut, P., Cuny, G., et al. (2006). Wild fauna as a probable animal reservoir for *Trypanosoma brucei* gambiense in Cameroon. *Infect. Genet. Evol.* 6, 147–153. doi: 10.1016/j.meegid.2005.04.003
70. Njiokou, F., Simo, G., Nkinin, S. W., Laveissière, C., and Herder, S. (2004). Infection rate of *Trypanosoma brucei* s.l., *T. vivax*, *T. congolense* "forest type," and *T. simiae* in small wild vertebrates in south Cameroon. *Acta Trop.* 92, 139–146. doi: 10.1016/j.actatropica.2004.04.011
71. Nkinin, S. W., Njiokou, F., Penchenier, L., Grébaut, P., Simo, G., and Herder, S. (2002). Characterization of *Trypanosoma brucei s.l* subspecies by izoenzymes in domestic pigs from the Fontem sleeping sickness focus of Cameroon. *Acta Trop.* 81, 225–232. doi: 10.1016/S0001-706X(01)00213-3
72. Pawlowski, J., Christen, R., Lecroq, B., Bachar, D., Shahbazkia, H. R., Amaral-Zettler, L., et al. (2011). Eukaryotic richness in the abyss: insights from pyrotag sequencing. *PLoS ONE* 6:e18169. doi: 10.1371/journal.pone.0018169
73. Poinar, G. O. Jr, Wassink, H. J., Leegwater-van der Linden, M. E., and van der Geest, L. P. (1979). *Serratia marcescens* as a pathogen of tsetse flies. *Acta Trop.* 36, 223–227.
74. Porter, T. M., Shokralla, S., Baird, D., Golding, G. B., and Hajibabaei, M. (2016). Ribosomal, DNA, and plastid markers used to sample fungal and plant communities from wetland soils reveals complementary biotas. *PLoS ONE* 11:e0142759. doi: 10.1371/journal.pone.0142759
75. Quast, C., Pruesse, E., Yilmaz, P., Gerken, J., Schweer, T., Yarza, P., et al. (2012). The SILVA ribosomal RNA gene database project: improved data processing and web-based tools. *Nucleic Acids Res.* 41, D590–D596. doi: 10.1093/nar/gks1219
76. Rani, A., Sharma, A., Rajagopal, R., Adak, T., and Bhatnagar, R. K. (2009). Bacterial diversity analysis of larvae and adult midgut microflora using culture-dependent and culture-independent methods in lab-reared and field-collected *Anopheles stephensi*-an Asian malarial vector. *BMC Microbiol.* 9:96. doi: 10.1186/1471-2180-9-96
77. Rio, R. V., Hu, Y., and Aksoy, S. (2004). Strategies of the home-team: symbioses exploited for vector-borne disease control. *Trends Microbiol.* 12, 325–336. doi: 10.1016/j.tim.2004.05.001
78. Rio, R. V. M., Symula, R. E., Wang, J., Lohs, C., Wu, Y. N., Snyder, A. K., et al. (2012). Insight into the transmission biology and species-specific functional capabilities of tsetse (Diptera: Glossinidae) obligate symbiont Wigglesworthia. *MBio* 3, e00240–e00211. doi: 10.1128/mBio.00240-11
79. Rose, C., Belmonte, R., Armstrong, S. D., Molyneux, G., Haines, L. R., Lehane, M. J., et al. (2014). An investigation into the protein composition of the teneral *Glossina morsitans* morsitans peritrophic matrix. *PLoS Negl. Trop. Dis.* 8:e2691. doi: 10.1371/journal.pntd.0002691
80. Segata, N., Waldron, L., Ballarini, A., Narasimhan, V., Jousson, O., and Huttenhower, C. (2012). Metagenomic microbial community profiling using unique clade-specific marker genes. *Nat. Methods* 9, 811–814. doi: 10.1038/nmeth.2066
81. Shaw, A. P., Torr, S. J., Waiswa, C., Cecchi, G., Wint, G. R., Mattioli, R. C., et al. (2013). Estimating the costs of tsetse control options: an example for Uganda. *Prev. Vet. Med.* 110, 290–303. doi: 10.1016/j.prevetmed.2012.12.014
82. Sievers, F., Wilm, A., Dineen, D., Gibson, T. J., Karplus, K., Li, W., et al. (2011). Fast, scalable generation of high-quality protein multiple sequence alignments using Clustal Omega. *Mol. Syst. Biol.* 7:539. doi: 10.1038/msb. 2011.75
83. Simo, G., Njiokou, F., Mbida Mbida, J. A., Njitchouang, G. R., Herder, S., Asonganyi, T., et al. (2008). Tsetse fly host preference from sleeping sickness foci in Cameroon. Epidemiological implications. *Infect. Genet. Evol.* 8, 34–39. doi: 10.1016/j.meegid.2007.09.005
84. Solano, P., Salou, E., Rayaisse, J.-B., Ravel, S., Gimonneau, G., Traore, I., et al.

(2015). "Do tsetse flies only feed on blood?" *Infect. Genet. Evol.* 36, 184–189. doi: 10.1016/j.meegid.2015.09.016

85. Tchioffo, M. T., Boissière, A., Abate, L., Nsango, S. E., Bayibéki, A. N., Awono-Ambéné, P. H., et al. (2016). Dynamics of bacterial community composition in the malaria mosquito's Epithelia. *Front. Microbiol.* 6:1500. doi: 10.3389/fmicb.2015.01500
86. Tchouomene-Labou, J., Nana-Djeunga, H., Simo, G., Njitchouang, G. R., Cuny, G., Asonganyi, T., et al. (2014). Spatial and temporal variations relevant to tsetse control in the Bipindi focus of southern Cameroon. *Parasit. Vectors* 6:193. doi: 10.1186/1756-3305-6-193
87. Terenius, O., Lindh, J. M., Eriksson-Gonzales, K., Bussière, L., Laugen, A. T., Bergquist, H., et al. (2012). Midgut bacterial dynamics in *Aedes aegypti*. *FEMS Microbiol. Ecol.* 80, 556–565. doi: 10.1111/j.1574-6941.2012.01317.x
88. Vickerman, K., Tetley, L., Hendry, A., and Turner, C. M. (1988). Biology of African trypanosomes in the tsetse fly. *Biol. Cell* 64, 109–119. doi: 10.1016/0248-4900(88)90070-6
89. Wang, J., Wu, Y., Yang, G., and Aksoy, S. (2009). Interactions between mutualist Wigglesworthia and tsetse peptidoglycan recognition protein (PGRP- LB) influence trypanosome transmission. *Proc. Natl. Acad. Sci. U.S.A.* 106, 12133–12138. doi: 10.1073/pnas.0901226106
90. Weiss, B. L., Savage, A. F., Griffith, B. C., Wu, Y., and Aksoy, S. (2014). The peritrophic matrix mediates differential infection outcomes in the tsetse fly gut following challenge with commensal, pathogenic, and parasitic microbes. *J. Immunol.* 193, 773–782. doi: 10.4049/jimmunol.14 00163
91. Weiss, B. L., Wang, J., and Aksoy, S. (2011). Tsetse immune system maturation requires the presence of obligate symbionts in larvae. *PLoS Biol.* 9:e1000619. doi: 10.1371/journal.pbio.1000619
92. Weiss, B. L., Wang, J., Maltz, M. A., Wu, Y., and Aksoy, S. (2013). Trypanosome infection establishment in the tsetse fly gut is influenced by microbiome-regulated host immune barriers. *PLoS Pathog.* 9:e1003318. doi: 10.1371/journal.ppat.1003318
93. Welburn, S. C., and Maudlin, I. (2012). Priorities for the elimination of sleeping sickness. *Adv. Parasitol.* 79, 299–337. doi: 10.1016/B978-0-12-398457-9.00004-4
94. Welburn, S. C., Maudlin, I., and Molyneux, D. H. (1994). Midgut lectin activity and sugar specificity in teneral and fed tsetse. *Med. Vet. Entomol.* 8, 81–87. doi: 10.1111/j.1365-2915.1994.tb00391.x
95. Zélé, F., Nicot, A., Berthomieu, A., Weill, M., Duron, O., and Rivero, A. (2014). Wolbachia increases susceptibility to Plasmodium infection in a natural system. *Proc. Biol. Sci.* 281:20132837. doi: 10.1098/rspb.2013.2837
96. Zhang, J., Kobert, K., Flouri, T., and Stamatakis, A. (2014). PEAR: a fast and accurate Illumina Paired-End reAd mergeR. *Bioinformatics* 30, 614–620. doi: 10.1093/bioinformatics/btt593
97. Zouache, K., Raharimalala, F. N., Raquin, V., Tran-Van, V., Raveloson,
98. L. H., Ravelonandro, P., et al. (2011). Bacterial diversity of field-caught mosquitoes, *Aedes albopictus* and *Aedes aegypti*, from different geographic regions of Madagascar. *FEMS Microbiol. Ecol.* 75, 377–389. doi: 10.1111/j.1574-6941.2010.01012.x

18

Transcriptional Profiling of Midguts Prepared from *Trypanosoma/T. congolense*-Positive *Glossina palpalis palpalis* Collected from Two Distinct Cameroonian Foci: Coordinated Signatures of the Midguts' Remodeling as *T. congolense*-Supportive Niches

*Jean M. Tsagmo Ngoune[1,2], Flobert Njiokou[1], Béatrice Loriod[3], Ginette Kame-Ngasse[1], Nicolas Fernandez-Nunez[3], Claire Rioualen[3], Jacques van Helden[3] and Anne Geiger[2]**

[1] Faculty of Science, University of Yaoundé I, Yaoundé, Cameroon, [2] UMR 177, IRD-CIRAD, CIRAD TA A-17/G, Campus International de Baillarguet, Montpellier, France, [3] Aix-Marseille University, INSERM, TAGC, Technological Advances for Genomics and Clinics, UMR S 1090, Marseille, France

***Correspondence:**
Anne Geiger
anne.geiger@ird.fr

Our previous transcriptomic analysis of *Glossina palpalis gambiensis* experimentally infected or not with *Trypanosoma brucei gambiense* aimed to detect differentially expressed genes (DEGs) associated with infection. Specifically, we selected candidate genes governing tsetse fly vector competence that could be used in the context of an anti-vector strategy, to control human and/or animal trypanosomiasis. The present study aimed to verify whether gene expression in field tsetse flies (*G. p. palpalis*) is modified in response to natural infection by trypanosomes (*T. congolense*), as reported when insectary-raised flies (*G. p. gambiensis*) are experimentally infected with *T. b. gambiense*. This was achieved using the RNA-seq approach, which identified 524 DEGs in infected vs. non-infected tsetse flies, including 285 downregulated genes and 239 upregulated genes (identified using DESeq2). Several of these genes were highly differentially expressed, with log2 fold change values in the vicinity of either +40 or −40. Downregulated genes were primarily involved in transcription/translation processes, whereas encoded upregulated genes governed amino acid and nucleotide biosynthesis pathways. The BioCyc metabolic pathways associated with infection also revealed that downregulated genes were mainly involved in fly immunity processes. Importantly, our study demonstrates that data on the molecular cross-talk between the host and the parasite (as well as the always present fly microbiome) recorded from an experimental biological model has a counterpart in field flies, which in turn validates the use of experimental host/parasite couples.

Keywords: field tsetse fly, Cameroonian foci, RNAseq, vector control, trypanosomiasis

INTRODUCTION

Human African trypanosomiasis [HAT or sleeping sickness; (1)] and animal African trypanosomiasis [AAT or nagana; (2)] are two vector-borne diseases that inflict heavy social and economic burdens on sub-Saharan African populations. Although the number of newly diagnosed HAT cases is decreasing (<10,000 per year) (3), more than 60 million people living in endemic areas are at risk of infection (4). In addition, AAT causes a large amount of livestock loss, which has been estimated as high as US$ 4.5 billion per year (5). HAT is due to either *Trypanosoma brucei gambiense* (Tbg; the chronic form of the disease in West and Central Africa) or *T. b. rhodesiense* (the acute form of the disease in East Africa), which are, respectively, transmitted by *Glossina palpalis* and *G. morsitans*. In contrast, AAT is caused by *T. b. brucei*, *T. congolense* (Tc; the forest or savannah type), or *T. vivax*, and is transmitted by *G. palpalis* or *G. morsitans*.

Despite differences between Tc and Tbg [reviewed in Ref. (6)], the parasites share several important characteristics. In particular, they are digenetic, meaning that they need to successively infect two different hosts to achieve their life cycle. One of these hosts, a *Glossina* fly, is the vector, whereas the other host is a vertebrate, typically a mammal. These parasites must accomplish a crucial part of their life cycle within their vector, namely their multiplication and maturation into the infectious form that can be transmitted to the vertebrate host while the tsetse fly ingests its blood meal. More specifically, Tc and Tbg undergo sequential differentiations after their ingestion by the fly, from the ingested blood stream form to the vertebrate-infective metacyclic form. The latter differentiation occurs either in the proboscis (for Tc) or in the salivary glands (for Tbg) (7), which is the basis for their respective classification into two different subgenera, *Nannomonas* and *Trypanozoon* (8). They also share the ability to excrete/secrete a number of proteins, some of which are considered to be involved in their establishment in the tsetse midgut and/or in the pathogenic process developed within the vertebrate host (9–12). Finally, the establishment of both Tc and Tbg in the *G. palpalis* vector is reported to be favored by *Sodalis glossinidius*, the secondary symbiont inhabitant of the tsetse gut (13). This finding demonstrates the occurrence in naturally infected field tsetse flies of a tripartite interaction (fly/trypanosome/gut bacteria) already reported to occur in experimentally infected insectary flies (14–18).

Another similarity between the parasites is that their mantle, which consists of a variant surface glycoprotein, allows them to evade the host's immune system by means of antigenic variations (19–21), thus rendering ineffective any vaccine approaches to fight HAT or AAT. Nevertheless, progress has been made in rapid diagnosis (22) and therapy that uses a nifurtimox–elfornitine combination in the treatment of the second phase of HAT (23). Furthermore, besides the use of trypanocidal drugs, the incidence of AAT can be lowered by introducing trypanotolerant cattle into AAT-infected area or through the antibody-mediated inhibition of trypanosome-secreted proteins involved in the parasite pathogenic process (24, 25).

Another approach to fight HAT or AAT is by vector control. Diverse strategies are available, including the application of pesticides, the use of sterile males, and the development of paratransgenic approaches (26–32).

The normal status of tsetse flies is considered to be refractory to trypanosome infection, given that artificial or natural infection rates are always low (28, 33–36). Recently, a global transcriptomic analysis was performed (15–17) in the context of an anti-vector strategy, aimed at deciphering the molecular cross-talk occurring between the different participants involved in tsetse infection: the fly, the trypanosome, and the fly gut bacteria, especially the primary (*Wigglesworthia glossinidia*) and secondary (*S. glossinidius*) symbionts. The authors also focused on identifying differentially expressed genes (DEGs) associated with fly susceptibility or refractoriness as a result of fly infection by the trypanosome. These investigations were performed on insectary-raised *G. p. gambiensis* (Gpg) flies that were artificially infected (or not) by Tbg. This study raised the question of whether the results recorded under these experimental conditions could be transposed to what actually occurs under natural conditions in HAT and AAT foci.

To address this question we have conducted similar transcriptomic analyses on *G. p. palpalis* (Gpp) flies infected or not with Tc, collected in two HAT foci in southern Cameroon. Our experimental design involved a different host vector/parasite couple (Gpp/Tc) from what was used in the previous insectary-raised approach. However, as shown above and in support of this approach, several notable characteristics are shared between the Gpp/Tc couple and the previously used Gpg/Tbg couple, including life cycle, sequential differentiation within the vector, transmission modalities, host immune response escape, and pathological effects on susceptible vertebrate hosts, among others. Thus, the objectives of this study were to determine whether or not field-collected tsetse flies react to trypanosome infection under natural conditions similar to insectary flies under experimental conditions, and whether or not Tc induces molecular disruptions in Gpp similar to those provoked by Tbg in Gpg. Importantly, our approach provides novel evidence that validates the use of experimental host/parasite couples in the context of investigating anti-vector strategies.

MATERIALS AND METHODS

Sampling Areas

Tsetse flies were sampled in May and June 2015 in two active HAT foci (Campo and Bipindi), located in the Ocean Division of the southern region of Cameroon. The Campo focus (2°20′N, 9°52′E) is located on the Atlantic coast and extends along the Ntem river. The HAT National Control Program that visits Campo once per year diagnosed 61 novel HAT cases between 2001 and 2011. The passive identification of two cases in 2012 (37) indicates that HAT is still present. The Bipindi focus (3°2′N, 10°22′E) has a typical forest bioecological environment, including equatorial forest and farmland along roads and around villages. This focus has been recognized since 1920 (38) and includes several villages. Sleeping sickness is still present, since approximately 83 HAT cases were identified by the National Control Program in this focus between 1998 and 2011 (Ebo'o Eyenga, personal communication). In addition to HAT cases that involve *G. palpalis* and Tbg, regular global surveys have identified the presence of several other *Glossina* (including Gpp) and *Trypanosoma* species (including Tc) in both foci. Surveys have also identified a variety of domestic and wild animals that serve as reservoirs for diverse *Trypanosoma* species (39–42). As described below, flies were trapped in these areas in order to select non-infected and Tc-infected individuals.

Fly Sampling, Dissection, and Subsequent RNA Preservation

The May 2015 tsetse fly trapping campaign was conducted in three Campo villages (Ipono, Mabiogo, and Campo-Beach), and the June 2015 campaign was conducted in three Bipindi villages (Lambi, Bidjouka, and Ebiminbang). The geographical positions of the sampling sites were determined by GPS. Tsetse flies were captured using pyramidal traps (43) placed in suitable tsetse fly biotopes. Each trap was installed for four consecutive days, and the flies were collected twice per day.

Prior to handling samples, work stations and dissecting instruments were cleaned with RNase away (Ambion) in order to eliminate any RNases that could degrade sample RNA. Furthermore, tsetse flies were dissected alive to prevent RNA degradation by normal *post mortem* degradation processes. The first step in sample processing consisted in identifying the collected tsetse flies to the species level on the basis of morphological criteria and adapted taxonomic keys (44). Next, the samples were separated into two groups of teneral and non-teneral flies. The non-teneral Gpp flies were dissected in a drop of sterile 0.9% saline solution, according to the midgut dissection protocol developed by Penchenier and Itard (45). The organs were immediately transferred to tubes containing RNAlater (Ambion) for DNA and RNA extraction. These samples were then used for parasite identification by specific PCR amplification, and ultimately for transcriptomic analysis. All tools were carefully cleaned after the dissection of each fly to prevent cross-contamination. During field manipulations, the tubes containing the organs were stored at −20°C for 5 days; subsequently, they were stored in the laboratory at −80°C until use.

DNA and RNA Extraction

To prepare for extraction, samples stored at −80°C were thawed and RNAlater was removed. The midguts were treated with the NucleoSpin TriPrep extraction kit (Macherey-Nagel) according to the manufacturer's instructions, which allow the separate extraction of DNA and RNA. RNase free water (40 µl) was added to elute the RNA, and 100 µl of DNA elute solution was added to recover the DNA. RNA quality and the absence of any DNA contamination were checked on an Agilent RNA 6000 Bioanalyzer and quantified using the Agilent RNA 6000 Nano kit (Agilent Technologies, France).

PCR Amplification

To identify which trypanosome species had infected the sampled tsetse flies, the isolated DNA samples stored at −80°C were thawed and used as a template for PCR amplification with specific primers (**Table 1**). PCR amplification of parasites was performed as described by Herder et al. (46) and consisted of a denaturing step at 94°C (5 min) followed by 44 amplification cycles, each comprising a denaturing step at 94°C (30 s), annealing at 55°C (30 s), and an extension step at 72°C (1 min). A final extension was performed at 72°C for 10 min. The amplified products were separated on a 2% agarose gel containing ethidium bromide and visualized under UV illumination. Positive (2 ng of reference DNA) and negative controls were included in each PCR amplification experiment. PCR amplifications that gave a positive result were repeated once for confirmation.

RNA-Seq Processing

Preparation of cDNA Libraries

Total RNA from 10 Gpp flies (5 non-infected flies and 5 flies infected by Tc s.l.) was assayed using the TruSeq mRNA-seq Stranded v2 Kit (Illumina), according to the manufacturer's instructions. Briefly, 4 µg of total RNA were used for poly(A)-selection to generate 120–210 bp cDNA fragments (mean size: 155 bp) after an 8-min elution-fragmentation incubation. Each library was barcoded using TruSeq Single Index (Illumina), according to the manufacturer's instructions. After library preparation, Agencourt AMPure XP (Beckman Coulter, Inc.) was used to select 200- to 400-bp size libraries. Each library size distribution was examined using the Bioanalyzer with a High Sensitivity DNA chip (Agilent) to ensure that the samples had the proper size and that they were devoid of any adaptor contamination. The sample concentration was quantified on Qubit with the Qubit® dsDNA HS Assay Kit (Life Technologies). Each library was then diluted to 4 nM and pooled at an equimolar ratio.

NextSeq-500 Sequencing

For sequencing, 5 µL of pooled libraries (4 nM) were denatured with 5 µl NaOH (0.2 N) according to the manufacturer's instructions. Following a 5-min incubation, 5 µl of Tris–HCl (200 mM; pH 7) were added, and 20 pM of the pooled libraries were diluted with HT1 to a 1.6-pM final concentration. As a sequencing

TABLE 1 | Primers used for PCR amplification of trypanosomes.

Species	Primer sequence	Amplified product (bp)	Reference
T. brucei s.l.	5′-CGAATGAATATTAAACAATGCGCAG-3′ 5′-AGAACCATTTATTAGCTTTGTTGC-3′	164	Masiga et al. (47)
T. congolense ("forest" type)	5′-CGAATGAATATTAAACAATGCGCAG-3′ 5′-AGAACCATTTATTAGCTTTGTTGC-3′	350	Masiga et al. (47)
T. congolense ("savannah" type)	5′-CGAATGAATATTAAACAATGCGCAG-3′ 5′-AGAACCATTTATTAGCTTTGTTGC-3′	341	Moser et al. (48)

T, Trypanosoma; s.l., sensu lato.

control, a PhiX library was denatured and diluted according to the manufacturer's instructions, and 1.2 µl were added to the sample of denatured and diluted pooled libraries before loading. Finally, the libraries were sequenced on a high-output flow cell (400M clusters) using the NextSeq® 500/550 High Output Kit v2 (150 cycles; Illumina) in paired-end 75/75 nt mode, according to the manufacturer's instructions.

Datasets for the reads are available from the NCBI, GEO submission, accession number GSE98989.

Bioinformatics Analysis

Workflow

The successive tasks of the bioinformatics analysis were managed using a Snakemake workflow (49). This workflow enables the reproduction of all analyses from the raw read files and is available from the supporting Web site.[1]

Reference Genomes

The *G. palpalis* genomic sequences (Glossina-palpalis-IAEA_SCAFFOLDS_GpapI1.fa) and annotations (Glossina-palpalis-IAEA_BASEFEATURES_GpapI1.1.gff3) were downloaded from VectorBase (50). For the annotation of Tc genes, the reference genome (TriTrypDB-9.0_TcongolenseIL3000.gff) was downloaded from TriTrypDB (51), whereas the *Drosophila melanogaster* reference genome (Drosophila_melanogaster.BDGP6.30.gff3) was downloaded from Flybase (52).

Lane Merging

Since each sample was sequenced on four lanes, the original fastq-formatted read files were merged to produce two files per sample (one for each paired-end extremity).

Read Quality Control

FastQC[2] was run on the raw reads in order to check their quality.

Read Mapping

Raw reads were mapped onto the genome with the local alignment algorithm Subread-align (53) in paired-ends mode with at most 10 mismatches. Read mapping statistics were computed using samtools flagstats (54) and are summarized in Table S1 in Supplementary Material.

Read Counts per Gene

The number of read pairs (fragments) per gene was counted using the featureCounts tool from the Subread package (55), including the option "feature type" to only count reads overlapping transcripts.

Visualization

Genome maps were generated using the Integrative Genomic Viewer (56).

[1]https://github.com/rioualen/gene-regulation.
[2]http://www.bioinformatics.babraham.ac.uk/projects/fastqc/.

Detection of DEGs

Differential gene expression analysis was performed using the SARTools R package (57), which separately runs DESeq2 (58) and egdeR (59) as well as generates readable reports.

Identification of Orthologs between Gpp and *D. melanogaster*

Because the *G. palpalis* genome is inadequately assembled and annotated, our functional interpretation of the DEGs relied on a comparative genomics approach. This was based on the identification of bidirectional best hits (BBH) between all sequences of *G. palpalis* and *D. melanogaster* (assembly BDGP6). BBH were identified using blastp (60) and the BLOSUM45 substitution matrix, and by setting a threshold of 10^{-5} on the expected score.

Functional Enrichment of DEGs

Identification of functions associated with the DEGs was based on *Drosophila* orthologs of the DEGs (ortho-DEG). Functional enrichment was separately performed using the DAVID (61) and g:Profiler (62) tools. The Bonferroni correction was used to obtain the enrichments of these functions, with a threshold set at 10^{-3}.

Pathway Mapping of DEGs

Drosophila orthologs of the DEGs were loaded into the metabolic cellular overview of BioCyc (63) in order to highlight the pathways affected by the infection.

Statistical Treatment of Entomological Data

Entomological data, as well as all other calculations, were evaluated using the statistical package SPSS version 2.0. Spreadsheets were made using Microsoft Office Excel 2007.

RESULTS

Entomological Data

A total of 1,991 tsetse flies were collected during the entomological survey (775 flies from Campo and 1,216 flies from Bipindi). The Campo fly population was composed of Gpp (95.61%), *Glossina caliginea* (2.06%), *Glossina palicera* (1.87%), and *Glossina nigrofusca* (0.52%). Two tsetse fly species were identified at the Bipindi focus: Gpp (99.34%) and *G. palicera* (0.66%). The mean apparent density was 4.24 flies per trap per day; however, this parameter was highly variable between the different villages and was higher in Bipindi (8.1) than in Campo (3.52) (**Table 2**). The frequency of teneral flies was typically low in both Bipindi (0.08%) and Campo (1.16%). These data are roughly in line with data recorded in 2007/2008 (13), although the rate of teneral flies was much lower in the present study. Only 1,245 of the trapped 1,991 tsetse flies were dissected, since 10 flies were teneral and 736 flies were desiccated.

PCR Identification of Trypanosome Species in the Tsetse Midgut

The number of flies carrying single or mixed trypanosome infections is presented in **Table 3**. Of the 337 Campo flies analyzed, 25 (7.41%) were infected by the Tc "forest" type, 16 (4.74%) by the

TABLE 2 | Entomological field data from the Bipindi and Campo foci.

Focus	Village	Number of traps	Number of tsetse flies captured	ADT	Number of teneral tsetse flies (%)	Number of tsetse flies dissected
Campo	Ipono	15	161	2.68	4 (2.48)	110
	Beach	15	341	4.55	3 (0.87)	264
	Mabiogo	18	273	3.21	2 (0.73)	228
	Total Campo	48	775	3.52	9 (1.16)	602
Bipindi	Bidjouka	23	608	5.28	1 (0.16)	278
	Lambi	12	486	8.1	0 (0)	303
	Ebimimbang	15	122	1.74	0 (0)	72
	Total Bipindi	50	1,216	4.96	1 (0.50)	653
Total		98	1,991	4.24	10 (0.50)	1,255

ADT, apparent density per trap per day.

TABLE 3 | Number of *Trypanosoma congolense* s.l. simple and mixed infections by village.

Focus	Village	Number of tsetse flies analyzed	Number of flies infected with TcF	Number of flies infected with TcS	Number of flies carrying a mixed infection
Campo	Ipono	63	2	1	1
	Beach	170	15	8	7
	Mabiogo	104	8	7	6
	Total Campo	337	25	16	14
Bipindi	Bidjouka	40	1	0	0
	Lambi	33	5	0	0
	Ebimimbang	11	1	0	0
	Total Bipindi	84	7	0	0
Total		421	32	16	14

TcF, T. congolense "forest" type; TcS, T. congolense "savannah" type.

Tc "savanah" type, and 14 (4.15%) by both parasites. In contrast, Bipindi flies only carried the Tc "forest" type (8.33%). Table S1 in Supplementary Material details the characteristics of the different samples including those used for transcriptomic analyses.

Raw Data

The sequencing of libraries produced a total of 400 million reads (theoretically 40 million reads per sample), which represent a satisfactory sequencing depth for subsequent differential gene expression analysis (**Figure 1**). Out of the 328 raw clusters generated, 77.6% were successfully filtered, with each sample producing 50–72 million clusters (mean: 61 million clusters) (**Figure 1**). Sequencing also revealed a total of 31,320 contigs distributed in 3,926 scaffolds with a mean size of 96,817 bp (varying in size from 545 bp to 3.6 Mb).

Mapping on Gpp

RNA-seq sequencing produced an average of 124 million reads per sample. From this, 111.45 million reads (83.6%) were mapped onto the genome of Gpp, 103.68 M (73.7%) of which were properly paired (**Table 4**).

Mapping on Tc

Reads were also mapped onto the trypanosome genome in order to validate the infection status of the samples, as well as to investigate the role played by the trypanosome in this molecular dialog. Since trypanosome cells represented a small fraction of the analyzed material, only a smaller fraction of the reads could be mapped. Specifically, 300,302.5 (0.24%) reads were mapped from an average of 124 million reads per sample. This resulted in 137,305.4 (0.11%) properly paired reads and 157,712.5 (0.12%) singletons (**Table 4**).

DEGs between Infected and Non-Infected Flies

We used DESeq2 (**Table 5**) to detect genes that were differentially expressed between the five infected and five non-infected samples. When a Benjamini–Hochberg corrected p-value lower than 0.05 was applied, 524 genes were observed to be significantly differentially expressed in infected vs. non-infected flies, among which 285 genes were downregulated and 239 were upregulated. A similar DEG analysis was performed using edgeR (**Table 5**), which identified only 20 downregulated genes and 53 upregulated genes. **Figure 2** presents the volcano plots produced by DESeq2 (**Figure 2A**) and edgeR (**Figure 2B**); genes that were significantly (p-value <0.05) differentially expressed and with a fold change of log2 (fold change) >2 (i.e., upregulated genes) or log2 (fold change) <−2 (i.e., downregulated genes) were considered relevant.

Functional Annotation

To understand the roles of DEGs associated with tsetse fly infection by Tc, identifiers of the *Drosophila* orthologs of the *Glossina* DEGs were examined using the DAVID-functional enrichment tool. Separately, we analyzed the 290 downregulated and 213 upregulated genes reported by DESeq2 and identified 207 *Drosophila* best hits (121 downregulated and 86 upregulated genes). The same analysis by edgeR only resulted in 25 DEG orthologs (6 downregulated and 19 upregulated genes). This reduced number of orthologs could possibly be due to the incomplete assembly and annotation of the *Glossina* genome and/or the high stringency of the BBH criterion (which discards the case where several tsetse fly proteins have the same closest hit in *Drosophila*). These DEGs were examined using DAVID, which compares the list of input genes with a variety of functional annotations. This analysis was focused on the three primary categories of the Gene

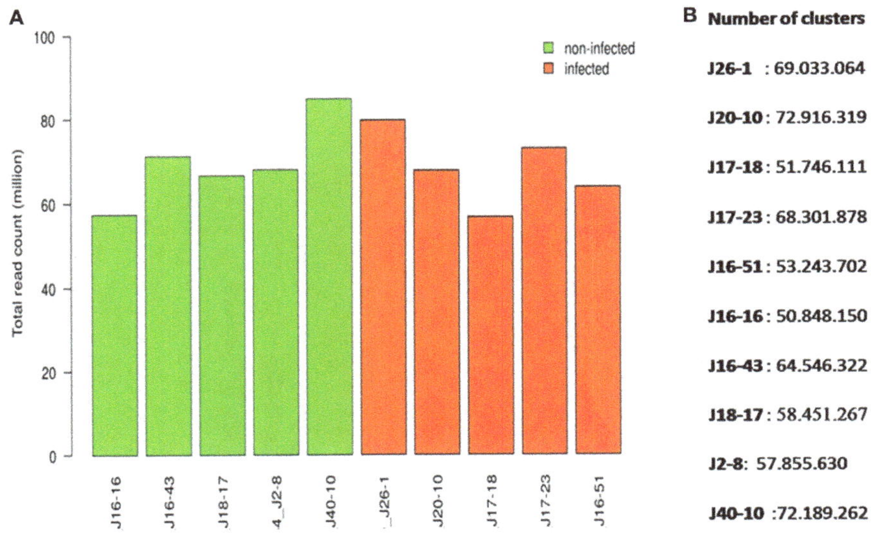

FIGURE 1 | The score quality of different sequences of clusters, presented base by base. Green indicates a good quality. **(A)** Total read count per sample (millions). **(B)** Number of clusters per sample.

TABLE 4 | Read mapping statistics.

Mapping on	Mapped reads (%)	Properly paired reads (%)	Singleton reads (%)	QC-passed reads
Glossina	111.45 M (89.87)	103.68 M (83.61)	3.62 M (2.92)	123.8 M
Trypanosoma	0.3 M (0.24)	0.13 M (0.11)	0.15 M (0.12)	123.8 M

M, millions of reads.

TABLE 5 | Differentially expressed genes.

	Downregulated	Upregulated	Total
DESeq2	285	239	524
edgeR	20	53	73
Common	20	46	66
Total	285	246	531

Ontology annotation: biological process (BP), molecular function (MF), and cellular component (CC). The list of different features is provided in **Table 6**.

The 285 downregulated genes identified by DESeq2 in flies infected with Tc mainly belonged to the BP category, in which the major functional classes were RNA processing (58 genes; 23.48%), ribosome biogenesis (24 genes; 9.71%), and translation (13 genes; 5.26%); the other genes corresponded to several poorly represented classes. The MF category included the functional RNA binding classes (20 genes; 8.09%) and catalytic activity (25 genes; 10.12%). Finally, the CC category included the intracellular lumen (48 genes; 19.43%), non-membrane-bound organelle (34 genes; 13.75%), and ribonucleoprotein complex (25 genes; 10.12%) functional classes (**Figure 3**).

In addition, 239 DEGs were overexpressed in Tc-infected tsetse flies. These DEGs encoded proteins corresponding to the same three primary ontology categories. The BP category include the neuron morphogenesis functional class (83 genes; 38.96%), amino acid biosynthesis (24 genes; 11.26%), and carboxylic acid biosynthesis (10 genes; 4.7%). The MF category included the iron binding (64 genes, 30%) and catalytic activity (24 genes; 11.26%) functional classes. Finally, the CC category only included the mitochondrion functional class (8 genes; 3.75%).

As already shown for DEGs, edgeR provides a much lower number of functional annotations than DESeq2. Here, using edgeR, fly genes that displayed an increased expression in response to Tc infection were found to belong to the MF category, with only three functional classes: phospholipase activity (2 genes; 10.5%), lipase activity (2 genes; 10.5%), and carboxylesterase activity (2 genes; 10.5%). Finally, expression was decreased for only two genes belonging to the one-carbon metabolic process term (BP category).

Functional Enrichment of DEGs

To make our analysis more focused and efficient, a functional enrichment was performed to refine the list of tsetse fly DEGs in which expression was influenced by Tc infection. We therefore combined fold enrichment and the *p*-value at a 5% threshold, which allowed applying a Bonferroni correction to eliminate false positives. The Bonferroni correction threshold was fixed at $\alpha = 10^{-2}$, and all functionality with a Bonferroni value below this threshold was considered to be due to trypanosome infection.

Following this correction, 16 functional classes were found to be selectively altered by trypanosome infection. These classes are mainly involved in the transcription process, including (a) RNA related processes (rRNA processing, rRNA metabolic process, ncRNA processing, ncRNA metabolic processes, and RNA processing), involving 63 DEGs; (b) monitoring processes related to the synthesis of the ribonucleoprotein complex (ribonucleoprotein complex biogenesis and ribonucleoprotein

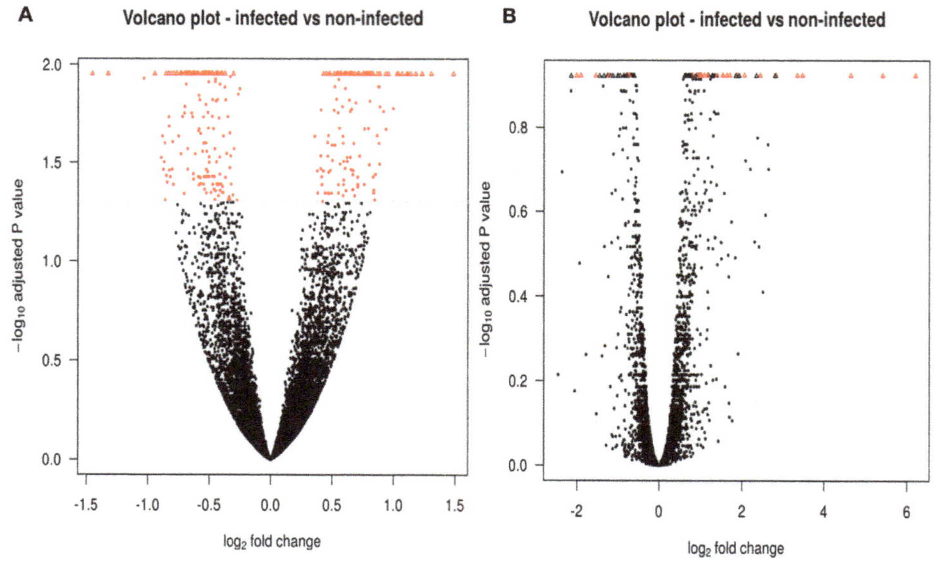

FIGURE 2 | Comparisons of significantly differentially expressed genes. DESeq2 **(A)** and edgeR **(B)** results are illustrated by volcano plots, in which the differentially expressed features are shown in red. Upregulated genes are thus observed as positive values, and downregulated genes as negative values. Triangles correspond to features where the log of the adjusted *p*-value is too low or too high to be displayed on the plot.

complex), involving 29 DEGs; (c) RNA binding, involving 24 DEGs; (d) nucleolus biogenesis (nucleolus and nuclear lumen), involving 23 DEGs; (e) ribosome synthesis, involving 17 DEGs; and (f) eukaryotic translation factor 3 complex, involving 4 DEGs. In contrast to the transcription process, which involved 160 DEGs, the BPs of organic acid synthesis (amine biosynthetic process, cellular amino acid biosynthetic process, carboxylic acid biosynthetic process, and organic acid biosynthetic process) that were found to be activated by trypanosome infection only involved 21 DEGs (**Table 7**).

Associated Metabolic Pathways

The BioCyc metabolic map (**Figure 4**) and **Table 8** illustrate the different pathways that the DEGs are involved in. Among these, the amino acid biosynthesis pathway (which includes the biosynthesis of L-glutamine, L-glutamate, L-serine, L-asparagine, L-aspartate, etc.) is controlled by genes that were shown to be overexpressed following trypanosome infection in the flies. Similarly, DEGs associated with the nucleotide biosynthesis pathway were overexpressed following trypanosome infection, especially uridine monophosphate, an RNA monomer. In contrast, genes involved in the pentose phosphate pathway, namely those implicated in the synthesis of D-ribose 5-phosphate, were downregulated. Phosphorylated pentose is converted by ribose phosphate diphosphokinase into phosphoribosylpyrophosphate, a precursor of nucleotide synthesis. Finally, regarding the carbohydrate biosynthesis pathway, we observed an overexpression of genes encoding malate dehydrogenase, which converts malate into pyruvate.

Interestingly, a large number of up- and downregulated DEGs were related to a given biosynthetic process meaning that upregulated DEGs encoding amino acids (such as tyrosine, serine, glutamine, and several others) were found in the amino acid synthesis pathway. Other overexpressed genes that were identified are involved in the biosynthesis of galactosyltransferase, *N*-acetylglucosamine, and beta-1,4-manosylglycolipide, which are all molecules that interact with the immune system of the tsetse fly (64–66). In contrast, genes involved in the biosynthesis of cytokines were downregulated in trypanosome-infected flies, as compared to non-infected flies. Similarly, genes involved in folate metabolism (e.g., the biosynthesis of formyltetrahydrofolate dehydrogenase), the main source of energy in flies, were downregulated.

Finally, DEGs involved in the transport of several molecules from the extracellular space toward the cytosol compartment were upregulated. This transport includes molecules with a role in cell nutrition, and nutrients such as lipids, but also ATP, succinate, and L-carnitine (which participates in the degradation of fats).

DISCUSSION

Understanding the mechanisms involved in tsetse fly susceptibility or refractoriness to trypanosome infection is crucial for developing a novel anti-vector based strategy to control the spread of sleeping sickness and nagana. One recent study was performed within this context to identify genes in Gpg associated with its susceptibility or refractoriness to Tbg infection, using an RNA-seq approach (17). The underlying hypothesis was that some of the genes involved in controlling fly susceptibility/resistance to trypanosome infection could be targeted in order to increase the refractoriness of the fly, thereby decreasing its vector competence while enabling the development of an anti-vector strategy against

TABLE 6 | Functional annotation of differentially expressed genes (DEGs).

Category	Term	Number of DEG	*p*-value	Log2 (fold enrichment)
DEGs identified with DESeq2				
GOTERM_BP_FAT	Amine biosynthetic process	6	2.80E−05	15.70
SP_PIR_KEYWORDS	Amino acid biosynthesis	3	2.00E−03	42.80
GOTERM_MF_FAT	ATPase activity, uncoupled	5	9.10E−02	−2.90
GOTERM_MF_FAT	ATP-dependent helicase activity	4	5.80E−02	−4.50
GOTERM_MF_FAT	ATP-dependent RNA helicase activity	4	1.10E−02	−8.40
GOTERM_BP_FAT	Axon guidance	6	2.90E−03	5.90
GOTERM_BP_FAT	Axonal defasciculation	2	8.70E−02	21.50
GOTERM_BP_FAT	Axonogenesis	6	1.20E−02	4.20
GOTERM_BP_FAT	Carboxylic acid biosynthetic process	5	9.90E−04	10.80
GOTERM_MF_FAT	Cation binding	18	6.10E−02	1.50
GOTERM_BP_FAT	Cell morphogenesis	7	8.10E−02	2.20
GOTERM_BP_FAT	Cell morphogenesis involved in differentiation	6	5.70E−02	2.80
GOTERM_BP_FAT	Cell morphogenesis involved in neuron differentiation	6	5.00E−02	2.90
GOTERM_BP_FAT	Cell motion	6	5.20E−02	2.90
GOTERM_BP_FAT	Cell part morphogenesis	6	7.60E−02	2.60
GOTERM_BP_FAT	Cell projection morphogenesis	6	7.20E−02	2.60
GOTERM_BP_FAT	Cell recognition	3	4.40E−02	8.70
GOTERM_BP_FAT	Cellular amino acid biosynthetic process	5	5.40E−05	22.40
GOTERM_BP_FAT	Chemical homeostasis	3	7.70E−02	6.30
GOTERM_MF_FAT	Coenzyme binding	4	6.40E−02	4.30
GOTERM_CC_FAT	Cytosol	6	9.30E−02	−2.40
INTERPRO	DEAD-like helicase, N-terminal	4	6.20E−02	−4.30
GOTERM_BP_FAT	Defasciculation of motor neuron axon	2	6.20E−02	30.70
SMART	DEXDc	4	4.30E−02	−4.90
GOTERM_BP_FAT	Di-, tri-valent inorganic cation transport	3	3.40E−02	10.10
INTERPRO	DNA/RNA helicase, C-terminal	4	6.20E−02	−4.30
INTERPRO	DNA/RNA helicase, DEAD/DEAH box type, N-terminal	4	1.60E−02	−7.40
GOTERM_MF_FAT	Electron carrier activity	5	2.50E−02	4.40
GOTERM_MF_FAT	Enzyme inhibitor activity	3	9.90E−02	5.50
GOTERM_CC_FAT	Eukaryotic translation initiation factor 3 complex	4	4.40E−04	−24.50
GOTERM_MF_FAT	Glutamate synthase activity	2	2.10E−02	93.60
GOTERM_BP_FAT	Glutamine family amino acid biosynthetic process	2	9.50E−02	19.60
GOTERM_BP_FAT	Glutamine family amino acid metabolic process	3	1.50E−02	15.40
GOTERM_BP_FAT	Glutamine metabolic process	2	6.20E−02	30.70
SP_PIR_KEYWORDS	Helicase	4	6.80E−02	−4.20
INTERPRO	Helicase, superfamily 1 and 2, ATP-binding	4	6.00E−02	−4.40
SMART	HELICc	4	4.30E−02	−4.90
SP_PIR_KEYWORDS	Heme	3	8.40E−02	6.10
GOTERM_MF_FAT	Heme binding	4	2.90E−02	5.90
GOTERM_BP_FAT	Homeostatic process	4	8.90E−02	3.70
SP_PIR_KEYWORDS	Hydrolase	14	6.20E−02	1.70
SP_PIR_KEYWORDS	Initiation factor	3	3.40E−02	−10.10
GOTERM_CC_FAT	Intracellular non-membrane-bounded organelle	17	3.60E−03	−2.00
GOTERM_CC_FAT	Intracellular organelle lumen	12	1.00E−02	−2.30
GOTERM_MF_FAT	Ion binding	18	6.40E−02	1.50
GOTERM_MF_FAT	Iron ion binding	6	1.10E−02	4.30
KEGG_PATHWAY	Limonene and pinene degradation	3	6.60E−02	6.60
GOTERM_MF_FAT	Lipase activity	3	9.30E−02	5.70
SP_PIR_KEYWORDS	Lipid-binding	2	4.80E−02	39.90
GOTERM_CC_FAT	Membrane-enclosed lumen	12	1.20E−02	−2.20
GOTERM_MF_FAT	Metal ion binding	18	5.10E−02	1.50
INTERPRO	Mitochondrial substrate carrier	3	3.10E−02	10.60
INTERPRO	Mitochondrial substrate/solute carrier	3	3.30E−02	10.20
GOTERM_CC_FAT	Mitochondrion	8	6.00E−02	2.10
GOTERM_BP_FAT	Mitotic spindle elongation	4	6.50E−02	−4.20
GOTERM_MF_FAT	mRNA binding	6	3.70E−02	−3.20
GOTERM_BP_FAT	ncRNA metabolic process	12	3.10E−07	−7.50
GOTERM_BP_FAT	ncRNA processing	12	6.00E−09	−10.80
GOTERM_BP_FAT	Neuron development	6	9.30E−02	2.40
GOTERM_BP_FAT	Neuron projection development	6	5.00E−02	2.90
GOTERM_BP_FAT	Neuron projection morphogenesis	6	4.90E−02	2.90
GOTERM_BP_FAT	Neuron recognition	3	4.40E−02	8.70
GOTERM_BP_FAT	Nitrogen compound biosynthetic process	6	1.10E−02	4.20

(Continued)

TABLE 6 | Continued

Category	Term	Number of DEG	*p*-value	Log2 (fold enrichment)
GOTERM_CC_FAT	Non-membrane-bounded organelle	17	3.60E−03	−2.00
GOTERM_CC_FAT	Nuclear lumen	12	4.10E−04	−3.30
GOTERM_CC_FAT	Nucleolus	11	2.20E−09	−13.50
SP_PIR_KEYWORDS	Nucleus	18	1.90E−02	−1.80
GOTERM_CC_FAT	Organelle lumen	12	1.00E−02	−2.30
GOTERM_BP_FAT	Organic acid biosynthetic process	5	9.90E−04	10.80
GOTERM_BP_FAT	Oxidation reduction	8	3.10E−02	2.50
GOTERM_MF_FAT	Phospholipase activity	3	3.60E−02	9.70
SP_PIR_KEYWORDS	Phosphoprotein	16	4.90E−02	−1.70
GOTERM_BP_FAT	Positive regulation of protein kinase cascade	2	8.50E−02	−22.30
GOTERM_CC_FAT	Preribosome	3	3.40E−03	−31.50
SP_PIR_KEYWORDS	Protein biosynthesis	5	1.70E−02	−5.00
GOTERM_BP_FAT	Pseudouridine synthesis	2	9.90E−02	−19.10
GOTERM_MF_FAT	Purine NTP-dependent helicase activity	4	5.80E−02	−4.50
GOTERM_BP_FAT	Regulation of translational initiation	3	1.10E−02	−18.20
SP_PIR_KEYWORDS	Ribonucleoprotein	6	1.30E−02	−4.20
GOTERM_CC_FAT	Ribonucleoprotein complex	13	6.50E−05	−3.70
GOTERM_BP_FAT	Ribonucleoprotein complex biogenesis	12	2.80E−09	−11.60
GOTERM_BP_FAT	Ribosome biogenesis	12	7.10E−11	−16.00
SP_PIR_KEYWORDS	Ribosome biogenesis	5	1.20E−04	−18.60
GOTERM_MF_FAT	RNA binding	14	9.00E−05	−3.60
GOTERM_MF_FAT	RNA helicase activity	4	1.50E−02	−7.50
INTERPRO	RNA helicase, ATP-dependent, DEAD-box, conserved site	3	4.20E−02	−9.00
INTERPRO	RNA helicase, DEAD-box type, Q motif	4	6.50E−03	−10.20
GOTERM_BP_FAT	RNA modification	3	7.10E−02	−6.70
GOTERM_BP_FAT	RNA processing	14	1.40E−05	−4.30
SP_PIR_KEYWORDS	RNA-binding	10	2.20E−05	−6.40
GOTERM_MF_FAT	RNA-dependent ATPase activity	4	1.10E−02	−8.40
GOTERM_BP_FAT	rRNA metabolic process	10	2.10E−10	−22.30
GOTERM_BP_FAT	rRNA modification	2	9.90E−02	−19.10
GOTERM_BP_FAT	rRNA processing	10	2.10E−10	−22.30
SP_PIR_KEYWORDS	rRNA processing	5	1.50E−04	−17.70
COG_ONTOLOGY	Secondary metabolites biosynthesis, transport, and catabolism	3	3.40E−02	8.60
GOTERM_CC_FAT	Small nuclear ribonucleoprotein complex	4	1.80E−02	−6.80
GOTERM_CC_FAT	Small nucleolar ribonucleoprotein complex	4	4.20E−05	−49.00
GOTERM_CC_FAT	Small-subunit processome	3	1.70E−03	−44.10
GOTERM_BP_FAT	Spindle elongation	4	6.70E−02	−4.20
GOTERM_MF_FAT	Tetrapyrrole binding	4	2.90E−02	5.90
GOTERM_BP_FAT	Translation	9	2.10E−02	−2.60
GOTERM_BP_FAT	Translational initiation	4	1.80E−02	−7.00
SP_PIR_KEYWORDS	Transport	7	5.60E−02	2.50
SP_PIR_KEYWORDS	WD repeat	7	1.00E−02	−3.80
SMART	WD40	7	8.30E−03	−3.80
INTERPRO	WD40 repeat	7	1.80E−02	−3.30
INTERPRO	WD40 repeat, conserved site	5	5.30E−02	−3.50
INTERPRO	WD40 repeat, region	6	2.60E−02	−3.60
INTERPRO	WD40 repeat, subgroup	7	7.80E−03	−4.00
INTERPRO	WD40/YVTN repeat-like	8	5.90E−03	−3.60
DEGs identified with DESeq2				
GOTERM_BP_FAT	One-carbon metabolic process	2	6.00E−02	−27.2
GOTERM_MF_FAT	Carboxylesterase activity	2	8.40E−02	20.4
GOTERM_MF_FAT	Lipase activity	2	7.90E−02	21.7
GOTERM_MF_FAT	Phospholipase activity	2	4.80E−02	36.6

Categories: GOTERM_BP_FAT, biological process; GOTERM_CC_FAT, cellular component; GOTERM_MF_FAT, molecular function.
SMART & INTERPRO, protein domains; SPIR_KEYWORD, protein information resource provided by SWISSPROT and UniProt.
CDG_ONTOLOGY, cluster orthology group.
Black fonts: downregulated DEGs; red fonts: upregulated DEGs.

the disease. As this analysis was performed with insectary flies artificially infected with trypanosomes, it was necessary to verify that similar molecular events occur in field flies naturally infected by trypanosome vs. non-infected flies. To accomplish this, we have chosen the Gpp/Tc couple, whose prevalence (even in HAT foci) is often higher than observed with the Gpp/Tbg couple.

As in the previous study (17), we employed an RNA-seq approach. This provided satisfactory results regarding the

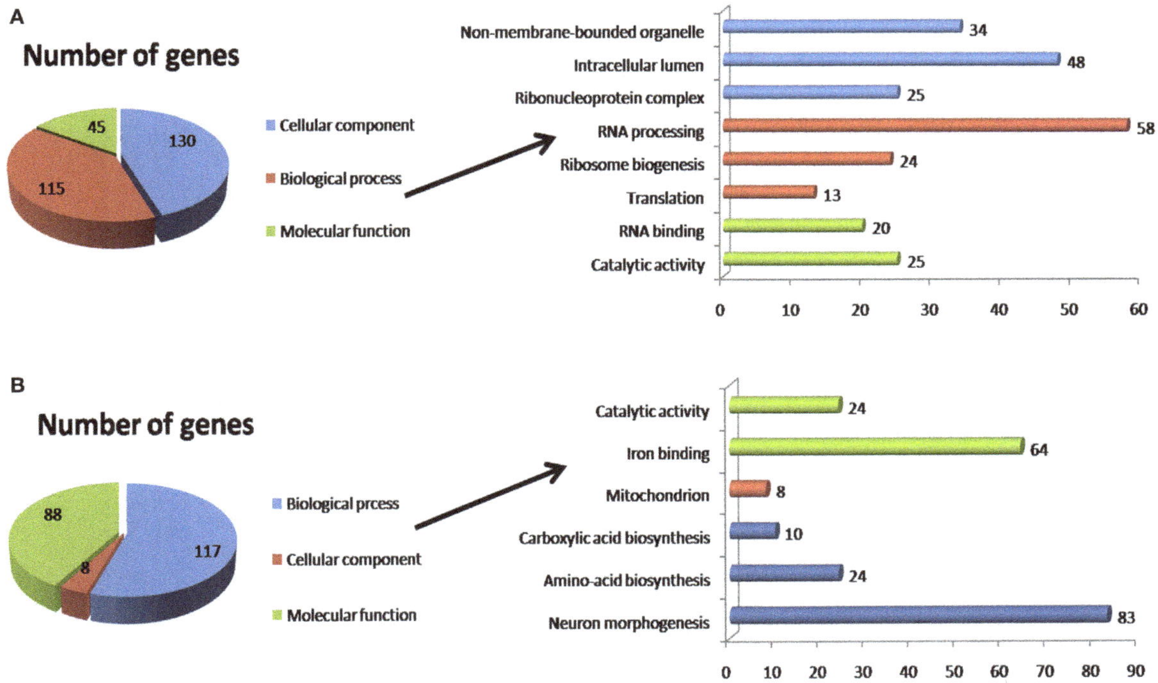

FIGURE 3 | Functional annotation of differentially expressed genes using DAVID. **(A)** Downregulated genes identified by DESeq2. **(B)** Upregulated genes identified by DESeq2. The *x*-axis indicates the number of genes enriched for the term, and the *y*-axis indicates the functional classes that were differentially expressed.

TABLE 7 | Bonferroni correction for differentially expressed genes (DEGs) enriched functionalities.

Category	Term	Number of DEGs	Bonferroni
	Downregulated DESEQ2		
GOTERM_BP_FAT	Ribosome biogenesis	12	3.90E−08
GOTERM_BP_FAT	rRNA processing	10	5.80E−08
GOTERM_BP_FAT	rRNA metabolic process	10	5.80E−08
GOTERM_BP_FAT	Ribonucleoprotein complex biogenesis	12	5.10E−07
GOTERM_BP_FAT	ncRNA processing	12	8.30E−07
GOTERM_BP_FAT	ncRNA metabolic process	12	3.40E−05
GOTERM_BP_FAT	RNA processing	14	1.20E−03
GOTERM_CC_FAT	Nucleolus	11	2.00E−07
GOTERM_CC_FAT	Small nucleolar ribonucleoprotein complex	4	1.90E−03
GOTERM_CC_FAT	Ribonucleoprotein complex	13	2.00E−03
GOTERM_CC_FAT	Nuclear lumen	12	9.40E−03
GOTERM_CC_FAT	Eukaryotic transl. initiation factor 3 complex	4	8.00E−03
GOTERM_MF_FAT	RNA binding	14	1.40E−02
SP_PIR_KEYWORDS	RNA-binding	10	1.80E−03
SP_PIR_KEYWORDS	Ribosome biogenesis	5	4.70E−03
SP_PIR_KEYWORDS	rRNA processing	5	4.00E−03
	Upregulated DESEQ2		
GOTERM_BP_FAT	Amine biosynthetic process	6	8.80E−03
GOTERM_BP_FAT	Cellular amino acid biosynthetic process	5	8.50E−03
GOTERM_BP_FAT	Carboxylic acid biosynthetic process	5	9.90E−02
GOTERM_BP_FAT	Organic acid biosynthetic process	5	9.90E−02

Categories: GOTERM_BP_FAT, biological process; GOTERM_CC_FAT, cellular component; GOTERM_MF_FAT, molecular function. SMART & INTERPRO, protein domains; SPIR_KEYWORD, protein information resource provided by SWISSPROT and UniProt.

mapping of reads on the fly genome, since nearly 75% of the 124 million reads (mean number per sample) were properly paired. However, this was not the case for the Tc genome, which displayed an average of less than 1% of properly mapped reads. This result is not surprising, given that our pre-sequencing manipulations did not target the trypanosome genome. Other contributing factors include the preparation of libraries, which was based on poly(a) selection using Oligo(dT) beads (67) and

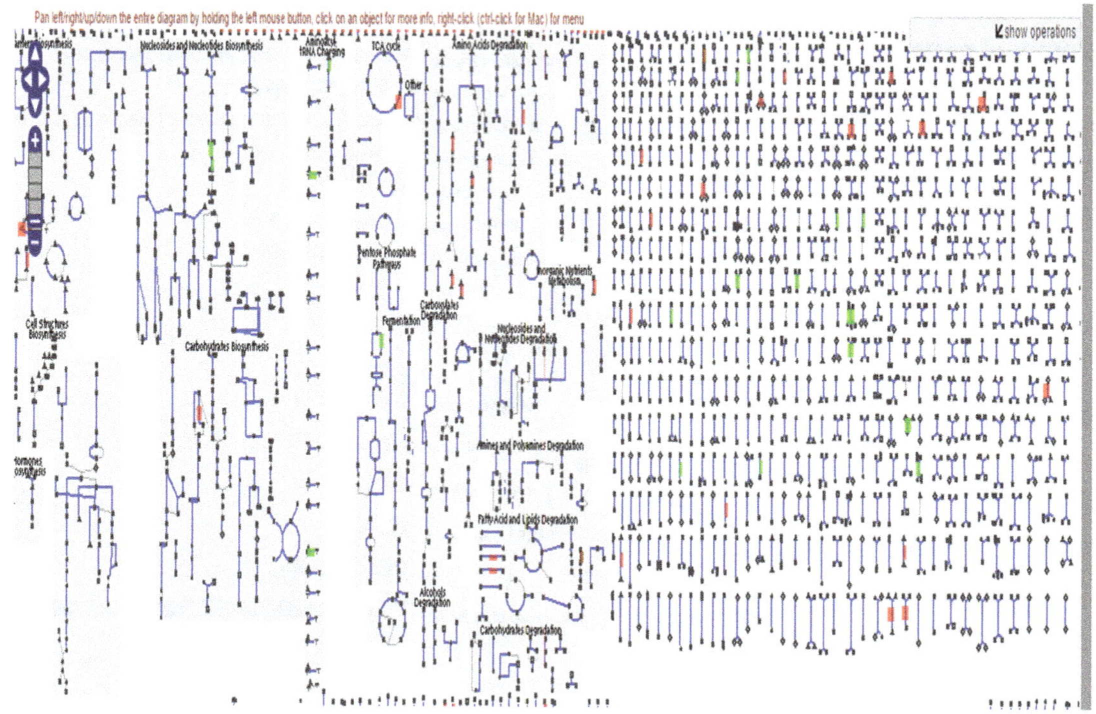

FIGURE 4 | BioCyc metabolic map illustrating the different differentially expressed genes involved in tsetse fly metabolic pathways. The genes activated by the infection are displayed in red, whereas the repressed genes are displayed in green.

the *Trypanosoma* genome, which is organized in polycistron units (68).

The infection duration in artificial infection experiments was monitored in the previous report, revealing that the levels of over- or under-expression in DEGs at 3, 10, or 20 days after infection can vary largely (17). In contrast, the present study was performed on tsetse flies sampled in the field, thus neither their age- nor the time-elapsed post-fly infection could be measured. Consequently, the recorded results represent an average level of DEG expression in Gpp flies that may have been infected by trypanosomes (Tc) recently or in the past several days. Similarly, it is possible that non-infected samples could group together flies that were truly never infected with flies that have eliminated their ingested trypanosomes (i.e., "self-cured" or "refractory" flies).

Despite this uncertainty, the results clearly demonstrate a very strong interaction between the parasite and its host/vector, resulting in major transcriptomic changes in the fly. For instance, the level of the "rRNA processing" function in infected vs. non-infected flies was as low as $\log2 = -22.3$. In other words, when the infected flies were captured and dissected, the "rRNA processing" function was $2^{22.3} = 5.16 \times 10^6$ fold lower than the value recorded in non-infected flies sampled at the same time and in the same areas. This indicates that the "rRNA processing" function was not effective at that time, and that at least 1 of the 10 DEGs shown to be involved in this function was essentially no longer expressed; however, this does not mean that it could not be reactivated at a later point in a fly's life.

In this study, we reported that 290 fly genes were downregulated and 213 were upregulated. This type of imbalance is expected to be induced either by a parasite or a symbiont, and to result in disturbing the host metabolism in such a way as to facilitate microorganism establishment (69, 70). In agreement with this, we observed the repression or non-activation of transcription genes that may allow the trypanosome to alter its host's transcription steps. Furthermore, certain metabolic pathways were downregulated that can prevent the host from synthesizing factors (proteins or metabolites) needed to fight infection (71). In this context and concerning the "Biological Process," "Cellular Component," and "Molecular Function" categories, most of the functional classes were associated with the host transcription/translation machinery (translation, RNA binding, ribonucleoprotein complex, ribosome processing helicase, etc.). Only 10% of the DEGs were related to "Catalytic activities." In contrast, overexpressed DEGs were involved with catalytic activities, cellular activities (morphogenesis, motion, and cell recognition) and, surprisingly, neuron activities (neuron development and neuron recognition). This is coherently illustrated in **Table 6**, where those "terms" that were over- or under-represented in DEGs (equal to or higher than a fourfold change) and that were identified through functional annotation on the *D. melanogaster* database have been alphabetically classified.

Our identification of the metabolic pathways associated with infection (**Table 8**) highlights the importance of the amino acid

TABLE 8 | Metabolic pathways associated with fly infection.

Pathways	Functions
Amino acid biosynthesis pathway	Synthesis of L-glutamine
	Synthesis of L-glutamate
	Synthesis of L-serine
	Synthesis of L-asparagine
	Synthesis of L-aspartate
	Synthesis of L-valine
	Synthesis of L-proline
	Synthesis of L-isoleucine
Nucleotide biosynthesis pathway	Biosynthesis of uridine monophosphate
Pentose phosphate pathway	Repression of D-ribose-5-phosphate
	Synthesis of orotidine
	Synthesis of pyruvate
Carbohydrate biosynthesis pathway	Biosynthesis of pyruvate
Isolated reactions	Synthesis of tyrosine
	Synthesis of serine
	Synthesis of L-glutamine
	Synthesis of L-glutamate
	Synthesis of L-serine
	Synthesis of L-asparagine
	Synthesis of L-methionine
	Synthesis of L-aspartate
	Synthesis of L-valine
	Synthesis of L-isoleucine
	Synthesis of *N*-acetylglucosamine
	Synthesis of galactosyltransferase
	Synthesis of beta-1,4-manosylglycolipid
	Synthesis of S-adenosyl-L-homocysteine
	Repression of immune cytokines
	Repression of formyltetrahydrofolate DH
Transport	Transport of lipids
	Transport of ATP
	Transport of succinate
	Transport of L-carnitine
	Transport of GTP
	Transport of acid dicarboxylic
	Transport of acid monocarboxylic
	Transport of L-tyrosine
	Transport of L-serine
	Transport of Ca^{2+}
	Transport of nucleotide
	Transport of Cyclic GMP
	Transport of proteinogenic amino acid
	Transport of NAD^{+}
	Transport of L-fructose
	Transport of GDP
	Transport of fatty acid
	Transporter activity
	Calcium ion binding

biosynthesis pathway. This provides the parasite with a broad range of amino acids that serve as a valuable source of energy, as previously reported for *T. cruzi*, the parasite causing Chagas disease (72), and microsporidia, a parasite of fishes (73). One such amino acid that we identified is proline, whose synthesis was overexpressed in Gpg infected with Tbg in comparison to non-infected flies (17). We also observed an increase in the biosynthesis of *N*-acetyl-glucosamine, a molecule that can affix itself to lectins that possess a sugar recognition area (74). This process inactivates tsetse fly lectins that are otherwise lethal to procyclic forms of trypanosomes (65), which consequently favor trypanosome installation in the fly vector. Interestingly, this mechanism has also been reported in Gpg infected with Tbg.

As reported in experimental Gpg insectary flies infected with Tbg, we have shown that field-collected Gpp naturally infected with Tc exhibit a strong cytokine repression in comparison to uninfected tsetse flies. This result indicates that strong alteration of the immune system occurred in infected flies, favoring parasite installation. In addition, *Trypanosoma* infection repressed 34 DEGs encoding non-membrane-bound organelles and 48 DEGs encoding expression of the intracellular lumen (an organelle consisting of chromatin). This type of scenario has also been described for the herpes simplex virus type 1, which can modify the structure and dynamics of chromatin through posttranscriptional modification of histone or other chromatin-forming proteins, contributing to their establishment within the host (75).

This is the first study to evaluate the transcriptomic events associated with infection by the Tc trypanosome in field Gpp tsetse flies. Our results establish that field flies naturally infected by trypanosomes display disruptions in their gene expression that result in either overexpression or under-expression of certain fly genes, as similarly observed in experimentally infected insectary flies. Furthermore, molecular disruptions occur in Gpp when infected with Tc, just as in Gpg that have been artificially infected with Tbg. Importantly, these findings indicate that different *Glossina* species infected with different trypanosome species under different conditions display comparable molecular reactions, which validate the use of experimental host/parasite couples for future research programs.

AUTHOR CONTRIBUTIONS

AG conceived and designed the experiments. JMTN, FN, BL, GK-N, and NF-N performed the experiments. JMTN, CR, JH, and AG analyzed the data. BL and AG contributed reagents/materials/analysis tools. JMTN, FN, JH, and AG wrote the paper.

REFERENCES

1. Buguet A, Bert J, Tapie P, Bogui P, Doua F, Mouanga G, et al. The distribution of sleep and wakefulness in human African trypanosomiasis. *Bull Soc Pathol Exot* (1994) 87:362–7.
2. Mehlitz D, Brinkmann U, Haller L. Epidemiological studies on the animal reservoir of gambiense sleeping sickness. Part I. Review of literature and description of the study areas. *Tropenmed Parasitol* (1981) 32:129–33.
3. Simarro PP, Diarra A, Postigo JAR, Franco JR, Jannin JG. The human African trypanosomiasis control and surveillance programme of the World Health Organization 2000–2009: the way forward. *PLoS Negl Trop Dis* (2011) 5:e1007. doi:10.1371/journal.pntd.0001007
4. Louis FJ, Simarro PP, Lucas P. Sleeping sickness: one hundred years of control strategy evolution. *Bull Soc Pathol Exot* (2002) 95:331–6.
5. Reinhardt E. *Travailler ensemble: la mouche tsé-tsé et la pauvreté rurale.* Chronique ONU (2002). Available from: www.un.org/french/pubs/chronique/2002/numero2/0202p17_la_mouche_tsetse.html
6. Gibson W, Kay C, Peacock L. *Trypanosoma congolense*: molecular toolkit and resources for studying a major livestock pathogen and model trypanosome. *Advances in Parasitology*. (Vol. 98) (2017). doi:10.1016/bs.apar.2017.03.002
7. Van den Abbeele J, Claes Y, Bockstaele D, Ray D, Coosemans M. *Trypanosoma brucei* spp. development in the tsetse fly: characterization of the post-mesocyclic stages in the foregut and proboscis. *Parasitology* (1999) 118:469–78. doi:10.1017/S0031182099004217
8. Peacock L, Cook S, Ferris V, Bailey M, Gibson W. The life cycle of *Trypanosoma (Nannomonas) congolense* in the tsetse fly. *Parasit Vectors* (2012) 5:109. doi:10.1186/1756-3305-5-109
9. Holzmuller P, Grébaut P, Peltier JB, Brizard JP, Perrone T, Gonzatti M, et al. Secretome of animal trypanosomes. *Ann N Y Acad Sci* (2008) 1149:337–42. doi:10.1196/annals.1428.097
10. Grébaut P, Chuchana P, Brizard JP, Demettre E, Seveno M, Bossard G, et al. Identification of total and differentially expressed excreted-secreted proteins from *Trypanosoma congolense* strains exhibiting different virulence and pathogenicity. *Int J Parasitol* (2009) 39:1137–50. doi:10.1016/j.ijpara.2009.02.018
11. Atyame Nten CM, Sommerer N, Rofidal V, Hirtz C, Rossignol M, Cuny G, et al. Excreted/secreted proteins from trypanosome procyclic strains. *J Biomed Biotechnol* (2010) 2010:212817. doi:10.1155/2010/212817
12. Geiger A, Hirtz C, Bécue T, Bellard E, Centeno D, Gargani D, et al. Exocytosis and protein secretion in *Trypanosoma*. *BMC Microbiol* (2010) 10:20. doi:10.1186/1471-2180-10-20
13. Farikou O, Njiokou F, Mbida Mbida JA, Njitchouang GR, Djeunga HN, Asonganyi T, et al. Tripartite interactions between tsetse flies, *Sodalis glossinidius* and trypanosomes—An epidemiological approach in two historical human African trypanosomiasis foci in Cameroon. *Infect Genet Evol* (2010) 10:115–21. doi:10.1016/j.meegid.2009.10.008
14. Geiger A, Ravel S, Mateille T, Janelle J, Patrel D, Cuny G, et al. Vector competence of *Glossina palpalis gambiensis* for *Trypanosoma brucei* s.l. and genetic diversity of the symbiont *Sodalis glossinidius*. *Mol Biol Evol* (2007) 24:102–9. doi:10.1093/molbev/msl135
15. Hamidou Soumana I, Tchicaya B, Simo G, Geiger A. Comparative gene expression of *Wigglesworthia* inhabiting non-infected and *Trypanosoma brucei gambiense*-infected *Glossina palpalis gambiensis* flies. *Front Microbiol* (2014) 5:620. doi:10.3389/fmicb.2014.00620
16. Hamidou Soumana I, Loriod B, Ravel S, Tchicaya B, Simo G, Rihet P, et al. The transcriptional signatures of *Sodalis glossinidius* in the *Glossina palpalis gambiensis* flies negative for *Trypanosoma brucei gambiense* contrast with those of this symbiont in tsetse flies positive for the parasite: possible involvement of a *Sodalis*-hosted prophage in fly *Trypanosoma* refractoriness? *Infect Genet Evol* (2014) 24:41–56.
17. Hamidou Soumana I, Klopp C, Ravel S, Nabihoudine I, Tchicaya B, Parrinello H, et al. RNA-seq de novo assembly reveals differential gene expression in *Glossina palpalis gambiensis* infected with *Trypanosoma brucei gambiense* vs. non-infected and self-cured flies. *Front Microbiol* (2015) 6:1259. doi:10.3389/fmicb.2015.01259
18. Hamidou Soumana I, Tchicaya B, Rialle S, Parinello H, Geiger A. Comparative genomics of *Glossina palpalis gambiensis* and *G. morsitans morsitans* to reveal gene orthologs involved in infection by *Trypanosoma brucei gambiense*. *Front Microbiol* (2017) 8:540. doi:10.3389/fmicb.2017.00540
19. Matthews KR. 25 years of African trypanosome research: from description to molecular dissection and new drug discovery. *Mol Biochem Parasitol* (2015) 200:30–40. doi:10.1016/j.molbiopara.2015.01.006
20. Mugnier MR, Stebbins CE, Papavasiliou FN. Masters of disguise: antigenic variation and the VSG coat in *Trypanosoma brucei*. *PLoS Pathog* (2016) 12:e1005784. doi:10.1371/journal.ppat.1005784
21. Tiengwe C, Muratore KA, Bangs JD. Surface proteins, ERAD and antigenic variation in *Trypanosoma brucei*. *Cell Microbiol* (2016) 18:1673–88. doi:10.1111/cmi.12605
22. Odongo S, Sterckx YGJ, Stijlemans B, Pillay D, Baltz T, Muyldermans S, et al. An anti-proteome nanobody library approach yields a specific immunoassay for *Trypanosoma congolense* diagnosis targeting glycosomal aldolase. *PLoS Negl Trop Dis* (2016) 10:e0004420. doi:10.1371/journal.pntd.0004420
23. WHO. *The World Health Report – Working Together for Health*. (2006). Available from: http://www.who.int/whr/2006/en/
24. Authié E, Boulangé A, Muteti D, Lalmanach G, Gauthier F, Musoke AJ. Immunisation of cattle with cysteine proteinases of *Trypanosoma congolense*: targetting the disease rather than the parasite. *Int J Parasitol* (2001) 31:1429–33. doi:10.1016/S0020-7519(01)00266-1
25. Huson LE, Authié E, Boulangé AF, Goldring JP, Coetzer TH. Modulation of the immunogenicity of the *Trypanosoma congolense* cysteine protease, congopain, through complexation with alpha(2)-macroglobulin. *Vet Res* (2009) 40:52. doi:10.1051/vetres/2009036
26. Aksoy S, Weiss B, Attardo G. Paratransgenesis applied for control of tsetse transmitted sleeping sickness. In: Aksoy S, editor. *Transgenesis and the Management of Vector-Borne Disease, Advances in Experimental Medicine and Biology*. New York: Springer (2008). p. 35–48.
27. Matetovici I, Caljon G, Van Den Abbeele J. Tsetse fly tolerance to *T. brucei* infection: transcriptome analysis of trypanosome-associated changes in the tsetse fly salivary gland. *BMC Genomics* (2016) 17:971. doi:10.1186/s12864-016-3283-0
28. Rio RVM, Hu Y, Aksoy S. Strategies of the home-team: symbioses exploited for vector-borne disease control. *Trends Microbiol* (2004) 12:325–36. doi:10.1016/j.tim.2004.05.001
29. Abd-Alla AMM, Bergoin M, Parker AG, Maniania NK, Vlak JM, Bourtzis K, et al. Improving Sterile Insect Technique (SIT) for tsetse flies through research on their symbionts and pathogens. *J Invertebr Pathol* (2013) 112:S2–10. doi:10.1016/j.jip.2012.07.009
30. Vreysen MJB, Saleh KM, Ali MY, Abdulla AM, Zhu Z-R, Juma KG, et al. *Glossina austeni* (Diptera: Glossinidae) eradicated on the island of Unguja, Zanzibar, using the sterile insect technique. *J Econ Entomol* (2000) 93:123–35. doi:10.1603/0022-0493-93.1.123
31. Geiger A, Ponton F, Simo G. Adult blood-feeding tsetse flies, trypanosomes, microbiota and the fluctuating environment in sub-Saharan Africa. *ISME J* (2015) 9:1496–507. doi:10.1038/ismej.2014.236
32. Geiger A, Bossard G, Sereno D, Pissarra J, Lemesre JL, Vincendeau P, et al. Escaping deleterious immune response in their hosts: lessons from trypanosomatids. *Front Immunol* (2016) 7:212. doi:10.3389/fimmu.2016.00212
33. Frezil J-L, Cuisance D. Trypanosomiases, maladies d'avenir: leurs perspectives et leurs inconues. Trypanosomiasis, diseases with future: prospects and uncertainty. *Bull Soc Pathol Exot* (1994) 87:391–3.
34. Aksoy S, Gibson WC, Lehane MJ. Interactions between tsetse and trypanosomes with implications for the control of trypanosomiasis. *Adv Parasitol* (2003) 53:1–83. doi:10.1016/S0065-308X(03)53002-0
35. Lehane MJ, Aksoy S, Gibson W, Kerhornou A, Berriman M, Hamilton J, et al. Adult midgut expressed sequence tags from the tsetse fly *Glossina morsitans morsitans* and expression analysis of putative immune response genes. *Genome Biol* (2003) 4:R63. doi:10.1186/gb-2003-4-10-r63
36. Lehane MJ, Gibson W, Lehane SM. Differential expression of fat body genes in *Glossina morsitans morsitans* following infection with *Trypanosoma brucei brucei*. *Int J Parasitol* (2008) 38:93–101. doi:10.1016/j.ijpara.2007.06.004
37. Grébaut P, Melachio T, Nyangmang S, Eyenga VE, Njitchouang GR, Ofon E, et al. Xenomonitoring of sleeping sickness transmission in Campo (Cameroon). *Parasit Vectors* (2016) 9:201. doi:10.1186/s13071-016-1479-4
38. Grebaut P, Bodo JM, Assona A, Foumane Ngane V, Njiokou F, Ollivier G, et al. Risk factors for human African trypanosomiasis in the Bipindi region of Cameroon. *Med Trop Rev Corps Sante Colon* (2001) 61:377–83.

39. Farikou O, Njiokou F, Simo G, Asonganyi T, Cuny G, Geiger A. Tsetse fly blood meal modification and trypanosome identification in two sleeping sickness foci in the forest of southern Cameroon. *Acta Trop* (2010) 116:81–8. doi:10.1016/j.actatropica.2010.06.002
40. Njiokou F, Simo G, Nkinin SW, Laveissière C, Herder S. Infection rate of *Trypanosoma brucei* s.l., *T. vivax*, *T. congolense* "forest type", and *T. simiae* in small wild vertebrates in south Cameroon. *Acta Trop* (2004) 92:139–46. doi:10.1016/j.actatropica.2004.04.011
41. Njiokou F, Laveissière C, Simo G, Nkinin S, Grébaut P, Cuny G, et al. Wild fauna as a probable animal reservoir for *Trypanosoma brucei gambiense* in Cameroon. *Infect Genet Evol* (2006) 6:147–53. doi:10.1016/j.meegid.2005.04.003
42. Simo G, Njiokou F, Mbida Mbida JA, Njitchouang GR, Herder S, Asonganyi T, et al. Tsetse fly host preference from sleeping sickness foci in Cameroon: epidemiological implications. *Infect Genet Evol* (2008) 8:34–9. doi:10.1016/j.meegid.2007.09.005
43. Lancien J. Description du piège monoconique utilisé pour l'élimination des glossines en République Populaire du Congo. *Ent Méd Parasitol* (1981) 19:235–8.
44. Grébaut P, Mbida JAM, Kondjio CA, Njiokou F, Penchenier L, Laveissiére C. Spatial and temporal patterns of human African trypanosomosis (HAT) transmission risk in the bipindi focus, in the forest zone of southern Cameroon. *Vector Borne Zoonotic Dis* (2004) 4:230–8. doi:10.1089/vbz.2004.4.230
45. Penchenier L, Itard J. Une nouvelle technique de dissection rapide des glandes salivaires et de l'intestin de glossines. *Ent Méd Parasitol* (1981) 19:55–7.
46. Herder S, Simo G, Nkinin S, Njiokou F. Identification of trypanosomes in wild animals from southern Cameroon using the polymerase chain reaction (PCR). *Parasite* (2002) 9:345–9. doi:10.1051/parasite/2002094345
47. Masiga DK, Smyth AJ, Ayes P, Bromidge TJ, Gibson WC. Sensitive detection of trypanosomes in tsetse flies by DNA amplification. *Int J Parasitol* (1992) 22:909–18. doi:10.1016/0020-7519(92)90047-O
48. Moser DR, Cook GA, Ochs DE, Bailey CP, McKane MR, Donelson JE. Detection of *Trypanosoma congolense* and *Trypanosoma brucei* subspecies by DNA amplification using the polymerase chain reaction. *Parasitology* (1989) 99:57–66. doi:10.1017/S0031182000061023
49. Köster J, Rahmann S. Snakemake – a scalable bioinformatics workflow engine. *Bioinformatics* (2012) 28:2520–2. doi:10.1093/bioinformatics/bts480
50. Giraldo-Calderón GI, Emrich SJ, MacCallum RM, Maslen G, Dialynas E, Topalis P, et al. VectorBase: an updated bioinformatics resource for invertebrate vectors and other organisms related with human diseases. *Nucleic Acids Res* (2015) 43:D707–13. doi:10.1093/nar/gku1117
51. Aslett M, Aurrecoechea C, Berriman M, Brestelli J, Brunk BP, Carrington M, et al. TriTrypDB: a functional genomic resource for the *Trypanosomatidae*. *Nucleic Acids Res* (2010) 38:D457–62. doi:10.1093/nar/gkp851
52. Attrill H, Falls K, Goodman JL, Millburn GH, Antonazzo G, Rey AJ, et al. FlyBase: establishing a gene group resource for *Drosophila melanogaster*. *Nucleic Acids Res* (2016) 44:D786–92. doi:10.1093/nar/gkv1046
53. Liao Y, Smyth GK, Shi W. The subread aligner: fast, accurate and scalable read mapping by seed-and-vote. *Nucleic Acids Res* (2013) 41:e108. doi:10.1093/nar/gkt214
54. Li H, Handsaker B, Wysoker A, Fennell T, Ruan J, Homer N, et al. The sequence alignment/map format and SAMtools. *Bioinformatics* (2009) 25:2078–9. doi:10.1093/bioinformatics/btp352
55. Liao Y, Smyth GK, Shi W. FeatureCounts: an efficient general purpose program for assigning sequence reads to genomic features. *Bioinformatics* (2014) 30:923–30. doi:10.1093/bioinformatics/btt656
56. Robinson JT, Thorvaldsdóttir H, Winckler W, Guttman M, Lander ES, Getz G, et al. Integrative genomics viewer. *Nat Biotechnol* (2011) 29:24–6. doi:10.1038/nbt.1754
57. Varet H, Brillet-Guéguen L, Coppée J-Y, Dillies M-A. SARTools: a DESeq2- and EdgeR-based R pipeline for comprehensive differential analysis of RNA-Seq data. *PLoS One* (2016) 11:e0157022. doi:10.1371/journal.pone.0157022
58. Love MI, Huber W, Anders S. Moderated estimation of fold change and dispersion for RNA-seq data with DESeq2. *Genome Biol* (2014) 15:550. doi:10.1186/s13059-014-0550-8
59. Robinson MD, McCarthy DJ, Smyth GK. edgeR: a Bioconductor package for differential expression analysis of digital gene expression data. *Bioinformatics* (2010) 26:139–40. doi:10.1093/bioinformatics/btp616
60. Altschul SF, Madden TL, Schäffer AA, Zhang J, Zhang Z, Miller W, et al. Gapped BLAST and PSI-BLAST: a new generation of protein database search programs. *Nucleic Acids Res* (1997) 25:3389–402. doi:10.1093/nar/25.17.3389
61. Huang DW, Sherman BT, Lempicki RA. Systematic and integrative analysis of large gene lists using DAVID bioinformatics resources. *Nat Protoc* (2009) 4:44–57. doi:10.1038/nprot.2008.211
62. Reimand J, Kull M, Peterson H, Hansen J, Vilo J. g:Profiler—a web-based toolset for functional profiling of gene lists from large-scale experiments. *Nucleic Acids Res* (2007) 35:W193–200. doi:10.1093/nar/gkm226
63. Caspi R, Billington R, Ferrer L, Foerster H, Fulcher CA, Keseler IM, et al. The MetaCyc database of metabolic pathways and enzymes and the BioCyc collection of pathway/genome databases. *Nucleic Acids Res* (2016) 44:D471–80. doi:10.1093/nar/gkv1164
64. Maudlin I, Ellis DS. Association between intracellular *Rickettsia*-like infections of midgut cells and susceptibility to trypanosome infection in *Glossina* spp. *Z Parasitenkd* (1985) 71:683–7. doi:10.1007/BF00925601
65. Welburn SC, Maudlin I. Tsetse–trypanosome interactions: rites of passage. *Parasitol Today* (1999) 15:399–403. doi:10.1016/S0169-4758(99)01512-4
66. Dale C, Welburn SC. The endosymbionts of tsetse flies: manipulating host-parasite interactions. *Int J Parasitol* (2001) 31:628–31. doi:10.1016/S0020-7519(01)00151-5
67. Koch H, Raabe M, Urlaub H, Bindereif A, Preußer C. The polyadenylation complex of *Trypanosoma brucei*: characterization of the functional poly(A) polymerase. *RNA Biol* (2016) 13:221–31. doi:10.1080/15476286.2015.1130208
68. Kolev NG, Franklin JB, Carmi S, Shi H, Michaeli S, Tschudi C. The transcriptome of the human pathogen *Trypanosoma brucei* at single-nucleotide resolution. *PLoS Pathog* (2010) 6:e1001090. doi:10.1371/journal.ppat.1001090
69. Martinson EO, Wheeler D, Wright J, Mrinalini Siebert AL, Werren JH. *Nasonia vitripennis* venom causes targeted gene expression changes in its fly host. *Mol Ecol* (2014) 23:5918–30. doi:10.1111/mec.12967
70. Snyder AK, Rio RVM. "Wigglesworthia morsitans" folate (vitamin b9) biosynthesis contributes to tsetse host fitness. *Appl Environ Microbiol* (2015) 81:5375–86. doi:10.1128/AEM.00553-15
71. Zhang Q, Lai M-M, Lou Y-Y, Guo B-H, Wang H-Y, Zheng X-Q. Transcriptome altered by latent human cytomegalovirus infection on THP-1 cells using RNA-seq. *Gene* (2016) 594:144–50. doi:10.1016/j.gene.2016.09.014
72. Barisón MJ, Damasceno FS, Mantilla BS, Silber AM. The active transport of histidine and its role in ATP production in *Trypanosoma cruzi*. *J Bioenerg Biomembr* (2016) 48:437–49. doi:10.1007/s10863-016-9665-9
73. Dean P, Hirt RP, Embley TM. *Microsporidia*: why make nucleotides if you can steal them? *PLoS Pathog* (2016) 12:e1005870. doi:10.1371/journal.ppat.1005870
74. Kanost MR, Jiang H, Yu X-Q. Innate immune responses of a lepidopteran insect, *Manduca sexta*. *Immunol Rev* (2004) 198:97–105. doi:10.1111/j.0105-2896.2004.0121.x
75. Kent JR, Zeng P-Y, Atanasiu D, Gardner J, Fraser NW, Berger SL. During lytic infection herpes simplex virus type 1 is associated with histones bearing modifications that correlate with active transcription. *J Virol* (2004) 78:10178–86. doi:10.1128/JVI.78.18.10178-10186.2004

19

Circulating Plasma MicroRNA-208a as Potential Biomarker of Chronic Indeterminate Phase of Chagas Disease

*Leandra Linhares-Lacerda[1,2], Alessandra Granato[1], João Francisco Gomes-Neto[1], Luciana Conde[1], Leonardo Freire-de-Lima[3], Elisangela O. de Freitas[4], Celio G. Freire-de-Lima[3], Shana P. Coutinho Barroso[5], Rodrigo Jorge de Alcântara Guerra[5], Roberto C. Pedrosa[6], Wilson Savino[2,7] and Alexandre Morrot[8,9]**

[1] Departamento de Imunologia, Instituto de Microbiologia, Universidade Federal do Rio de Janeiro, Rio de Janeiro, Brazil, [2] Instituto Oswaldo Cruz, Fundação Oswaldo Cruz (FIOCRUZ), Rio de Janeiro, Brazil, [3] Instituto de Biofísica Carlos Chagas Filho, Universidade Federal do Rio de Janeiro, Rio de Janeiro, Brazil, [4] Departamento de Análises Clínicas e Toxicológicas, Faculdade de Ciências Farmacêuticas, Universidade de São Paulo, São Paulo, Brazil, [5] Instituto de Pesquisas Biomédicas, Hospital Naval Marcílio Dias, Marinha do Brasil, Rio de Janeiro, Brazil, [6] Instituto do Coração Edson Saad, Hospital Universitário Clementino Fraga Filho, Universidade Federal do Rio de Janeiro, Rio de Janeiro, Brazil, [7] National Institute of Science and Technology on Neuroimmunomodulation (INCT-NIM), Rio de Janeiro, Brazil, [8] Faculdade de Medicina, Centro de Pesquisas em Tuberculose, Universidade Federal do Rio de Janeiro, Rio de Janeiro, Brazil, [9] Laboratório de Imunopatologia, Instituto Oswaldo Cruz, Fundação Oswaldo Cruz (FIOCRUZ), Rio de Janeiro, Brazil

***Correspondence:**
Alexandre Morrot
alexandre.lima@ioc.fiocruz.br;
morrot@micro.ufrj.br

Chagas cardiomyopathy is the most severe clinical manifestation of chronic Chagas disease. The disease affects most of the Latin American countries, being considered one of the leading causes of morbidity and death in the continent. The pathogenesis of Chagas cardiomyopathy is very complex, with mechanisms involving parasite-dependent cytopathy, immune-mediated myocardial damage and neurogenic disturbances. These pathological changes eventually result in cardiac myocyte hypertrophy, arrhythmias, congestive heart failure and stroke during chronic infection phase. Herein, we show that miR-208a, a microRNA that is a key factor in promoting cardiovascular dysfunction during cardiac hypertrophy processes of heart failure, has its circulating levels increased during chronic indeterminate phase when compared to cardiac (CARD) clinical forms in patients with Chagas disease. In contrast, we have not found altered serum levels of miR-34a, a microRNA known to promote pro-apoptotic role in myocardial infarction during degenerative process of cardiac injuries thus indicating intrinsic differences in the nature of the mechanisms underlying the heart failure triggered by *Trypanosoma cruzi* infection. Our findings support that the chronic indeterminate phase is a progressive phase involved in the genesis of chagasic cardiopathy and point out the use of plasma levels of miR-208a as candidate biomarker in risk-prediction score for the clinical prognosis of Chagas disease.

Keywords: Chagas disease, *Trypanosoma cruzi*, infectious heart disease, microRNA, disease biomarkers

INTRODUCTION

Chagas disease or American trypanosomiasis is a tropical parasitic disease caused by the protozoan *Trypanosoma cruzi* and transmitted mainly by insects of the subfamily Triatominae (Rassi et al., 2010). It is estimated that more than seven million people, especially in Mexico, Central America and South America, have Chagas disease. This has resulted in about 12,500 deaths per year since 2006. Large-scale population movements have expanded the areas where cases of Chagas disease are found, including now many countries in Europe and North America (World Health Organization, 2017). In the endemic areas, the vector consists the main mechanism of human transmission through host contact with feces and urine of infected vectors, mainly of the genera *Triatoma*, *Rhodnius*, and *Panstrongylus*. The insect vector acquires *Trypanosoma cruzi* parasite by feeding blood from infected animals or humans (Noireau et al., 2009).

Within the invertebrate vector, the parasite multiplies under epimastigote forms that later differentiate into trypomastigotes in the digestive tract of triatomine. The trypomastigote forms are the infecting stages of vertebrate host, being released in the feces of triatomine during bloodfeeding, and transmitted when host scratches contaminated feces into the wound (Kollien and Schaub, 2000). Once inside the host, the trypomastigote invades the cells near the inoculation, in the first line resident macrophages, where they differentiate into intracellular amastigotes (Burleigh and Andrews, 1995). The amastigotes multiply by binary division and differentiate into trypomastigotes, which are released into the bloodstream, infecting cells of various tissues, and this cycle is repeated several times, due to its ability to persist prolonged periods in the host tissues mainly as dividing amastigote forms inside tissue cells and pseudocysts by subverting humoral and cell-mediated immunity. The clinical manifestations in humans are the result of this infectious cycle and may include, at early stages of infection, symptoms such as fever, lymphadenitis, or local swelling of the biting site (Burleigh and Andrews, 1995; Kollien and Schaub, 2000; Andrade and Andrews, 2005).

After an asymptomatic acute phase in 90% of infected individuals, the infection persists and enters its chronic indeterminate phase, in which 60–80% of patients will never develop clinical symptoms, although parasitism remains in balance with host immune responses. During the intermediate phase there is a cumulative progression to diffuse myocardial damage in about 20–40% of the chronic patients developing cardiac and/or digestive problems (Teixeira et al., 2011). The pathogenesis of Chagas disease is due to an intense inflammatory lesion and fibrosis induced to the tissues and organs involved in the infectious cycle of the parasite (Machado et al., 2000; Lepletier et al., 2014). If left untreated, Chagas disease can be fatal, in most cases by damaging cardiac muscle tissue (Marin-Neto et al., 2007). The cytopathic effects induced by the parasite and the host immune responses against the intracellular amastigote harm the intramural neurons of the autonomic nervous system of the gut and heart, leading to megacolon and cardiac aneurysms, respectively (Zhang and Tarleton, 1999; Campos et al., 2016).

The nature of Chagas disease lesions induced by parasitism is intrinsically related to the perpetuation of the parasite in the affected tissues (Rassi et al., 2009). The chronicity of infection is associated with profound changes in the molecular levels of the affected organs, as it has been shown that myocardial gene expression patterns are altered in advanced forms of chronic disease (Ferreira et al., 2014). Although the molecular mechanisms underlying the myocardial gene expression are not well elucidated, studies have shown that microRNAs involved in the genetic regulation process of heart development and cardiovascular disorders have their expression disregulated in advanced forms of chagasic chronic heart disease (Eulalio et al., 2012). These studies were performed in patients with more advanced forms of chagasic heart disease and their comparisons with normal healthy individuals (Eulalio et al., 2012). However, studies in the earliest forms of chronic infection, using patients in the indeterminate phase of the disease, would allow us to explore the use of cardiac microRNAs as a potential biomarker to predict/diagnose, in the indeterminate phase of disease, the patients that will develop cardiomyopathy (20–40%).

Along these lines, we investigated herein the modulation of potential heart disease-specific miRNA biomarkers in chagasic patients at early chronic infection to be used as a risk predictor for clinical prognosis in *Trypanosoma cruzi*-induced cardiomyopathy. Our research include analysis of cross-sectional studies from chronic chagasic patients at the indeterminate (IND) as compared to cardiac (CARD) clinical forms of Chagas disease, or non-infected control individuals to profile the plasma expression of cardiac miRNA biomarkers of two extreme processes involved in the cardiovascular dysfunction. In degenerative cardiovascular diseases, microRNAs (miRNAs) are crucial regulators of cardiac function (Filipowicz et al., 2008; Boon et al., 2013). Endogenous miRNAs were shown to regulate gene expression at the post-transcriptional level either through translation repression or mRNA degradation affecting independent processes resulting in degeneration of the cardiac tissue (Callis et al., 2009).

MiR-208a is one of the most important heart-specific miRNA playing a critical role in the heart failure and has been considered as a potential biomarker of myocardial injuries (Cunha-Neto et al., 2005; Wang et al., 2013; Doka et al., 2015; Shyu et al., 2015; Zhang et al., 2017). The miR-208a is encoded by an intronic region of the alpha-cardiac muscle myosin heavy chain gene (Myh6) regulating the myosin heavy chain isoform switch (Cunha-Neto et al., 2005). Under pathophysiologic conditions, miR-208a is critical to induce arrhythmias, cardiac remodeling, expression of hypertrophy pathway components and the cardiac conduction system (Cunha-Neto et al., 2005). Studies on mice lacking miR-208a have indicated that this microRNA is required for expression of the homeodomain-only protein (HOP), which is required to modulate cardiac growth and development, in addition to GATA4 and the Gap junction alpha-5 protein (GJA5), also known as connexin 40 (Cx40). These factors are determinants in the induction of heart injuries associated with cardiac conduction (Shyu et al., 2015).

In a different aspect of the mechanisms capable of promoting heart injury, miR-34a is shown to contribute to the age-dependent deterioration of cardiac function, contributing to cardiomyocyte death following acute myocardial infarction (Filipowicz et al., 2008). Studies have identified the PPP1R10 gene (also known as PNUTS) as a direct miR-34a target, whose inhibition promotes telomere shortening and cardiomyocyte apoptosis. The anti-apoptotic role of PNUTS and its counter-regulation by age-induced expression of miR-34a has a direct effect on the processes that regulate cardiac contractile function and functional cardiac recovery after acute myocardial infarction (Filipowicz et al., 2008). In the present study we attempted to clarify whether changes in the circulating levels of miR-208a and miR-34a in the blood is associated with the development of severe cardiac clinical form of human chronic Chagas disease.

MATERIALS AND METHODS

Ethics Statement

All the protocols for animal (IMPPG038-05/16) and human (CAAE No. 46502615.1.0000.5257) studies were approved by the Research Ethics Committee of Federal University of Rio de Janeiro. Experimental mice infections and assay procedures with *T. cruzi* were performed in biosafety area recommended for activities with infective stages of the parasites, in accordance with the terms of the Brazilian and international guidelines for the welfare regulations.

Study Population

Healthy volunteers and *T. cruzi* chronic chagasic patients were recruited from Chagas Cardiomyopathy clinic of Hospital Universitário Clementino Fraga Filho of Universidade Federal do Rio de Janeiro, HUCFF-UFRJ, Brazil. All individuals analyzed in this study, including chronic infected patients and non-infected individuals with ages ranging from 30 to 64 years, confirmed the diagnosis for *T. cruzi* infection in serological tests. The selected individuals included 10 seropositive cases of cardiac chronic-infected patients showed dilated cardiomyopathy diagnosed based in a detailed clinical examination, electrocardiography (ECG), and unidimensional/bidimensional echocardiography with Doppler (ECHO). Additionally, we included 10 patients in the indeterminate forms of Chagas disease, without any cardiac alterations detected. Twenty donors, age and sex matched-non-infected controls were included in the study. The research was approved by the Research Ethics Committee (CEP) and all patients signed a free and informed consent form in accordance with current legislation and the regulations of the HUCFF-UFRJ (CAAE No. 46502615.1.0000.5257).

Quantification of Human Plasma Levels of microRNA

Human plasma samples were collected using heparin-coated tubes and frozen at −80°C. RNA from 200 μl of human plasma were isolated with miRNeasy Serum/Plasma Kit (Qiagen) according to manufacturer instructions. Synthetic *C. elegans* miR-39 mimic (Qiagen) was spiked-in to all samples before RNA isolation to control for proper isolation. We performed miRNA expression profiling using the Taqman miRNA Assays for miR-34a (hsa-miR-34a-5p; ID number 000426), miR-208a (hsa-miR-208a-3p; ID number 000511), miR-221 (hsa-miR-221-3p; ID number 000524), miR-484 (hsa-miR-484; ID number 001821), and miR-39 (cel-miR-39; ID number 000200) in technical triplicate and the Taqman miRNA Reverse Transcription kit and Taqman Universal Master Mix II, no UNG according to the manufacturer's instructions (ThermoFisher) in a Step ONE Plus Fast Real Time PCR System (Applied Biosystems). The data were analyzed by fitting four-parameter sigmoid curves to the Rn data using the qPCR library (Ritz and Spiess, 2008) for the R statistical package version 2.922. The gene-stability measurement was determined by the optimal number of control genes required for normalization using average pairwise variation ($V_{n/n+1}$) analysis between the normalization factors NF_n and NF_{n+1} by geNorm method (Vandesompele et al., 2002). An adaptation of this method was used to assay the cel-miR-39 (spike-in) for the average expression stability of reference genes, beside the non-related hsa-miR-221-3p and hsa-miR-484 endogenous genes. Based on our analysis we selected hsa-miR-221-3p and hsa-miR-484 as most stable miRNA in our samples, since they are below the recommended threshold for pairwise variation V of 0.15 (between the normalization factors NF_n and NF_{n+1}) and used them for normalization. The comparison of the means of the normalized gene expression values between the groups was performed by a non-parametric one-way ANOVA with 1,000 unrestricted permutations, followed by *post-hoc* pair-wise comparisons with a Bonferroni adjustment using a non-parametric *t*-test, also with 1,000 permutations (Basso et al., 2009).

Animals, Infection, Parasite Load, Detection of Creatine Kinase Cardiac Isoenzyme and Intra-Cardiac Levels of miR-34a

Male C57BL/6 mice, aged 4–8 weeks, were housed and maintained in IMPPG-Federal University of Rio de Janeiro animal facility for experimental infection experiments. Chronic *T. cruzi* infection was performed by inoculating the 6-week-old mice intraperitoneally with 2×10^3 blood-derived trypomastigote forms of Y strain of *T. cruzi*. The parasitemia was monitored by counting blood parasites using Neubauer's chambers, and animals were bled and sacrificed at 30 days post-infection (DPI). To test the creatine kinase cardiac isoenzyme (CK-MB), plasma samples were collected at 14 DPI from *T. cruzi* infected and non-infected mice, and the CK-MB activity was measured by the commercial kit CK-MB Liquiform (Labtest) as described by the manufacturer. The assays were read in a microplate spectrophotometer (SpectraMax® Plus 384 Microplate Reader, Molecular devices) allowing the analysis of small quantities of mouse plasma according to manufacturer's recommendation. The optical density at 340 nm was recorded every 1 min (A_1) at 37°C, for 5 min (A_2). Calibration and quality control of the equipment were performed according to the recommended protocol. To assess the intracardiac parasite load, hearts were collected at

14 DPI, minced and 100 mg of tissue were homogenized in 1 mL of TRIzol® (Invitrogen) for DNA extraction, following manufacturer's instructions. The concentrations of extracted total DNA were measured using NanoDrop-1000 (Thermo Scientific). Each PCR reaction contained 50 ng of the genomic DNA, 0.25mM *T. cruzi* 195-bp repeat DNA-specific primers: TCZ-F: 5′-GCTCTTGCCCACAAGGGTGC-3′, and TCZ-R: 5′-CCAAGCAGCGGATAGTTCAGG-3′, amplified with SYBR Green® PCR Master Mix (Qiagen) and PCR-grade H_2O (Qiagen) on a Step One Real Time PCR System (Applied Biosystems). For loading controls, we used reactions containing 50 ng of the genomic DNA, 0.25 mM of murine-specific tumor necrosis factor-a (TNF-a) gene primers TNF-α-F: 5′-CCTGGAGGAGAAGAGGAAAGAGA-3′ and TNF-α-R: 5′-TTGAGGACCTCTGTGTATTTGTCAA-3′. To determine the intracardiac levels of mir-34a expression, high-purity miRNA was obtained from heart tissue by using standard protocol (Faragó et al., 2011). Quantitative real-time PCR analysis were performed using miScript SYBR Green PCR Kit for mouse mir-34a (Quiagen) at the same conditions as described above.

Statistical Analysis

Statistical analyses were performed with GraphPad Prism 5 software. Statistical differences between groups were compared by a non-parametrical test (Mann–Whitney Rank Sum Test). Results were expressed as mean ± standard deviation (S.D.), and differences between control and treated group were considered statistically significant when $p \leq 0.05$.

RESULTS

To evaluate whether changes in the plasma-circulating levels of cardiac-specific miRNAs is correlated with Chagas heart disease severity, we first aimed at normalizing the gene-expression levels by selected stable internal control gene in order to remove any non-specific variation of the target miRNAs in our analysis. To validate the genetic expression analyzes of the RT-qPCR data we should normalize the gene expression profiles of the cardiac-specific miRNA genes that are supposed to be modulated in the process of infectious cardiopathy with respect to stably expressed endogenous reference genes not related to the disease. However, it has been demonstrated that stable microRNAs derived from plasma/serum are likely disease-specific, and miRNA control genes for Chagas disease have not yet been identified. To address this question, beside using a spike with a micro RNA control which only controls for proper isolation and processing of miRNA samples we also used irrelevant microRNA genes known to be highly regulated in our donor sample collection study, as reference genes.

To this end, the expression ratios of both cardiac-specific miR-208a and miR-34a were assessed as the pairwise variation with the non-related internal hsa-mir-221-3p genes and hsa-miR-484 used as endogenous controls for other infectious diseases such as Hepatitis B and breast cancer were defined from internal control gene-stability measure analysis (Hu et al., 2012; Li et al., 2015). We first performed the expression stability of two internal control non-related genes in all samples (**Figure 1A**) and the algorithm for the normalization of the endogenous microRNAs was more stable than using the cel-miR-39 spike-in control (**Figure 1B**). Based on our findings, we decided to normalize the expression profile of cardiac-miRNA genes using a geometric mean of miR-221 and miR-484 expression as described in the methods section. In fact normalyzation analysis of cardiac-specific miR-208a and miR-34a related to spike-in control did not have significant differences among the groups as determined to access proper sample isolation for comparison between samples (**Figure 2**).

Using this averaging of the control genes in order to measure expression levels accurately, we next investigate whether the myocardial damage induced by *T. cruzi* infection is associated with the expression of miR-208a, a key factor in promoting cardiac hypertrophy during cardiovascular dysfunction. Based on our results, we found significant increased levels of circulating plasma miR-208a in cross-sectional studies (**Table 1**) of chronic chagasic patients at the indeterminate (IND) as compared

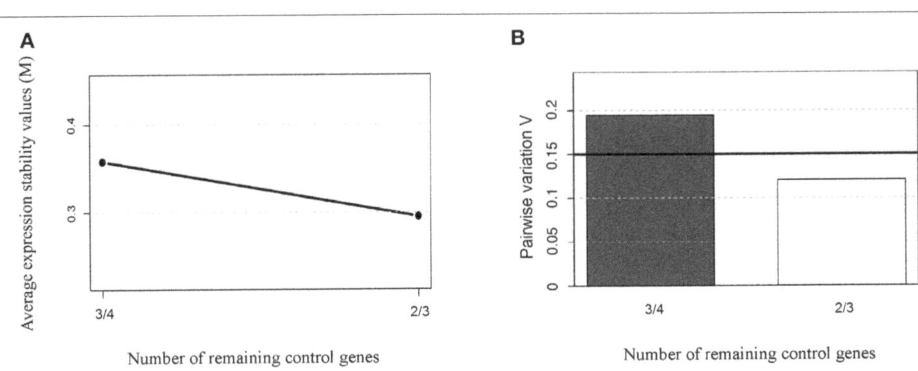

FIGURE 1 | Average expression stability of endogenous miRNAs. Ranking of the gene expression stability (M) performed in all samples analyzed in the study during stepwise exclusion **(A)**. A lower *M*-value indicates more stable expression. The least stable genes are on the left using the spike-in cel-miR-39 control gene; and the most stable genes are represented on the right using the expression of endogenous hsa-miR-221-3p and hsa-miR-484 as references. The non-related microRNAs hsa-mir-221-3p and hsa-miR-484 were used for relative normalization as endogenous controls. The optimal number of control genes was determined for normalization by Pairwise variation **(B)**, as described in section Materials and Methods.

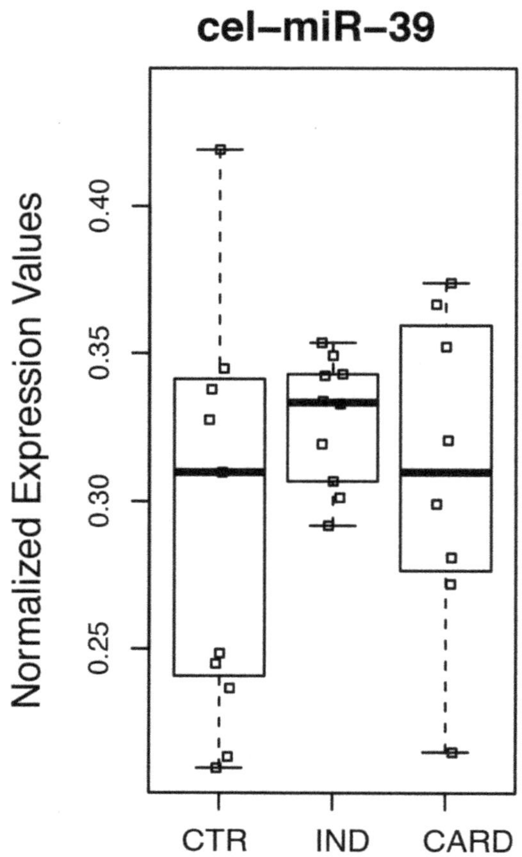

FIGURE 2 | Normalyzation analysis of cardiac-specific miR-208a and miR-34a related to cel-miR-39 spike-in gene. Spike-in control using external control miRNA gene expressed in *C. elegans* (cel-miR-39) was determined to access proper sample isolation for accurate comparison between samples. Real-time quantitative PCR was performed on total miRNA purified from plasma of non-infected individuals (CTR), patients at the indeterminate (IND), and cardiac (CARD) clinical forms of Chagas disease. Twenty donors, age, and sex matched-individuals were included for each group. Groups were compared by Mann-Whitney non-parametric test.

to cardiac (CARD) clinical forms of Chagas disease or non-infected control individuals (**Figure 3A**). However, we did not find any significant difference across the clinical groups in the expression levels of circulating miR-34a, a key regulator promoting cardiomyocyte cell death associated to heart failure (**Figure 3B**).

Although our goal is to investigate the plasma levels of cardiac miRNAs as potential candidate biomarkers of risk-predicting for patients in clinical prognosis, in fact some tissue-specific miRNA do not present satisfactory circulating levels in biomarkers analyzes.

We next ruled out the possibility that the absence of this modulation is due to an intrinsic characteristic of miR-34a being differentially expressed in cardiac tissues. We then measured the levels of intracardiac expression of this miRNA using an experimental Chagas' infection model. The murine models of heart disease share at different levels some of the pathophysiological changes seen in patients with chronic heart disease, such as extra-cellular deposition of fibronectin in the heart tissue and severe alterations of the heart's electrical activity (Pereira et al., 2014). These parameters are characteristic of more advanced forms of chronic human disease, so the murine model is not useful for studying the potential pathophisiological changes observed in the human chronic indeterminate phase of Chagas disease.

Therefore, using the murine experimental model of *Trypanosoma cruzi* infection-induced cardiomyopathy, by intraperitoneally injecting C57BL/6 mice with 2×10^3 bloodstream trypomastigotes of Y strain parasites, we observed a precocious blood parasitemia at day 8 post-infection (**Supplementary Figure 1A**), which further induced severe parasitism in the heart tissues as the infection continued (**Supplementary Figure 1B**). The heart parasitism intensity in this model is associated with cardiac muscle damage and can be monitored by measuring the release of CK-MB isoform of creatine kinase by heart muscle. This cardiac marker resides in the cytosol and facilitates the movement of high energy phosphates required for mitochondrial physiology.

Since CK-MB isoform has a short duration, its plasma levels can be used to access the level of heart tissue damage during the cardiopathy process (Adams et al., 1993; Pereira et al., 2014). As expected, we found a marked increase in the levels of CK-MB present in the peripheral blood circulation of *T. cruzi*-infected mice at 14 DPI (**Supplementary Figure 1C**). Our data indicated that this level of myocardial damage induced by *T. cruzi* infection is not associated with differences in the intracardiac expression of miR-34a as compared to non-infected controls (**Supplementary Figure 1D**), further indicating that the heart injury induced in the context of *T. cruzi* infection is not associated with upregulation of miR-34a pathway-dependent decline in cardiac activity. This finding corroborates the previous results showing unaltered plasma levels of miR-34a in the patients groups thus indicating that pro-apoptotic role of this cardiac miRNA is not involved in the heart injuries associated to chagas cardiomyopathy.

DISCUSSION

Chagas cardiomyopathy is the most severe and life-threatening manifestation of human disease caused by the protozoan parasite *Trypanosoma cruzi* (Marin-Neto et al., 2007). The knowledge of pathological changes in Chagas heart disease is largely derived from necropsy studies and endomyocardial biopsy of humans and observations in several experimental models that reasonably reproduce the various stages of the disease (Higuchi Mde et al., 1986; de Souza et al., 2001). The clinical manifestations and the tissue damage itself are closely associated with parasite multiplication and the consequent immunological reaction triggered in the parasitized myocardium (Marin-Neto et al., 2007). Thus, it is plausible to speculate that even if the parasitism is low-level, it may represent a mechanism of permanent antigenic activation and may constitute an

TABLE 1 | Circulating plasma miRNA in cross-sectional studies of chronic chagasic patients.

	Global *p*-value	log2(1ND/CTR)	*p*-value	log2(CARDC/CTR)	*p*-value	log2(CARDC/IND)	*p*-value
hsa-miR-208a-3p	0.008	0.942057053	0.005982038	0.1998333	0.923464	−0.742223753	0.18242931
hsa-miR-34a-5p	0.083	0.848200376	0.095676453	0.663184964	0.32519	−0.185015411	0.967330108

CTR, control group; IND, indeterminate group; CARD, cardiac clinical form of Chagas disease group.

essential pathogenic factor of immunological alteration in the chronic phase of Chagas disease (Rossi et al., 2010; Tarleton, 2015).

With the remission of parasitemia and systemic inflammatory reactions, it is believed that during the indeterminate stage the process of focal active myocarditis is more frequent, leading to the cumulative destruction of myocardial fibers, associated with microvascular disorders, intense neuronal depopulation, and the establishment of a gradual process of reparative fibrosis of cardiac tissue (Marin-Neto et al., 2007; Machado et al., 2012). Several studies using human and experimental models have shed light on the cellular and molecular mechanisms underlined in the pathogenesis of chronic manifestation of Chagas diseases. The heart infection by *T. cruzi* causes an intense inflammatory reaction resulting in leukocyte infiltration of the organ with an severely altered pattern of inflammatory-mediated factors in the infected tissues as seen by the increased expression levels of pro-inflammatory cytokines, chemokines, nitric oxide and vasoactive mediators in the cardiovascular system, with the predominance of CD8 T cells among lymphocyte populations in the chronic chagasic cardiomyopathy (Machado et al., 2012; Tarleton, 2015).

At the cellular and tissue level, the inflammatory injury of the cardiac tissue is characterized by the presence of parasitic pseudocysts associated with myonecrosis and vasculitis, with an intense accumulation of extracellular collagen affecting the function of cardiac muscle fibers (Machado et al., 2012). It has been shown that transforming growth factor-beta (TGF-β) participates in the fibrosis and heart remodeling during infection influencing the development of myocardiopathy in Chagas disease (Araújo-Jorge et al., 2002). Activation of fibrosis processes occurs through assessment of TGF-β-induced Smad2/3 and p38/ERK signaling (Zhang et al., 2006; Kolosova et al., 2011). The chagasic myocardial damage is disseminated throughout the heart, leading to electrocardiogram (ECG) abnormalities due to arrhythmias, conduction disturbances and also repolarization changes. Those alterations are representative of the widespread cardiac tissue damage (Elizari and Chiale, 1993; Machado et al., 2012). The nature of this injury process is considered an important feature of the mechanisms associated with pathogenesis of Chagasic cardiovascular disease (Machado et al., 2012).

In the present study we demonstrated that the human chronic indeterminate phase of Chagas disease results in increased levels of circulating miR-208a, an essential regulator of the genes involved in cardiac hypertrophy and fibrosis (Cunha-Neto et al., 2005; Wang et al., 2013; Doka et al., 2015; Shyu et al., 2015; Zhang et al., 2017). MiR-208a is encoded by an intronic region of the Myh6 gene that encodes α-myosin heavy chain, the prevalent heavy-chain contractile protein in the developed adult heart (Cunha-Neto et al., 2005). Alterations in the miR-208a expression levels are frequently associated with pathological heart dysfunctions, such as hypertrophy, fibrosis, arrhythmias, contractile dysfunction and conduction abnormalities (Cunha-Neto et al., 2005; Wang et al., 2013; Doka et al., 2015; Shyu et al., 2015; Zhang et al., 2017). Indeed, overexpression of miR-208a is associated with coronary heart disease (Zhang et al., 2017), and its therapeutic inhibition leads to recovery of cardiac function during heart disease (Doka et al., 2015). It has been shown that transforming growth factor-β (TGF-β) activates mirR-208a to regulate hypertrophic-related genes and the effect of neutralizing TGF-β antibody attenuates miR-208a induced-expression in cardiomyocyte hypertrophy (Wang et al., 2013).

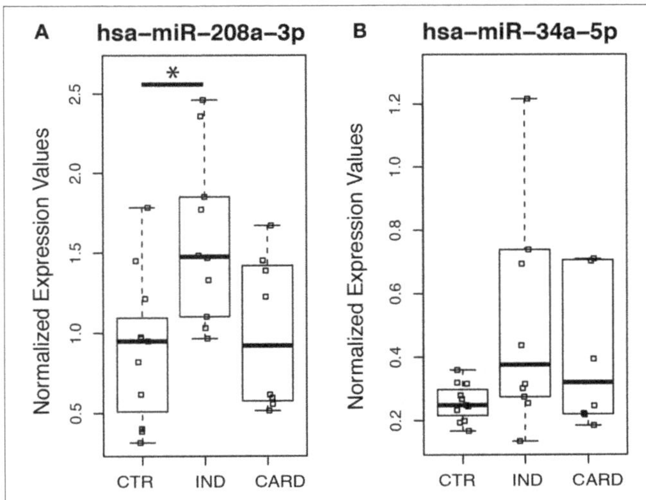

FIGURE 3 | Expression profiling of the heart-specific miR-34a and mir-208a in peripheral blood from chronic chagasic patients using endogenous miRNAs. Quantitative PCR was performed on total miRNA purified from plasma of normal control individuals (CTR), patients at the indeterminate (IND), and cardiac (CARD) clinical forms of Chagas disease. Individual and median values of relative expression of **(A)** hsa-miR-208a-3p or **(B)** hsa-miR-34a-5p normalized by the geometric mean of endogenous non-related hsa-mir-221-3p and hsa-miR-484 expression. Twenty donors, age, and sex matched-individuals were included for each group. Groups were compared by Mann-Whitney non-parametric test and the differences were considered significant at $^{*}p < 0.05$.

In fact the TGF-β signaling pathway has been shown to potentiate *T. cruzi* infection and heart damage in both human and experimental murine models (Araújo-Jorge et al., 2002, 2008, 2012; Waghabi et al., 2009). This suppressor cytokine is implicated in several aspects of host-parasite interplay. TGF-β is responsible for disarming the intracellular defense responses of *T. cruzi*-infected cells, thus potentiating the parasitic burden not only on macrophages but also on cardiac fibroblasts and cardiomyocytes (Araújo-Jorge et al., 2012); regulate the pro-inflammatory immune responses against *T. cruzi* (Gutierrez et al., 2009); and induction of fibrosis and heart injury during the chronicity of the disease (Araújo-Jorge et al., 2002, 2008; Waghabi et al., 2009). Indeed, circulating levels of TGF-β progressively increase during the chronicity of indeterminate stages for the cardiac, presenting a correlation with cardiac dysfunction and progressive fibrosis in Chagas disease (Araújo-Jorge et al., 2002). The regulation of targets by miRNAs is subject to various levels of control, and recent developments have shown that their targets can reciprocally control the level and function of miRNAs (Pasquinelli, 2012). Our data show that during the indeterminate phase of chronic infection, circulating levels of miR-208a are significantly increased. It is possible that there is a mutual regulation of miR-208a and its target genes, preceding the process of progressive fibrosis in Chagas disease during chronic infection.

Our findings therefore suggest a participation of the miR-208a in the early-onset events responsible for activation of the fibrosis and cardiac dysfunction processes in Chagas disease. Furthermore, our findings demonstrate that active myocardial inflammation promoted by *T. cruzi* infection does not yield altered levels of circulating miR-34a. MiR-34a negatively regulates the transcription of the anti-apoptotic factor PNUTS, and its response results in the induction processes of cardiac tissue degeneration (Filipowicz et al., 2008). Recent works have shown that miR-34a is an inducer of cardiomyocyte apoptosis, and its activation is determinant in cardiac senescence processes resulting in the induction of myocardial infarction processes (Filipowicz et al., 2008; Matsumoto et al., 2013). These findings suggest the participation of different mechanisms and signaling pathways of cardiac injury processes in *T. cruzi*-induced cardiomyopathy.

At present, the techniques of risk prediction in patients in the indeterminate phase of Chagas disease are based on the detection of cardiac wall motion abnormalities associated with functional and electrical defects. The presence of echocardiographic abnormalities in association with high interleukin-6 concentrations as a marker of myocardial injury has been highly predictive to screen patients for risk stratification (López et al., 2006). In this line, our findings demonstrating increased expression levels of circulating miR-208a during chronic indeterminate phase of Chagas disease should call attention to its predictive marker to identify patients at risk of developing chagasic heart disease. Subsequent translational studies should determine the levels of miR-208a in the course of chronic infection in order to determine its use as candidate biomarkers to be used in risk-prediction score for patients with Chagas cardiomyopathy.

AUTHOR CONTRIBUTIONS

AM: Conceived and designed the experiments; LL-L, AG, JG-N, and LC: Performed the experiments; LL-L, AG, JG-N, and LC: Analyzed the data; LF, CF, EF, SC, RA, RP, WS, and AM: Contributed reagents, materials, analysis tools; AG, RP, and AM: Wrote the paper.

ACKNOWLEDGMENTS

This work was supported by grants from Conselho Nacional de Desenvolvimento Científico e Tecnológico do Brasil (CNPq), Fundação de Amparo à Pesquisa do Estado do Rio de Janeiro (FAPERJ) and Focem/Mercosur.

SUPPLEMENTARY MATERIAL

Supplementary Figure 1 | Intra-cardiac levels of miR-34a expression in *T. cruzi*-induced myocarditis. **(A)** C57BL/6 mice were infected via *i.p.* with 2×10^3 blood-derived trypomastigote forms of Y strain of *T. cruzi* and the parasitemia for each mouse was determined during infection. The values are represented as the mean ± the standard deviation (*SD*) ($n = 5$). **(B)** DNA was extracted from heart tissue at 14 days post-infection and the parasite load was evaluated by quantitative PCR. **(C)** CK-MB levels were analyzed from serum at 14 DPI by enzymatic activity at 37°C. **(D)** MicroRNA-34a levels were measured from serum from non-infected control and *T. cruzi*-infected animals at 14 days post-infection by quantitative RT-PCR. Data are means ± *SD*. and represent the results of three independent experiments performed with 5 mice per treatment. Differences between between the groups were considered significant ***$p < 0.001$.

REFERENCES

1. Adams, J. E., Abendschein, D. R., and Jaffe, A. S. (1993). Biochemical markers of myocardial injury. Is MB creatine kinase the choice for the 1990s? *Circulation* 88, 750–763. doi: 10.1161/01.CIR.88.2.750
2. Andrade, L. O., and Andrews, N. W. (2005). The Trypanosoma cruzi-host- cell interplay: location, invasion, retention. *Nat. Rev. Microbiol.* 3, 819–823. doi: 10.1038/nrmicro1249
3. Araújo-Jorge, T. C., Waghabi, M. C., Bailly, S., and Feige, J. J. (2012). The TGF- β pathway as an emerging target for Chagas disease therapy. *Clin. Pharmacol. Ther.* 92, 613–621. doi: 10.1038/clpt.2012.102
4. Araújo-Jorge, T. C., Waghabi, M. C., Hasslocher-Moreno, A. M., Xavier, S. S., Higuchi Mde, L., Keramidas, M., et al. (2002). Implication of transforming growth factor-beta1 in Chagas disease myocardiopathy. *J. Infect. Dis.* 186, 1823–1828. doi: 10.1086/345882
5. Araújo-Jorge, T. C., Waghabi, M. C., Soeiro Mde, N., Keramidas, M., Bailly, S., and Feige, J. J. (2008). Pivotal role for TGF-β in infectious heart disease: the case of *Trypanosoma cruzi* infection and consequent Chagasic myocardiopathy. *Cytokine Growth Factor Rev.* 19, 405–413. doi: 10.1016/j.cytogfr.2008.08.002
6. Basso, D., Pesarin, F., Salmaso, L., and Solari, A. (2009). "Nonparametric one- way ANOVA," in *Permutation Tests for Stochastic Ordering and ANOVA. Theory and Applications with R* (New York, NY: Springer), 133–172. doi: 10.1007/978-0-387-85956-9
7. Boon, R. A., Iekushi, K., Lechner, S., Seeger, T., Fischer, A., Heydt, S., et al. (2013). MicroRNA-34a regulates cardiac ageing and function. *Nature* 495, 107–110. doi: 10.1038/nature11919
8. Burleigh, B. A., and Andrews, N. W. (1995). The mechanisms of *Trypanosoma cruzi* invasion of mammalian cells. *Annu. Rev. Microbiol.* 49, 175–200. doi: 10.1146/annurev.mi.49.100195.001135

9. Callis, T. E., Pandya, K., Seok, H. Y., Tang, R. H., Tatsuguchi, M., Huang, Z. P., et al. (2009). MicroRNA-208a is a regulator of cardiac hypertrophy and conduction in mice. *J. Clin. Invest.* 119, 2772–2786. doi: 10.1172/JCI 36154
10. Campos, C. F., Cangussú, S. D., Duz, A. L., Cartelle, C. T., Noviello, Mde L., Veloso, V. M., et al. (2016). Enteric neuronal damage, intramuscular denervation and smooth muscle phenotype changes as mechanisms of chagasic megacolon: long-term murine model of *Tripanosoma cruzi* infection. *PLoS ONE* 11:e0153038. doi: 10.1371/journal.pone.0153038
11. Cunha-Neto, E., Dzau, V. J., Allen, P. D., Stamatiou, D., Benvenutti, L., Higuchi, M. L., et al. (2005). Cardiac gene expression profiling provides evidence for cytokinopathy as a molecular mechanism in Chagas' disease cardiomyopathy. *Am. J. Pathol.* 167, 305–313. doi: 10.1016/S0002-9440(10)6 2976-8
12. de Souza, M. M., Franco, M., Almeida, D. R., Diniz, R. V., Mortara, R. A., da Silva, S., et al. (2001). Comparative histopathology of endomyocardial biopsies in chagasic and non-chagasic heart transplant recipients. *J. Heart Lung Transp.* 20, 534–543. doi: 10.1016/S1053-2498(00)00320-X
13. Dóka, G., Radik, M., Krenek, P., Kyselovic, J., and Klimas, J. (2015). 1a.02: microrna-208a and its host gene cardiac myosin heavy chain Myh6 are involved in hypertrophic heart dysfunction. *J. Hypertens* 33(Suppl. 1), e1. doi: 10.1097/01.hjh.0000467352.59037.c9
14. Elizari, M. V., and Chiale, P. A. (1993). Cardiac arrhythmias in Chagas' heart disease. *J. Cardiovasc. Electrophysiol.* 4, 596–608. doi: 10.1111/j.1540-8167.1993.tb01247.x
15. Eulalio, A., Mano, M., Dal Ferro, M., Zentilin, L., Sinagra, G., Zacchigna, S., et al. (2012). Functional screening identifies miRNAs inducing cardiac regeneration. *Nature* 492, 376–381. doi: 10.1038/nature11739
16. Faragó, N., Zvara, A., Varga, Z., Ferdinandy, P., and Puskás, L. G. (2011). Purification of high-quality micro RNA from the heart tissue. *Acta Biol. Hung.* 62, 413–425. doi: 10.1556/ABiol.62.2011.4.7
17. Ferreira, L. R., Frade, A. F., Santos, R. H., Teixeira, P. C., Baron, M. A., Navarro, I. C., et al. (2014). MicroRNAs miR-1, miR-133a, miR-13 miR-208a and miR-208b are dysregulated in chronic Chagas disease cardiomyopathy. *Int. J. Cardiol.* 175, 409–417. doi: 10.1016/j.ijcard.2014.05.019
18. Filipowicz, W., Bhattacharyya, S. N., and Sonenberg, N. (2008). Mechanisms of post-transcriptional regulation by microRNAs: are the answers in sight? *Nat. Rev. Genet.* 9, 102–114. doi: 10.1038/nrg2290
19. Gutierrez, F. R., Mineo, T. W., Pavanelli, W. R., Guedes, P. M., and Silva, J. S. (2009). The effects of nitric oxide on the immune system during *Trypanosoma cruzi* infection. *Mem. Inst. Osw. Cruz* 104(Suppl. 1), 236–245. doi: 10.1590/S0074-02762009000900030
20. Higuchi Mde, L., Lopes, E. A., Saldanha, L. B., Barretto, A. C., Stolf, N. A., Bellotti, G., et al. (1986). Immunopathologic studies in myocardial biopsies of patients with Chagas' disease and idiopathic cardiomyopathy. *Rev. Inst. Med. Trop. Sao Paulo* 28, 87–90. doi: 10.1590/S0036-46651986000200004
21. Hu, Z., Dong, J., Wang, L. E., Ma, H., Liu, J., Zhao, Y., et al. (2012). Serum microRNA profiling and breast cancer risk: the use of miR-484/191 as endogenous controls. *Carcinogenesis* 33, 828–834. doi: 10.1093/carcin/bgs030
22. Kollien, A. H., and Schaub, G. A. (2000). The development of Trypanosoma cruzi in triatominae. *Parasitol. Today* 16, 381–387. doi: 10.1016/S0169-4758(00)0 1724-5
23. Kolosova, I., Nethery, D., and Kern, J. A. (2011). Role of Smad2/3 and p38 MAP kinase in TGF-β1-induced epithelial-mesenchymal transition of pulmonary epithelial cells. *J. Cell. Physiol.* 226, 1248–1254. doi: 10.1002/jcp. 22448
24. Lepletier, A., de Almeida, L., Santos, L., da Silva Sampaio, L., Paredes, B., González, F. B., et al. (2014). Early double-negative thymocyte export in *Trypanosoma cruzi* infection is restricted by sphingosine receptors and associated with human Chagas disease. *PLoS Negl. Trop. Dis.* 8:e3203. doi: 10.1371/journal.pntd.0003203
25. Li, Y., Zhang, L., Liu, F., Xiang, G., Jiang, D., and Pu, X. (2015). Identification of endogenous controls for analyzing serum exosomal miRNA in patients with hepatitis B or hepatocellular carcinoma. *Dis. Mark.* 2015:893594. doi: 10.1155/2015/893594
26. López, L., Arai, K., Giménez, E., Jiménez, M., Pascuzo, C., Rodríguez-Bonfante, C., et al. (2006). C-reactive protein and interleukin-6 serum levels increase as Chagas disease progresses towards cardiac failure. *Rev. Esp. Cardiol.* 59, 50–56. doi: 10.1157/13083649
27. Machado, F. S., Jelicks, L. A., Kirchhoff, L. V., Shirani, J., Nagajyothi, F., Mukherjee, S., et al. (2012). Chagas heart disease: report on recent developments. *Cardiol. Rev.* 20, 53–65. doi: 10.1097/CRD.0b013e31823efde2
28. Machado, F. S., Martins, G. A., Aliberti, J. C., Mestriner, F. L., Cunha, F. Q., and Silva, J. S. (2000). *Trypanosoma cruzi*-infected cardiomyocytes produce chemokines and cytokines that trigger potent nitric oxide-dependent trypanocidal activity. *Circulation* 102, 3003–3008. doi: 10.1161/01.CIR.102.24.3003
29. Marin-Neto, J. A., Cunha-Neto, E., Maciel, B. C., and Simões, M. V. (2007). Pathogenesis of chronic Chagas heart disease. *Circulation* 115, 1109–1123. doi: 10.1161/CIRCULATIONAHA.106.624296
30. Matsumoto, S., Sakata, Y., Suna, S., Nakatani, D., Usami, M., Hara, M., et al. (2013). Circulating p53-responsive microRNAs are predictive indicators of heart failure after acute myocardial infarction. *Circ. Res.* 113, 322–326. doi: 10.1161/CIRCRESAHA.113.301209
31. Noireau, F., Diosque, P., and Jansen, A. M. (2009). *Trypanosoma cruzi*: adaptation to its vectors and its hosts. *Vet. Res.* 40:26. doi: 10.1051/vetres/2009009
32. Pasquinelli, A. E. (2012). MicroRNAs and their targets: recognition, regulation and an emerging reciprocal relationship. *Nat. Rev. Genet.* 13, 271–282. doi: 10.1038/nrg3162
33. Pereira, I. R., Vilar-Pereira, G., Silva, A. A., and Lannes-Vieira, J. (2014). Severity of chronic experimental Chagas' heart disease parallels tumour necrosis factor and nitric oxide levels in the serum: models of mild and severe disease. *Mem. Inst. Oswaldo Cruz* 109, 289–298. doi: 10.1590/0074-0276140033
34. Rassi, A. Jr., Rassi, A., and Marin-Neto, J. A. (2009). Chagas heart disease: pathophysiologic mechanisms, stratification. *Mem. Inst. Oswaldo Cruz* 104(Suppl. 1), 152–158. doi: 10.1590/S0074-02762009000900021
35. Rassi, A. Jr., Rassi, A., and Marin-Neto, J. A. (2010). Chagas disease. *Lancet* 375, 1388–1402. doi: 10.1016/S0140-6736(10)60061-X
36. Ritz, C., and Spiess, A. N. (2008). qpcR: an R package for sigmoidal model selection in quantitative real-time polymerase chain reaction analysis. *Bioinformatics* 24, 1549–1551. doi: 10.1093/bioinformatics/btn227
37. Rossi, M. A., Tanowitz, H. B., Malvestio, L. M., Celes, M. R., Campos, E. C., Blefari, V., et al. (2010). Coronary microvascular disease in chronic Chagas cardiomyopathy including an overview on history, pathology, and other proposed pathogenic mechanisms. *PLoS Negl. Trop. Dis.* 4:e674. doi: 10.1371/journal.pntd.0000674
38. Shyu, K. G., Wang, B. W., Cheng, W. P., and Lo, H. M. (2015). MicroRNA-208a increases myocardial endoglin expression and myocardial fibrosis in acute myocardial infarction. *Can. J. Cardiol.* 31, 679–690. doi: 10.1016/j.cjca.2014.12.026
39. Tarleton, R. L. (2015). CD8+ T cells in *Trypanosoma cruzi* infection. *Semin. Immunopathol.* 37, 233–238. doi: 10.1007/s00281-015-0481-9
40. Teixeira, A. R., Hecht, M. M., Guimaro, M. C., Sousa, A. O., and Nitz, N. (2011). Pathogenesis of chagas' disease: parasite persistence and autoimmunity. *Clin. Microbiol. Rev.* 24, 592–630. doi: 10.1128/CMR.00063-10
41. Vandesompele, J., De Preter, K., Pattyn, F., Poppe, B., Van Roy, N., De Paepe, A., et al. (2002). Accurate normalization of real-time quantitative RT-PCR data by geometric averaging of multiple internal control genes. *Genome Biol.* 3:research0034.1. doi: 10.1186/gb-2002-3-7-research0034
42. Waghabi, M. C., de Souza, E. M., de Oliveira, G. M., Keramidas, M., Feige, J. J., Araújo-Jorge, T. C., et al. (2009). Pharmacological inhibition of transforming growth factor beta signaling decreases infection and prevents heart damage in acute Chagas' disease. *Antim. Agents Chemother.* 53, 4694–4701. doi: 10.1128/AAC.00580-09
43. Wang, B. W., Wu, G. J., Cheng, W. P., and Shyu, K. G. (2013). Mechanical stretch via transforming growth factor-beta1 activates microRNA-208a to regulate hypertrophy in cultured rat cardiac myocytes. *J. Formosan Med. Assoc.* 112, 635–643. doi: 10.1016/j.jfma.2013.01.002
44. World Health Organization (2017). *Chagas Disease (American Trypanosomiasis). Fact Sheet.* Geneva.

45. Zhang, L., and Tarleton, R. L. (1999). Parasite persistence correlates with disease severity and localization in chronic Chagas' disease. *J. Infect. Dis.* 180, 480–486. doi: 10.1086/314889
46. Zhang, M., Fraser, D., and Phillips, A. (2006). ERK, p38, and Smad signaling pathways differentially regulate transforming growth factor-beta1 autoinduction in proximal tubular epithelial cells. *Am. J. Pathol.* 169, 1282–1293. doi: 10.2353/ajpath.2006.050921
47. Zhang, Y., Li, H. H., Yang, R., Yang, B. J., and Gao, Z. Y. (2017). Association between circulating microRNA-208a and severity of coronary heart disease. *Scand. J. Clin. Lab. Invest.* 77, 379–384. doi: 10.1080/00365513.2017.1328740

20

L-Arginine Uptake by Cationic Amino Acid Transporter Promotes Intra-Macrophage Survival of *Leishmania donovani* by Enhancing Arginase-Mediated Polyamine Synthesis

*Abhishek Mandal[1], Sushmita Das[2], Ajay Kumar[1], Saptarshi Roy[3], Sudha Verma[1], Ayan Kumar Ghosh[1], Ruby Singh[1], Kumar Abhishek[1], Savita Saini[1,4], Abul Hasan Sardar[1†], Bidyut Purkait[1], Ashish Kumar[1], Chitra Mandal[3] and Pradeep Das[1]**

[1] *Department of Molecular Biology, Rajendra Memorial Research Institute of Medical Sciences (ICMR), Patna, India,*
[2] *Department of Microbiology, All India Institute of Medical Sciences (AIIMS), Patna, India,* [3] *Cancer Biology and Inflammatory Disorder Division, CSIR-Indian Institute of Chemical Biology, Kolkata, India,* [4] *Department of Biotechnology, National Institute of Pharmaceutical Education and Research, Hajipur, India*

Correspondence:
Pradeep Das
drpradeep.das@gmail.com

The survival of intracellular protozoan parasite, *Leishmania donovani,* the causative agent of Indian visceral leishmaniasis (VL), depends on the activation status of macrophages. L-Arginine, a semi-essential amino acid plays a crucial regulatory role for activation of macrophages. However, the role of L-arginine transport in VL still remains elusive. In this study, we demonstrated that intra-macrophage survival of *L. donovani* depends on the availability of extracellular L-arginine. Infection of THP-1-derived macrophage/human monocyte-derived macrophage (hMDM) with *Leishmania*, resulted in upregulation of L-arginine transport. While investigating the involvement of the transporters, we observed that *Leishmania* survival was greatly impaired when the transporters were blocked either using inhibitor or siRNA-mediated downregulation. CAT-2 was found to be the main isoform associated with L-arginine transport in *L. donovani*-infected macrophages. L-arginine availability and its transport regulated the host arginase in *Leishmania* infection. Arginase and inducible nitric oxide synthase (iNOS) expression were reciprocally regulated when assayed using specific inhibitors and siRNA-mediated downregulation. Interestingly, induction of iNOS expression and nitric oxide production were observed in case of inhibition of arginase in infected macrophages. Furthermore, inhibition of L-arginine transport as well as arginase resulted in decreased polyamine production, limiting parasite survival inside macrophages. L-arginine availability and transport regulated Th1/Th2 cytokine levels in case of *Leishmania* infection. Upregulation of L-arginine transport, induction of host arginase, and enhanced polyamine production were correlated with increased level of IL-10 and decreased level of IL-12 and TNF-α in *L. donovani*-infected macrophages. Our findings provide clear evidence for targeting the metabolism of L-arginine and L-arginine-metabolizing enzymes as an important therapeutic and prophylactic strategy to treat VL.

Keywords: macrophage, *Leishmania*, L-arginine, CAT-2, arginase, nitric oxide, polyamine, cytokine

INTRODUCTION

Leishmania donovani, the causative agent of Indian visceral leishmaniasis (VL) exhibit a dimorphic life cycle, transmitted by a *Phlebotomine* sand fly vector as flagellated promastigotes and inhabit within mammalian macrophages (MΦs) as amastigotes. The destiny of intracellular amastigotes relies predominantly on the MΦ-activation status, which is largely affected by different cytokines and chemokines (1–3).

While diverse molecules and characteristics of macrophages are reciprocally or mutually exclusively related to the activation status of macrophages, the dichotomous regulation of L-arginine metabolism is at the center of the different functions that are associated with classically or alternatively activated macrophages. Classically activated MΦs can generate anti-microbicidal molecules and oxidative mediators and eliminate parasites successfully, whereas "alternatively" activated MΦs augment parasite persistence (4, 5). Although two apparent types of MΦ activation can lead to antithetical outcomes of infection, these two pathways employ L-arginine as a common substrate for their enzymatic activities.

L-Arginine is a non-essential amino acid for healthy adult human, but it has to be supplemented during growth or various disease states (6, 7) and has thus been characterized as a semi- or conditionally essential amino acid. Mammalian L-arginine metabolism is critical both at the level of the whole organism (6, 7) and at the level of the discrete cell types (8). In macrophages, L-arginine is an antecedent for principally two crucial metabolic pathways: it is metabolized either by inducible nitric oxide synthase (iNOS) to nitric oxide (NO) and citrulline or it is hydrolyzed by arginase to ornithine and urea. Arginase has two isoforms (arginase 1 and arginase 2), which catalyze the alike biochemical reaction but vary in cellular expression, cell-type-specific regulation, and subcellular localization one being cytosolic and the other mitochondrial, respectively (9, 10). The availability of L-arginine regulates the expression of different genes (7) and it is reported that L-arginine from the extracellular milieu is vital for iNOS-mediated NO production (11, 12). Furthermore, it is documented that the extent of arginase activities are indicators of disease extremity in human VL and in HIV infections (13–15).

Ornithine, the downstream molecule of L-arginine metabolism, is metabolized by ornithine decarboxylase, a rate-limiting enzyme, to produce polyamines which regulate several cellular processes like DNA replication, protein translation, cellular growth, and differentiation (16, 17). It is reported that polyamines enhance the growth of intracellular *Leishmania* amastigotes inside murine macrophages (18) and arginase-expressing granulocytes (13, 14). However, little is known about the role of polyamines in immune regulation. Therefore, macrophage L-arginine metabolism may have wide ranging implications for the type and outcome of immune responses.

Importance of L-arginine have been investigated considerably in cancer, trauma (19), and several other infectious diseases, including *Trypanosoma cruzi* (20), *Toxoplasma gondii* (21), *Pseudomonas aeruginosa* (22), *Plasmodium falciparum* (23), *Listeria monocytogenes* (24), and *Mycobacterium tuberculosis* (25) infections, but role of L-arginine in host immune responses against *L. donovani* infection and its biological relevance to disease outcome is obscure. Previous studies reported that trypanosomatids lack a biosynthetic route for L-arginine (26). *Leishmania* parasite cannot synthesize L-arginine *de novo*, indicating that its metabolism depends on extracellular supplies, making L-arginine, an essential amino acid for the growth and survival of the parasite (27, 28). Krassner and Flory reported that L-arginine is an important molecule for the growth of *Leishmania* parasites (29), and these parasites import this amino acid from *in vitro* culture media (29, 30) for their survival. Nonetheless, how the Leishmania parasite utilizes L-arginine inside macrophages and promotes its growth has yet not been clearly elucidated. Polyamine biosynthesis in *Leishmania* parasites takes a convoluted pathway, beginning with the L-arginine scavenged from the host, then translocated to glycosomes by an as yet unexplored permeation process (26). Furthermore, it has also been documented that *in vitro* cultured *Leishmania* parasites can directly attain and employ L-arginine from the extracellular milieu for polyamine production (26, 31). Previously, Castilho-Martins et al. reported that in *L. (L.) amazonensis*, arginine uptake is controlled by transporter-coding mRNA levels and they suggested a mechanism that senses internal arginine concentrations and regulates uptake of L-arginine by augmenting expression of arginine transporter (32). Later, Goldman-Pinkovich et al. reported that parasites respond to the inadequacy of L-arginine by elevating expression and activity of the *Leishmania* arginine transporter (LdAAP3) in addition to numerous other transporters and they proposed that the arginine deprivation response is mediated through a mitogen-activated protein kinase-2-dependent signaling cascade (33). However, the involvement of host pathways by which *Leishmania* can acquire the L-arginine pool within the MΦs remain obscure. Boitz et al. recently reported that arginase is essential for polyamine biosynthesis *de novo* and for promastigote growth in unsupplemented media but not for intracellular amastigotes suggesting that *L. donovani* amastigotes in the parasitophorous vacuole scavenge ornithine and spermidine for their survival (34).

Several mammalian L-arginine transport systems, encompassing systems y+, Bo+, bo+, and y + L, have been reported (35). The basal level of L-arginine is retained mainly through the y + L system in non-activated MΦs, while transport through the y+ system exacerbates considerably in activated MΦs (36). The cationic amino acid transporter family (CAT) belongs to the y+ system transporter family that comprises four members, CAT-1 to CAT-4, encoded by the *Slc7A1* to *-4* genes, respectively (35). Arginine is transported by the first three members (CAT-1, -2, and -3) of the CAT family (37). CAT-1 is ubiquitously expressed excluding in liver while CAT-3 is rendered only in brain. CAT-2 exists in two isoforms, with CAT-2A being basically expressed in the liver and muscle cells (38) and CAT-2B in the macrophages (39). CAT-2B is induced by cytokines in several cell types, including MΦs and plays a critical role in the modulation of iNOS and arginase activities (40). However, there is limited knowledge on how this transporter directly determines the outcome of *Leishmania* infection. It is reported that in MΦs with impairing L-arginine transporter, NO and polyamine synthesis were diminished upon activation with Th1 and Th2 cytokines, respectively

(36), demonstrating that L-arginine accessibility is the impediment control step for both iNOS and arginase.

In the present study, we deciphered the involvement of CAT for the transport of L-arginine in *Leishmania*-infected macrophages and tried to understand the pathways by which L-arginine is utilized. Our study indicated that intra-macrophage survival of *L. donovani* depends on the availability and transport of extracellular L-arginine because intra-macrophage parasite burden was reduced upon inhibition of L-arginine availability and transport either by pharmacological inhibitor or by siRNA-mediated downregulation of the transporter. Furthermore, CAT-2 was observed to be the major isoform associated with L-arginine transport in *L. donovani*-infected macrophages. L-arginine supply regulated the host arginase in *Leishmania* infection. Simultaneously, inhibition of L-arginine transport as well as arginase leads to decreased polyamine production, resulting in decreased parasite survival inside macrophages. Therefore, we hope that understanding the biological role played by arginine deficiency in case of *Leishmania* infection will lead to its early identification and to the design of new and novel treatments.

MATERIALS AND METHODS

Ethics Statement

All studies were approved by the Institutional Human Ethical Committee of the Rajendra Memorial Research Institute of Medical Sciences (Patna, India). Human monocyte-derived macrophages (hMDM) were isolated from healthy adult individuals after written, informed consent. Routine experimentation with animals was approved by the Institutional Animal Ethical Committee of the Rajendra Memorial Research Institute of Medical Sciences, Patna, India.

Reagents

THP-1 cell line was purchased from NCCS, Pune, India. Phorbol 12-myristate 13-acetate (PMA), L-arginine, *N*-Ethylmaleimide (NEM; inhibitor of L-arginine transport), L-N^6-(1-Iminoethyl) lysine dihydrochloride (L-NIL; inhibitor of iNOS), sulfanilamide (component of Griess reagent), and *N*-(1-Naphthyl) ethylenediamine dihydrochloride (NED; component of Griess reagent) were purchased from Sigma-Aldrich (St. Louis, MO, USA). (S)-(2-Boronoethyl)-L-cysteine, HCl (BEC; inhibitor of arginase), and Dansyl chloride were purchase from EMD Millipore, USA. Fetal bovine serum (FBS), OptiMEM, dialyzed FBS, and Lipofectamine RNAiMax reagent were purchased from Invitrogen, USA. siRNAs for CAT-1 (sc-44923), CAT-2 (sc-77441), Arg-1 (sc-29728), Arg-2 (sc-29729), and iNOS (sc-29417) were purchased from Santa Cruz Biotechnology, USA. PCR primers were designed from Avantor, IDT, USA. HRP-conjugated secondary antibodies were purchased from Jackson Laboratory, USA. [^{3}H] L-arginine was purchased from PerkinElmer, Singapore. Amersham™ ECL™ Prime Western Blotting Detection Reagent was purchased from GE Healthcare, UK.

Culture of Parasite

Leishmania donovani strain AG83 (MHOM/IN/1983/AG83), used in this study was maintained routinely in golden hamsters by repeated passage to sustain its virulence. Amastigotes were isolated from the spleen of infected hamster and were made to undergo transformation from amastigotes to promastigotes routinely, prior to infection as described earlier (41). *Leishmania* parasites were grown at 22°C in normal RPMI media (Invitrogen, USA) and supplemented with 10% heat-inactivated dialyzed FBS (Invitrogen, USA), 25 mM HEPES, pH 7.4, 4 mM $NaHCO_3$, 100 U/ml of penicillin G-sodium (Sigma-Aldrich), and 100 mg/ml of streptomycin (Sigma-Aldrich), and these parasites were used for our experimental purpose. Levels of LPS in parasite stock preparations were found to be below the limit of detection [<0.1 endotoxin U/ml (LAL-test; BioWhittaker, Inc., Walkersville, MD, USA)].

Cell Culture and Infection

THP-1 cells, an acute monocytic leukemia-derived human cell line, were maintained in RPMI-1640 (Invitrogen, USA) medium supplemented with 10% heat-inactivated FBS (Invitrogen, USA) and penicillin (100 U/ml), streptomycin (100 mg/ml), and gentamycin (20 µg/ml) at 37°C in humidified air containing 5% CO_2. The cells were treated with 20 nM phorbol 12-myristate 7-acetate (PMA) for 48 h so as to become matured macrophage-like phenotype and adhered with plastic. Non-adherent cells were removed by washing with RPMI without FBS. The cells were then further incubated in complete RPMI media containing no PMA for 24 h before using it for the experimental purpose.

Blood was collected from healthy donors in heparinized tubes and was processed within 10 min after blood collection. Mononuclear cells were isolated from peripheral blood by density gradient centrifugation over Ficoll-Paque Plus (GE Healthcare, Piscataway, NJ, USA) according to the manufacturer's instructions. The viability of the mononuclear cells was checked by trypan blue dye exclusion method (~95%). hMDMs were isolated by the method as described previously (42). Briefly, isolated monocytes were cultured overnight in 6-well plates at a density of 2×10^6 cells per well in the presence of macrophage colony-stimulating factor (M-CSF) (300 ng/ml) in RPMI medium with 10% FBS. Non-adherent cells were repeatedly washed, and cells were allowed to differentiate into MDMs in the presence of M-CSF and 10% FBS. Differentiated MDMs were harvested after 96 h.

The THP-1 or hMDMs were infected with *Leishmania* parasites for 6 hs at macrophage/parasite multiplicities of 1:10. The unbound parasites were removed by washing with RPMI without FBS followed by additional incubation of up to 48 h in complete RPMI medium. The cells were then fixed followed by staining with May-Grunwald Giemsa and observation under bright field microscope at 100× with oil immersion. Parasite load was determined by counting the number of amastigotes per 100 macrophages and percent infectivity was calculated by counting the number of infected cells (43). The results were expressed as mean ± SD of three independent experiments performed in triplicate.

Transfection

THP-1 cells (1×10^6) or hMDMs were seeded in 6-well plate. Fresh siRNA transfection reagent containing siRNA (final concentration 25 nM), optiMEM, and lipofectamine RNAiMax was prepared by the protocol as described previously (44). The above reagent (200 μl) was added to each well and cultured for 6 h. Then, the supernatant was aspirated and cells were further cultured with fresh complete growth medium for 12–15 h before any inhibitor treatment. Confirmation of siRNA-mediated downregulation of target gene was evaluated by western blot analysis. Control cells were without siRNA.

Measurement of Arginase Activity

Arginase activity in THP-1 or hMDM lysates were measured using a micromethod as described previously (45, 46). Briefly, after incubations, cells were lysed with 0.1% Triton X-100. After 30 min on a shaker, 25 mM Tris–HCl were added to the lysate. Then, to this lysate, 10 mM $MnCl_2$ were added, and the enzyme was activated by heating for 10 min at 56°C. Arginine hydrolysis was supervised by incubating the lysate with 0.5 M L-arginine (pH 9.7) for 15–20 min at 37°C. The reaction was stopped with H_2SO_4 (96%)/H_3PO_4 (85%)/H_2O (1/3/7, v/v/v) followed by addition of α-isonitrosopropiophenone (dissolved in 100% ethanol) and heating at 95°C for 30 min. The concentration of urea produced was quantified at 540 nm. Protein concentration was measured by BCA method [Pierce Thermo Fisher Scientific]. One unit of enzyme activity was defined as the amount of enzyme that catalyzes the formation of 1 μmol urea/min. BEC (200 μM) was used as an inhibitor of arginase as described previously (43, 47). Each measurement was performed in triplicate and the data were expressed as mean ± SD of three independent experiments.

Measurement of NO

Nitrite (NO_2^-) accumulation was used as an indicator of NO production and measured by using the Griess reagent (48). THP-1 or hMDM culture supernatants were collected after 48 h of incubation. Equal volume of supernatants and Griess reagent [1% sulphanilamide/0.1% *n*-(1-napthyl) ethylenediamine dihydrochloride/2.5% H_3PO_4] were mixed and incubated for 10 min at room temperature. Absorbance was recorded at 540 nm in a plate reader (Thermo Multiscan, USA). Nitrite concentration was estimated using $NaNO_2$ as standard. L-NIL (100 ng/ml) was used as an inhibitor of iNOS as described previously (49).

Semi-Quantitative RT-PCR and Quantitive Real-time PCR

RNA was extracted from macrophages (THP-1 and hMDM), and c-DNA was prepared from 20 μg of total RNA using c-DNA synthesis kit (Invitrogen). The c-DNAs were used in PCR amplification of L-arginine transporters, such as CAT-1, CAT-2A, CAT-2B, arginine metabolizing enzymes such as Arg-1, Arg-2, iNOS, and cytokines such as IL-10, IL-12 and TNF-α using gene-specific primers. After initial denaturation at 94°C for 5 min, targeted genes were amplified (94°C for 45 s, 56°C or 58°C for 30 s, and 72°C for 1 min) for 25 amplification cycles followed by a final extension at 72°C for 10 min. The PCR products were run on ethidium bromide stained 1.5% agarose gel and finally documented and quantified in gel documentation system (Bio-Rad) associated Quantity One software. All the PCR products were normalized with respect to GAPDH transcript and expressed as fold change. Each measurement was performed in triplicate and one of the representative gel image was shown. The data were expressed as mean ± SD of three independent experiments.

These semi-quantitative data were further validated by quantitative real-time PCR, which was performed in the LightCycler 480 (Roche) using SYBR green (Roche) chemistry as described previously (50). The cycling conditions were as follows: 1 cycle at 95°C for 3 min and 40 cycles of 95°C for 15 s (denaturation), 58°C for 30 s (annealing), and 72°C for 30 s (extension). The fluorescence signal was captured at the end of each cycle using the SYBR channel (490 nm wavelength for excitation and 525 nm wavelength for emission). Results were analyzed by LightCyclerR 480 relative quantification software (Roche) and expressed as the target/reference ratios of each sample, normalized by the target/reference ratio of the calibrator. Here, the target/reference value of uninfected macrophages was used as calibrator and GAPDH was used as reference. The primers used for both semi-quantitative RT-PCR and quantitative real-time PCR are summarized in Table S1 in Supplementary Material.

Western Blotting

After individual incubations were over, protein was isolated from MΦs (THP-1 and hMDM). 50 μg of each protein were separated by electrophoresis on 12% SDS-polyacrylamide gel and transferred onto PVDF membrane (43). Membrane was washed with 1× TBST solution thrice and blocked with 3% BSA for 2 h at room temperature. Blocked membrane was washed in TBST solution thrice and then was incubated with monoclonal primary antibody against CAT-1, CAT-2, Arg-1, Arg-2, and iNOS. Horseradish peroxidase-conjugated secondary antibody was used, and the protein band was visualized by enhanced chemiluminescence reaction, normalized with respect to GAPDH and expressed as fold change. Each measurement was performed in triplicate and one of the representative gel image was shown. The data were expressed as mean ± SD of three independent experiments.

Measurement of Polyamines

Poyamines (putrescine and spermidine) were identified and quantified by a prederivatization method using high performance liquid chromatography (HPLC) as described by Balaña-Fouce et al. (51). Briefly, after incubations, both uninfected and infected macrophages were harvested, washed twice with PBS (pH 7.4), and the last pellet was disintegrated with 5% trichloroacetic acid (w/v) overnight. The extracts were centrifuged (10,000 *g*, 15 min), and the supernatant was neutralized with a saturated $NaHCO_3$ solution. The mixture was incubated with a solution containing 20 mg dansyl chloride/ml (Merck) in acetone (Merck. HPLC grade) at 50°C for overnight. The dansylated polyamines were extracted twice with toluene (Merck, HPLC grade), evaporated under nitrogen stream and the precipitate was dissolved in 1 ml of acetonitrile (Merck, HPLC grade), before analysis by HPLC on a C^{18} reverse-phase column (Shimadzu, Japan). Dansylated polyamines were quantified with a spectrofluorimeter at excitation of 330 nm and emission at 510 nm. The peak areas, retention times were recorded and calculated by a PC Integration Pack Programme. The level of polyamines were expressed as nmol per

10^6 cells. There were three replicates in each test, and the data were the mean ± SD of three independent observations.

Measurement of L-Arginine Transport

Uptake of L-arginine in macrophages were measured using the protocol described elsewhere (32) with minor modifications. Briefly, after incubation, THP-1 or hMDM (1×10^6 macrophages/ml) were pelleted down and washed with cold Earle's Balanced Salt Solution (EBSS) containing 137 mM NaCl, 26 mM $NaHCO_3$, 5 mM KCl, 1.8 mM $CaCl_2$, 1 mM NaH_2PO_4, 0.8 mM $MgSO_4$, and 5.5 mM glucose twice followed by resuspension in [^{3}H]-L-arginine (5 μCi/ml) using stock from 1 mCi/ml (specific activity-51.5 Ci/mmole) (PerkinElmer, Singapore) at 25°C. Uptake was stopped after 8 min by adding 50 mM of ice-cold L-arginine (non-radioactive). Macrophages were then washed twice with EBSS, lysed in lysing solution (0.1% SDS, 100 mM NaOH). The incorporated radioactivity inside cell was estimated using liquid scintillation counter (Tri-Carb 2810 TR, PerkinElmer, USA). Uptake was expressed as nmol/10^6 cells/min. NEM (CAT specific inhibitor, 250 μM) was used as an inhibitor of L-arginine transport as described previously (52, 53). Each measurement was performed in triplicate and data were expressed as mean ± SD of three independent experiments.

ELISA

The level of cytokines IL-10, IL-12, and TNF-α in the supernatant of THP-1 macrophages were determined using commercial BD OptEIA ELISA kits (BD, San Jose, CA, USA) according to manufacturer's protocol as described previously (41). The BD OptEIA test is a solid phase sandwich enzyme-linked immunosorbent assay (ELISA). Required quantities of strips were taken and 50 μl of ELISA diluent was added to each well. After that, 100 μl of standard/sample was added and incubation at RT was done for 2 h followed by five times washing. 100 μl of detection antibody was then added followed by 1 h incubation. Washing was done seven times, and 100 μl of TMB One-Step Substrate was added. Incubation was done for 30 min at RT and then 50 μl of stop solution was added to stop the reaction and quantitative measurement was done by taking absorbance at 450 nm. Cytokine concentrations were estimated from respective standard curve and expressed as pg/ml.

Statistical Analysis

We analyzed our data using Graph Pad Prism (Version 6.0, GraphPad Software, USA). Each experiment was repeated three times in separate sets and the results were expressed as Mean ± SD. Statistical differences were determined using Mann–Whitney *U* test for comparing two groups or Kruskal–Wallis with Dunn's multiple comparison test for comparing three or more groups. $p \leq 0.05$ were considered significant.

RESULTS

L-Arginine Availability Regulates *Leishmania* Viability inside Macrophages

In our previous study, we have shown that L-arginine is an important amino acid for the survival of *Leishmania* promastigotes. In that study, we observed that the viability and the cell proliferation were greatly diminished when parasites were grown in L-arginine-depleted media (43). In the present study, the same phenomena were examined in *Leishmania* parasites inside macrophages. Macrophages (THP-1 and hMDM) were cultured in L-arginine-depleted and L-arginine-supplemented RMPI medium separately and then infected with *L. donovani* parasite. However, macrophages were never switched from L-arginine-replete to L-arginine-depleted conditions. It was observed that macrophage viability was not altered upon L-argininie deprivation (data not shown). Further, it was observed that both parasite load (**Figures 1A,B,D**) and percent infectivity (**Figures 1A,C,E**) was increased at 48 h when compared to 6 and 24 h. Simultaneously, both parasite load and percent infectivity was significantly higher in L-arginine-supplemented media compared to L-arginine-depleted media at 24 and 48 h ($p \leq 0.05$). However, no significant change in parasite load or percent infectivity were observed at 6 h time point upon L-arginine deprivation from the culture media. Parasite load was found to be significantly reduced (~2.04-fold at 24 h and ~2.27-fold at 48 h; $p \leq 0.05$) in case of THP-1 macrophages grown in L-arginine-depleted medium compared to L-arginine-supplemented medium (**Figures 1A,B**). Similarly, significant decrease in parasite load was also observed (~2.16-fold at 24 h and ~2.29-fold at 48 h; $p \leq 0.05$) when hMDM were cultured in L-arginine-depleted medium compared to L-arginine-supplemented medium (**Figure 1D**). On the other hand, percent infectivity was significantly reduced (~1.5-fold at 24 h and ~1.6-fold at 48 h $p \leq 0.05$) when THP-1 macrophages were grown in L-arginine-depleted medium compared to L-arginine-supplemented medium (**Figures 1A,C**). Simultaneously, in case hMDM, percent infectivity was found to be reduced by ~1.65-fold at 24 h and ~1.6-fold at 48 h when macrophages were cultured in L-arginine-depleted medium compared to L-arginine-supplemented medium (**Figure 1E**). Therefore, these findings suggested that the availability of L-arginine in the culture media promotes parasite survival inside macrophages. However, in its absence, parasite growth was significantly reduced indicating that L-arginine is an important amino acid for the survival of *Leishmania* inside macrophages.

Leishmania Infection Upregulates L-Arginine Transport through CAT-2 Transporter

In the present study, we wanted to observe the effect of L-arginine starvation from extracellular milieu on the expression of macrophage L-arginine transporters (CAT-1, CAT-2) in normal and infected condition. We also measured the amount of L-arginine transport during *Leishmania* infection in presence or absence of L-arginine in the culture medium. THP-1-derived macrophages and hMDM were cultured in L-arginine-depleted as well as L-arginine-supplemented RPMI media and infected with *L. donovani* parasite for 48 h. The expression of CAT-1 and CAT-2 (CAT-2A and CAT-2B) were checked at the transcript level by semi-quantitive RT-PCR as well as quantitive real-time PCR and translational level by western blot. No significant change in CAT-1

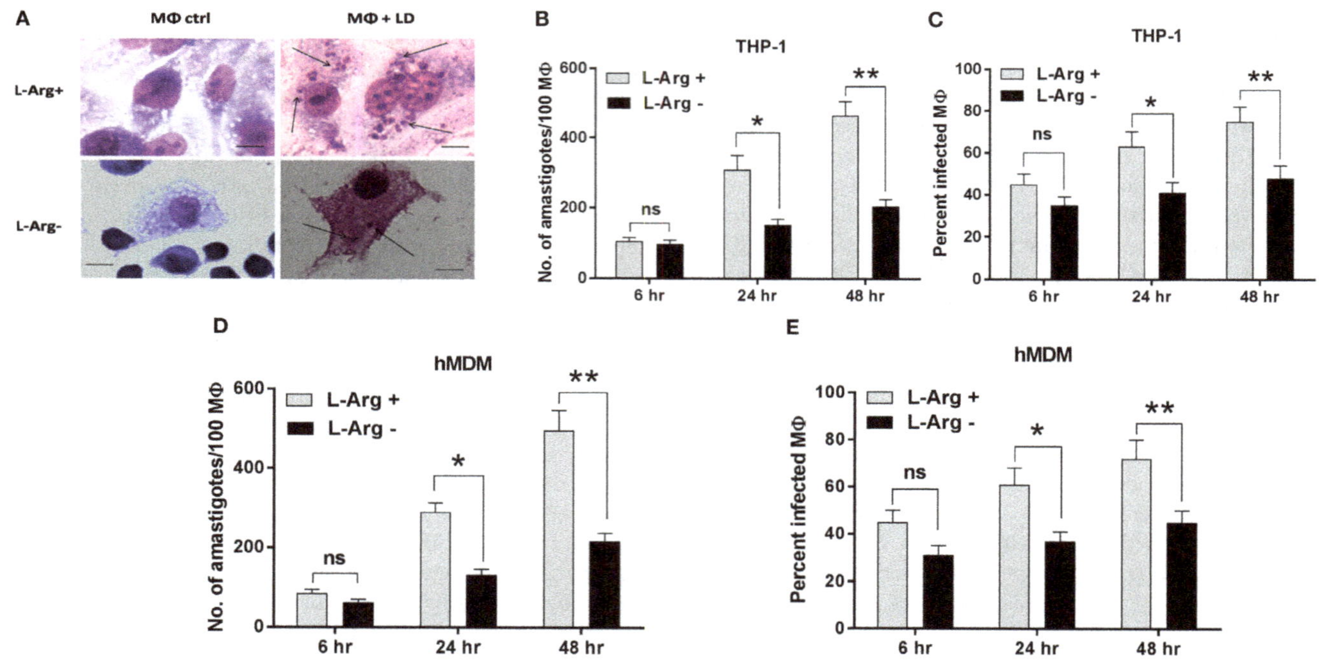

FIGURE 1 | Effect of L-arginine availability on survival of *Leishmania* parasite inside macrophages. THP-1 monocyte-derived MΦs **(A,B,C)** and human monocyte-derived macrophages (hMDM) **(D,E)** (5×10^4 cells/ml) were grown in L-arginine-supplemented and L-arginine-depleted RPMI medium followed by infection with *Leishmania donovani* (multiplicity of infection 1:10) for 6, 24, and 48 h. Intracellular parasites were visualized by staining the cells with Giemsa followed by optical microscopy at 100x oil immersion **(A)**. The horizontal bar indicates 5 µm size. The parasite load was measured by counting the number of intracellular amastigotes per 100 macrophages **(B,D)**. The rate of infection was analyzed by counting the percent infected macrophages **(C,E)**. Each experiment was repeated three times. Each determination was made in triplicate and the values were expressed as mean ± SD for three independent experiments. Mann–Whitney *U* test was used to evaluate statistical significance for comparing two groups; $^*p < 0.05$; $^{**}p < 0.005$.

or CAT-2A expression was observed in case of *Leishmania* infection either in L-arginine-depleted or L-arginine-supplemented condition (**Figures 2A–E**).

However, from the semi-quantitive PCR data, it was observed that in case of *Leishmania* infection to THP-1, the expression of CAT-2B transcript was increased by ~2.8-fold in L-arginine-supplemented condition and ~5.8-fold in L-arginine-depleted condition (**Figure 2A**). Similar results were observed when we checked the expression of CAT-2B by quantitive real-time PCR. In this case, the expression of CAT-2B transcript was increased by ~2.7-fold in L-arginine-supplemented condition and ~6.7-fold in L-arginine-depleted condition (**Figure 2B**). Comparative analysis indicated that CAT-2B transcript is significantly increased upon L-arginine deprivation (~2.1-fold, $p \leq 0.005$ in case of semi-QRT PCR and ~2.5-fold, $p \leq 0.005$ in case of quantitive real-time PCR) in case of *Leishmania* infection (**Figures 2A,B**). The expression of CAT-2B in *Leishmania*-infected hMDM was further checked by real-time PCR. It was observed that in case of *Leishmania* infection, the expression of CAT-2B transcript was increased by ~2.5-fold in L-arginine-supplemented condition and ~5.8-fold in L-arginine-depleted condition (**Figure 2C**). Comparative analysis indicated that L-arginine deprivation led to significant increase (~2.3-fold, $p \leq 0.005$) in CAT-2B transcript in *Leishmania*-infected macrophages compared to L-arginine supplementation (**Figure 2C**). Simultaneously, from the western blot data, it was also observed that deprivation of L-arginine led to significant increase (~2.8-fold, $p \leq 0.005$) in CAT-2 in *Leishmania*-infected macrophages when compared to L-arginine supplementation (**Figure 2D**).

The expression of CAT-2 in *Leishmania*-infected hMDM were also checked by western blot and comparative analysis indicated that CAT-2 is significantly increased in case of *Leishmania* infection upon L-arginine deprivation (~2.1-fold, $p \leq 0.005$) compared to L-arginine supplementation (**Figure 2E**).

The expression of CAT-1 and CAT-2 was further assessed in *Leishmania*-infected macrophages pretreated with inhibitor of L-arginine transport (NEM) both at the transcript and translational level. Surprisingly, no significant change in CAT-1 or CAT-2 expression was observed in case of NEM pretreatment either at the transcript or protein level (**Figures 3A–E**).

Uptake of L-arginine in uninfected and infected THP-1 and hMDM were measured by radioactivity incorporation. It was observed that in case of *Leishmania* infection to THP-1, L-arginine transport was increased by ~2.7-fold in normal condition and ~4.2-fold in case of L-arginine deprivation (**Figure 4A**). However, at the same time, comparative analysis indicated that L-arginine deprivation leads to significant increase (~2.3-fold, $p \leq 0.005$) in L-arginine transport in *Leishmania*-infected THP-1 (**Figure 4A**).

Simultaneously, when we measured L-arginine transport in *Leishmania*-infected hMDM, it was observed that in case of

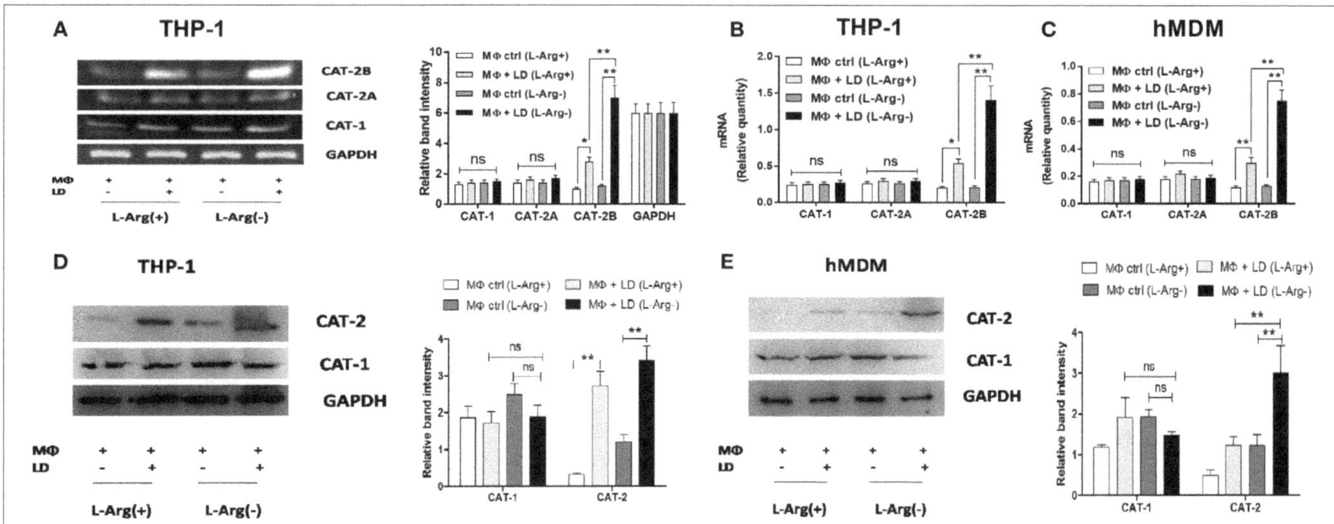

FIGURE 2 | Effect of *Leishmania* infection on expression of CAT-1 and CAT-2. THP-1 monocyte-derived MΦs **(A,B,D)** and human monocyte-derived macrophages (hMDM) **(C,E)** (1×10^6 cells/ml) were grown in L-arginine-supplemented and L-arginine-depleted RPMI medium followed by infection with *Leishmania donovani* (multiplicity of infection 1:10) for 48 h. The expression of CAT-1 and CAT-2 (CAT-2A and CAT-2B) were evaluated at the transcript level by semi-quantitative RT-PCR **(A)** and real-time PCR **(B,C)** and protein level by western blotting **(D,E)**. The intensity of the bands were quantified by densitometry in Quantity one software. Each experiment was repeated three times. Semi-QRT PCR gel images and western blots are representative of three experiments. Densitometric plots are shown adjacent to the gel images. Data are mean ± SD ($n = 3$) (*$p < 0.05$; **$p < 0.001$; ns, non-significant) (Mann–Whitney *U* test).

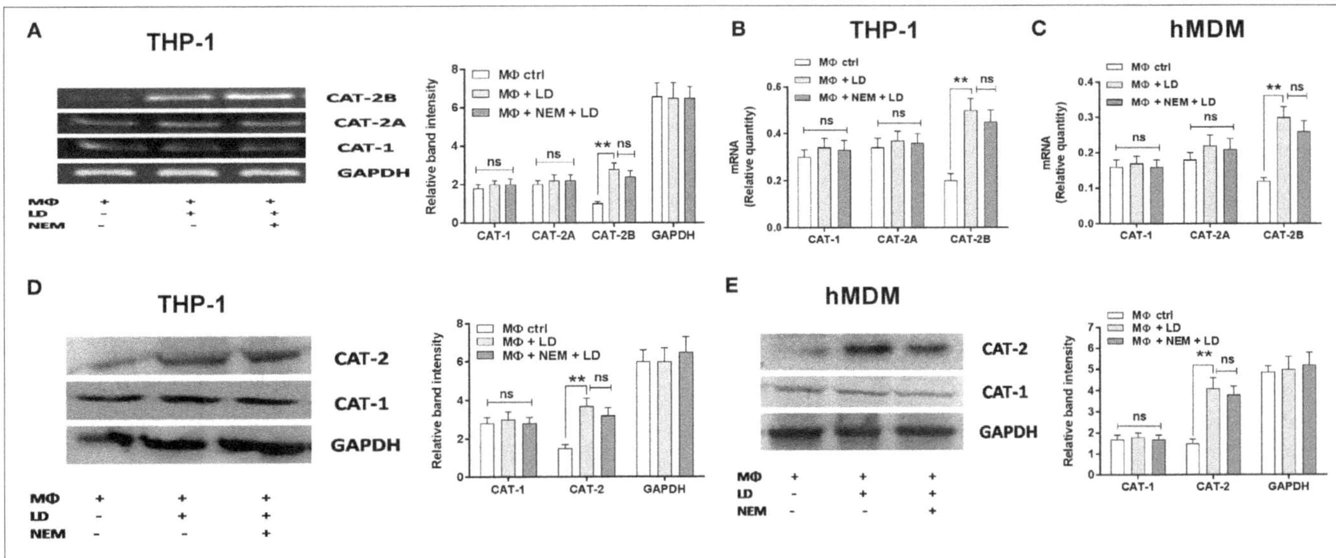

FIGURE 3 | Effect of NEM on expression of CAT-1 and CAT-2 in *Leishmania donovani*-infected macrophages. THP-1 MΦs **(A,B,D)** and human monocyte-derived macrophages (hMDM) **(C,E)** were left untreated or preincubated with NEM (250 μM) for 10 min followed by infection with *L. donovani* for 48 h. The expression of CAT-1 and CAT-2 (CAT-2A and CAT-2B) were evaluated at the transcript level by semi-quantitative RT-PCR **(A)** and real-time PCR **(B,C)** and protein level by western blotting **(D,E)**. The intensity of the bands were quantified by densitometry in Quantity one software. Each experiment was repeated three times. Semi-QRT PCR gel images and western blots are representative of three experiments. Densitometric plots are shown adjacent to the gel images. Data are mean ± SD ($n = 3$) (*$p < 0.05$; **$p < 0.001$; ns, non-significant) (Mann–Whitney *U* test).

Leishmania infection, L-arginine transport was increased by ~2.3-fold in normal condition and ~3.6-fold in case of L-arginine deprivation condition (**Figure 4B**). Furthermore, comparative analysis indicated that L-arginine transport is significantly increased in case of *Leishmania* infection upon L-arginine deprivation (~1.8-fold, $p \leq 0.005$) compared to L-arginine-supplemented condition (**Figure 4B**).

The effect of NEM on macrophage L-arginine transport was further checked. It was observed that NEM pretreatment decreased L-arginine transport by ~2.4-fold in *Leishmania*-infected

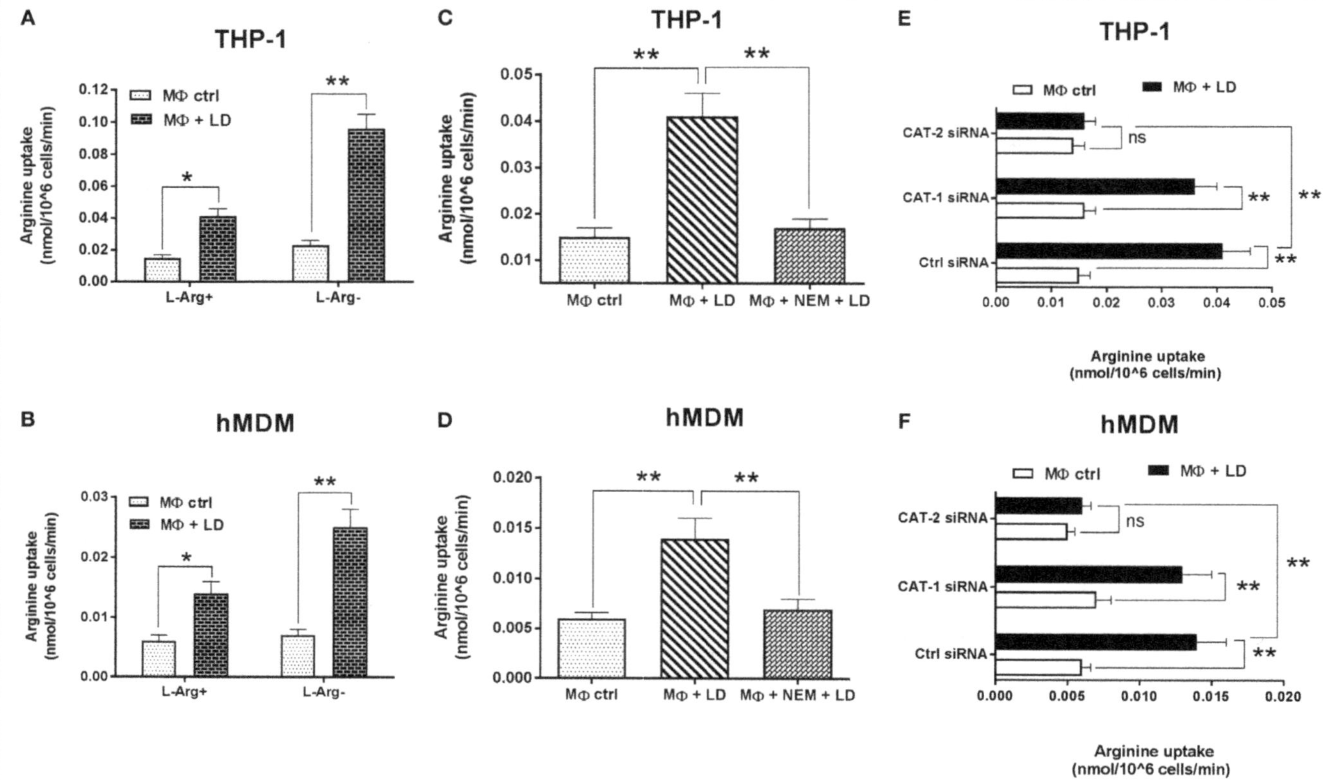

FIGURE 4 | Effect of *Leishmania* infection on L-arginine transport. THP-1 monocyte-derived MΦs **(A)** and human monocyte-derived macrophages (hMDM) **(B)** (1 × 10^6 cells/ml) were grown in L-arginine-supplemented and L-arginine-depleted RPMI medium followed by infection with *Leishmania donovani* (multiplicity of infection 1:10) for 48 h. In another experiment, THP-1 MΦs **(C)** and hMDM **(D)** were left untreated or preincubated with NEM (250 μM) for 10 min followed by infection with *L. donovani* for 48 h. In a separate experiment, THP-1 MΦs **(E)** and hMDM **(F)** (1 × 10^6 cells/ml) were transfected with control siRNA, CAT-1 or CAT-2 siRNA followed by infection with *L. donovani* for 48 h. Arginine transport was measured after incubating the cells with 1 μCi/ml of [^{3}H] L-arginine uptake solution for 8 min followed by counting the incorporation of [^{3}H] L-arginine in liquid scintillation counter **(A–F)**. Each experiment was repeated three times. Each determination was made in triplicate and the values were expressed as mean ± SD for three independent experiments. Kruskal–Wallis with Dunn's multiple comparison test was used to evaluate statistical significance for comparing three or more groups; *$p < 0.05$; **$p < 0.005$; ns, non-significant.

THP-1 macrophages (**Figure 4C**) and ~2.0-fold in *Leishmania*-infected hMDM (**Figure 4D**).

Further, to confirm that CATs are the main transporters for L-arginine in macrophages, we downregulated macrophage CAT-1 and CAT-2 by siRNA-mediated transfection and then infected with *Leishmania* parasite. It was observed that silencing of CAT-1 or CAT-2 had no significant effect on L-arginine transport in uninfected macrophages (**Figures 4E,F**). Simultaneously, CAT-1 knock down showed no significant decrease in L-arginine transport in *Leishmania*-infected THP-1 macrophages or hMDM. On the other hand, CAT-2 silencing leads to significant decrease (~2.6-fold; $p \leq 0.005$) in L-arginine transport in *Leishmania*-infected macrophages compared to normal infected macrophage (**Figures 4E,F**). Hence, our results suggested that CAT-2 is the main isoform associated with L-arginine transport in *Leishmania*-infected macrophages. Our study pointed out that as *Leishmania* is auxotroph for L-arginine, it modulates the host to upregulate the expression of CAT, thereby increases L-arginine uptake and utilizes this amino acid for their survival inside macrophages.

Inhibition of Macrophage L-Arginine Transport Limits *Leishmania* Survival inside Macrophages

Further, we studied the effect of inhibition of L-arginine transport upon survival of *Leishmania* parasite inside macrophages. For this, we pretreated both THP-1 macrophages and hMDM with NEM (250 μM) and infected with *Leishmania* parasite for 48 h and measured the parasite load and percent infectivity. A ~2.4-fold reduction in parasite load (**Figures 5A,B**) and ~2.3-fold reduction in percent infectivity (**Figures 5A,C**) was observed when THP-1 macrophages were pretreated with NEM. Similar results were observed with the use of hMDM. In this case ~2.8-fold reduction in parasite load (**Figure 5B**) and ~2.7-fold reduction in percent infectivity (**Figure 5C**) was observed when hMDM were pretreated with NEM.

Parasite load and percent infectivity were further measured in CAT-1 and CAT-2 siRNA transfected *Leishmania*-infected THP-1 macrophages and hMDM. It was observed that silencing of CAT-1 had no significant effect on parasite load and percent

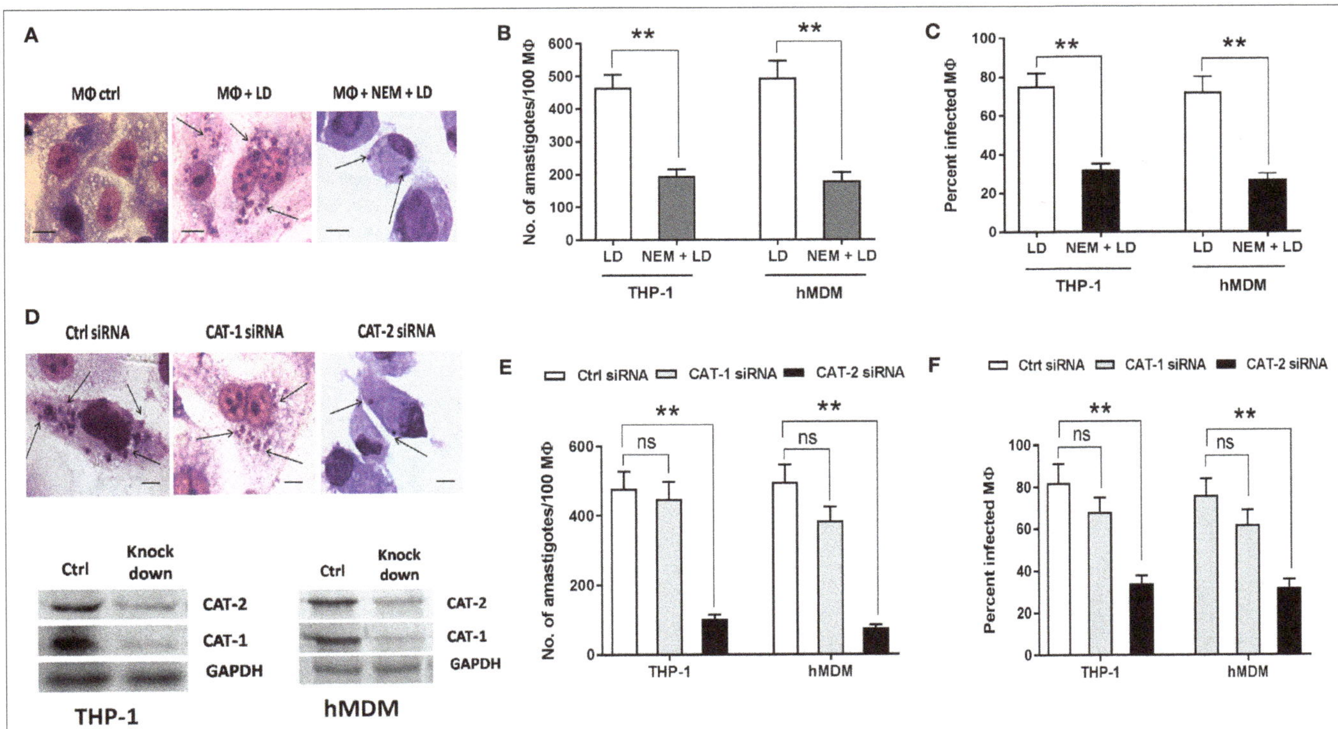

FIGURE 5 | Effect of inhibition of macrophage L-arginine transport on survival of *Leishmania* inside MΦ. THP-1 monocyte-derived MΦs **(A–C)** and human monocyte-derived macrophages (hMDM) **(B,C)** (5×10^4 cells/ml) were either left untreated or preincubated with 250 μM NEM for 10 min followed by infection with *Leishmania donovani* (multiplicity of infection 1:10) for 48 h. In a separate experiment, THP-1 MΦs **(D,E,F)** and hMDM **(E,F)** (1×10^6 cells/ml) were transfected with control siRNA, CAT-1 or CAT-2 siRNA followed by infection with *L. donovani* for 48 h. Intracellular parasites were visualized by staining the cells with Giemsa followed by optical microscopy at 100x oil immersion **(A,D)**. The horizontal bar indicates 5 μm size. The parasite load was measured by counting the number of intracellular amastigotes per 100 macrophages **(B,E)**. The rate of infection was analyzed by counting the percent infected macrophages **(C,F)**. Each experiment was repeated three times. Each determination was made in triplicate and the values were expressed as mean ± SD for three independent experiments. Mann–Whitney *U* test was used to evaluate statistical significance for comparing two groups. Kruskal–Wallis with Dunn's multiple comparison test was used to evaluate statistical significance for comparing three or more groups; *$p < 0.05$; **$p < 0.005$; ns, non-significant.

infectivity. However, CAT-2 knock down decreased the parasite load by ~4.7-fold (**Figures 5D,E**) and percent infectivity by ~2.4-fold (**Figures 5D,F**) in *Leishmania*-infected THP-1 macrophages compared to control siRNA transfected macrophages. Significant reduction in parasite load and percent infectivity were also observed in case of hMDM CAT-2 knock down (**Figures 5E,F**). Therefore, our study indicated that L-arginine transport is critically involved in the regulation of parasite survival inside macrophages.

L-Arginine Availability Regulates Expression of Arginase and iNOS in Infected Macrophages

The effect of L-arginine availability in regulation of arginase–iNOS balance in *Leishmania*-infected macrophages was investigated. We cultured THP-1 macrophages and hMDM in L-arginine-depleted as well as L-arginine-supplemented RPMI media, infected with *L. donovani* parasite for 48 h and checked the expression of Arg-1, Arg-2, and iNOS at the transcript level by semi-quantitive RT-PCR and quantitive real-time PCR. The expression of macrophage Arg-1 and Arg-2 was increased by ~2.3-fold and ~1.8-fold, respectively, upon *Leishmania* infection in case of normal (L-arginine supplementation) condition (**Figure 6A**). However, in case of L-arginine deprivation, no significant increase in Arg-1 or Arg-2 expression was observed upon *Leishmania* infection (**Figure 6A**). Comparative analysis indicated significant decrease in Arg-1 (~2.7-fold; $p \leq 0.005$) and Arg-2 (~1.8-fold; $p \leq 0.05$) expression in infected macrophages upon L-arginine deprivation (**Figure 6A**). However, no significant change in iNOS expression was observed upon L-arginine deprivation in case of *Leishmania* infection. Similar results were observed when the expression of these genes was studied by real-time PCR (**Figure 6B**).

The expression of these genes were further checked by limiting L-arginine availability through blockade of L-arginine transporter (CATs) by NEM (CAT specific inhibitor) and siRNA-mediated downregulation. NEM pretreatment decreased the expression of Arg-1 by ~2.0-fold and Arg-2 by ~1.5-fold in infected macrophages (**Figure 6C**). Similar results were observed when the expression of these genes were studied by real-time PCR (**Figure 6D**).

Furthermore, silencing of CAT-1 decreased the expression of Arg-1 by ~1.96-fold and had no significant effect

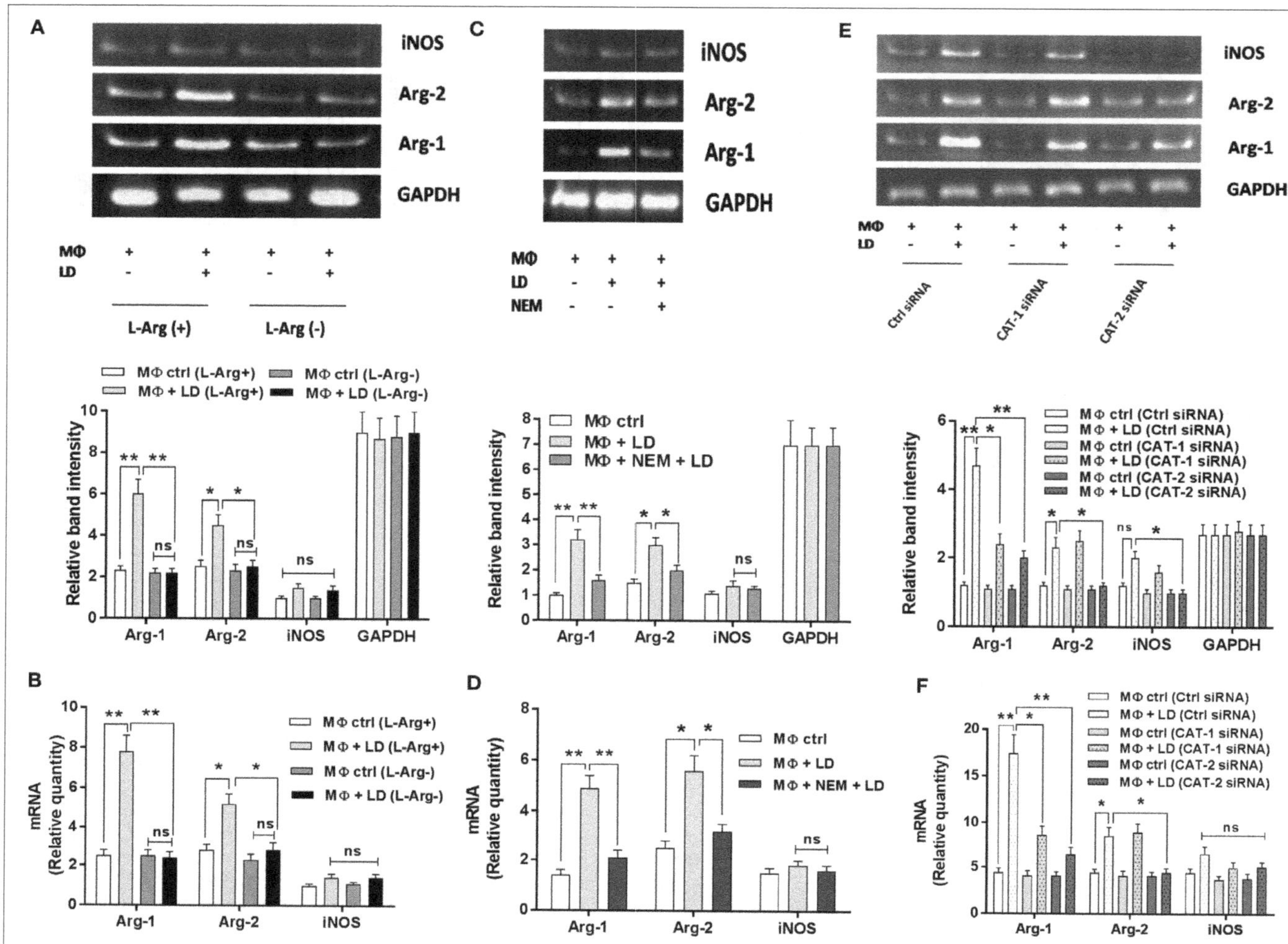

FIGURE 6 | Effect of inhibition of L-arginine availability on Arg-1, Arg-2, and inducible nitric oxide synthase (iNOS) expression in case of *Leishmania* infection. THP-1 monocyte-derived MΦs (1×10^6 cells/ml) were grown in L-arginine-supplemented and L-arginine-depleted RPMI medium followed by infection with *Leishmania donovani* (multiplicity of infection 1:10) for 48 h **(A,B)**. In another experiment, THP-1 monocyte-derived MΦs (1×10^6 cells/ml) were left untreated or preincubated with NEM (250 μM) for 10 min followed by infection with *L. donovani* for 48 h **(C,D)**. In a separate experiment, THP-1 monocyte-derived MΦs (1×10^6 cells/ml) were transfected with control siRNA, CAT-1, or CAT-2 siRNA followed by infection with *L. donovani* for 48 h **(E,F)**. The expression of Arg-1, Arg-2, and iNOS were determined at the transcript level by semi-quantitative RT-PCR **(A,C,E)** and real-time PCR **(B,D,F)**. The intensity of the bands was quantified by densitometry using Quantity one software. Each experiment was repeated three times. Each determination was made in triplicate and the values were expressed as mean ± SD for three independent experiments. Semi-QRT PCR gel images are representative of three experiments. Densitometric plots are shown below the gel images. Kruskal–Wallis with Dunn's multiple comparison test was used to evaluate statistical significance for comparing three or more groups; $^*p < 0.05$; $^{**}p < 0.005$; ns, non-significant.

on expression of Arg-2 and iNOS in *Leishmania*-infected macrophages. However, CAT-2 knock down decreased Arg-1 expression by ~2.3-fold, Arg-2 expression by ~1.9-fold, and iNOS expression by ~2.0-fold in *Leishmania*-infected macrophages compared to control siRNA transfected macrophages (**Figure 6E**). Simultaneously, when we checked the expression of these genes by real-time PCR, we also observed that silencing of CAT-1 decreased Arg-1 expression by ~2.0-fold whereas it had no significant effect on Arg-2 and iNOS expression in *Leishmania*-infected macrophages. On the other hand, CAT-2 knock down decreased the expression of Arg-1 by ~2.7-fold and Arg-2 by ~1.9-fold in *Leishmania*-infected macrophages (**Figure 6F**). Therefore, our results indicated that L-arginine availability and transport is critically involved in the regulation of Arg-1, Arg-2, and iNOS expression in *Leishmania*-infected macrophages.

The reciprocal regulation of arginase and iNOS in case of *Leishmania* infection was further evaluated at the transcript and translational level using an inhibitor of arginase (BEC) and iNOS (L-NIL). From the semi-quantitive RT-PCR data, it was observed that inhibition of iNOS increased Arg-1 transcript by ~1.9-fold and Arg-2 by ~1.9-fold, whereas, arginase inhibition upregulated iNOS transcript by ~4.6-fold in infected macrophages (**Figure 7A**). Simultaneously, real-time PCR data further confirmed that inhibition of iNOS led to significant increase in Arg-1 (~1.7-fold; $p \leq 0.05$) and Arg-2 (~1.7-fold; $p \leq 0.05$) transcript, whereas, arginase inhibition led to increased iNOS (~4.6-fold; $p \leq 0.05$) transcript in *Leishmania*-infected macrophages (**Figure 7B**).

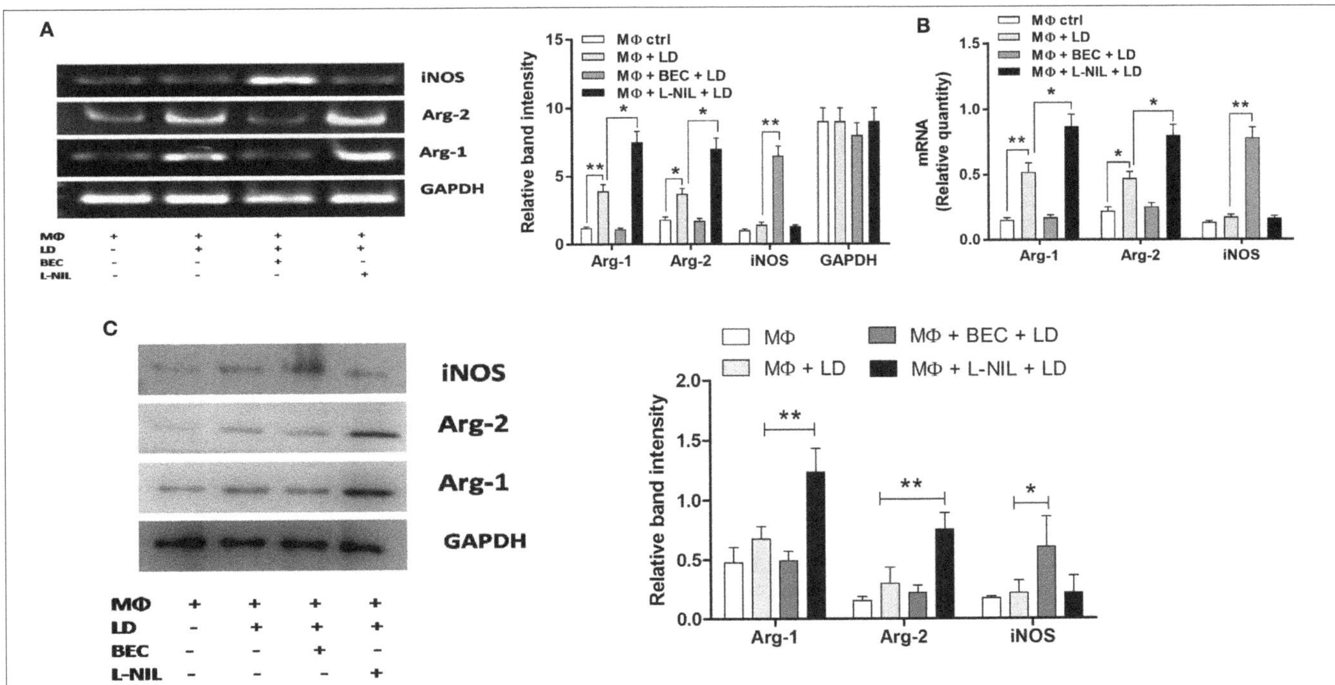

FIGURE 7 | Regulation of Arg-1, Arg-2, and inducible nitric oxide synthase (iNOS) expression in case of *Leishmania donovani* infection. THP-1 monocyte-derived MΦs (1 × 10^6 cells/ml) were either left untreated or preincubated with BEC (200 µM) or L-NIL (100 ng/ml) for 3 h followed by infection with *L. donovani* for 48 h **(A–C)**. The expression of Arg-1, Arg-2, and iNOS was determined at the transcript level by semi-quantitative RT-PCR **(A)** and real-time PCR **(B)** and protein level by western blotting **(C)**. The intensity of the bands was quantified by densitometry using Quantity one software. Each experiment was repeated three times. Each determination was made in triplicate and the values were expressed as mean ± SD for three independent experiments. Semi-QRT PCR gel images and western blots are representative of three experiments. Densitometric plots are shown adjacent to the gel images. Kruskal–Wallis with Dunn's multiple comparison test was used to evaluate statistical significance for comparing three or more groups; *$p < 0.05$; **$p < 0.005$.

In accordance with the semiQ-RT PCR and real-time PCR result, when we measured the protein level by western blot, we observed that the expression of Arg-1 was increased by ~2.5-fold and Arg-2 by ~2.1-fold upon *Leishmania* infection (**Figure 7C**). Arginase inhibition increased the iNOS expression by ~2.1-fold, whereas, inhibition of iNOS increased Arg-1 expression by ~1.6-fold and Arg-2 by ~1.8-fold in *Leishmania*-infected macrophages compared to normal infected macrophages (**Figure 7C**). Therefore, our study indicated that both Arg-1 and Arg-2 are upregulated at the transcript and translational level in case of *Leishmania* infection and Arg-1 is the major isoform associated with *L. donovani* infection. As downregulation of Arg-1 and Arg-2 increased the iNOS level, it is obvious that Arg-1/Arg-2-iNOS balance play a crucial role in regulation of each other and thereby determining the outcome of *Leishmania* infection.

Arginase activity at the enzymatic level was further measured in case of *Leishmania* infection upon L-arginine deprivation. Arginase activity was found to be increased by ~2.7- and ~1.6-fold in *Leishmania*-infected THP-1 macrophages compared to uninfected macrophages in case of L-arginine supplementation condition and L-arginine depletion condition, respectively (**Figure 8A**). Further, comparative analysis indicated significant decrease in arginase activity (~2.7-fold; $p \leq 0.005$) in *Leishmania*-infected THP-1 macrophages upon L-arginine deprivation (**Figure 8A**). Similar results were observed with hMDM. In this case, significant decrease in arginase activity (~2.1-fold; $p \leq 0.005$) was also observed in infected macrophages upon L-arginine deprivation (**Figure 8A**).

Simultaneously, inhibition of L-arginine transport by NEM decreased arginase activity by ~2.4-fold and ~2.43-fold in infected THP-1macrophages and hMDM, respectively, when compared to untreated infected macrophages (**Figure 8B**).

Arginase activity was further measured in CAT-1 and CAT-2 knock down *Leishmania*-infected macrophages. Our results indicated that silencing of CAT-1 had no significant effect on arginase activity in both *Leishmania*-infected THP-1 and hMDM (**Figure 8C**). On the other hand, CAT-2 knock down led to significant decrease in arginase activity (~2.3-fold; $p \leq 0.005$ in THP-1 and ~2.6-fold; $p \leq 0.005$ in hMDM) in infected macrophages compared to control siRNA transfected *Leishmania*-infected macrophages (**Figure 8C**).

However, while measuring the NO level, no significant change in NO level was observed in case of *Leishmania* infection upon L-arginine deprivation (**Figure 8D**). Pretreatment of NEM also had no significant effect on NO level in *Leishmania*-infected macrophages (**Figure 8E**). NO level was further measured in CAT-1 and CAT-2 siRNA transfected *Leishmania*-infected macrophages and similar results were observed (**Figure 8F**). Therefore, our results confirmed that L-arginine availability and transport is critically involved in the regulation of arginase

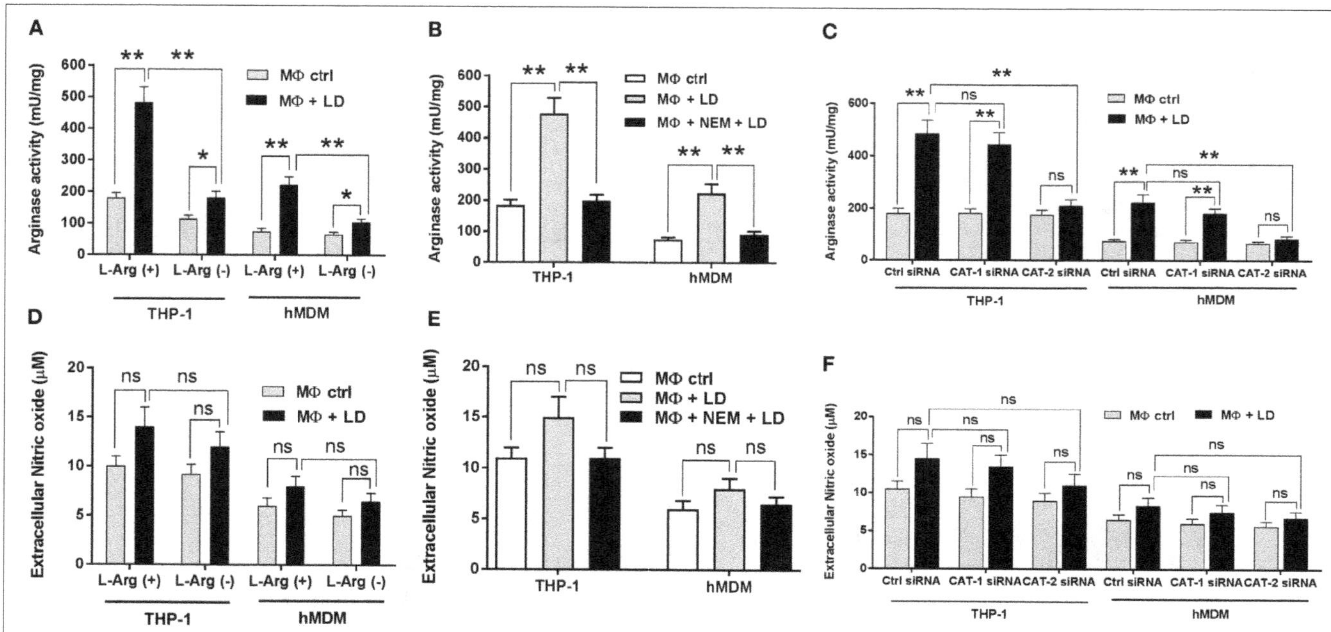

FIGURE 8 | Effect of inhibition of L-arginine availability on regulation of arginase activity and nitric oxide production in macrophages infected with *Leishmania donovani*. THP-1 monocyte-derived MΦs and human monocyte-derived macrophages (hMDM) (1 × 10[6] cells/ml) were grown in L-arginine-supplemented and L-arginine-depleted RPMI medium followed by infection with *L. donovani* (multiplicity of infection 1:10) for 48 h **(A,D)**. In a separate experiment, both THP-1 monocyte-derived MΦs and hMDM (1 × 10[6] cells/ml) were left untreated or preincubated with 250 μM NEM for 10 min followed by infection with *L. donovani* for 48 h **(B,E)**. In another experiment, both THP-1 monocyte-derived MΦs and hMDM (1 × 10[6] cells/ml) were transfected with control siRNA, CAT-1, or CAT-2 siRNA followed by infection with *L. donovani* for 48 h **(C,F)**. Arginase activity in MΦs was assessed spectrophotometrically by the method as described in Section "Materials and Methods." The protein content was measured by BCA method, and the enzyme activity was expressed as mU/mg protein **(A–C)**. Extracellular nitrite level was measured by Griess method using $NaNO_2$ as standard **(D–F)**. Each experiment was repeated three times. Each determination was made in triplicate and the values were expressed as mean ± SD for three independent experiments. Kruskal–Wallis with Dunn's multiple comparison test was used to evaluate statistical significance for comparing three or more groups; *$p < 0.05$; **$p < 0.005$; ns, non-significant.

activity without altering NO production in *Leishmania*-infected macrophages.

L-Arginine Availability and Transport Regulates Polyamine Production

Leishmania parasites and all other members of the trypanosomatid family depend on polyamines for growth and survival. As, L-arginine is the precursor molecule for synthesis of polyamines, trypanothiones, and tryparedoxin, the effect of L-arginine availability and transport on regulation of polyamine production for survival of *Leishmania* parasite inside macrophages was investigated. So, we cultured THP-1 macrophages in both L-arginine-depleted and L-arginine-supplemented RPMI media, infected with *L. donovani* and measured the putrescine and spermidine content. Putrescine level was found to be increased by ~3.0-fold and ~1.5-fold in *Leishmania*-infected macrophages compared to uninfected macrophages grown in L-arginine-supplemented and L-arginine-depleted media, respectively (**Figure 9A**). At the same time, spermidine level was increased by ~2.1-fold and ~1.6-fold (**Figure 9B**) upon L-arginine supplementation and L-arginine depletion condition, respectively, in infected macrophages. Simultaneously, when we compared the level of polyamines, we observed that putrescine (**Figure 9A**) and spermidine levels (**Figure 9B**) were significantly decreased (~2.8-fold, $p \leq 0.05$ for putrescine and for spermidine ~1.8-fold; $p \leq 0.05$) in L-arginine-depleted infected macrophages compared to L-arginine-supplemented macrophages.

Polyamine level was further measured in *Leishmania*-infected macrophages pretreated with L-arginine transporter inhibitor. It was observed that NEM pretreatment decreased putrescine level by ~2.8-fold (**Figure 9C**) and spermidine level by ~1.9-fold (**Figure 9D**) in infected macrophages compared to untreated infected macrophages. Putrescine level was found to be increased by ~3.0-fold, ~3.1–fold, and ~1.5-fold (**Figure 9E**) while spermidine level by ~2.2-fold, ~2.0–fold, and ~1.6-fold (**Figure 9F**) in control siRNA transfected, CAT-1 siRNA transfected, and CAT-2 siRNA transfected infected macrophages, respectively, in comparison to uninfected macrophages. Simultaneously, it was observed that knock down of CAT-1 had no significant effect on macrophage putrescine and spermidine level. However, CAT-2 knock down decreased the putrescine level by ~2.7-fold (**Figure 9E**) and spermidine level by ~1.9-fold (**Figure 9F**) in *Leishmania*-infected macrophages compared to control siRNA transfected infected macrophages. Therefore, our results showed clear decrease in the level of polyamines in infected macrophages in both L-arginine deprivation as well as during inhibition of L-arginine transport.

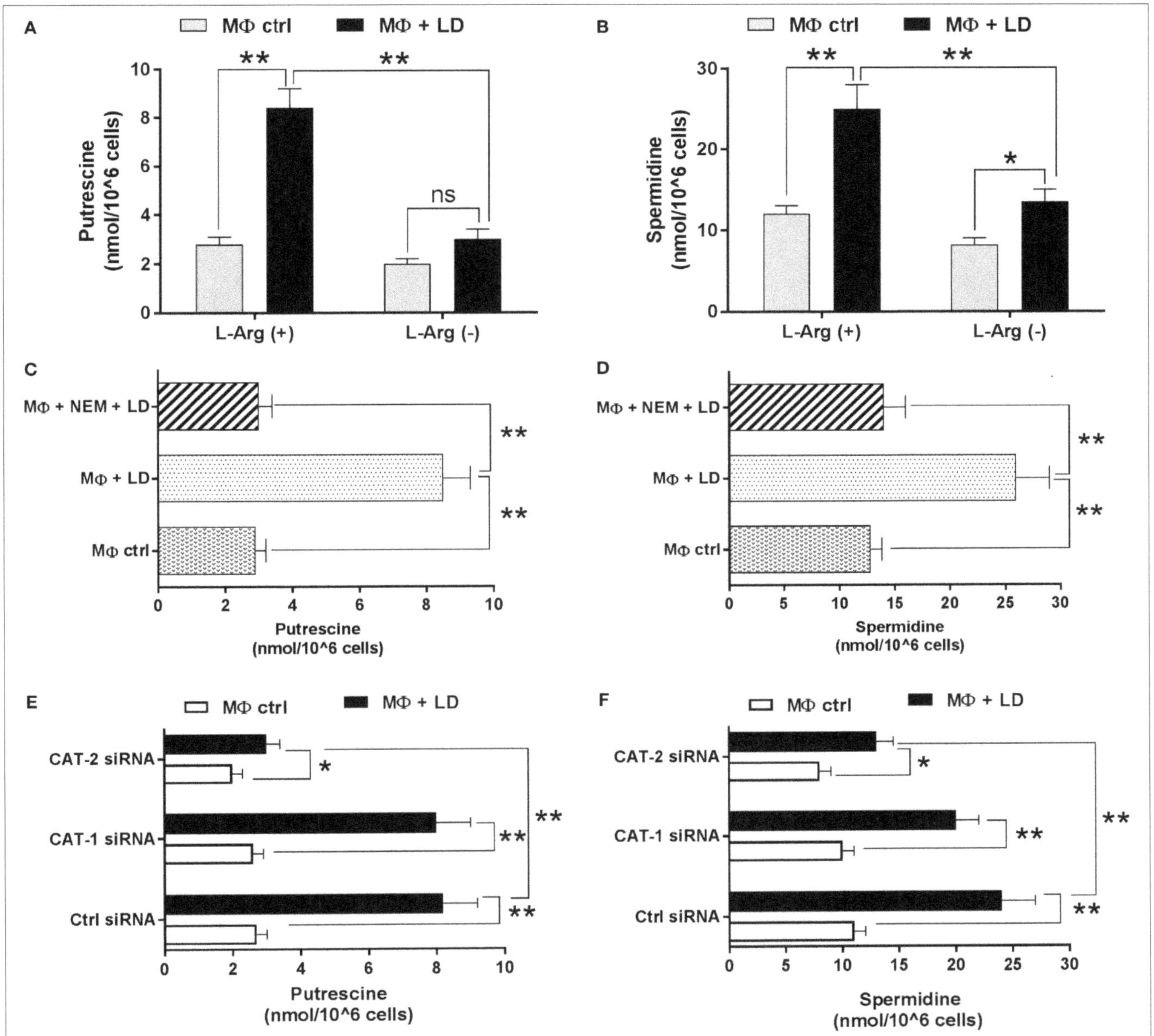

FIGURE 9 | Effect of inhibition of L-arginine availability on regulation of polyamine production in *Leishmania donovani*-infected macrophages. THP-1 monocyte-derived MΦs (1×10^6 cells/ml) were grown in L-arginine-supplemented and L-arginine-depleted RPMI medium followed by infection with *L. donovani* (multiplicity of infection 1:10) for 48 h **(A,B)**. In a seperate experiment, THP-1 MΦs (1×10^6 cells/ml) were either left untreated or preincubated with 250 µM NEM for 10 min followed by infection with *L. donovani* for 48 h **(C,D)**. In another experiment, THP-1 MΦs (1×10^6 cells/ml) were transfected with control siRNA, CAT-1 or CAT-2 siRNA followed by infection with *L. donovani* for 48 h **(E,F)**. The polyamines (putrescine and spermidine) were extracted by TCA precipitation followed by dansyl chloride derivatization, separation by reverse-phase high performance liquid chromatography as described in "Materials and Methods." Dansylated putrescine **(A,C,E)** and dansylated spermidine **(B,D,F)** were quantified by fluorescence spectrometry. Each experiment was repeated three times. Each determination was made in triplicate and the values were expressed as mean ± SD for three independent experiments. Kruskal–Wallis with Dunn's multiple comparison test was used to evaluate statistical significance for comparing three or more groups; $^{*}p < 0.05$; $^{**}p < 0.005$; ns, non-significant.

Significance of Arginase–iNOS Expression in the Survival of *Leishmania* inside Macrophages

Arginase–iNOS expression critically regulates the outcome of infection. In this study, we wanted to explore the role of arginase and iNOS in the regulation of *Leishmania* infection. It was observed that arginase inhibition decreased the parasite load by ~3.8-fold, whereas, iNOS inhibition increased the parasite load by ~1.7-fold (**Figure 10A**). Similar observation was found in case of measurement of percent infectivity. Arginase inhibition led to a decreased percent infectivity by ~1.9-fold (**Figure 10B**).

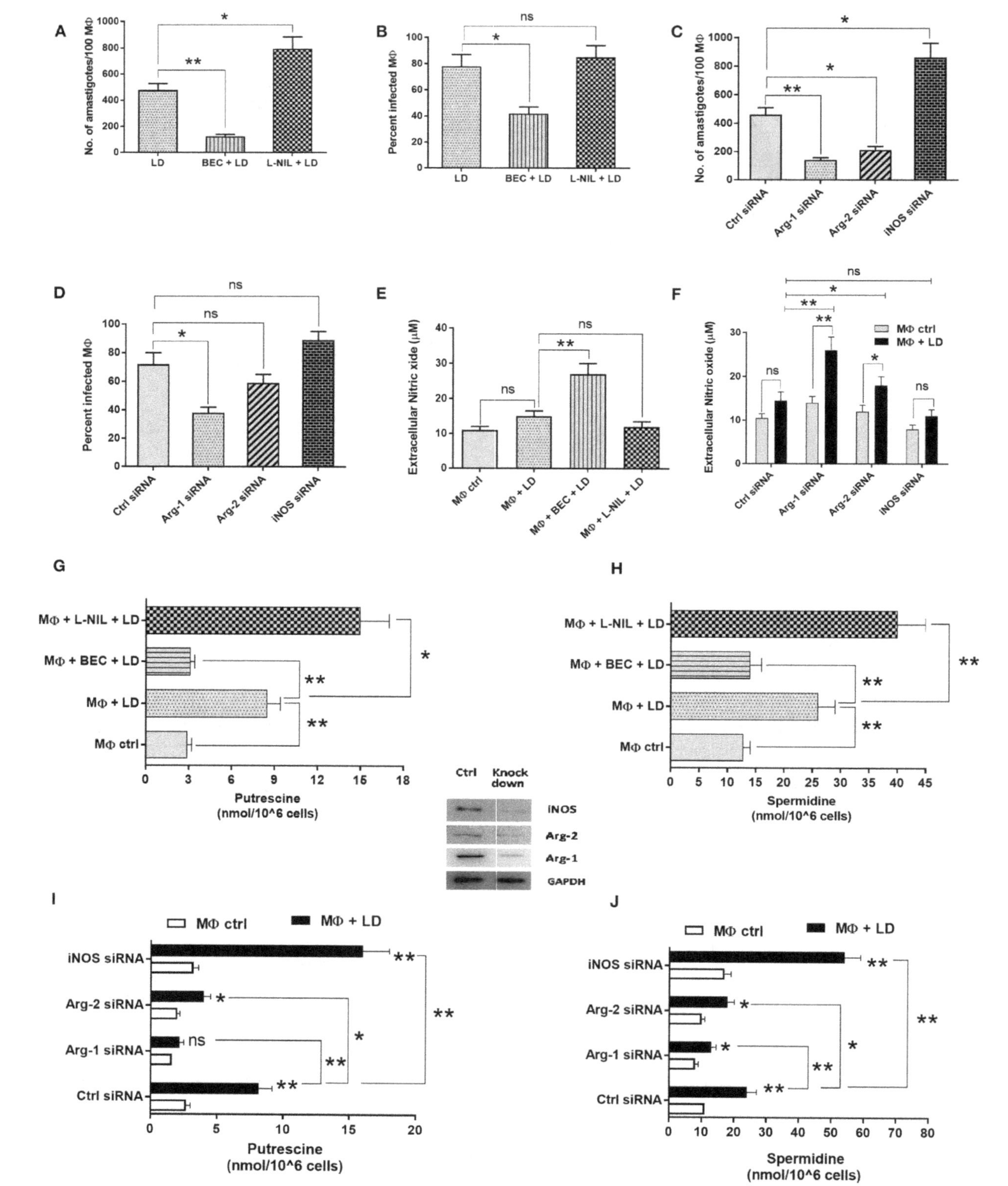

FIGURE 10 | Continued

FIGURE 10 | Continued
Effect of regulation of arginase-inducible nitric oxide synthase (iNOS) balance in *Leishmania donovani* survival inside macrophages. THP-1 monocyte-derived MΦs were either left untreated or preincubated with BEC (200 μM) or L-NIL (100 ng/ml) for 3 h followed by infection with *L. donovani* for 48 h **(A,B,E,G,H)**. In another experiment, THP-1 MΦs were transfected with control siRNA, Arg-1, Arg-2, or iNOS siRNA followed by infection with *L. donovani* for 48 h **(C,D,F,I,J)**. Intracellular parasites were visualized by staining the cells with Giemsa followed by optical microscopy at 100x oil immersion. The parasite load was measured by counting the number of intracellular amastigotes per 100 macrophages **(A,C)**. The rate of infection was analyzed by counting the percent infected macrophages **(B,D)**. Extracellular nitrite level was measured by Griess method using $NaNO_2$ as standard **(E,F)**. The polyamines (putrescine and spermidine) were extracted by TCA precipitation followed by dansyl chloride derivatization, separation by reverse-phase high performance liquid chromatography as described in "Materials and Methods." Dansylated putrescine **(G,I)** and dansylated spermidine **(H,J)** were quantified by fluorescence spectrometry. Each experiment was repeated three times. Each determination was made in triplicate and the values were expressed as mean ± SD for three independent experiments. Kruskal–Wallis with Dunn's multiple comparison test was used to evaluate statistical significance for comparing three or more groups; *$p < 0.05$; **$p < 0.005$; ns, non-significant.

Parasite load and percent infectivity was further measured in Arg-1, Arg-2, and iNOS siRNA transfected and *Leishmania*-infected macrophages. It was observed that silencing of Arg-1 decreased the parasite load by ~3.3-fold (**Figure 10C**) and percent infectivity by ~1.9-fold (**Figure 10D**) in comparison to control siRNA transfected macrophages. On the other hand, silencing of Arg-2 decreased the parasite load by ~2.1-fold (**Figure 10C**) when compared to control siRNA transfected macrophages. However, in case of Arg-2 knock down percent infectivity was not significantly altered (**Figure 10D**). However, silencing of iNOS increased the parasite load by ~1.9-fold (**Figure 10C**). Therefore, our results indicated that arginase expression is critically involved in promoting parasite survival inside macrophages.

Simultaneously, inhibition of arginase activity by BEC also resulted in ~1.8-fold increased NO level in infected macrophages (**Figure 10E**). Silencing of macrophage Arg-1 and Arg-2 also increased the NO level in *Leishmania*-infected macrophages by ~1.8-fold and ~1.3–fold, respectively (**Figure 10F**).

Further, polyamines were also measured in *Leishmania*-infected macrophages pretreated with inhibitor of arginase and iNOS. It was observed that BEC pretreatment decreased the putrescine level by ~2.7-fold (**Figure 10G**) and spermidine level by ~1.9-fold (**Figure 10H**) in infected macrophages when compared to untreated infected macrophages. However, pretreatment of L-NIL increased the putrescine level by ~1.8-fold (**Figure 10G**) and spermidine level by ~1.6-fold (**Figure 10H**) in infected macrophages when compared to untreated infected macrophages. Polyamine level was also measured in Arg-1, Arg-2, and iNOS downregulated *Leishmania*-infected macrophages. Putrescine level was found to be decreased by ~3.7-fold and ~2.0-fold (**Figure 10I**) and spermidine level by ~1.8-fold and ~1.3-fold (**Figure 10J**), respectively, in Arg-1 and Arg-2 siRNA transfected *Leishmania*-infected macrophages. However, iNOS knock down increased the putrescine level by ~1.9-fold (**Figure 10I**) and spermidine level by ~2.2-fold (**Figure 10J**) in *Leishmania*-infected macrophages compared to control siRNA transfected infected macrophages. These findings possibly suggest that arginase and iNOS expression are reciprocally regulated in case of *Leishmania* infection and the balance between these two enzymes regulate production of NO and polyamines and thereby determines the fate of *Leishmania* survival inside macrophages.

L-Arginine Availability and Transport Regulates Host Th1/Th2 Cytokine Response in Infected Macrophages

The involvement of L-arginine transport in regulation of Th1/Th2 balance in *Leishmania* infection was assessed by measuring cytokines at the transcript level by semi-quantitive RT-PCR as well as quantitive real-time PCR and released level by sandwich ELISA. The expression of Th2 cytokine, IL-10 was increased by ~3.2-fold in *Leishmania*-infected macrophages when compared to uninfected macrophages in L-arginine-supplemented media (**Figure 11A**). Simultaneously, IL-10 expression in infected macrophages was found to be reduced significantly in L-arginine deprived condition when compared to L-arginine-supplemented condition (**Figures 11A,B**). However, L-arginine deprivation had no significant effect on Th1 cytokine production in infected macrophages (**Figures 11A,B**). Cytokine expressions were further measured in *Leishmania*-infected macrophages in presence or absence of NEM. IL-10 level was found to be decreased by ~4.6-fold in NEM pretreated infected macrophages when compared to untreated infected macrophages (**Figure 11C**). However, pretreatment of macrophage with NEM had no significant effect on IL-12 and TNF-α level in infected macrophages (**Figures 11C,D**). The expression of cytokines was further checked in CAT-1 and CAT-2 siRNA transfected *Leishmania*-infected macrophages. Silencing of CAT-1 decreased the IL-10 level by ~1.9-fold in infected macrophages. However, CAT-2 knock down decreased the IL-10 expression by ~2.8-fold in *Leishmania*-infected macrophages when compared to control siRNA transfected macrophages (**Figure 11E**). Moreover, CAT-2 knock down decreased the IL-12 level by ~1.3-fold and had no significant effect on expression of TNF-α in infected macrophages (**Figure 11E**). Our real-time PCR data further validate the results of semi-quantitive RT-PCR (**Figure 11F**).

To further validate our semi-quantitative data, we measured the concentration of cytokines at the released level by sandwich ELISA. Th2 cytokine, IL-10 level was increased by ~2.1-fold in *Leishmania*-infected macrophages when compared to uninfected macrophages in normal condition (**Figure 12A**). However, when Th2 cytokine released by *Leishmania*-infected macrophages in L-arginine deprivation and L-arginine supplementation condition was compared, significant decrease in IL-10 level (~1.9-fold; $p \leq 0.005$) was observed in case of L-arginine deprivation. Moreover, L-arginine deprivation had no significant effect on

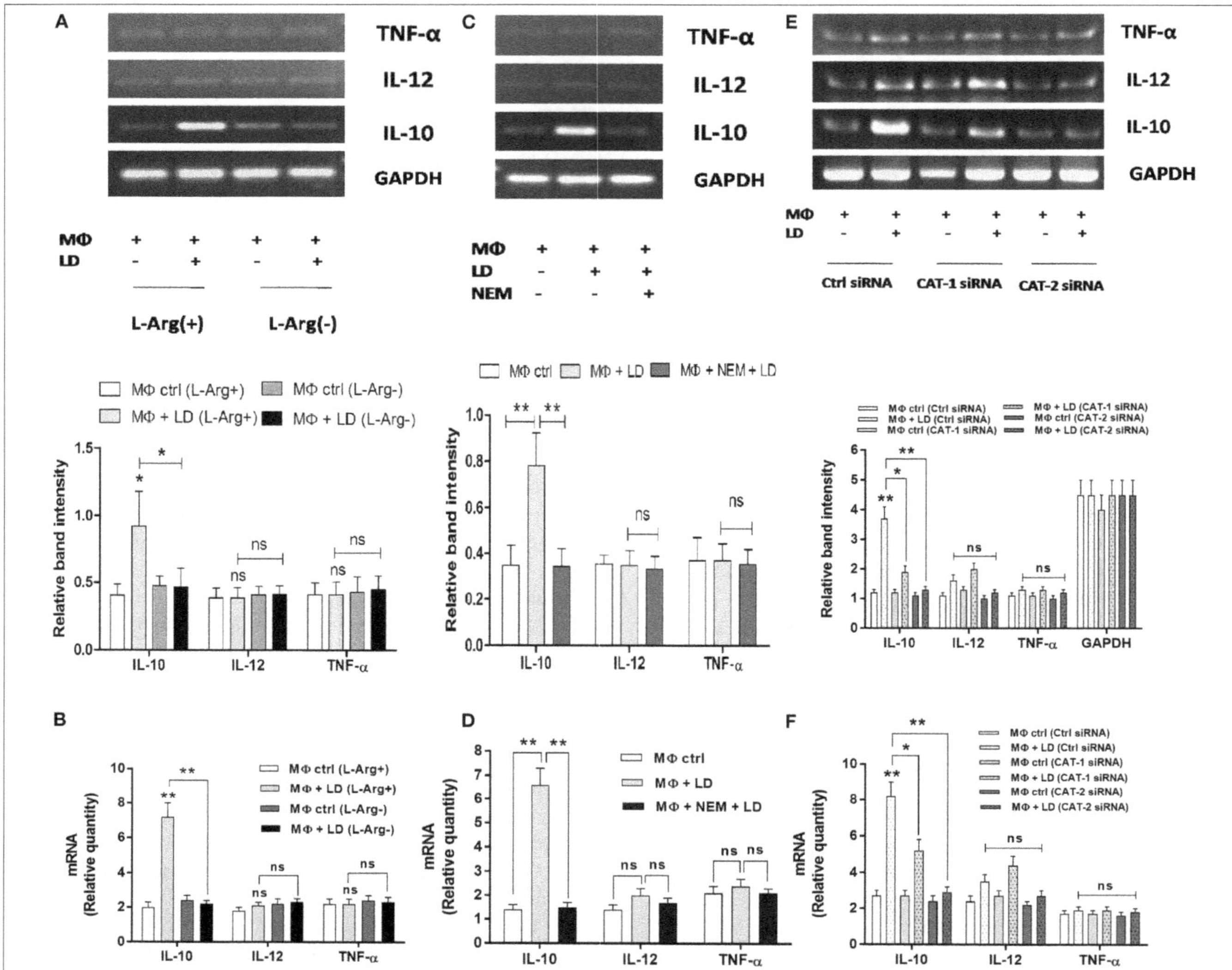

FIGURE 11 | L-Arginine availability and transport regulate expression of pro-inflammatory and anti-inflammatory cytokines in infected macrophages. THP-1 monocyte-derived MΦs (1 × 10^6 cells/ml) were grown in L-arginine-supplemented and L-arginine-depleted RPMI medium followed by infection with *Leishmania donovani* (multiplicity of infection 1:10) for 48 h **(A,B)**. In a separate experiment, THP-1 MΦs (1 × 10^6 cells/ml) were either left untreated or preincubated with 250 μM NEM for 10 min followed by infection with *L. donovani* for 48 h **(C,D)**. In another experiment, THP-1 MΦs (1 × 10^6 cells/ml) were transfected with control siRNA, CAT-1, or CAT-2 siRNA followed by infection with *L. donovani* for 48 h **(E,F)**. The expression of IL-10, IL-12, and TNF-α were determined at the transcript level by semi-quantitative RT-PCR **(A,C,E)** and quantitative real-time PCR **(B,D,F)**. The intensity of the bands was quantified by densitometry in Quantity one software. Each experiment was repeated three times. Each determination was made in triplicate and the values were expressed as mean ± SD for three independent experiments. Semi-QRT PCR gel images are representative of three experiments. Densitometric plots are shown below the gel images. Kruskal–Wallis with Dunn's multiple comparison test was used to evaluate statistical significance for comparing three or more groups; *$p < 0.05$; **$p < 0.005$; ns, non-significant.

Th1 cytokine production in infected macrophages (**Figure 12A**). Cytokines were further measured in *Leishmania*-infected macrophages in presence or absence of NEM. It was observed that IL-10 level was decreased by ~1.9-fold in NEM pretreated infected macrophages compared to untreated infected macrophages (**Figure 12B**). However, pretreatment of macrophages with NEM had no significant effect on IL-12 and TNF-α level in infected macrophages.

The level of cytokines in CAT-1 and CAT-2 siRNA transfected *Leishmania*-infected macrophages was also measured. It was observed that silencing of CAT-1 had no significant effect on cytokine release in infected macrophages. CAT-2 silencing decreased the IL-10 level by ~2.0-fold in *Leishmania*-infected macrophages compared to control siRNA transfected macrophages (**Figure 12C**). However, CAT-2 knock down had no significant effect on release of IL-10 and TNF-α in infected macrophages (**Figure 12C**). These findings clearly indicate that *Leishmania* infection is characterized by significant increased level of IL-10 cytokine. Inhibition of L-arginine transport decreased IL-10 level resulting in decreased parasite survival inside macrophages.

DISCUSSION

Arginine is one of the metabolic and signaling molecule required for protein synthesis by macrophages and their growth (54). Macrophages require exogenous arginine to meet their metabolic

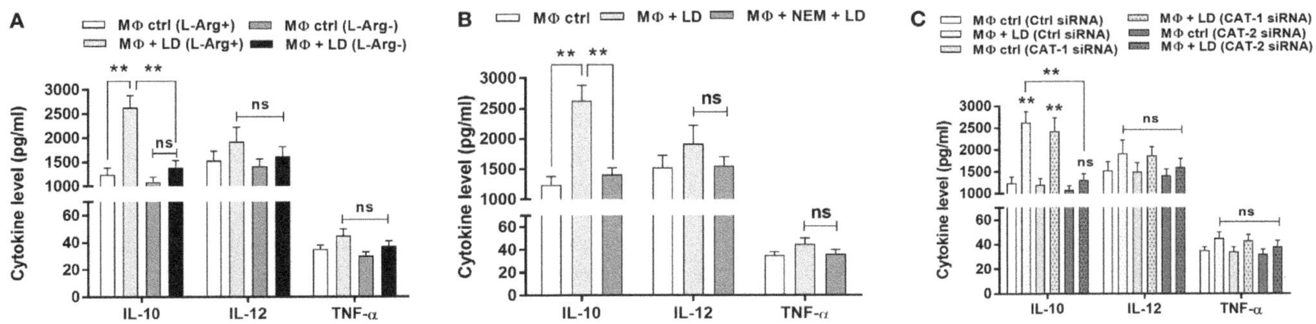

FIGURE 12 | L-Arginine availability and transport regulate release of pro-inflammatory and anti-inflammatory cytokines in *Leishmania*-infected macrophages. THP-1 monocyte-derived MΦs (1×10^6 cells/ml) were grown in L-arginine-supplemented and L-arginine-depleted RPMI medium followed by infection with *Leishmania donovani* (multiplicity of infection 1:10) for 48 h **(A)**. In a separate experiment, THP-1 MΦs (1×10^6 cells/ml) were either left untreated or preincubated with 250 μM NEM for 10 min followed by infection with *L. donovani* for 48 h **(B)**. In another experiment, THP-1 MΦs (1×10^6 cells/ml) were transfected with control siRNA, CAT-1, or CAT-2 siRNA followed by infection with *L. donovani* for 48 h **(C)**. Level of IL-10, IL-12, and TNF-α in the macrophage culture supernatants were quantified by sandwich ELISA **(A–C)**. Each experiment was repeated three times. Each determination was made in triplicate and the values were expressed as mean ± SD for three independent experiments. Kruskal–Wallis with Dunn's multiple comparison test was used to evaluate statistical significance for comparing three or more groups; $^*p < 0.05$; $^{**}p < 0.005$; ns, non-significant.

demands and it is also the key amino acid which signals M1 and M2 activation (55, 56). It is documented that when *Leishmania* enters inside the macrophage, instead of being classically activated, macrophage becomes alternatively activated and this ultimately promotes *Leishmania* survival inside macrophages. Simultaneously, inside the phagolysosome, the parasite has to face relatively carbohydrate sparse environment and, therefore, possibly uptakes fatty acids and amino acids as alternate energy sources for their survival and other activities (57–59). In our previous report, we have shown that L-arginine is crucial for the survival of *L. donovani* promastigotes *in vitro* (43). However, the role of L-arginine in the intra-macrophage survival of *L. donovani* is yet not properly elucidated. In the present study, we have investigated how *L. donovani* utilizes host L-arginine metabolic pathway and survives inside macrophages. Our results showed that the parasite load and percent infectivity was significantly reduced upon removal of L-arginine from the culture medium indicating the importance of L-arginine for the survival of *L. donovani* inside macrophages. Similar observations were reported by Sans-Fons et al. who demonstrated that the availability of L-arginine critically regulates macrophage activation and thereby promoting susceptibility to *L. major* infection (60).

Previously, Darlyuk et al. reported that starvation resulted in increase in L-arginine uptake in *Leishmania* promastigotes after amino acid depletion, along with concomitant increase of LdAAP3 at both mRNA and protein levels (61). In our previous study, we also observed that L-arginine deprivation led to its increased uptake in *Leishmania* promastigotes (43). Therefore, although the role of *Leishmania* L-arginine transporters for their survival was reported earlier (61), there are few reports regarding the involvement of macrophage L-arginine transporters for intracellular survival of *Leishmania*. Wanasen et al. previously reported the involvement of mouse cationic amino acid transporter 2B (mCAT-2B) in case of *L. braziliensis* infection (62). Later, Sans-Fons et al. also reported that the growth enhancement of *L. major* amastigotes inside macrophages was associated with CAT-2-mediated L-arginine transport (60). In this study, we also observed that the expression of CAT-2 is specifically increased in case of *L. donovani* infection. CAT-2 level was found to be further increased upon L-arginine deprivation during *Leishmania* infection. Therefore, we hypothesized that upon sensing low L-arginine availability, *L. donovani* modulates the expression of macrophage L-arginine transporters particularly CAT-2 and increases the uptake of L-arginine for its survival and growth. However, as we observed that even in case of knock down of CAT-2, macrophage L-arginine transport is not decreased in normal condition, it is evident that L-arginine is transported by CAT-1 transporter in normal resting condition. Simultaneously, from the parasite load and percent infectivity data in case of CAT-1 and CAT-2 downregulation, we observed that CAT-2 downregulation had more pronounced effect than CAT-1 in decreasing parasite survival inside macrophages. Therefore, we hypothesize that when the amount of L-arginine required by *Leishmania* for intra-macrophage survival is not sufficient by CAT-1 mediated transport, then the parasite upregulates host CAT-2 expression, and utilizes CAT-2 mediated L-arginine supply. Further, we observed that when L-arginine transporters were blocked either by inhibitor or siRNA treatment, *L. donovani* survival was greatly reduced indicating the importance of L-arginine transport for their survival inside macrophages. Therefore, our results are in agreement with the study of Wanasen et al (62).

Previous studies have demonstrated that pathogens take up extracellular L-arginine and compete with iNOS for L-arginine substrate to evade host defense (63). In this study, we observed that deprivation of L-arginine did not impair the upregulation of macrophage iNOS and arginase in normal condition. Similar results were reported in peritoneal exudate MΦ by Choi et al., where they have shown that MΦ activation and biological functions are not altered by the lack of L-arginine (64). However, our results are in contrary to the findings of El-Gayar et al. who showed that the presence of arginine is requisite for adequate translation of iNOS (65). In this study, we observed that host arginase is induced upon *Leishmania* infection and its expression is regulated by L-arginine availability in extracellular milieu and upon expression of CAT-2. Our study is the first to report that L-arginine transport is a critical factor for *L. donovani* infection *ex vivo* and this transport differentially regulate the expression of arginase in infected macrophages. However, as we observed that even in case of knock down of CAT-1, the expression of Arg-1 was decreased at the transcript level, we assume that CAT-1 mediated L-arginine transport might also have a role in regulation of arginase activity in *L. donovani*-infected macrophages. Our observation indicates that induction of host arginase is important for the survival of *L. donovani* parasite inside macrophages. In contrary to our observation, Wanasen et al. described that the L-arginine dependent intra-macrophage *L. amazonensis* survival was independent of arginase–iNOS activities (62). However, our findings is correlated with the studies by Boitz et al. who have recently shown that leishmanial arginase is not essential for proliferation of intracellular amastigotes, indicating that the parasites utilize host arginase pathway for their survival inside macrophages (34).

The conversion of L-arginine to L-ornithine and urea and its participation in polyamine production has been reported to stimulate growth of many pathogens, including *Leishmania* spp. (18, 26)., *Trypanosoma* spp. (20)., *Helicobacter pylori* (66) and *Mycobacterium bovis* (67). Several organisms, including *Leishmania* spp., can both synthesize polyamines *de novo* and salvage them by transport across their plasma membranes. In the present study, we observed that polyamine production was greatly diminished due to L-arginine deprivation or blockade of L-arginine transport ultimately resulting in decreased parasite survival inside macrophages.

The metabolism of arginine by iNOS or arginase 1 produces radically different biological products (68). It is reported that iNOS generates NO in large quantities and under physiological conditions plays an important role in killing parasites (69) whereas arginase 1 in turn regulates NO through depletion of arginine availability (68). In the present study, we wanted to understand how the expressions of iNOS and/or arginase are regulated in macrophages after *L. donovani* infection. We observed that iNOS and arginase are reciprocally regulated. If arginase is inhibited, iNOS expression is increased resulting in increased production of NO. In contrast, if iNOS is inhibited, arginase activity got increased favoring *Leishmania* survival inside macrophages. Elevated arginase activity has also been documented by multiple investigators in animal models of cancer (70, 71) and recently in human (72, 73). Thus, it is possible that increased arginase 1 expression may downregulate the production of NO as it limits arginine accessibility for iNOS. The present study for the first time revealed that L-arginine transport is a crucial factor for *L. donovani* infection *ex vivo* and that this transport system could moderately explain the differential

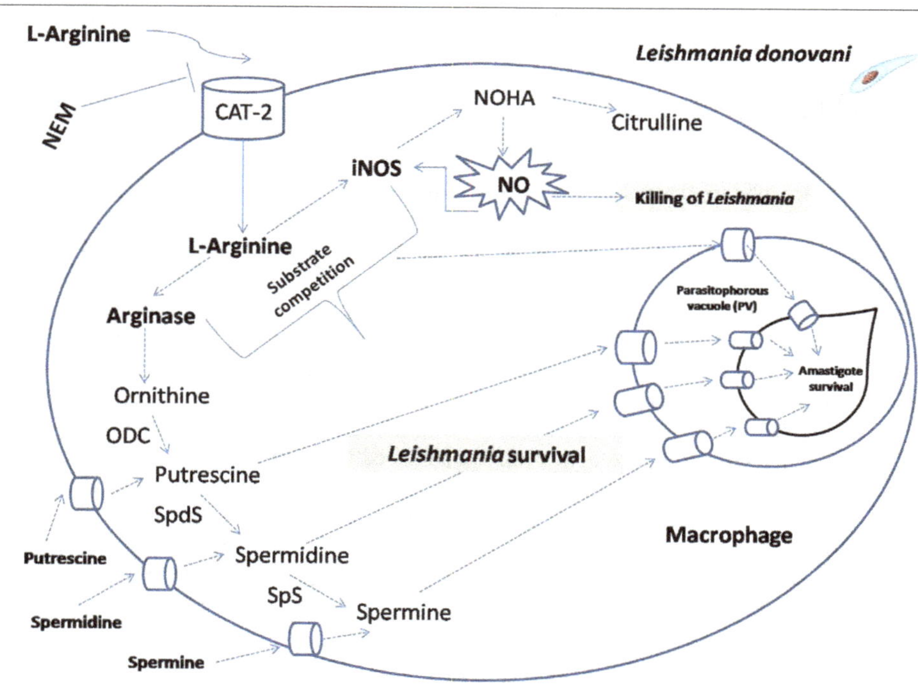

FIGURE 13 | Schematic representation demonstrating the role of L-arginine availability and transport in the modulation of host immune response and *Leishmania* survival inside macrophages. The model illustrates that the fate of *Leishmania* parasites inside macrophages depend on the availability of extracellular L-arginine and activation status of macrophages. If L-arginine is available, it is taken up from the external medium by cationic amino acid transporters (CAT-2) and metabolized by arginase and other polyamine biosynthetic and thiol metabolic pathway enzymes, such as ornithine decarboxylase (ODC), spermidine synthase (SpdS), spermine synthase (Sps) to produce L-ornithine, putrescine, spermidine, and spermine. *Leishmania* acquires either arginine or polyamines by the transporters present on the membrane of the parasitophorous vacuole which promotes amastigote proliferation and cell growth. Simultaneously, L-arginine can also be utilized by inducible nitric oxide synthase (iNOS) to produce nitric oxide (NO) that would kill *Leishmania* parasites. *Leishmania* infection modulate the host to downregulate this pathway for their survival.

expression of arginase and iNOS in infected macrophages. Our experiments point to a link between reduced L-arginine transport and decreased *L. donovani* growth. The data presented here provide a new explanation for the intracellular parasite replication in *L. donovani* infections.

The catabolism of L-arginine by macrophages plays a crucial role in regulation of the immune response, in several parasitic diseases including *L. major* infection (74). It is reported that to evade immune responses, some pathogens induce arginase expression in the host (75, 76) and that high level of arginase production blocks the immune response by local depletion of L-arginine (77). In this study, we investigated the involvement of L-arginine transport in regulation of Th1/Th2 balance in *L.* donovani infection. Our findings clearly indicated that *Leishmania* infection is associated with increase in IL-10 level and inhibition of L-arginine transport significantly decreased IL-10 level resulting in decreased parasite survival inside macrophages. Our findings are in agreement with the studies of Hesse et al. (56). Therefore, we propose that the IL-10 released by the macrophages in case of L-arginine availability in extracellular milieu induce the host arginase pathway leading to polyamine production and thereby promoting *L. donovani* survival inside macrophages.

In conclusion, our results decipher that L-arginine availability and transport plays a crucial regulatory role for survival of *L. donovani* parasite inside macrophages. *L. donovani* upregulates host L-arginine transport and controls L-arginine metabolism resulting in increased production of polyamines and skewed immune response for their survival inside macrophages (**Figure 13**). Our study is the first report describing the importance of CAT-2 mediated L-arginine transport for survival of *L. donovani* inside macrophages. The findings presented here further increase our knowledge about the pathways by which L-arginine deprivation regulates host immune response and promotes *Leishmania* survival inside macrophages. Therefore, targeting the metabolism of L-arginine and the macrophage cells expressing L-arginine-metabolizing enzymes is likely to constitute an important therapeutic and prophylactic approach to treat VL.

AUTHOR CONTRIBUTIONS

Conceived and designed the experiments: AM, SD, and PD. Performed the experiments: AM, AjayK, SR, SV, AG, SS, RS, and KA. Analyzed the data: AM, SD, AG, CM, and PD. Contributed reagents/materials/analysis tools: SR, AS, BP, AshishK, CM, and PD. Wrote the paper: AM, SD, and PD.

ACKNOWLEDGMENTS

This work was supported by an intramural grant (INT-76-BAS) from the Indian Council of Medical Research (ICMR), Ministry of Health and Family Welfare, Government of India. The funders have no role in study design, data collection and analysis, decision to publish, or preparation of the manuscript. AM was supported by Senior Research Fellowship from ICMR, Government of India. The authors are grateful to Dr. Sujoy Das Gupta, Professor, Deptartment of Microbiology and Swaroop Biswas, Bose Institute, Kolkata for providing HPLC facility. The authors are thankful to Mrs. Joyshree Karmakar, UGC-JRF for her support in transport experiments. The authors are also thankful to Subhash Kumar for providing technical assistance for this study.

REFERENCES

1. Kane MM, Mosser DM. The role of IL-10 in promoting disease progression in leishmaniasis. *J Immunol* (2001) 166:1141–7. doi:10.4049/jimmunol.166.2.1141
2. Teixeira MJ, Teixeira CR, Andrade BB, Barral-Netto M, Barral A. Chemokines in host-parasite interactions in leishmaniasis. *Trends Parasitol* (2006) 22:32–40. doi:10.1016/j.pt.2005.11.010
3. Vasquez RE, Soong L. CXCL10/gamma interferon-inducible protein 10-mediated protection against *Leishmania amazonensis* infection in mice. *Infect Immun* (2006) 74:6769–77. doi:10.1128/IAI.01073-06
4. Noel W, Raes G, Hassanzadeh GG, De Baetselier P, Beschin A. Alternatively activated macrophages during parasite infections. *Trends Parasitol* (2004) 20:126–33. doi:10.1016/j.pt.2004.01.004
5. Kreider T, Anthony RM, Urban JF Jr, Gause WC. Alternatively activated macrophages in helminth infections. *Curr Opin Immunol* (2007) 19:448–53. doi:10.1016/j.coi.2007.07.002
6. Boger RH, Bode-Boger SM. The clinical pharmacology of L-arginine. *Annu Rev Pharmacol Toxicol* (2001) 41:79–99. doi:10.1146/annurev.pharmtox.41.1.79
7. Morris SM Jr. Arginine: beyond protein. *Am J Clin Nutr* (2006) 83:508S–12S.
8. Wu G, Morris SM Jr. Arginine metabolism: nitric oxide and beyond. *Biochem J* (1998) 336:1–17. doi:10.1042/bj3360001
9. Munder M. Arginase: an emerging key player in the mammalian immune system. *Br J Pharmacol* (2009) 158:638–51. doi:10.1111/j.1476-5381.2009.00291.x
10. Jenkinson CP, Grody WW, Cederbaum SD. Comparative properties of arginases. *Comp Biochem Physiol B Biochem Mol Biol* (1996) 114:107–32. doi:10.1016/0305-0491(95)02138-8
11. Granger DL, Hibbs JB Jr, Perfect JR, Durack DT. Metabolic fate of L-arginine in relation to microbiostatic capability of murine macrophages. *J Clin Invest* (1990) 85:264–73. doi:10.1172/JCI114422
12. Hrabak A, Idei M, Temesi A. Arginine supply for nitric oxide synthesis and arginase is mainly exogenous in elicited murine and rat macrophages. *Life Sci* (1994) 55:797–805. doi:10.1016/0024-3205(94)00563-X
13. Abebe T, Takele Y, Weldegebreal T, Cloke T, Closs E, Corset C, et al. Arginase activity – a marker of disease status in patients with visceral leishmaniasis in ethiopia. *PLoS Negl Trop Dis* (2013) 7:e2134. doi:10.1371/journal.pntd.0002134

14. Takele Y, Abebe T, Weldegebreal T, Hailu A, Hailu W, Hurissa Z, et al. Arginase activity in the blood of patients with visceral leishmaniasis and HIV infection. *PLoS Negl Trop Dis* (2013) 7:e1977. doi:10.1371/journal.pntd.0001977
15. Cloke TE, Garvey L, Choi BS, Abebe T, Hailu A, Hancock M, et al. Increased level of arginase activity correlates with disease severity in HIV-seropositive patients. *J Infect Dis* (2010) 202:374–85. doi:10.1086/653736
16. Tabor CW, Tabor H. Polyamines. *Annu Rev Biochem* (1984) 53:749–90. doi:10.1146/annurev.bi.53.070184.003533
17. Pegg AE. Mammalian polyamine metabolism and function. *IUBMB Life* (2009) 61:880–94. doi:10.1002/iub.230
18. Kropf P, Fuentes JM, Fahnrich E, Arpa L, Herath S, Weber V, et al. Arginase and polyamine synthesis are key factors in the regulation of experimental leishmaniasis in vivo. *FASEB J* (2005) 19:1000–2. doi:10.1096/fj.04-3416fje
19. Popovic PJ, Zeh HJ, Ochoa JB. Arginine and immunity. *J Nutr* (2007) 137:1681S–6S.
20. Peluffo G, Piacenza L, Irigoin F, Alvarez MN, Radi R. L-arginine metabolism during interaction of *Trypanosoma cruzi* with host cells. *Trends Parasitol* (2004) 20:363–9. doi:10.1016/j.pt.2004.05.010
21. Fox BA, Gigley JP, Bzik DJ. *Toxoplasma gondii* lacks the enzymes required for de novo arginine biosynthesis and arginine starvation triggers cyst formation. *Int J Parasitol* (2004) 34:323–31. doi:10.1016/j.ijpara.2003.12.001
22. Everett J, Turner K, Cai Q, Gordon V, Whiteley M, Rumbaugh K. Arginine is a critical substrate for the pathogenesis of *Pseudomonas aeruginosa* in burn wound infections. *MBio* (2017) 8:e2160–2116. doi:10.1128/mBio.02160-16
23. Brussee JM, Yeo TW, Lampah DA, Anstey NM, Duffull SB. Pharmacokinetic-pharmacodynamic model for the effect of L-arginine on endothelial function in patients with moderately severe falciparum malaria. *Antimicrob Agents Chemother* (2016) 60:198–205. doi:10.1128/AAC.01479-15
24. Cheng C, Dong Z, Han X, Sun J, Wang H, Jiang L, et al. *Listeria monocytogenes* 10403S arginine repressor ArgR finely tunes arginine metabolism regulation under acidic conditions. *Front Microbiol* (2017) 8:145. doi:10.3389/fmicb.2017.00145
25. Rapovy S, Zhao J, Bricker RL, Schmidt SM, Setchell KDR, Qualls JE, et al. Differential requirements for L-citrulline and L-arginine during anti-mycobacterial macrophage activity. *J Immunol* (2015) 195:3293–300. doi:10.4049/jimmunol.1500800
26. Roberts SC, Tancer MJ, Polinsky MR, Gibson KM, Heby O, Ullman B. Arginase plays a pivotal role in polyamine precursor metabolism in *Leishmania*. Characterization of gene deletion mutants. *J Biol Chem* (2004) 279:23668–78. doi:10.1074/jbc.M402042200
27. Ivens AC, Peacock CS, Worthey EA, Murphy L, Aggarwal G, Berriman M, et al. The genome of the kinetoplastid parasite, *Leishmania major*. *Science* (2005) 309:436–42. doi:10.1126/science.1112680
28. Shaked-Mishan P, Suter-Grotemeyer M, Yoel-Almagor T, Holland N, Zilberstein D, Rentsch D. A novel high-affinity arginine transporter from the human parasitic protozoan *Leishmania donovani*. *Mol Microbiol* (2006) 60:30–8. doi:10.1111/j.1365-2958.2006.05060.x
29. Krassner SM, Flory B. Essential amino acids in the culture of *Leishmania tarentolae*. *J Parasitol* (1971) 57:917–20. doi:10.2307/3277829
30. Steiger RF, Meshnick SR. Amino-acid and glucose utilization of *Leishmania donovani* and *L. braziliensis*. *Trans R Soc Trop Med Hyg* (1977) 5:441–3. doi:10.1016/0035-9203(77)90049-9
31. Kandpal M, Fouce RB, Pal A, Guru PY, Tekwani BL. Kinetics and molecular characteristics of arginine transport by *Leishmania donovani* promastigotes. *Mol Biochem Parasitol* (1995) 71:193–201. doi:10.1016/0166-6851(95)00042-Y
32. Castilho-Martins EA, Laranjeira da Silva MF, dos Santos MG, Muxel SM, Floeter-Winter LM. Axenic *Leishmania amazonensis* promastigotes sense both the external and internal arginine pool distinctly regulating the two transporter-coding genes. *PLoS One* (2011) 6:e27818. doi:10.1371/journal.pone.0027818
33. Goldman-Pinkovich A, Balno C, Strasser R, Zeituni-Molad M, Bendelak K, Rentsch D, et al. An arginine deprivation response pathway is induced in *Leishmania* during macrophage invasion. *PLoS Pathog* (2016) 12:e1005494. doi:10.1371/journal.ppat.1005494
34. Boitz JM, Gilroy CA, Olenyik TD, Paradis D, Perdeh J, Dearman K, et al. Arginase is essential for survival of *Leishmania donovani* promastigotes but not intracellular amastigotes. *Infect Immun* (2017) 85:e554–516. doi:10.1128/IAI.00554-16
35. Verrey F, Closs EI, Wagner CA, Palacin M, Endou H, Kanai Y. CATs and HATs: the SLC7 family of amino acid transporters. *Pflugers Arch* (2004) 447:532–42. doi:10.1007/s00424-003-1086-z
36. Yeramian A, Martin L, Serrat N, Arpa L, Soler C, Bertran J, et al. Arginine transport via cationic amino acid transporter 2 plays a critical regulatory role in classical or alternative activation of macrophages. *J Immunol* (2006) 176:5918–24. doi:10.4049/jimmunol.176.10.5918
37. Deves R, Boyd CA. Transporters for cationic amino acids in animal cells: discovery, structure, and function. *Physiol Rev* (1998) 78:487–545.
38. Closs EI, Albritton LM, Kim JW, Cunningham JM. Identification of a low affinity, high capacity transporter of cationic amino acids in mouse liver. *J Biol Chem* (1993) 268:7538–44.
39. MacLeod CL. Regulation of cationic amino acid transporter (CAT) gene expression. *Biochem Soc Trans* (1996) 24:846–52. doi:10.1042/bst0240846
40. Nicholson B, Manner CK, Kleeman J, MacLeod CL. Sustained nitric oxide production in macrophages requires the arginine transporter CAT2. *J Biol Chem* (2001) 276:15881–5. doi:10.1074/jbc.M010030200
41. Das S, Pandey K, Kumar A, Sardar AH, Purkait B, Kumar M, et al. TGF-β1 re-programs TLR4 signaling in *L. donovani* infection: enhancement of SHP-1 and ubiquitin-editing enzyme A20. *Immunol Cell Biol* (2012) 90:640–54. doi:10.1038/icb.2011.80
42. Singh AK, Pandey RK, Siqueira-Neto JL, Kwon Y-J, Freitas-Junior LH, Shaha C, et al. Proteomic-based approach to gain insight into reprogramming of THP-1 cells exposed to *Leishmania donovani* over an early temporal window. *Infect Immun* (2015) 83:1853–68. doi:10.1128/IAI.02833-14
43. Mandal A, Das S, Roy S, Ghosh AK, Sardar AH, Verma S, et al. Deprivation of L-arginine induces oxidative stress mediated apoptosis in *Leishmania donovani* promastigotes: contribution of the polyamine pathway. *PLoS Negl Trop Dis* (2016) 10(1):e0004373. doi:10.1371/journal.pntd.0004373
44. Gantier MP, Tong S, Behlke MA, Xu D, Phipps S, Foster PS, et al. TLR7 is involved in sequence-specific sensing of single-stranded RNAs in human macrophages. *J Immunol* (2008) 180(4):2117–24. doi:10.4049/jimmunol.180.4.2117
45. Corraliza IM, Campo ML, Soler G, Modolell M. Determination of arginase activity in macrophages: a micromethod. *J Immunol Methods* (1994) 174:231–5. doi:10.1016/0022-1759(94)90027-2
46. Reguera RM, Balaña-Fouce R, Showalter M, Hickerson S, Beverley SM. *Leishmania major* lacking arginase (ARG) are auxotrophic for polyamines but retain infectivity to susceptible BALB/c mice. *Mol Biochem Parasitol* (2009) 165:48–56. doi:10.1016/j.molbiopara.2009.01.001
47. Rileya E, Roberts SC, Ullman B. Inhibition profile of *Leishmania mexicana* arginase reveals differences with human arginase I. *Int J Parasitol* (2011) 41:545–52. doi:10.1016/j.ijpara.2010.12.006
48. Kropf P, Brunson K, Etges R, Müller I. The leishmaniasis model. *Immunol Infect* (1998) 25:419–58. doi:10.1016/S0580-9517(08)70688-3
49. Schluter D, Deckert-Schluter M, Lorenz E, Meyer T, Rollinghoff M, Bogdan C. Inhibition of inducible nitric oxide synthase exacerbates chronic cerebral toxoplasmosis in *Toxoplasma gondii*-susceptible C57BL/6 mice but does not reactivate the latent disease in *T. gondii*-resistant BALB/c mice. *J Immunol* (1999) 162:3512–8.
50. Purkait B, Kumar A, Nandi N, Sardar AH, Das S, Kumar S, et al. Mechanism of amphotericin B resistance in clinical isolates of *Leishmania donovani*. *Antimicrob Agents Chemother* (2012) 56:1031–41. doi:10.1128/AAC.00030-11
51. Balaña-Fouce R, Escribano MI, Alunda JM. *Leishmania infantum*: polyamine biosynthesis and levels during the growth of promastigotes. *Int J Biochem* (1991) 23:1213–7. doi:10.1016/0020-711X(91)90218-C
52. Bozkus CC, Elzey BD, Crist SA, Ellies LG, Ratliff TL. Expression of cationic amino acid transporter 2 is required for myeloid-derived suppressor cell-mediated control of T cell immunity. *J Immunol* (2015) 195:5237–50. doi:10.4049/jimmunol.1500959
53. Williams D, Venardos KM, Byrne M, Joshi M, Horlock D, Lam NT, et al. Abnormal mitochondrial L-arginine transport contributes to the pathogenesis of heart failure and rexoygenation injury. *PLoS One* (2014) 9(8):e104643. doi:10.1371/journal.pone.0104643
54. Yeramian A, Martin L, Arpa L, Bertran J, Soler C, McLeod C, et al. Macrophages require distinct arginine catabolism and transport systems for proliferation and for activation. *Eur J Immunol* (2006) 36:1516–26. doi:10.1002/eji.200535694

55. Gordon S. Alternative activation of macrophages. *Nat Rev Immunol* (2003) 3:23–35. doi:10.1038/nri978
56. Hesse M, Modolell M, La Flamme AC, Schito M, Fuentes JM, Cheever AW, et al. Differential regulation of nitric oxide synthase-2 and arginase-1 by type 1/type 2 cytokines in vivo: granulomatous pathology is shaped by the pattern of L-arginine metabolism. *J Immunol* (2001) 167:6533–44. doi:10.4049/jimmunol.167.11.6533
57. Burchmore RJ, Barrett MP. Life in vacuoles – nutrient acquisition by *Leishmania* amastigotes. *Int J Parasitol* (2001) 31(12):1311–20. doi:10.1016/S0020-7519(01)00259-4
58. McConville MJ, de Souza D, Saunders E, Likic VA, Naderer T. Living in a phagolysosome; metabolism of *Leishmania* amastigotes. *Trends Parasitol* (2007) 23:368–75. doi:10.1016/j.pt.2007.06.009
59. Naderer T, McConville MJ. The *Leishmania*-macrophage interaction: a metabolic perspective. *Cell Microbiol* (2008) 10(2):301–8. doi:10.1111/j.1462-5822.2007.01096.x
60. Sans-Fons MG, Yeramian A, Pereira-Lopes S, Santamaría-Babi LF, Modolell M, Lloberas J, et al. Arginine transport is impaired in C57Bl/6 mouse macrophages as a result of a deletion in the promoter of Slc7a2 (CAT2), and susceptibility to *Leishmania* infection is reduced. *J Infect Dis* (2013) 207:1684–93. doi:10.1093/infdis/jit084
61. Darlyuk I, Goldman A, Roberts SC, Ullman B, Rentsch D, Zilberstein D. Arginine homeostasis and transport in the human pathogen *Leishmania donovani*. *J Biol Chem* (2009) 284:19800–7. doi:10.1074/jbc.M901066200
62. Wanasen N, MacLeod CL, Ellies LG, Soong L. L-arginine and cationic amino acid transporter 2B regulate growth and survival of *Leishmania amazonensis* amastigotes in macrophages. *Infect Immun* (2007) 75(6):2802–10. doi:10.1128/IAI.00026-07
63. Eckmann L, Laurent F, Langford TD, Hetsko ML, Smith JR, Kagnoff MF, et al. Nitric oxide production by human intestinal epithelial cells and competition for arginine as potential determinants of host defense against the lumen-dwelling pathogen *Giardia lamblia*. *J Immunol* (2000) 164:1478–87. doi:10.4049/jimmunol.164.3.1478
64. Choi BS, Martinez-Falero IC, Corset C, Munder M, Modolell M, Müller I, et al. Differential impact of L-arginine deprivation on the activation and effector functions of T cells and macrophages. *J Leukoc Biol* (2009) 85(2):268–77. doi:10.1189/jlb.0508310
65. El-Gayar S, Thüring-Nahler H, Pfeilschifter J, Röllinghoff M, Bogdan C. Translational control of inducible nitric oxide synthase by IL-13 and arginine availability in inflammatory macrophages. *J Immunol* (2003) 171:4561–8. doi:10.4049/jimmunol.171.9.4561
66. Bussiere FI, Chaturvedi R, Cheng Y, Gobert AP, Asim M, Blumberg DR, et al. Spermine causes loss of innate immune response to *Helicobacter pylori* by inhibition of inducible nitric-oxide synthase translation. *J Biol Chem* (2005) 280:2409–12. doi:10.1074/jbc.C400498200
67. Talaue MT, Venketaraman V, Hazbon MH, Peteroy-Kelly M, Seth A, Colangeli R, et al. Arginine homeostasis in J774.1 macrophages in the context of *Mycobacterium bovis* BCG infection. *J Bacteriol* (2006) 188:4830–40. doi:10.1128/JB.01687-05
68. Morris SM Jr. Enzymes of arginine metabolism. *J Nutr* (2004) 134 (Suppl 10):S2743–7.
69. Bogdan C. Nitric oxide and the immune response. *Nat Immunol* (2001) 2:907–16. doi:10.1038/ni1001-907
70. Serafini P, Borrello I, Bronte V. Myeloid suppressor cells in cancer: recruitment, phenotype, properties, and mechanisms of immune suppression. *Semin Cancer Biol* (2006) 16:53–65. doi:10.1016/j.semcancer.2005.07.005
71. Kusmartsev S, Gabrilovich DI. Role of immature myeloid cells in mechanisms of immune evasion in cancer. *Cancer Immunol Immunother* (2006) 55:237–45. doi:10.1007/s00262-005-0048-z
72. Zea AH, Rodriguez PC, Atkins MB, Hernandez C, Signoretti S, Zabaleta J, et al. Arginase producing myeloid suppressor cells in renal cell carcinoma patients: a mechanism of tumor evasion. *Cancer Res* (2005) 65:3044–8. doi:10.1158/0008-5472.CAN-04-4505
73. Bronte V, Kasic T, Gri G, Gallana K, Borsellino G, Marigo I, et al. Boosting antitumor responses of T lymphocytes infiltrating human prostate cancers. *J Exp Med* (2005) 201:1257–68. doi:10.1084/jem.20042028
74. Vincendeau P, Gobert AP, Daulouede S, Moynet D, Mossalayi MD. Arginases in parasitic diseases. *Trends Parasitol* (2003) 19:9–12. doi:10.1016/S1471-4922(02)00010-7
75. El Kasmi KC, Qualls JE, Pesce JT, Smith AM, Thompson RW, Henao-Tamayo M, et al. Toll-like receptor-induced arginase 1 in macrophages thwarts effective immunity against intracellular pathogens. *Nat Immunol* (2008) 9:1399–406. doi:10.1038/ni.1671
76. Qualls JE, Neale G, Smith AM, Koo MS, DeFreitas AA, Zhang H, et al. Arginine usage in mycobacteria infected macrophages depends on autocrine-paracrine cytokine signaling. *Sci Signal* (2010) 3:ra62. doi:10.1126/scisignal.2000955
77. Modolell M, Choi BS, Ryan RO, Hancock M, Titus RG, Abebe T, et al. Local suppression of T cell responses by arginase-induced L-arginine depletion in nonhealing leishmaniasis. *PLoS Negl Trop Dis* (2009) 3:e480. doi:10.1371/journal.pntd.0000480

21

Plasmodium falciparum Secretome in Erythrocyte and Beyond

*Rani Soni, Drista Sharma and Tarun K. Bhatt**

Department of Biotechnology, School of Life Sciences, Central University of Rajasthan, Rajasthan, India

***Correspondence:**
Tarun K. Bhatt
tarun@curaj.ac.in

Plasmodium falciparum is the causative agent of deadly malaria disease. It is an intracellular eukaryote and completes its multi-stage life cycle spanning the two hosts viz, mosquito and human. In order to habituate within host environment, parasite conform several strategies to evade host immune responses such as surface antigen polymorphism or modulation of host immune system and it is mediated by secretion of proteins from parasite to the host erythrocyte and beyond, collectively known as, malaria secretome. In this review, we will discuss about the deployment of parasitic secretory protein in mechanism implicated for immune evasion, protein trafficking, providing virulence, changing permeability and cyto-adherence of infected erythrocyte. We will be covering the possibilities of developing malaria secretome as a drug/vaccine target. This gathered information will be worthwhile in depicting a well-organized picture for host-pathogen interplay during the malaria infection and may also provide some clues for the development of novel anti-malarial therapies.

Keywords: plasmodium, secretome, cytoadherence, immune modulation, anti-malarial therapy

INTRODUCTION

World Health Organization report summarized that about 198 million cases and 0.58 million deaths occurred in year 2013 (World Health Organization [WHO], 2014). Amongst different species of *Plasmodium*, *P. falciparum* is the most dangerous and responsible for severe complexities during infection like multi-organ failure, cerebral malaria, coma, and death (Miller et al., 1994; Mendis and Carter, 1995). *P. falciparum* completes its life cycle spanning two alternate host, human, and mosquito. Within the human host, parasite undergoes series of developmental stages in the liver and erythrocytes (RBCs). The intra-erythrocytic cycle is found to be important as it is responsible for patho-physiology of the disease (Miller et al., 2002). Within the erythrocyte, the parasite proceeds through the different morphological stages such as ring, trophozoite, and schizont (Bannister et al., 2000; Florens et al., 2002). After completion of infection cycle, erythrocyte gets ruptured, and merozoites are released into the host bloodstream. The released merozoites initiate next round of erythrocytic cycle by infecting fresh erythrocytes (Gilson and Crabb, 2009). The survival of parasite inside the host cell is difficult, ascribed to which *Plasmodium* adapts various strategies to avoid the host immune response (Miller et al., 1994; Hisaeda et al., 2005). The strategies encompass the secretion of hitherto of proteins against infected RBC (iRBC) surface and beyond it into the host plasma (Singh et al., 2009). Infected erythrocyte surface remodeling is an example of such phenomena, involving the insertion of secreted proteins into the iRBC membrane (Deitsch and Wellems, 1996; Parker et al., 2004). Remodeling assists in cyto-adherence of iRBCs to the endothelial lining of blood vessels and thus averting them from splenic clearance (Newbold et al., 1999; Cooke et al., 2001; Rowe et al., 2009). Host immune modulation is another phenomenon involving the release of secretory proteins before or along with rupture of iRBCs. The released proteins interact with the components of the host immune system to provide conducive environment for merozoites before they invade new erythrocytes (Singh et al., 2009). The entire set of secreted proteins is known as 'Secretome.' These proteins are implicated in the processes essential for parasite survival such as host–parasite interactions and immune modulation (Ranganathan and Garg, 2009). Hence, in this review we will be focusing on parasite secretome and its significance in the malaria biology.

IDENTIFICATION OF MALARIA PARASITE'S SECRETOME

The export of secretory proteins from various species including *P. falciparum* has been thoroughly studied (van Ooij et al., 2008). Transport of secretory proteins follows a complicated route due to the presence of three membranes of parasite and vacuole inside the host cell (Martin et al., 2009). There must be a defined mechanism or recognizable sequence motifs behind such complex transport. Advent of bioinformatics tools facilitates the prediction of such conserved signal sequences responsible for the export and localization of the secretory proteins (Hiller et al., 2004; Marti et al., 2004, 2005).

The identification of sequence motifs necessary for export of parasite proteins is required for unearthing the complete secretome of the parasite. The first report proposed the presence of host targeting signal (HT motif) (Hiller et al., 2004) or *Plasmodium* export element (PEXEL motif) (Marti et al., 2004) in the sequence that is a requisite for the export of secretory proteins from parasitophorous vacuole (PV). The HT/PEXEL motif, present in more than 400 parasitic proteins, comprises short amino-terminal sequence, 'R/KxLxE/Q'. The role of motif in the export of both soluble and surface-associated protein is determined by green fluorescent protein (GFP) and yellow fluorescent protein (YFP) assays involving the fusion of secretory proteins such as Knob associated histidine rich protein (KAHRP), *Pf*EMP-1 (with PEXEL like motif), Glycophorin binding protein (GBP130), and members of repetitive interspersed family (rifin). Mutation or truncation of the PEXEL motif interrupted the transport of proteins and rendered their accumulation in PV itself (Marti et al., 2004; van Ooij et al., 2008). Prior to the secretion of PEXEL containing proteins to destination, N-terminus is processed in endoplasmic reticulum (ER) by protease enzyme plasmepsin V (PMV), followed by N-acetylation of the cleaved product (Chang et al., 2008; Boddey et al., 2010; Russo et al., 2010). The decisive role of PMV in export of proteins is also demonstrated by identification of transition state (TS) inhibitor, WEHI-916 (Walter and Eliza Hall Institute of Medical Research). The WEHI-916 inhibitor is found to compete with the PEXEL containing substrate resulting in blocking of activity of PMV and ultimately lead to the cessation of parasite growth at the trophozoite stage. Knockdown studies of PMV further supported the inhibitory role on PMV. Indirect hindrance of export of PfEMP-1 and the loss of virulence and cytoadherence of iRBC has been observed due to inhibitory activity of WEHI-916 (Sleebs et al., 2014a,b). Recently, another inhibitor of PMV, WEHI-842 has been identified. The inhibitory role of WEHI-842 is assessed through the immunoblotting of GFP tagged PEXEL containing PfEMP-3. It is found to be more effective in comparison to WEHI-916 (Hodder et al., 2015). The presence of PEXEL motif leads to identification of first set of parasite secretome. However, HT/PEXEL is found missing in various secretory proteins (Lingelbach and Przyborski, 2006). Analysis of such sequences showed the presence of a hydrophobic stretch in the internal region of trans-membrane proteins which helps in crossing the Parasitophorous Vacuolar Membrane (PVM). Immune localization experiments and GFP-tagged approach investigated that first 20 amino acids of N-terminus along with hydrophobic residues in trans-membrane domain are common features of all PEXEL negative export proteins (PNEPs). Thus PNEPs have further expanded the secretome repertoire of the parasite (Spielmann et al., 2006; Spielmann and Gilberger, 2010; Heiber et al., 2013).

Apart from sequence-motifs based approach, other approaches are used to predict secretory proteins of *Plasmodium*. A Position-Specific Scoring Matrix (PSSM) profile based method is adapted that employs phylogenetic relationship derived through PSI–Blast against the non-redundant database. Based on these data, web server called '*Plasmodium* Secretory and Infected erythrocyte Associated Protein prediction' (PSEApred) is developed to predict the secretory nature of *plasmodium* proteins (Verma et al., 2008). Similarly, the presence of N-myristoylation site, a cysteine S-palmitoylation site and some basic residues at N-terminus of parasite proteins are found to be responsible for the targeting to PVM and beyond (Gunaratne et al., 2000; Ma et al., 2012; Thavayogarajah et al., 2015; Wetzel et al., 2015). Together, both classical and non-classical path of secretion of proteins from parasite to the host cell have enhanced the secretome of the parasite. However, there is a possibility of appending more proteins to the growing secretome of parasite by identifying new signatures and patterns of secretion.

TRAFFICKING PATHWAY OF SECRETOME

The protein containing PEXEL motif moves from ER after cleavage by PMV to the PV either in the form of vesicular cargo (Barnwell, 1989) or through the secretory apparatus (Hinterberg et al., 1994; Taraschi et al., 2003). Proteins that are not cleaved by PMV have been shown to bind with phosphatidylinositol 3-phosphate (PI3-P) in the ER and proceed for further trafficking pathway (Bhattacharjee et al., 2012). The PNEP proteins require transmembrane domain for their transport (Heiber et al., 2013). All the proteins in the PV are found to be exported through *Plasmodium* Translocon of Exported protein (PTEX) complex (de Koning-Ward et al., 2009; Beck et al., 2014; Elsworth et al., 2014). These proteins undergo unfolding for their translocation across PV (Charpian and Przyborski, 2008; Gehde et al., 2009; Gruring et al., 2012). *P. falciparum* has developed a membranous structure in the cytoplasm of the host cell called 'Maurer's cleft'. It is a secondary organelle and required for the export of the proteins involved in virulence, modification of host cell environment (Trager et al., 1966; Rudzinska and Trager, 1968) and for trafficking of membrane localized proteins (Przyborski et al., 2003; Lanzer et al., 2006; Mundwiler-Pachlatko and Beck, 2013). The exported proteins from PV are found to reside in the Maurer's cleft (Haldar et al., 2002). Knock-down studies of Maurer's cleft residing proteins like Membrane-Associated Histidine-Rich Protein (MAHRP1) and Skeletal binding protein-1 (SBP-1) proved its vitality in protein sorting (Epp and Deitsch, 2006; Maier et al., 2007; Spycher et al., 2008). In addition, most of the known secretory proteins including three antigenic families of parasite proteins (Stevor, Rifin, and Var) are localized in the Maurer's cleft (Cheng et al., 1998) via PTEX export system (de Koning-Ward et al., 2009). PTEX export system, found exclusively in the genus *Plasmodium*, is responsible for the translocation of proteins targeted beyond the vacuolar membrane of the parasite (de Koning-Ward et al., 2009; Desai and Miller, 2014). It is a complex of five proteins including PTEX150, Heat shock protein 101 (HSP101), exported protein 2 (EXP2), PTEX88, and thioredoxin 2 (TRX2). The passage for directing proteins toward the cytosol of host erythrocyte is formed by EXP2 (de Koning-Ward et al., 2009). TRX 2 is found to be involved in unfolding of proteins destined to pass through the PTEX. Inhibition of HSP101 leads to the obstruction in protein export and eventually the accumulation of proteins such as Ring Infected Erythrocyte Surface Antigen (RESA), Ring Exported Protein 3 (REX3), Histidine Rich Protein-1 (HRP1), and KAHRP in parasitic compartment (Beck et al., 2014). It is observed that deletion of PTEX components prevent proteins from crossing PVM, resulting in interference of parasitic growth at the ring and trophozoite stage (Elsworth et al., 2014). However, mode of recognition between proteins to be exported and those to be retained by the PTEX complex still remains unclear. The mechanism of unfolding during protein export is also not defined and therefore it opens a new window of opportunity for scientists to explore and explain the facts related to PTEX system. In addition, the presence of this export system exclusively in *Plasmodium* genus makes it a captivating drug target (de Koning-Ward et al., 2009).

HOST CELL REMODELING

In order to make opportune environment within host, parasite makes substantial modifications in the host erythrocytes (Haldar and Mohandas, 2007). The modifications are predominantly mediated by secretion of parasite proteins across the PVM (Charpian and Przyborski, 2008; Maier et al., 2009; Goldberg and Cowman, 2010; Marti and Spielmann, 2013; Elsworth et al., 2014). The process of erythrocyte remodeling includes.

Cytoadherence

To circumvent immune clearance in spleen, infected erythrocytes get adhered to endothelial wall, which is mediated through various cell adhesion molecules like ICAMs, CD36 on blood vessels (Gardner et al., 1996; Ho and White, 1999; Bhalla et al., 2015). Some events during adhesion process such as rosette formation with fresh erythrocyte (Udomsangpetch et al., 1989), auto-agglutination due to clumping of iRBCs and platelets (Pain et al., 2001) leads to severe disease pathologies (Rowe et al., 1995, 2002; Newbold et al., 1999). *P. falciparum* erythrocytic membrane protein-1 (*Pf*EMP-1) is major virulent factor present on surface of erythrocyte (Magowan et al., 1988; Chen et al., 1998). A study regarding transgenic lines of *P. falciparum* with altered *Pf*EMP-1 expression shows strong immune response targeted against *Pf*EMP-1 (Chan et al., 2012). Alteration in functioning of B-cells during parasite infection comprehends the interaction between cysteine-rich inter-domain region 1α (CIDRα) of *Pf*EMP-1 and B-cells. The complex formed causes the activation of NF-kB pathway resulting in functional impairment of B-cells (Simone et al., 2011). Multiple *Pf*EMP-1 proteins of *P. falciparum* bind to Fc portion of IgM (Jeppesen et al., 2015; Stevenson et al., 2015a) and found to be involved in rosette formation (Stevenson et al., 2015a,b). In addition to *Pf*EMP-1, sub-telomeric variant open reading frame (STEVOR) and RIFIN members also play decisive role in rosette formation (Cheng et al., 1998; Kyes et al., 1999; Niang et al., 2014). The antigenic variation of proteins allows the parasite to escape host immune response (Bull et al., 1998). A protruding structure on the surface of erythrocyte namely 'knob' is found to be essential in adhesion process of iRBCs (Crabb et al., 1997). Some proteins localized to knob interact with surface proteins of erythrocytes. Interactions include binding of KAHRP with ankyrin R and pro-coagulant glucosaminoglycans (Waller et al., 1999; Wickham et al., 2001; Rug et al., 2006; Weng et al., 2014) and binding of *Plasmodium* helical interspersed sub-telomeric domain (PHIST) to *Pf*EMP-1 (Oberli et al., 2014). In case of cerebral malaria, *Pf*14_075, member of PHIST family is found to be highly up-regulated and binds to human brain endothelial cell line (HBEC-5i). The study indicates its mantle in cyto-adherence (Claessens et al., 2012). Proteins such as erythrocyte membrane protein 3 (*Pf*EMP3), Mature parasite-infected Erythrocyte Surface Antigen (MESA; Lustigman et al., 1990), RESA, *Pf*EMP-1 (Sharma, 1997; Horrocks et al., 2005), KAHRP (Rug et al., 2006) and *Pf*EMP3 (Knuepfer et al., 2005) are involved in knob formation. Merozoites Surface Protein-1 (MSP-1), another knob protein, shows interaction with RBC surface proteins like Band 3 and Glycophorin A (GPA). A study of mouse model deficient in GPA-Band3 complex described the role of knob formation in cyto-adherence. (Goel et al., 2003; Baldwin et al., 2015).

Membrane Permeability

Secretory proteins make astonishing alterations in the permeability of iRBCs membrane for ions and nutrient exchange. (Homewood and Neame, 1974; Ginsburg et al., 1983; Kutner et al., 1983). The presence of ion channels such as *Plasmodium* Surface Anion Channel (PSAC) is responsible for induction of drug resistance. The identification of structural composition of this complex would contribute to better understanding of pathogenic interaction and drug resistance mechanism and therefore suggested for therapeutic intervention (Lisk et al., 2008; Desai, 2012). Cytoadherence-linked antigen3 (Clag3) protein, found on the host membrane is appraised to be associated with PSAC in ion and nutrient transport through channels (Nguitragool et al., 2011; Pillai et al., 2012; Sharma et al., 2015). Secretory proteins involved in regulation of net flux of Na^+, K^+, and other ions are on the focus (Kirk, 2015). For instance, P-type ATP4 (*Pf*ATP4), regulating the transport of Na^+ ions is contemplated as a potential drug target (Spillman et al., 2013). Membrane permeabilization is found to be a necessary event for egress of parasites from iRBCs. Cysteine proteases have been shown to play cardinal role in rupture of erythrocyte membrane for the release of parasite (Hadley et al., 1983; Dluzewski et al., 1986; McKerrow et al., 1993; Raphael et al., 2000; Lee and Fidock, 2008). One of the members of this class, falcipian 2 is responsible for the cleavage of ankyrin and protein 4.1 of erythrocytic cytoskeleton (Dua et al., 2001). It has been evident through the gene disruption studies that expression of *Plasmodium* perforin like protein 2 (PPLP2) is paramount for membrane permeabilization during the gametocyte release from infected erythrocytes. It had been illustrated that gametocytes are unable to release from PPLP2 (−) lines of parasite, thereby reducing the transfer of gametocyte to vector (Wirth et al., 2014). MSP-1 has also been demonstrated to interact with host cytoskeleton spectrin causing the membrane destabilization and thereby enabling the release of merozoites from iRBC (Das et al., 2015).

Membrane Rigidity

Apart from cytoadherence, membrane rigidness or loss of deformability is also responsible for the sequestration of iRBCs (Bull et al., 1998). It has been clarified that knobs are liable for causing stiffness and hardening of the iRBCs (Zhang et al., 2015). Deformability of parasitized RBC is reduced due to association of RESA with spectrin (Mills et al., 2007). *Pf*332 exported on the membrane is directly involved in membrane rigidity and adhesion (Glenister et al., 2009). The KAHRP along with the membrane skeleton imparts rigidity to infected cell and will eventually obstruct blood flow (Waller et al., 1999; Pei et al., 2005). PHIST protein increases membrane rigidity by binding to membrane skeleton (Parish et al., 2013). Thus, it can be surmised that proteins responsible for rigidity are directly linked to virulence, providing an evidence for secretome in establishment of infection.

SECRETORY PROTEIN EXPORTED BEYOND THE ERYTHROCYTE

Most of the data reported with respect to secretome is related to proteins secreted into the erythrocytes cytosol or membrane. Interestingly, some proteins, which are not restricted to iRBCs membrane rather squeeze out from iRBCs membrane and get secreted out. First experimental evidence (Singh et al., 2009) identified secretion of 27 novel proteins beyond the erythrocyte membrane before it gets ruptured. Immune localization and immune electron microscopic studies confirmed the secretion of proteins beyond iRBC (Singh et al., 2009). Some of them are functionally characterized. The protein containing Sel-1 functional domain is found to be involved in regulating 'Notch signaling pathway' which in turn has been hypothesized to influence the T cell differentiation (Grant and Greenwald, 1996; Singh et al., 2009). In most protozoan parasites, to evade host immune response, common mechanism includes altered T-helper cell differentiation (Zambrano-Villa et al., 2002; Rodrigues et al., 2014). Some proteins, closely associated with highly polymorphic genes, contribute to antigenic determinants of parasite (Singh et al., 2009). Secretory protein with LCCL (Limulus clotting factor C) domain, conserved across apicomplexan parasite, assumed to have role in immune evasion mechanism, (Claudianos et al., 2002; Dessens et al., 2004), defense mechanism and shows binding with lipid A of lipopolysaccharides. CRISPLD2 (Cysteine-Rich Secretory Protein LCCL Domain containing 2), an example of LCCL domain containing protein, has an anti-inflammatory function and is related to disease pathology (Vásárhelyi et al., 2014).

Sequence similarity studies suggested that some proteins viz, virulent immuno-reactive protein (specific to bacteria and virus), PFB0765w (uncharacterized protein), rhoptry neck protein (RON4), moving junction protein and MAL13P1.39 (uncharacterized protein) are involved in modulation of host immune response (Singh et al., 2009). Domain analysis demonstrated the presence of extracellular domain responsible for the interaction with other proteins, speculative of being involved in host–parasite interactions. [**Table 1**: Domains identified by CDD (Conserved Domain Database), NCBI]. It is depicted through flowcytometery and confocal microscopy that translationally controlled tumor protein (TCTP) analog released by *Plasmodium* in host serum is responsible for release of histamine and IL-8 from basophils and eosinophils, respectively, (MacDonald et al., 2001) and reduction in B-cell immune response. In another study, a canonical tyrosyl-tRNA synthetase (*Pf*TyrRS) from *Plasmodium* is evidenced to be secreted out from the iRBCs and involved in non-canonical function of immune cell binding and modulation (Bhatt et al., 2011). Likewise in other intracellular pathogens such as *Mycobacterium tuberculosis* immune modulation ability is found in secretory proteins (Giacomini et al., 2001). During infection, secretome is also charged for causing alteration in functioning of antigen-presenting cells and dendritic cells (Sacks and Sher, 2002; Langhorne et al., 2004; Millington et al., 2006; Sponaas et al., 2006; Teirlinck et al., 2015). The presence of proteins on the surface or in secretion implicate their role in host–parasite interactions and probably in immune modulation for better survival of parasite and it would be fascinating to have information related to the 'Interactome' of the secretory proteins. *In-silico* knock-out studies and graphical analysis of protein–protein interaction network (PPIN) explored newer approach in order to identify the interacting partners vital to parasite during host–parasite interaction (Bhattacharyya and Chakrabarti, 2015). Nevertheless,

TABLE 1 | Some secretory protein exported out from the iRBC.

Sr. No	Gene name	Domain description/protein name	Reference
1	MAL7P1.138	–	Singh et al., 2009
2	MAL8P1.126	Serine protease DegP	Singh et al., 2009
3	MAL13P1.24	–	Singh et al., 2009
4	MAL13P1.39	–	Singh et al., 2009
5	*PF*07_0074	–	Singh et al., 2009
6	*PF*07_0086	Uncharacterized protein with domain 1. TATA element modulatory factor 1 2. DNA repair protein RAD18	Singh et al., 2009
7	*PF*07_0113	–	Singh et al., 2009
8	GBP-*PF*10_0159	1. Glycophorin-binding protein	Singh et al., 2009
9	*PF*10_0318	1. Uncharacterized / ACR, YagE family domain	Singh et al., 2009
10	*PF*10_0380	Trophozoite antigen R45, putative	Singh et al., 2009
11	*PF* EP *PF*11_0139	Protein tyrosine phosphates	Singh et al., 2009
12	RON4 *PF*11_0168	Moving junction protein	Singh et al., 2009
13	TKL-2 *PF*11_0220	Protein Kinase	Singh et al., 2009
14	*PF*11_0324	Uncharacterized protein	Singh et al., 2009
15	*PF*11_0369	Uncharacterized protein	Singh et al., 2009
16	*PF*11_0381	Subtilisin-like protease 2	Singh et al., 2009
18	*PF*13_0198	Reticulocyte-binding protein 2 homolog a	Singh et al., 2009
19	*PF*14_0462	SEL-1 protein, putative	Singh et al., 2009
20	CCP1 *PF*14_0723	LCCL domain containing protein CCP1	Singh et al., 2009
21	*PF*A018w	1. L-seryl-tRNA(Sec) kinase, 2. Predicted nucleotide kinase	Singh et al., 2009
22	*PF*B0190c	Conserved *Plasmodium* protein with domain 1. Sel1-like repeats 2. TPR repeat, SEL1 subfamily	Singh et al., 2009
23	*PF*B0315w	Uncharacterized protein *PF*B0315w	Singh et al., 2009
24	*PF*b0465c	Monocarboxylate transporter, putative with domain 1. The Major Facilitator Super family (MFS) 2. Oxalate/formate antiporter family transporter. 3. Monocarboxylate transporter	Singh et al., 2009
25	*PF*B0655c	Conserved *Plasmodium* protein	Singh et al., 2009
26	*PF*B0750w	Vacuolar protein-sorting protein VPS45, putative	Singh et al., 2009
27	*PF*B0765w	Uncharacterized protein *PF*B0765w with domain 1. Chromosome segregation ATPases 2. Myosin class II heavy chain [Cytoskeleton]	Singh et al., 2009
28	*PF*E0245c	Uncharacterized protein with domain 1. Dos2-interacting transcription regulator of RNA-Pol-II 2. DNA repair/transcription protein Mms19 3. Ultrahigh sulfur keratin-associated protein	Singh et al., 2009
29	*PF*E0440w	Uncharacterized	Singh et al., 2009
30	*PF*L0030c	Erythrocyte membrane protein 1 (*PF*EMP1)	Singh et al., 2009
31	*PF*I1150w	HRP II/I II domain	Singh et al., 2009
32	*PF*L2405c	Chromosome segregation protein SMC (structural maintenance of chromosomes) *PF*G377 protein	Singh et al., 2009
33	*PF*TyrRS	Tyrosyl-tRNA synthetase	Bhatt et al., 2011
34	*PF*TCTP	*Plasmodium falciparum* translationally controlled tumor protein	MacDonald et al., 2001; Calderon-Perez et al., 2014

some more studies are required to understand the role of secretory proteins in regulating host pathways. The role of secretory proteins of the parasite could have larger impact on malaria biology. Besides available knowledge, there is a need to identify signature motif or pattern responsible for secretion of proteins outside iRBCs. The identification of marker responsible for the localization of proteins to infected erythrocyte membrane and their export will be highly beneficial in interaction studies. There is a requirement of classifying secretome in terms of cellular localization and expression during developmental stages of parasite in order to understand its role in better way. It would be interesting to explore trafficking pathway of protein exported beyond the iRBCs membrane.

SECRETOME AS POTENTIAL DRUG/VACCINE TARGET

The intracellular parasite adapts different strategies for protein export in order to survive in host environment. As the secretome is intimately associated with disease pathology and parasite survival is reliant on them, any interference in the secretory pathway or inhibition of secretory proteins itself would jeopardize the parasite. In addition, utilization of information of secretome available shall provide clues to certain strategies involved in host–parasite interaction at molecular level (Ranganathan and Garg, 2009). The function of these proteins can be annotated by comparing with homologous protein of known function in other organisms. Homology modeling of secretory proteins could also provide a starting point for the lead identification in the process of drug development. Vaccine and drug development against the secretory protein is in progress in various other pathogens like *H. pylori* (Lower et al., 2008), Helminths parasite (Hewitson et al., 2009) etc. Till date, various parasite proteins involved in secretory pathway have been characterized and may be critical in anti-malarial drug targeting such as inhibition of PTEX complex. Another important drug target capturing the interest in context of drug development area is PMV (plasmepsin V). Indispensability of PMV in virulence, cytoadherence, and parasitic growth makes PMV an attractive anti-malarial drug target (Sleebs et al., 2014a,b). Structural determination of PMV–WEHI 842 inhibitor complex provides an insight for interaction between active site residue and inhibitor. This study paves the way for developing potent anti-malarial by blocking export machinery of parasite (Hodder et al., 2015).

Taken together, the functional characterization of secretory proteins and proteins involved in their export, implicated in knob formation, involved in trafficking pathway, or those involved in host pathogenic interaction and invasion of host immune system, are all indispensible for parasite survival or pathogenicity. Therefore, complete investigation and characterization of secretome may provide us better understanding to get effective therapies for malaria disease. Allelic replacement and GFP tagging revealed the importance of PMV in protein export and parasite survival thus making it an attractive target for anti malarial drugs.

CONCLUSION

Export of secretory parasite proteins into host cytoplasm will lead to apprehension of host cell functions required for parasite growth and survival by modulating crucial phenomena of malaria biology such as immune evasion and virulence. Deep understanding and investigation of role played by malaria secretome will be not only beneficial in deciphering host–pathogen interactions but it may also lead to better therapeutic intervention for malaria disease.

AUTHOR CONTRIBUTIONS

RS and DS provided data and TB wrote the manuscript.

REFERENCES

1. Baldwin, M. R., Li, X., Hanada, T., Liu, S.-C., and Chishti, A. H. (2015). Merozoite surface protein 1 recognition of host glycophorin A mediates malaria parasite invasion of red blood cells. *Blood* 125, 2704–2711. doi: 10.1182/blood-2014-11- 611707
2. Bannister, L. H., Hopkins, J. M., Fowler, R. E., Krishna, S., and Mitchell, G. H. (2000). A Brief illustrated guide to the ultrastructure of *Plasmodium falciparum* asexual blood stages. *Parasitol. Today* 16, 427–433. doi: 10.1016/ S0169- 4758(00)01755-5
3. Barnwell, J. (1989). Vesicle-mediated transport of membrane and proteins in malaria-infected erythrocytes. *Blood Cells* 16, 379–395.
4. Beck, J. R., Muralidharan, V., Oksman, A., and Goldberg, D. E. (2014). PTEX component HSP101 mediates export of diverse malaria effectors into host erythrocytes. *Nature* 511, 592–595. doi: 10.1038/nature 13574
5. Bhalla, K., Chugh, M., Mehrotra, S., Rathore, S., Tousif, S., Prakash Dwivedi, V., et al. (2015). Host ICAMs play a role in cell invasion by *Mycobacterium tuberculosis* and *Plasmodium falciparum*. *Nat. Commun.* 6:6049. doi: 10.1038/ncomms7049
6. Bhatt, T. K., Khan, S., Dwivedi, V. P., Banday, M. M., Sharma, A., Chandele, A., et al. (2011). Malaria parasite tyrosyl-tRNA synthetase secretion triggers pro-inflammatory responses. *Nat. Commun.* 2:530. doi: 10.1038/ ncomm s1522
7. Bhattacharjee, S., Stahelin, R. V., Speicher, K. D., Speicher, D. W., and Haldar, K. (2012). Endoplasmic reticulum PI(3)P lipid binding targets malaria proteins to the host cell. *Cell* 148, 201–212. doi: 10.1016/j.cell.2011. 10.051
8. Bhattacharyya, M., and Chakrabarti, S. (2015). Identification of important interacting proteins (IIPs) in *Plasmodium falciparum* using large-scale interaction network analysis and in-silico knock-out studies. *Malar. J.* 14:70. doi: 10.1186/s12936-015-0562-1
9. Boddey, J. A., Hodder, A. N., Gunther, S., Gilson, P. R., Patsiouras, H., Kapp, E. A., et al. (2010). An aspartyl protease directs malaria effector proteins to the host cell. *Nature* 463, 627–631. doi: 10.1038/nature08728
10. Bull, P. C., Lowe, B. S., Kortok, M., Molyneux, C. S., Newbold, C. I., and Marsh, K. (1998). Parasite antigens on the infected red cell surface are targets for naturally acquired immunity to malaria. *Nat. Med.* 4, 358–360. doi: 10.1038/nm 0398-358
11. Calderon-Perez, B., Xoconostle-Cazares, B., Lira-Carmona, R., Hernandez- Rivas, R., Ortega-Lopez, J., and Ruiz-Medrano, R. (2014). The *Plasmodium falciparum* translationally controlled tumor protein (TCTP) is incorporated more efficiently into B cells than its human homologue. *PLoS ONE* 9:e85514. doi: 10.1371/journal.pone.00 85514
12. Chan, J.-A., Howell, K. B., Reiling, L., Ataide, R., Mackintosh, C. L., Fowkes, F. J. I., et al. (2012). Targets of antibodies against *Plasmodium falciparum*–infected erythrocytes in malaria immunity. *J. Clin. Invest.* 122, 3227–3238. doi: 10.1172/JCI62182

13. Chang, H. H., Falick, A. M., Carlton, P. M., Sedat, J. W., DeRisi, J. L., and Marletta, M. A. (2008). N-terminal processing of proteins exported by malaria parasites. *Mol. Biochem. Parasitol.* 160, 107–115. doi: 10.1016/j.molbiopara.2008. 04.011
14. Charpian, S., and Przyborski, J. M. (2008). Protein transport across the parasitophorous vacuole of *Plasmodium falciparum*: into the great wide open. *Traffic* 9, 157–165. doi: 10.1111/j.1600-0854.2007.00648.x
15. Chen, Q., Barragan, A., Fernandez, V., Sundström, A., Schlichtherle, M., Sahlén, A., et al. (1998). Identification of *Plasmodium falciparum* erythrocyte membrane protein 1 (PfEMP1) as the rosetting ligand of the malaria parasite *P. falciparum*. *J. Exp. Med.* 187, 15–23. doi: 10.1084/jem.187.1.15
16. Cheng, Q., Cloonan, N., Fischer, K., Thompson, J., Waine, G., Lanzer, M., et al. (1998). stevor and rif are *Plasmodium falciparum* multicopy gene families which potentially encode variant antigens. *Mol. Biochem. Parasitol.* 97, 161–176. doi: 10.1016/S0166-6851(98)00144-3
17. Claessens, A., Adams, Y., Ghumra, A., Lindergard, G., Buchan, C. C., Andisi, C., et al. (2012). A subset of group A-like var genes encodes the malaria parasite ligands for binding to human brain endothelial cells. *Proc. Natl. Acad. Sci. U.S.A.* 109, E1772–E1781. doi: 10.1073/pnas.1120461109
18. Claudianos, C., Dessens, J. T., Trueman, H. E., Arai, M., Mendoza, J., Butcher, G. A., et al. (2002). A malaria scavenger receptor-like protein essential for parasite development. *Mol. Microbiol.* 45, 1473–1484. doi: 10.1046/j.1365- 2958.2002.03118.x
19. Cooke, B. M., Mohandas, N., and Coppel, R. L. (2001). The malaria-infected red blood cell: structural and functional changes. *Adv. Parasitol.* 50, 1–86. doi: 10.1016/S0065-308X(01)50029-9
20. Crabb, B. S., Cooke, B. M., Reeder, J. C., Waller, R. F., Caruana, S. R., Davern, K. M., et al. (1997). Targeted gene disruption shows that knobs enable malaria-infected red cells to cytoadhere under physiological shear stress. *Cell* 89, 287–296. doi: 10.1016/S0092-8674(00)80207-X
21. Das, S., Hertrich, N., Perrin A. J., Withers-Martinez, C., Collins, C. R., Jones, M. L., et al. (2015). Processing of *Plasmodium falciparum* merozoite surface protein msp1 activates a spectrin-binding function enabling parasite egress from RBCs. *Cell Host Microbe* 18, 433–444. doi: 10.1016/j.chom.2015.09.007
22. Deitsch, K. W., and Wellems, T. E. (1996). Membrane modifications in erythrocytes parasitized by *Plasmodium falciparum*. *Mol. Biochem. Parasitol.* 76, 1–10. doi: 10.1016/0166-6851(95)02575-8
23. de Koning-Ward, T. F., Gilson, P. R., Boddey, J. A., Rug, M., Smith, B. J., Papenfuss, A. T., et al. (2009). A novel protein export machine in malaria parasites. *Nature* 459, 945–949. doi: 10.1038/nature08104
24. Desai, S. A. (2012). Ion and nutrient uptake by malaria parasite-infected erythrocytes. *Cell Microbiol.* 14, 1003–1009. doi: 10.1111/j.1462-5822.2012.01790.x
25. Desai, S. A., and Miller, L. H. (2014). Malaria: protein-export pathway illuminated. *Nature* 511, 541–542. doi: 10.1038/nature13646
26. Dessens, J. T., Sinden, R. E., and Claudianos, C. (2004). LCCL proteins of apicomplexan parasites. *Trends Parasitol.* 20, 102–108. doi: 10.1016/j.pt.2004.01.002
27. Dluzewski, A. R., Rangachari, K., Wilson, R. J. M., and Gratzer, W. B. (1986). *Plasmodium falciparum*: protease inhibitors and inhibition of erythrocyte invasion. *Exp. Parasitol.* 62, 416–422. doi: 10.1016/0014-4894(86)90050-0
28. Dua, M., Raphael, P., Sijwali, P. S., Rosenthal, P. J., and Hanspal, M. (2001). Recombinant falcipain-2 cleaves erythrocyte membrane ankyrin and protein 4.1. *Mol. Biochem. Parasitol.* 116, 95–99. doi: 10.1016/S0166-6851(01) 00306-1
29. Elsworth, B., Matthews, K., Nie, C. Q., Kalanon, M., Charnaud, S. C., Sanders, P. R., et al. (2014). PTEX is an essential nexus for protein export in malaria parasites. *Nature* 511, 587–591. doi: 10.1038/nature13555
30. Epp, C., and Deitsch, K. (2006). Deciphering the export pathway of malaria surface proteins. *Trends Parasitol.* 22, 401–404. doi: 10.1016/j.pt.2006.07.002
31. Florens, L., Washburn, M. P., Raine, J. D., Anthony, R. M., Grainger, M., Haynes, J. D., et al. (2002). A proteomic view of the *Plasmodium falciparum* life cycle. *Nature* 419, 520–526. doi: 10.1038/nature01107
32. Gardner, J. P., Pinches, R. A., Roberts, D. J., and Newbold, C. I. (1996). Variant antigens and endothelial receptor adhesion in *Plasmodium falciparum*. *Proc. Natl. Acad. Sci. U.S.A.* 93, 3503–3508. doi: 10.1073/pnas.93.8.3503
33. Gehde, N., Hinrichs, C., Montilla, I., Charpian, S., Lingelbach, K., and Przyborski, J. M. (2009). Protein unfolding is an essential requirement for transport across the parasitophorous vacuolar membrane of *Plasmodium falciparum*. *Mol. Microbiol.* 71, 613–628. doi: 10.1111/j.1365-2958.2008.06552.x
34. Giacomini, E., Iona, E., Ferroni, L., Miettinen, M., Fattorini, L., Orefici, G., et al. (2001). Infection of human macrophages and dendritic cells with *Mycobacterium tuberculosis* induces a differential cytokine gene expression that modulates T cell response. *J. Immunol.* 166, 7033–7041. doi: 10.4049/jimmunol.166.12.7033
35. Gilson, P. R., and Crabb, B. S. (2009). Morphology and kinetics of the three distinct phases of red blood cell invasion by *Plasmodium falciparum* merozoites. *Int. J. Parasitol.* 39, 91–96. doi: 10.1016/j.ijpara.2008.09.007
36. Ginsburg, H., Krugliak, M., Eidelman, O., and Ioav Cabantchik, Z. (1983). New permeability pathways induced in membranes of *Plasmodium falciparum* infected erythrocytes. *Mol. Biochem. Parasitol.* 8, 177–190. doi: 10.1016/0166- 6851(83)90008-7
37. Glenister, F. K., Fernandez, K. M., Kats, L. M., Hanssen, E., Mohandas, N., Coppel, R. L., et al. (2009). Functional alteration of red blood cells by a megadalton protein of *Plasmodium falciparum*. *Blood* 113, 919–928. doi: 10.1182/blood- 2008-05-157735
38. Goel, V. K., Li, X., Chen, H., Liu, S.-C., Chishti, A. H., and Oh, S. S. (2003). Band 3 is a host receptor binding merozoite surface protein 1 during the *Plasmodium falciparum* invasion of erythrocytes. *Proc. Natl. Acad. Sci. U.S.A.* 100, 5164–5169. doi: 10.1073/pnas.0834959100
39. Goldberg, D. E., and Cowman, A. F. (2010). Moving in and renovating: exporting proteins from *Plasmodium* into host erythrocytes. *Nat. Rev. Microbiol.* 8, 617–621. doi: 10.1038/nrmicro2420
40. Grant, B., and Greenwald, I. (1996). The *Caenorhabditis elegans* sel-1 gene, a negative regulator of lin-12 and glp-1, encodes a predicted extracellular protein. *Genetics* 143, 237–247.
41. Gruring, C., Heiber, A., Kruse, F., Flemming, S., Franci, G., Colombo, S. F., et al. (2012). Uncovering common principles in protein export of malaria parasites. *Cell Host Microbe* 12, 717–729. doi: 10.1016/j.chom.2012.09.010
42. Gunaratne, R. S., Sajid, M., Ling, I. T., Tripathi, R., Pachebat, J. A., and Holder, A. A. (2000). Characterization of N-myristoyltransferase from *Plasmodium falciparum*. *Biochem. J.* 348(Pt 2), 459–463. doi: 10.1042/bj3480459
43. Hadley, T., Aikawa, M., and Miller, L. H. (1983). *Plasmodium knowlesi*: studies on invasion of rhesus erythrocytes by merozoites in the presence of protease inhibitors. *Exp. Parasitol.* 55, 306–311. doi: 10.1016/0014-4894(83) 90027-9
44. Haldar, K., and Mohandas, N. (2007). Erythrocyte remodeling by malaria parasites. *Curr. Opin. Hematol.* 14, 203–209. doi: 10.1097/MOH.0b013e3280f31b2d
45. Haldar, K., Mohandas, N., Samuel, B. U., Harrison, T., Hiller, N. L., Akompong, T., et al. (2002). Protein and lipid trafficking induced in erythrocytes infected by malaria parasites. *Cell Microbiol.* 4, 383–395. doi: 10.1046/j.1462- 5822.2002.00204.x
46. Heiber, A., Kruse, F., Pick, C., Gruring, C., Flemming, S., Oberli, A., et al. (2013). Identification of new PNEPs indicates a substantial non-PEXEL exportome and underpins common features in *Plasmodium falciparum* protein export. *PLoS Pathog.* 9:e1003546. doi: 10.1371/journal.ppat.1003546
47. Hewitson, J. P., Grainger, J. R., and Maizels, R. M. (2009). Helminth immunoregulation: the role of parasite secreted proteins in modulating host immunity. *Mol. Biochem. Parasitol.* 167, 1–11. doi: 10.1016/j.molbiopara.2009.04.008
48. Hiller, N. L., Bhattacharjee, S., van Ooij, C., Liolios, K., Harrison, T., Lopez- Estrano, C., et al. (2004). A host-targeting signal in virulence proteins reveals a secretome in malarial infection. *Science* 306, 1934–1937. doi: 10.1126/science.1102737
49. Hinterberg, K., Scherf, A., Gysin, J., Toyoshima, T., Aikawa, M., Mazie, J. C., et al. (1994). *Plasmodium falciparum*: the Pf332 antigen is secreted from the parasite by a brefeldin A-dependent pathway and is translocated to the erythrocyte membrane via the Maurer's clefts. *Exp. Parasitol.* 79, 279–291. doi: 10.1006/expr.1994.1091

50. Hisaeda, H., Yasutomo, K., and Himeno, K. (2005). Malaria: immune evasion by parasites. *Int. J. Biochem. Cell Biol.* 37, 700–706. doi: 10.1016/j.biocel.2004.10.009
51. Ho, M., and White, N. J. (1999). Molecular mechanisms of cytoadherence in malaria. *Am. J. Physiol. Cell Physiol.* 276, C1231–C1242.
52. Hodder, A. N., Sleebs, B. E., Czabotar, P. E., Gazdik, M., Xu, Y., O'Neill, M. T., et al. (2015). Structural basis for plasmepsin V inhibition that blocks export of malaria proteins to human erythrocytes. *Nat. Struct. Mol. Biol.* 22, 590–596. doi: 10.1038/nsmb.3061
53. Homewood, C. A., and Neame, K. D. (1974). Malaria and the permeability of the host erythrocyte. *Nature* 252, 718–719. doi: 10.1038/252718a0
54. Horrocks, P., Pinches, R. A., Chakravorty, S. J., Papakrivos, J., Christodoulou, Z., Kyes, S. A., et al. (2005). PfEMP1 expression is reduced on the surface of knobless *Plasmodium falciparum* infected erythrocytes. *J. Cell Sci.* 118, 2507- 2518. doi: 10.1242/jcs.02381
55. Jeppesen, A., Ditlev, S. B., Soroka, V., Stevenson, L., Turner, L., Dzikowski, R., et al. (2015). Multiple *Plasmodium falciparum* erythrocyte membrane protein 1 variants per genome can bind IgM via Its Fc fragment fcmu. *Infect. Immun.* 83, 3972–3981.
56. Kirk, K. (2015). Ion regulation in the malaria parasite. *Annu. Rev. Microbiol.* 69, 341–359. doi: 10.1146/annurev-micro-091014-104506
57. Knuepfer, E., Rug, M., Klonis, N., Tilley, L., and Cowman, A. F. (2005). Trafficking determinants for PfEMP3 export and assembly under the *Plasmodium falciparum*-infected red blood cell membrane. *Mol. Microbiol.* 58, 1039–1053. doi: 10.1111/j.1365-2958.2005.04895.x
58. Kutner, S., Ginsburg, H., and Cabantchik, Z. I. (1983). Permselectivity changes in malaria (*Plasmodium falciparum*) infected human red blood cell membranes. *J. Cell. Physiol.* 114, 245–251. doi: 10.1002/jcp.1041140215
59. Kyes, S. A., Rowe, J. A., Kriek, N., and Newbold, C. I. (1999). Rifins: a second family of clonally variant proteins expressed on the surface of red cells infected with *Plasmodium falciparum*. *Proc. Natl. Acad. Sci. U.S.A.* 96, 9333–9338. doi: 10.1073/pnas.96.16.9333
60. Langhorne, J. R., Albano, F., Hensmann, M., Sanni, L., Cadman, E., Voisine, C., et al. (2004). Dendritic cells, pro-inflammatory responses, and antigen presentation in a rodent malaria infection. *Immunol. Rev.* 201, 35–47.
61. Lanzer, M., Wickert, H., Krohne, G., Vincensini, L., and Breton, C. B. (2006). Maurer's clefts: a novel multi-functional organelle in the cytoplasm of *Plasmodium falciparum*-infected erythrocytes. *Int. J. Parasitol.* 36, 23–36. doi: 10.1016/j.ijpara.2005.10.001
62. Lee, M. C. S., and Fidock, D. A. (2008). Arresting malaria parasite egress from infected red blood cells. *Nat. Chem. Biol.* 4, 161–162. doi: 10.1038/nchembio0308-161
63. Lingelbach, K., and Przyborski, J. M. (2006). The long and winding road: protein trafficking mechanisms in the *Plasmodium falciparum* infected erythrocyte. *Mol. Biochem. Parasitol.* 147, 1–8. doi: 10.1016/j.molbiopara.2006.01.014
64. Lisk, G., Pain, M., Gluzman, I. Y., Kambhampati, S., Furuya, T., Su, X.-Z., et al. (2008). Changes in the plasmodial surface anion channel reduce leupeptin uptake and can confer drug resistance in *Plasmodium falciparum*-infected erythrocytes. *Antimicrob. Agents Chemother.* 52, 2346–2354.
65. Lower, M., Weydig, C., Metzler, D., Reuter, A., Starzinski-Powitz, A., Wessler, S., et al. (2008). Prediction of extracellular proteases of the human pathogen *Helicobacter pylori* reveals proteolytic activity of the Hp1018/19 protein HtrA. *PLoS ONE* 3:e3510. doi: 10.1371/journal.pone.0003510
66. Lustigman, S., Anders, R. F., Brown, G. V., and Coppel, R. L. (1990). The mature-parasite-infected erythrocyte surface antigen (MESA) of *Plasmodium falciparum* associates with the erythrocyte membrane skeletal protein, band 4.1. *Mol. Biochem. Parasitol.* 38, 261–270. doi: 10.1016/0166-6851(90) 90029-L
67. Ma, J., Rahlfs, S., Jortzik, E., Schirmer, R. H., Przyborski, J. M., and Becker, K. (2012). Subcellular localization of adenylate kinases in *Plasmodium falciparum*. *FEBS Lett.* 586, 3037–3043. doi: 10.1016/j.febslet.2012.07.013
68. MacDonald, S. M., Bhisutthibhan, J., Shapiro, T. A., Rogerson, S. J., Taylor, T. E., Tembo, M., et al. (2001). Immune mimicry in malaria: *Plasmodium falciparum* secretes a functional histamine-releasing factor homolog in vitro and in vivo. *Proc. Natl. Acad. Sci. U.S.A.* 98, 10829–10832. doi: 10.1073/pnas.2011 91498
69. Magowan, C., Wollish, W., Anderson, L., and Leech, J. (1988). Cytoadherence by *Plasmodium falciparum*-infected erythrocytes is correlated with the expression of a family of variable proteins on infected erythrocytes. *J. Exp. Med.* 168, 1307–1320. doi: 10.1084/jem.168.4.1307
70. Maier, A. G., Cooke, B. M., Cowman, A. F., and Tilley, L. (2009). Malaria parasite proteins that remodel the host erythrocyte. *Nat. Rev. Microbiol.* 7, 341–354. doi: 10.1038/nrmicro2110
71. Maier, A. G., Rug, M., O'Neill, M. T., Beeson, J. G., Marti, M., Reeder, J., et al. (2007). Skeleton-binding protein 1 functions at the parasitophorous vacuole membrane to traffic PfEMP1 to the *Plasmodium falciparum*-infected erythrocyte surface. *Blood* 109, 1289–1297. doi: 10.1182/blood-2006-08-043364 Marti, M., Baum, J., Rug, M., Tilley, L., and Cowman, A. F. (2005). Signal-mediated export of proteins from the malaria parasite to the host erythrocyte. *J. Cell Biol.* 171, 587–592. doi: 10.1083/jcb.200508051
72. Marti, M., Good, R. T., Rug, M., Knuepfer, E., and Cowman, A. F. (2004). Targeting malaria virulence and remodeling proteins to the host erythrocyte. *Science* 306, 1930–1933. doi: 10.1126/science.1102452
73. Marti, M., and Spielmann, T. (2013). Protein export in malaria parasites: many membranes to cross. *Curr. Opin. Microbiol.* 16, 445–451. doi: 10.1016/j.mib.2013.04.010
74. Martin, R. E., Ginsburg, H., and Kirk, K. (2009). Membrane transport proteins of the malaria parasite. *Mol. Microbiol.* 74, 519–528. doi: 10.1111/j.1365- 2958.2009.06863.x
75. McKerrow, J. H., Sun, E., Rosenthal, P. J., and Bouvier, J. (1993). The proteases and pathogenicity of parasitic protozoa. *Annu. Rev. Microbiol.* 47, 821–853. doi: 10.1146/annurev.mi.47.100193.004133
76. Mendis, K. N., and Carter, R. (1995). Clinical disease and pathogenesis in malaria. *Parasitol. Today* 11, TI1–TI16. doi: 10.1016/0169-4758(95)80143-X
77. Miller, L. H., Baruch, D. I., Marsh, K., and Doumbo, O. K. (2002). The pathogenic basis of malaria. *Nature* 415, 673–679. doi: 10.1038/415673a
78. Miller, L. H., Good, M. F., and Milon, G. (1994). Malaria pathogenesis. *Science* 264, 1878–1883. doi: 10.1126/science.8009217
79. Millington, O. R., Di Lorenzo, C., Phillips, R. S., Garside, P., and Brewer, J. M. (2006). Suppression of adaptive immunity to heterologous antigens during *Plasmodium* infection through hemozoin-induced failure of dendritic cell function. *J. Biol.* 5:5. doi: 10.1186/jbiol34
80. Mills, J., Diez-Silva, M., Quinn, D., Dao, M., Lang, M., Tan, K., et al. (2007). Effect of plasmodial RESA protein on deformability of human red blood cells harboring *Plasmodium falciparum*. *Proc. Natl. Acad. Sci. U.S.A.* 104, 9213–9217. doi: 10.1073/pnas.0703433104
81. Mundwiler-Pachlatko, E., and Beck, H.-P. (2013). Maurer's clefts, the enigma of *Plasmodium falciparum*. *Proc. Natl. Acad. Sci. U.S.A.* 110, 19987–19994. doi: 10.1073/pnas.1309247110
82. Newbold, C., Craig, A., Kyes, S., Rowe, A., Fernandez-Reyes, D., and Fagan, T. (1999). Cytoadherence, pathogenesis and the infected red cell surface in *Plasmodium falciparum*. *Int. J. Parasitol.* 29, 927–937. doi: 10.1016/S0020-7519(99)00049-1
83. Nguitragool, W., Bokhari, A. A. B., Pillai, A. D., Rayavara, K., Sharma, P., Turpin, B., et al. (2011). Malaria parasite clag genes determine nutrient uptake channel activity on infected red blood cells. *Cell* 145, 665–677. doi: 10.1016/j.cell.2011.05.002
84. Niang, M., Bei A. K., Madnani, K. G., Pelly, S., Dankwa, S., Kanjee, U., et al. (2014). STEVOR is a *Plasmodium falciparum* erythrocyte binding protein that mediates merozoite invasion and rosetting. *Cell Host Microbe* 16, 81–93. doi: 10.1016/j.chom.2014.06.004
85. Oberli, A., Slater, L. M., Cutts, E., Brand, F., Mundwiler-Pachlatko, E., Rusch, S., et al. (2014). A *Plasmodium falciparum* PHIST protein binds the virulence factor PfEMP1 and comigrates to knobs on the host cell surface. *FASEB J.* 28, 4420–4433. doi: 10.1096/fj.14-256057
86. Pain, A., Ferguson, D. J., Kai, O., Urban, B. C., Lowe, B., Marsh, K., et al. (2001). Platelet-mediated clumping of *Plasmodium falciparum*-infected erythrocytes is a common adhesive phenotype and is associated with severe malaria. *Proc. Natl. Acad. Sci. U.S.A.* 98, 1805–1810. doi: 10.1073/pnas.98.4.1805
87. Parish, L. A., Mai, D. W., Jones, M. L., Kitson, E. L., and Rayner, J. C. (2013). A member of the *Plasmodium falciparum* PHIST family binds to the erythrocyte cytoskeleton component band 4.1. *Malar. J.* 12, 160–160. doi: 10.1186/1475- 2875-12-160

88. Parker, P. D., Tilley, L., and Klonis, N. (2004). *Plasmodium falciparum* induces reorganization of host membrane proteins during intraerythrocytic growth. *Blood* 103, 2404–2406. doi: 10.1182/blood-2003-08-2692
89. Pei, X., An, X., Guo, X., Tarnawski, M., Coppel, R., and Mohandas, N. (2005). Structural and functional studies of interaction between *Plasmodium falciparum* knob-associated histidine-rich protein (KAHRP) and erythrocyte spectrin. *J. Biol. Chem.* 280, 31166–31171. doi: 10.1074/jbc.M5052 98200
90. Pillai, A. D., Nguitragool, W., Lyko, B., Dolinta, K., Butler, M. M., Nguyen, S. T., et al. (2012). Solute restriction reveals an essential role for clag3-associated channels in malaria parasite nutrient acquisition. *Mol. Pharmacol.* 82, 1104– 1114. doi: 10.1124/mol.112.081224
91. Przyborski, J. M., Wickert, H., Krohne, G., and Lanzer, M. (2003). Maurer's clefts—a novel secretory organelle? *Mol. Biochem. Parasitol.* 132, 17–26. doi: 10.1016/S0166-6851(03)00212-3
92. Ranganathan, S., and Garg, G. (2009). Secretome: clues into pathogen infection and clinical applications. *Genome Med.* 1:113. doi: 10.1186/gm113
93. Raphael, P., Takakuwa, Y., Manno, S., Liu, S. C., Chishti, A. H., and Hanspal, M. (2000). A cysteine protease activity from *Plasmodium falciparum* cleaves human erythrocyte ankyrin. *Mol. Biochem. Parasitol.* 110, 259–272. doi: 10.1016/S0166- 6851(00)00283-8
94. Rodrigues, V., Cordeiro-da-Silva, A., Laforge, M., Ouaissi, A., Akharid, K., Silvestre, R., et al. (2014). Impairment of T cell function in parasitic infections. *PLoS Negl. Trop. Dis.* 8:e2567. doi: 10.1371/journal.pntd.0002567
95. Rowe, A., Obeiro, J., Newbold, C. I., and Marsh, K. (1995). *Plasmodium falciparum* rosetting is associated with malaria severity in Kenya. *Infect. Immun.* 63, 2323–2326.
96. Rowe, J. A., Claessens, A., Corrigan, R. A., and Arman, M. (2009). Adhesion of *Plasmodium falciparum*-infected erythrocytes to human cells: molecular mechanisms and therapeutic implications. *Expert Rev. Mol. Med.* 11:e16. doi: 10.1017/S1462399409001082
97. Rowe, J. A., Obiero, J., Marsh, K., and Raza, A. (2002). Short report: positive correlation between rosetting and parasitemia in *Plasmodium falciparum* clinical isolates. *Am. J. Trop. Med. Hyg.* 66, 458–460.
98. Rudzinska, M. A., and Trager, W. (1968). The fine structure of trophozoites and gametocytes in *Plasmodium coatneyi**. *J. Protozool.* 15, 73–88. doi: 10.1111/j.1550-7408.1968.tb02091.x
99. Rug, M., Prescott, S. W., Fernandez, K. M., Cooke, B. M., and Cowman, A. F. (2006). The role of KAHRP domains in knob formation and cytoadherence of *P. falciparum*-infected human erythrocytes. *Blood* 108, 370–378. doi: 10.1182/blood-2005-11-4624
100. Russo, I., Babbitt, S., Muralidharan, V., Butler, T., Oksman, A., and Goldberg, D. E. (2010). Plasmepsin V licenses Plasmodium proteins for export into the host erythrocyte. *Nature* 463, 632–636. doi: 10.1038/nature08726
101. Sacks, D., and Sher, A. (2002). Evasion of innate immunity by parasitic protozoa. *Nat. Immunol.* 3, 1041–1047. doi: 10.1038/ni1102-1041
102. Sharma, P., Rayavara, K., Ito, D., Basore, K., and Desai, S. A. (2015). A CLAG3 mutation in an amphipathic transmembrane domain alters malaria parasite nutrient channels and confers leupeptin resistance. *Infect. Immun.* 83, 2566– 2574. doi: 10.1128/IAI.02966-14
103. Sharma, Y. D. (1997). Knob proteins in falciparum malaria. *Indian J. Med. Res.* 106, 53–62.
104. Simone, O., Bejarano, M. T., Pierce, S. K., Antonaci, S., Wahlgren, M., Troye- Blomberg, M., et al. (2011). TLRs innate immunereceptors and *Plasmodium falciparum* erythrocyte membrane protein 1 (PfEMP1) CIDR1alpha- driven human polyclonal B-cell activation. *Acta Trop.* 119, 144–150. doi: 10.1016/j.actatropica.2011.05.005
105. Singh, M., Mukherjee, P., Narayanasamy, K., Arora, R., Sen, S. D., Gupta, S., et al. (2009). Proteome analysis of *Plasmodium falciparum* extracellular secretory antigens at asexual blood stages reveals a cohort of proteins with possible roles in immune modulation and signaling. *Mol. Cell. Proteom.* 8, 2102–2118. doi: 10.1074/mcp.M900029-MCP200
106. Sleebs, B. E., Gazdik, M., O'Neill, M. T., Rajasekaran, P., Lopaticki, S., Lackovic, K., et al. (2014a). Transition state mimetics of the *Plasmodium* export element are potent inhibitors of plasmepsin V from *P. falciparum* and *P. vivax*. *J. Med. Chem.* 57, 7644–7662. doi: 10.1021/jm500797g
107. Sleebs, B. E., Lopaticki, S., Marapana, D. S., O'Neill, M. T., Rajasekaran, P., Gazdik, M., et al. (2014b). Inhibition of Plasmepsin V activity demonstrates its essential role in protein export, PfEMP1 display, and survival of malaria parasites. *PLoS Biol* 12:e1001897. doi: 10.1371/journal.pbio.1001897
108. Spielmann, T., and Gilberger, T.-W. (2010). Protein export in malaria parasites: do multiple export motifs add up to multiple export pathways? *Trends Parasitol.* 26, 6–10. doi: 10.1016/j.pt.2009.10.001
109. Spielmann, T., Hawthorne, P. L., Dixon, M. W. A., Hannemann, M., Klotz, K., Kemp, D. J., et al. (2006). A cluster of ring stage–specific genes linked to a locus implicated in cytoadherence in *Plasmodium falciparum* codes for PEXEL- negative and PEXEL-positive proteins exported into the host cell. *Mol. Biol. Cell* 17, 3613–3624. doi: 10.1091/mbc.E06-04-0291
110. Spillman, N. J., Allen, R. J., McNamara, C. W., Yeung, B. K., Winzeler, E. A., Diagana, T. T., et al. (2013). Na+ regulation in the malaria parasite *Plasmodium falciparum* involves the cation ATPase PfATP4 and is a target of the spiroindolone antimalarials. *Cell Host Microbe* 13, 227–237. doi: 10.1016/j.chom.2012.12.006
111. Sponaas, A.-M., Cadman, E. T., Voisine, C., Harrison, V., Boonstra, A., O'Garra, A., et al. (2006). Malaria infection changes the ability of splenic dendritic cell populations to stimulate antigen-specific T cells. *J. Exp. Med.* 203, 1427–1433. doi: 10.1084/jem.20052450
112. Spycher, C., Rug, M., Pachlatko, E., Hanssen, E., Ferguson, D., Cowman, A. F., et al. (2008). The Maurer's cleft protein MAHRP1 is essential for trafficking of PfEMP1 to the surface of *Plasmodium falciparum*-infected erythrocytes. *Mol. Microbiol.* 68, 1300–1314. doi: 10.1111/j.1365-2958.2008. 06235.x
113. Stevenson, L., Huda, P., Jeppesen, A., Laursen, E., Rowe, J. A., Craig, A., et al. (2015a). Investigating the function of Fc-specific binding of IgM to *Plasmodium falciparum* erythrocyte membrane protein 1 mediating erythrocyte rosetting. *Cell Microbiol.* 17, 819–831. doi: 10.1111/cmi.12403
114. Stevenson, L., Laursen, E., Cowan, G. J., Bandoh, B., Barfod, L., Cavanagh, D. R., et al. (2015b). α 2-Macroglobulin can crosslink multiple *Plasmodium falciparum* erythrocyte membrane protein 1 (PfEMP1) molecules and may facilitate adhesion of parasitized erythrocytes. *PLoS Pathog.* 11:e1005022. doi: 10.1371/journal.ppat.1005022
115. Taraschi, T. F., O'Donnell, M., Martinez, S., Schneider, T., Trelka, D., Fowler, V. M., et al. (2003). Generation of an erythrocyte vesicle transport system by *Plasmodium falciparum* malaria parasites. *Blood* 102, 3420–3426. doi: 10.1182/blood-2003-05-1448
116. Teirlinck, A. C., Roestenberg, M., Bijker, E. M., Hoffman, S. L., Sauerwein, R. W., and Scholzen, A. (2015). *Plasmodium falciparum* infection of human volunteers activates monocytes and CD16+ dendritic cells and induces upregulation of CD16 and CD1c expression. *Infect. Immun.* 83, 3732–3739. doi: 10.1128/IAI.00473-15
117. Thavayogarajah, T., Gangopadhyay, P., Rahlfs, S., Becker, K., Lingelbach, K., Przyborski, J. M., et al. (2015). Alternative protein secretion in the malaria parasite *Plasmodium falciparum*. *PLoS ONE* 10:e0125191. doi: 10.1371/journal.pone.0125191
118. Trager, W., Rudzinska, M. A., and Bradbury, P. C. (1966). The fine structure of *Plasmodium falciparum* and its host erythrocytes in natural malarial infections in man. *Bull. World Health Organ.* 35, 883–885.
119. Udomsangpetch, R., Wahlin, B., Carlson, J., Berzins, K., Torii, M., Aikawa, M., et al. (1989). *Plasmodium falciparum*-infected erythrocytes form spontaneous erythrocyte rosettes. *J. Exp. Med.* 169, 1835–1840. doi: 10.1084/jem.169. 5.1835
120. van Ooij, C., Tamez, P., Bhattacharjee, S., Hiller, N. L., Harrison, T., Liolios, K., et al. (2008). The malaria secretome: from algorithms to essential function in blood stage infection. *PLoS Pathog.* 4:e1000084. doi: 10.1371/journal.ppat.10 00084
121. Vásárhelyi, V., Trexler, M., and Patthy, L. (2014). Both LCCL-domains of human CRISPLD2 have high affinity for lipid A. *Biochimie* 97, 66–71. doi: 10.1016/j.biochi.2013.09.021
122. Verma, R., Tiwari, A., Kaur, S., Varshney, G. C., and Raghava, G. P. (2008). Identification of proteins secreted by malaria parasite into erythrocyte using SVM and PSSM profiles. *BMC Bioinform.* 9:201. doi: 10.1186/1471-2105- 9-201
123. Waller, K. L., Cooke, B. M., Nunomura, W., Mohandas, N., and Coppel, R. L. (1999). Mapping the binding domains involved in the interaction between the *Plasmodium falciparum* knob-associated histidine-rich

protein (kahrp) and the cytoadherence ligand *P. falciparum* erythrocyte membrane protein 1 (PfEMP1). *J. Biol. Chem.* 274, 23808–23813. doi: 10.1074/jbc.274.34. 23808

124. Weng, H., Guo, X., Papoin, J., Wang, J., Coppel, R., Mohandas, N., et al. (2014). Interaction of *Plasmodium falciparum* knob-associated histidine-rich protein (KAHRP) with erythrocyte ankyrin R is required for its attachment to the erythrocyte membrane. *Biochim. Biophys. Acta* 1838, 185–192. doi: 10.1016/j.bbamem.2013.09.014
125. Wetzel, J., Herrmann, S., Swapna, L. S., Prusty, D., John Peter, A. T., Kono, M., et al. (2015). The role of palmitoylation for protein recruitment to the inner membrane complex of the malaria parasite. *J. Biol. Chem.* 290, 1712–1728. doi: 10.1074/jbc.M114.598094
126. World Health Organization [WHO] (2014). *World Malaria Report 2013*. Geneva: World Health Organization.
127. Wickham, M. E., Rug, M., Ralph, S. A., Klonis, N., McFadden, G. I., Tilley, L., et al. (2001). Trafficking and assembly of the cytoadherence complex in *Plasmodium falciparum*-infected human erythrocytes. *EMBO J.* 20, 5636–5649. doi: 10.1093/emboj/20.20.5636
128. Wirth, C. C., Glushakova, S., Scheuermayer, M., Repnik, U., Garg, S., Schaack, D., et al. (2014). Perforin-like protein PPLP2 permeabilizes the red blood cell membrane during egress of *Plasmodium falciparum* gametocytes. *Cell Microbiol.* 16, 709–733. doi: 10.1111/cmi. 12288
129. Zambrano-Villa, S., Rosales-Borjas, D., Carrero, J. C., and Ortiz-Ortiz, L. (2002). How protozoan parasites evade the immune response. *Trends Parasitol.* 18, 272–278. doi: 10.1016/S1471-4922(02)02289-4
130. Zhang, Y., Huang, C., Kim, S., Golkaram, M., Dixon, M. W., Tilley, L., et al. (2015). Multiple stiffening effects of nanoscale knobs on human red blood cells infected with *Plasmodium falciparum* malaria parasite. *Proc. Natl. Acad. Sci. U.S.A.* 112, 6068–6073. doi: 10.1073/pnas.1505 584112

Permissions

All chapters in this book were first published by Frontiers; hereby published with permission under the Creative Commons Attribution License or equivalent. Every chapter published in this book has been scrutinized by our experts. Their significance has been extensively debated. The topics covered herein carry significant findings which will fuel the growth of the discipline. They may even be implemented as practical applications or may be referred to as a beginning point for another development.

The contributors of this book come from diverse backgrounds, making this book a truly international effort. This book will bring forth new frontiers with its revolutionizing research information and detailed analysis of the nascent developments around the world.

We would like to thank all the contributing authors for lending their expertise to make the book truly unique. They have played a crucial role in the development of this book. Without their invaluable contributions this book wouldn't have been possible. They have made vital efforts to compile up to date information on the varied aspects of this subject to make this book a valuable addition to the collection of many professionals and students.

This book was conceptualized with the vision of imparting up-to-date information and advanced data in this field. To ensure the same, a matchless editorial board was set up. Every individual on the board went through rigorous rounds of assessment to prove their worth. After which they invested a large part of their time researching and compiling the most relevant data for our readers.

The editorial board has been involved in producing this book since its inception. They have spent rigorous hours researching and exploring the diverse topics which have resulted in the successful publishing of this book. They have passed on their knowledge of decades through this book. To expedite this challenging task, the publisher supported the team at every step. A small team of assistant editors was also appointed to further simplify the editing procedure and attain best results for the readers.

Apart from the editorial board, the designing team has also invested a significant amount of their time in understanding the subject and creating the most relevant covers. They scrutinized every image to scout for the most suitable representation of the subject and create an appropriate cover for the book.

The publishing team has been an ardent support to the editorial, designing and production team. Their endless efforts to recruit the best for this project, has resulted in the accomplishment of this book. They are a veteran in the field of academics and their pool of knowledge is as vast as their experience in printing. Their expertise and guidance has proved useful at every step. Their uncompromising quality standards have made this book an exceptional effort. Their encouragement from time to time has been an inspiration for everyone.

The publisher and the editorial board hope that this book will prove to be a valuable piece of knowledge for researchers, students, practitioners and scholars across the globe.

List of Contributors

Rosa T. Pinho and Paulo R. Z. Antas
Laboratório de Imunologia Clínica, Instituto Oswaldo Cruz, FIOCRUZ, Rio de Janeiro, Brazil

Mariana C. Waghabi
Laboratório de Genômica Funcional e Bioinformática, Instituto Oswaldo Cruz, FIOCRUZ, Rio de Janeiro, Brazil

Fabíola Cardillo
Centro de Pesquisa Gonçalo Muniz, FIOCRUZ, Salvador, Brazil

José Mengel
Laboratório de Imunologia Clínica, Instituto Oswaldo Cruz, FIOCRUZ, Rio de Janeiro, Brazil
Faculdade de Medicina de Petropolis (FMP-FASE), Petrópolis, Brazil

Laurent Rénia and Yun Shan Goh
Singapore Immunology Network, Agency for Science, Technology and Research (A*STAR), Singapore

Begoña Pérez-Cabezas, Pedro Cecílio and Ana Luisa Robalo
i3S - Instituto de Investigação e Inovação em Saúde, Universidade do Porto, Porto, Portugal
IBMC - Instituto de Biologia Molecular e Celular, Universidade do Porto, Porto, Portugal

Ricardo Silvestre
ICVS - Instituto de Investigação em Ciências da Vida e Saúde, Escola de Ciências da Saúde, Universidade do Minho, Braga, Portugal
ICVS/3B's - Laboratório Associado, Braga, Portugal

Eugenia Carrillo and Javier Moreno
WHO Collaborating Centre for Leishmaniasis, Centro Nacional de Microbiología, Instituto de Salud Carlos III, Madrid, Spain

Juan V. San Martín
Hospital Universitario de Fuenlabrada, Madrid, Spain

Rita Vasconcellos
Departamento de Imunobiologia, Instituto de Biologia, Universidade Federal Fluminense, Niterói, Brazil

Jyoti Bhardwaj
Division of Parasitology, Council of Scientific and Industrial Research-Central Drug Research Institute, Lucknow, Uttar Pradesh, India
Academy of Scientific and Innovative Research, Anusandhan Bhawan, New Delhi, India

Anabela Cordeiro-da-Silva
i3S - Instituto de Investigação e Inovação em Saúde, Universidade do Porto, Porto, Portugal
IBMC - Instituto de Biologia Molecular e Celular, Universidade do Porto, Porto, Portugal
Faculdade de Farmácia, Departamento de Ciências Biológicas, Universidade do Porto, Porto, Portugal

Alessandra Almeida Filardy, Kamila Guimarães-Pinto, Ketiuce Zukeram, Lara Fliess, Ludimila Pereira, Danielle Oliveira Nascimento and Luciana Conde
Department of Immunology, Paulo de Góes Microbiology Institute, Federal University of Rio de Janeiro, Rio de Janeiro, Brazil

Marise Pinheiro Nunes
Immunoparasitology Laboratory, Oswaldo Cruz Foundation, Oswaldo Cruz Institute, FIOCRUZ, Rio de Janeiro, Brazil

Alexandre Morrot
Immunoparasitology Laboratory, Oswaldo Cruz Foundation, Oswaldo Cruz Institute, FIOCRUZ, Rio de Janeiro, Brazil
Tuberculosis Research Center, Faculty of Medicine, Federal University of Rio de Janeiro, Rio de Janeiro, Brazil

Pollyanna S. Gomes and Alexandre Morrot
Departamento de Microbiologia Geral, Universidade Federal do Rio de Janeiro, Rio de Janeiro, Brazil

Juan Rivera-Correa
Division of Parasitology, Department of Microbiology, New York University School of Medicine, New York, NY, USA

Celio G. Freire-De-Lima
Instituto de Biofísica Carlos Chagas Filho, Universidade Federal do Rio de Janeiro, Rio de Janeiro, Brazil

Gabriela Minigo
Vaccine and Infectious Diseases Laboratory, Department of Immunology and Pathology, Monash University, Melbourne, VIC, Australia
Global and Tropical Health Division, Menzies School of Health Research, Charles Darwin University, Darwin, NT, Australia

Robyn M. Slattery
Diabetes Laboratory, Department of Immunology and Pathology, Monash University, Melbourne, VIC, Australia

Katie L. Flanagan
Vaccine and Infectious Diseases Laboratory, Department of Immunology and Pathology, Monash University, Melbourne, VIC, Australia
School of Medicine, University of Tasmania, Hobart, TAS, Australia

Magdalena Plebanski
Vaccine and Infectious Diseases Laboratory, Department of Immunology and Pathology, Monash University, Melbourne, VIC, Australia

Sarah de Athayde Couto Falcão and Cecília B. F. Favali
Department of Cell Biology, Biology Institute, University of Brasília, Brasília, Brazil
Núcleo de Medicina Tropical (NMT), University of Brasília, Brasília, Brazil

Tatiana M. G. Jaramillo, Daniela M. Bernardes and Jaime M. Santana
Department of Cell Biology, Biology Institute, University of Brasília, Brasília, Brazil

Luciana G. Ferreira
Núcleo de Medicina Tropical (NMT), University of Brasília, Brasília, Brazil

Liliana Maria Sanmarco, Natalia Eberhardt, Maria Cecilia Ramello, Nicolás Eric Ponce, Susana Gea and Maria Pilar Aoki
Centro de Investigaciones en Bioquímica Clínica e Inmunología CIBICI-CONICET, Facultad de Ciencias Químicas, Universidad Nacional de Córdoba, Córdoba, Argentina

Laura Marina Visconti, Natalia Beatriz Spitale, Maria Lola Vozza, Germán Andrés Bernardi and Angel Ramón Minguez
Hospital Nuestra Señora de la Misericordia del Nuevo Siglo, Córdoba, Argentina

Natalia Gil-Jaramillo, Izabela M. D. Bastos and Jaime M. Santana
Laboratório de Interação Patógeno-Hospedeiro, Instituto de Biologia, Universidade de Brasília, Brasília, Brazil

Flávia N. Motta
Laboratório de Interação Patógeno-Hospedeiro, Instituto de Biologia, Universidade de Brasília, Brasília, Brazil
Faculdade de Ceilândia, Universidade de Brasília, Brasília, Brazil

Cecília B. F. Faval
Laboratório de Biologia do Gene, Instituto de Biologia, Universidade de Brasília, Brasília, Brazil

Galia Ramírez-Toloza
Faculty of Veterinary Medicine and Livestock Sciences, University of Chile, Santiago, Chile

Paula Abello and Arturo Ferreira
Program of Immunology, Faculty of Medicine, Institute of Biomedical Sciences (ICBM), University of Chile, Santiago, Chile

Illiassou Hamidou Soumana, Bernadette Tchicaya and Anne Geiger
UMR 177, Institut de Recherche pour le Développement-CIRAD, CIRAD TA A-17/G, Montpellier, France

Stéphanie Rialle and Hugues Parrinello
Centre National de la Recherche Scientifique Unité Mixte de Recherche 5203, Institut de Génomique Fonctionnelle, Montpellier, France
Institut National de la Santé Et de la Recherche Médicale U661, Montpellier, France
Universités de Montpellier 1 and 2, UMR 5203, Montpellier, France
Montpellier GenomiX, c/o Institut de Génomique Fonctionnelle, Montpellier, France

Pollyanna S. Gomes
Departamento de Imunologia, Instituto de Microbiologia, Universidade Federal do Rio de Janeiro, Rio de Janeiro, Brazil

Daniel F. Feijó
Instituto Gonçalo Moniz, Fundação Oswaldo Cruz (Fiocruz), Salvador, Brazil

Alexandre Morrot
Departamento de Imunologia, Instituto de Microbiologia, Universidade Federal do Rio de Janeiro, Rio de Janeiro, Brazil
Instituto Oswaldo Cruz, Fiocruz, Rio de Janeiro, Brazil

Pedro Henrique Braz Mendonça, Raphael Francisco Dutra Barbosa da Rocha, Julliane Brito de Braz Moraes and Debora Decote-Ricardo
Instituto de Veterinária, Universidade Federal Rural do Rio de Janeiro, Rio de Janeiro, Brazil

Isabel Ferreira LaRocque-de-Freitas, Jorgete Logullo and Celio Geraldo Freire-de-Lima
Instituto de Biofísica Carlos Chagas Filho, Universidade Federal do Rio de Janeiro, Rio de Janeiro, Brazil

Marise Pinheiro Nunes
Instituto Oswaldo Cruz, FIOCRUZ, Rio de Janeiro, Brazil

Benoit Stijlemans
Laboratory of Cellular and Molecular Immunology, Vrije Universiteit Brussel (VUB), Brussels, Belgium
Myeloid Cell Immunology Lab, VIB-UGent Center for Inflammation Research, Ghent, Belgium

Magdalena Radwanska
Laboratory for Biomedical Research, Ghent University Global Campus, Yeonsu-Gu, Incheon, South Korea

Carl De Trez
Laboratory of Cellular and Molecular Immunology, Vrije Universiteit Brussel (VUB), Brussels, Belgium
Structural Biology Research Centre (SBRC), VIB, Brussels, Belgium

Stefan Magez
Laboratory of Cellular and Molecular Immunology, Vrije Universiteit Brussel (VUB), Brussels, Belgium
Laboratory for Biomedical Research, Ghent University Global Campus, Yeonsu-Gu, Incheon, South Korea

Débora Decote-Ricardo
Instituto de Veterinária, Universidade Federal Rural do Rio de Janeiro, Seropédica, Brazil

Marise P. Nunes
Instituto Oswaldo Cruz, Fundação Oswaldo Cruz, Rio de Janeiro, Brazil

Angélica Fernandes Arcanjo and Célio G. Freire-de-Lima
Instituto de Biofísica Carlos Chagas Filho, Universidade Federal do Rio de Janeiro, Rio de Janeiro, Brazil

Dirlei Nico, Gabriellen Menezes Migliani de Castro, Yasmin da Silva Fontes, Paula Saltarelli, Antônio Ferreira-Pereira and Clarisa B. Palatnik-de-Sousa
Departamento de Microbiologia Geral, Universidade Federal do Rio de Janeiro, Rio de Janeiro, Brazil

Debora Decote-Ricardo
Instituto de Veterinária, Universidade Federal Rural do Rio de Janeiro, Rio de Janeiro, Brazil

Alexandre Morrot
Instituto Oswaldo Cruz, Fiocruz, Rio de Janeiro, Brazil
Departamento de Imunologia, Instituto de Microbiologia, Universidade Federal do Rio de Janeiro, Rio de Janeiro, Brazil

Marise P. Nunes
Instituto Oswaldo Cruz, Fiocruz, Rio de Janeiro, Brazil

Franck Jacob, Anne Geiger and Geoffrey Gimonneau
UMR INTERTRYP, Institut de Recherche pour le Développement CIRAD, CIRAD TA A-17/G, Montpellier, France

Trésor T. Melachio, Guy R. Njitchouang and Flobert Njiokou
Parasitology and Ecology Laboratory, Department of Animal Biology and Physiology, Faculty of Science, University of Yaounde 1, Yaounde, Cameroon

Luc Abate
UMR MIVEGEC, Institut de Recherche pour le Développement 224-Centre National de la Recherche Scientifique 5390, Montpellier, France

Richard Christen
UMR 7138, Systématique Adaptation Evolution, Université de Nice-Sophia Antipolis, Nice, France

Julie Reveillaud
Institut National de la Recherche Agronomique, UMR 1309 ASTRE, Montpellier, France
CIRAD, UMR ASTRE, Montpellier, France

Jean M. Tsagmo Ngoune
Faculty of Science, University of Yaoundé I, Yaoundé, Cameroon
UMR 177, IRD-CIRAD, CIRAD TA A-17/G, Campus International de Baillarguet, Montpellier, France

Flobert Njiokou and Ginette Kame-Ngasse
Faculty of Science, University of Yaoundé I, Yaoundé, Cameroon

Béatrice Loriod, Nicolas Fernandez-Nunez, Claire Rioualen and Jacques van Helden
Aix-Marseille University, INSERM, TAGC, Technological Advances for Genomics and Clinics, UMR S 1090, Marseille, France

Anne Geiger
UMR 177, IRD-CIRAD, CIRAD TA A-17/G, Campus International de Baillarguet, Montpellier, France

Leandra Linhares-Lacerda
Departamento de Imunologia, Instituto de Microbiologia, Universidade Federal do Rio de Janeiro, Rio de Janeiro, Brazil,
Instituto Oswaldo Cruz, Fundação Oswaldo Cruz (FIOCRUZ), Rio de Janeiro, Brazil

Alessandra Granato, João Francisco Gomes-Neto and Luciana Conde
Departamento de Imunologia, Instituto de Microbiologia, Universidade Federal do Rio de Janeiro, Rio de Janeiro, Brazil

Elisangela O. de Freitas
Departamento de Análises Clínicas e Toxicológicas, Faculdade de Ciências Farmacêuticas, Universidade de São Paulo, São Paulo, Brazil

Shana P. Coutinho Barroso and Rodrigo Jorge de Alcântara Guerra
Instituto de Pesquisas Biomédicas, Hospital Naval Marcílio Dias, Marinha do Brasil, Rio de Janeiro, Brazil

Roberto C. Pedrosa
Instituto do Coração Edson Saad, Hospital Universitário Clementino Fraga Filho, Universidade Federal do Rio de Janeiro, Rio de Janeiro, Brazil

Wilson Savino
Instituto Oswaldo Cruz, Fundação Oswaldo Cruz (FIOCRUZ), Rio de Janeiro, Brazil
National Institute of Science and Technology on Neuroimmunomodulation (INCT-NIM), Rio de Janeiro, Brazil

Alexandre Morrot
Faculdade de Medicina, Centro de Pesquisas em Tuberculose, Universidade Federal do Rio de Janeiro, Rio de Janeiro, Brazil
Laboratório de Imunopatologia, Instituto Oswaldo Cruz, Fundação Oswaldo Cruz (FIOCRUZ), Rio de Janeiro, Brazil

Abhishek Mandal, Ajay Kumar, Sudha Verma, Ayan Kumar Ghosh, Ruby Singh, Kumar Abhishek Abul Hasan Sardar, Bidyut Purkait, Ashish Kumar and Pradeep Das
Department of Molecular Biology, Rajendra Memorial Research Institute of Medical Sciences (ICMR), Patna, India

Sushmita Das
Department of Microbiology, All India Institute of Medical Sciences (AIIMS), Patna, India

Saptarshi Roy and Chitra Mandal
Cancer Biology and Inflammatory Disorder Division, CSIR-Indian Institute of Chemical Biology, Kolkata, India

Savita Saini
Department of Molecular Biology, Rajendra Memorial Research Institute of Medical Sciences (ICMR), Patna, India
Department of Biotechnology, National Institute of Pharmaceutical Education and Research, Hajipur, India

Rani Soni, Drista Sharma and Tarun K. Bhatt
Department of Biotechnology, School of Life Sciences, Central University of Rajasthan, Rajasthan, India

Index

www.ingramcontent.com/pod-product-compliance
Lightning Source LLC
LaVergne TN
LVHW082147200926
848484LV00008B/2117
9798887400907